Development and Clinical Uses of Haemophilus b Conjugate Vaccines

INFECTIOUS DISEASE AND THERAPY

Series Editors

Brian E. Scully, M.B., B.Ch.
Harold C. Neu, M.D.

College of Physicians & Surgeons
Columbia University
New York, New York

1. Parasitic Infections in the Compromised Host, *edited by Peter D. Walzer and Robert M. Genta*
2. Nucleic Acid and Monoclonal Antibody Probes: Applications in Diagnostic Methodology, *edited by Bala Swaminathan and Gyan Prakash*
3. Opportunistic Infections in Patients with the Acquired Immunodeficiency Syndrome, *edited by Gifford Leoung and John Mills*
4. Acyclovir Therapy for Herpesvirus Infections, *edited by David A. Baker*
5. The New Generation of Quinolones, *edited by Clifford Siporin, Carl L. Heifetz, and John M. Domagala*
6. Methicillin-Resistant *Staphylococcus aureus*: Clinical Management and Laboratory Aspects, *edited by Mary T. Cafferkey*
7. Hepatitis B Vaccines in Clinical Practice, *edited by Ronald W. Ellis*
8. The New Macrolides, Azalides, and Streptogramins: Pharmacology and Clinical Applications, *edited by Harold C. Neu, Lowell S. Young, and Stephen H. Zinner*
9. Antimicrobial Therapy in the Elderly Patient, *edited by Thomas T. Yoshikawa and Dean C. Norman*
10. Viral Infections of the Gastrointestinal Tract: Second Edition, Revised and Expanded, *edited by Albert Z. Kapikian*
11. Development and Clinical Uses of Haemophilus b Conjugate Vaccines, *edited by Ronald W. Ellis and Dan M. Granoff*

Additional Volumes in Production

Herpesvirus Infections, *edited by Ronald Glaser and James F. Jones*

Immunotherapy of Infections, *edited by K. Noel Masihi*

Pseudomonas aeruginosa Infections and Treatment, *edited by Aldona L. Baltch and Raymond P. Smith*

Chronic Fatigue Syndrome, *edited by Stephen Straus*

To my wife, Danielle, and children, Jacob and Miriam, for their love, patience, and support

RWE

Development and Clinical Uses of Haemophilus b Conjugate Vaccines

edited by

Ronald W. Ellis
Merck Research Laboratories
West Point, Pennsylvania

Dan M. Granoff
Chiron Corporation
Emeryville, California
and Children's Hospital
Oakland Research Institute,
Oakland, California

Marcel Dekker, Inc. New York • Basel • Hong Kong

Library of Congress Cataloging-in-Publication Data
Development and clinical uses of haemophilus b conjugate vaccines /
edited by Ronald W. Ellis, Dan M. Granoff.
p. cm.—(Infectious disease and therapy ; v. 11)
Includes bibliographical references and index.
ISBN 0-8247-9186-X (alk. paper)
1. Influenza vaccines. 2. Synthetic vaccines. I. Ellis, Ronald
W. II. Granoff, Dan M. III. Series: Infectious disease
and therapy ; 11.
[DNLM: 1. Haemophilus Vaccines. W1 IN406HMN v.11 1994 / WC 200
D489 1994]
QR189.5.I5D48 1994
614.5′18—dc20
DNLM/DLC
for Library of Congress 94-302
CIP

The publisher offers discounts on this book when ordered in bulk quantities. For more information, write to Special Sales/Professional Marketing at the address below.

This book is printed on acid-free paper.

Marcel Dekker, Inc.
270 Madison Avenue, New York, New York 10016

Current printing (last digit):
10 9 8 7 6 5 4 3 2 1

PRINTED IN THE UNITED STATES OF AMERICA

Series Introduction

Marcel Dekker, Inc., has for many years specialized in the publication of high-quality monographs in tightly focused areas in a variety of medical disciplines. These have been of great value to both the practicing physician and the research scientist as sources of detailed and up-to-date information presented in an attractive format. During the last decade, there has been a veritable explosion in knowledge in the various fields related to infectious diseases and clinical microbiology. Antimicrobial resistance, antibacterial and antiviral agents, AIDS, Lyme disease, infections in immunocompromised patients, and parasitic diseases are but a few of the areas in which an enormous amount of significant work has been published. The Infectious Disease and Therapy series covers carefully chosen topics that should be of interest and value to the practicing physician, the clinical microbiologist, and the research scientist.

Brian E. Scully, M.B., B.Ch.
Harold C. Neu, M.D.

Preface

Invasive diseases caused by *Haemophilus influenzae* type b (Hib) have been a cause of significant mortality and morbidity in infants and young children. The serious sequelae of Hib meningitis include mental retardation and hearing loss. Thus, the medical community has been very interested for the last 25 years in the prevention through vaccination of this very serious childhood disease.

The Haemophilus b conjugate vaccines have several unique attributes among human vaccines: they are the world's first licensed vaccines in which the antigen is chemically linked (conjugated) to a carrier; they are the only vaccines that utilize process chemistry in their preparation; and they are the first new bacterial vaccines in four decades to become available and to be widely recommended for infants (along with diphtheria-tetanus-pertussis). In addition, whereas different vaccines that prevent a particular disease are generally similar for all types of other vaccines (e.g., measles, mumps, rubella, diphtheria, tetanus, whole-cell pertussis, oral polio, injected polio, hepatitis, and varicella), there are four licensed Haemophilus b conjugate vaccines of greatly different structure and distinct immunological properties. The table details the distinctive properties of these vaccines. Despite this tremendous diversity, each of the vaccines has been shown to be effective in preventing invasive Hib disease in different clinical studies.

The Distinct Properties of the Four Licensed Haemophilus b Conjugate Vaccines

	Product name			
Properties	PRP-D	HbOC[a]	PRP-OMPC	PRP-T
Trade name	ProHIBit®	HibTITER®[b]	PedvaxHIB®	ActHIB®[c]/OmniHIB®[d]
Manufacturer	Connaught	Lederle-Praxis	Merck	Pasteur-Mérieux
Indicated ages for vaccination (months)[e]	>15[f]	2,4,6,12–15	2,4,12–15	2,4,6,12–15
Carrier protein	Diphtheria toxoid	Mutant diphtheria toxoid[g]	Outer Membrane Protein Complex[h]	Tetanus toxoid
Polysaccharide dose (μg)	25	10	15[i]	10
Polysaccharide source	Heat-sized	Oligosaccharide	Native	Native
Protein dose (μg)	18	25	250[i]	20
Protein molecular weight (kilodaltons)	62	62	30,000–50,000	150
Chemical Linkage	Isourea	Amine	Thioether	Hydroxyl
Form	Liquid	Liquid	Lyophilized[i]	Lyophilized[j]
Preservative	Thimerosal	Thimerosal	Thimerosal	None
Adjuvant	None	None	Aluminum hydroxide	None

[a]Haemophilus b Oligosaccharide Conjugate.
[b]Also available in combination with diphtheria-tetanus-pertussis as TETRAMUNE®.
[c]Manufactured and distributed worldwide by Pasteur-Mérieux.
[d]Manufactured by Pasteur-Mérieux and distributed by SmithKline Beecham (U.S. only).
[e]In the U.S.; indicated ages are different in some other countries.
[f]3, 5, 7, 15 months in Germany and Iceland.
[g]CRM_{197} mutant.
[h]From *Neisseria meningitidis* serogroup B.
[i]Liquid 7.5 μg vaccine (125 μg carrier protein) and combinations of it in development.
[j]Liquid vaccine and combinations of it in development.

The first-generation Hib vaccine, consisting of purified Hib capsular polysaccharide (PRP), became available in the 1980s. Licensure of this vaccine helped lay the technical, clinical, and regulatory groundwork for Hib conjugate vaccines (Chapter 1). The development process undertaken by each vaccine company has integrated a broad range of activities in order to produce its vaccine. These include preclinical, clinical, process, analytical, regulatory, biostatistics, manufacturing, quality assurance, quality control, legal, and marketing (Chapter 2). Each of the four licensed vaccines is produced by a distinct process chemistry (Chapter 3) with polysaccharide and carrier proteins of different properties such that each conjugate vaccine has a unique immunological profile (Chapters 4 and 6). These vaccines are subject to rigorous quality control testing prior to their use in clinical trials and to their commercial distribution (Chapter 5).

For unknown reasons, the epidemiology of invasive Hib infections varies in different parts of the world (Chapters 11 and 12). Studies in developing countries have shown the difficulty associated with getting consistent, robust immune responses in such populations (Chapter 16). These differences in epidemiology may affect vaccine efficacy. Clinical studies of Hib conjugate vaccines have been designed to take into consideration differences in regional epidemiology as well as accepted principles for the proper conduct of such trials (Chapter 13). Seminal to the clinical trials and to the interpretation of immunogenicity data has been the development of standardized quantitative serological assays to evaluate immune responses after vaccination (Chapter 14). Studies in developed countries have included extensive comparative testing of the four licensed Hib conjugate vaccines and combination vaccine. Besides revealing immunological differences among the vaccines, these studies have revealed significant changes in the immunogenicity of commercial lots of two of the vaccines postlicensure, a result that highlights the technical challenge in the development and production of this entire class of vaccines (Chapter 15). Several large-scale protective efficacy studies have demonstrated the ability of these vaccines to protect against invasive Hib disease (Chapter 18). Vaccination has also been shown to decrease oropharyngeal carriage of Hib organisms, which may have contributed to the profound decrease in the incidence of Hib disease even before the widespread use of conjugate vaccines in infants (Chapter 22). It is possible to draw a range of immunological and epidemiological conclusions from all these trials as well as from the widespread use of these vaccines (Chapter 23). All the above considerations, including the development of immunological surrogates for evaluating vaccines, have become the basis for the licensure of the vaccines (Chapter 24).

There are several other important clinical issues related to Hib infection. A number of factors have been enumerated with respect to risk for colonization, transmission, and disease (Chapter 19). Despite the excellent control of disease by vaccination, questions remain regarding the pathogenesis of disease in infants and children and recommendations for optimal treatment (Chapter 20). The use of passively administered immune globulin enriched for antibodies against PRP has been shown to be effective in preventing disease and may be an alternative to active immunization of special high-risk groups of infants (Chapter 17). However, in adults, most infections are caused by nontypable *H. influenzae* strains, with Hib strains in the minority (Chapter 21).

The application of new methods for molecular analysis has had a strong influence on research in this entire field. The analysis of DNA, proteins, polysaccharides, and lipids has enabled detailed studies of molecular epidemiology of Hib strains worldwide (Chapter 7). The molecular genetics of numerous Hib structural antigens has contributed to understanding the pathogenesis of infection (Chapter 8). The electrophoretic analysis of allelic variants of *H. influenzae* metabolic enzymes has been the basis for studying the population genetics of these organisms worldwide (Chapter 9). From the point of view of the host, a variety of new techniques have been used to analyze the antibody genes responsible for immune responses to conjugate vaccines in order to determine the molecular basis for immunity for Hib (Chapter 10). In addition, as in all fields of biomedical research, there is interest in potential new strategies aimed at augmenting the immunogenicity of current vaccines, designing new Hib vaccines, and applying conjugate technology to develop effective vaccines against other pathogens (Chapter 25).

We hope that this book will become a comprehensive reference on all major aspects of Hib conjugate vaccines. Since vaccination remains a practical and most cost-effective means of disease control, the widespread use of Hib conjugate vaccines offers the long-term prospect of eradication of invasive Hib disease. Worldwide, the increased use of this vaccine is highly desirable for disease control. In this regard, the availability of the first combination vaccine and ongoing development of future combination vaccines containing Hib conjugates should help to ensure the increased use of these new vaccines concomitant with public policy initiatives to increase vaccination rates of infants and young children in different countries.

The editors owe many thanks to their friends and colleagues. Ronald W. Ellis is especially grateful to Kenneth R. Brown, Gary B. Calandra, John A. Ryan, and Edward M. Scolnick for their many stimulating discussions, and he is indebted to numerous colleagues at Merck for their collaboration over the years. The love and support of his wife, Danielle, and children, Jacob and Miriam, were very important to him throughout all phases of preparing this book. Special mention should go to Grayce Albanesius, who provided her expert assistance with this book, and to Jacob for helping to prepare the index. Dan M. Granoff is especially grateful to Alexander H. Lucas, Penelope G. Shackelford, Robert S. Munson, Jr., Michael T. Osterholm, and Trudy V. Murphy for many years of fruitful collaboration. A special debt is also owed to the many post-doctoral infectious disease fellows at Washington University, St. Louis, who participated in these investigations, for their enthusiasm, intelligence, hard work, and fresh insights as the field of Hib conjugate vaccine development evolved. Special mention should also go to Frances LoCascio, who provided expert and dedicated secretarial support for 13 years, and to Kathleen Lottenbach, who kept his laboratory operating in St. Louis from 1992 to 1993 while he was on sabbatical at the Children's Hospital Oakland Research Institute when this book was being prepared. His children, Jonathan and Jeffrey, were fortunate to be away attending university during this year, but Dr. Granoff is indebted to them for their understanding and patience, especially during the early years of his studies, and for their participation in the initial immunogenicity trials with the plain Hib polysaccharide vaccine.

Most importantly, we thank all the authors for their professional and insightful contributions which have made this book the key reference in the field of Haemophilus b conjugate vaccines.

Ronald W. Ellis
Dan M. Granoff

Contents

Contributors

Elisabeth E. Adderson Department of Pediatrics, University of Utah, Salt Lake City, Utah

Vincent I. Ahonkhai Anti-Infectives Division, Robert Wood Johnson Pharmaceutical Research Institute, Raritan, New Jersey

Henk A. Bijlmer Department of Medical Microbiology, Bronovo Hospital, The Hague, The Netherlands

William L. Carroll Department of Human Molecular Biology and Genetics, University of Utah, Salt Lake City, Utah

Janné Croll Center for American Indian and Alaskan Native Health, Department of International Health, The Johns Hopkins University, Baltimore, Maryland

Robert S. Daum Department of Pediatrics, University of Chicago, Chicago, Illinois

Renee Z. Dintzis Departments of Cell Biology and Anatomy, and Biophysics and Biophysical Chemistry, The Johns Hopkins University School of Medicine, Baltimore, Maryland

John J. Donnelly Virus and Cell Biology, Merck Research Laboratories, West Point, Pennsylvania

Ronald W. Ellis Virus and Cell Biology, Merck Research Laboratories, West Point, Pennsylvania

Juhani Eskola Department of Infectious Disease Epidemiology, National Public Health Institute, Helsinki, Finland

Carl E. Frasch Division of Bacterial Products, Center for Biologics Evaluation and Research, Bethesda, Maryland

Lallan Giri* Connaught Laboratories, Inc., Swiftwater, Pennsylvania

Dan M. Granoff** Washington University School of Medicine, St. Louis, Missouri

Brian M. Greenwood Medical Research Council Laboratories, Banjul, The Gambia

Richard A. Insel Department of Pediatrics and Microbiology and Immunology, University of Rochester School of Medicine and Dentistry, Rochester, New York

Sheldon L. Kaplan Department of Pediatrics, Baylor College of Medicine and Infectious Disease Service, Texas Children's Hospital, Houston, Texas

Vivek Kapur Department of Pathology, Baylor College of Medicine, Houston, Texas

Helena Käyhty Department of Bacterial Respiratory Infections, National Public Health Institute, Helsinki, Finland

Peter J. Kniskern Virus and Cell Biology, Merck Research Laboratories, West Point, Pennsylvania

John Simon Kroll Department of Paediatrics, Imperial College of Science, Technology and Medicine, St. Mary's Hospital Medical School, London, England

Paul Richard Langford Department of Paediatrics, Imperial College of Science, Technology and Medicine, St. Mary's Hospital Medical School, London, England

Margaret A. Liu Virus and Cell Biology, Merck Research Laboratories, West Point, Pennsylvania

Alexander H. Lucas Children's Hospital Oakland Research Institute, Oakland, California

---

**Present affiliation:* B.W. Manufacturing, Inc., West Greenwich, Rhode Island

***Present affiliation:* Biocine Clinical Research, Chiron Corporation, Emeryville, California, and Children's Hospital Oakland Research Institute, Oakland, California

P. Helena Mäkelä Department of Special Bacterial Pathogens, National Public Health Institute, Helsinki, Finland

Stephen Marburg Synthetic Chemical Research, Merck Research Laboratories, Rahway, New Jersey

E. Kim Mulholland Medical Research Council Laboratories, Banjul, The Gambia

Daniel Musher Departments of Medicine, Microbiology, and Immunology, Baylor College of Medicine and Infectious Disease Section, Veterans Affairs Medical Center, Houston, Texas

James M. Musser Department of Pathology, Microbiology, and Immunology, Section of Molecular Pathobiology, Baylor College of Medicine, Houston, Texas

Moon H. Nahm Departments of Pathology and Medicine, Washington University School of Medicine, St. Louis, Missouri

Heikki Peltola Children's Hospital, University of Helsinki, Helsinki, Finland

Raymond Reid Center for American Indian and Alaskan Native Health, Department of International Health, The Johns Hopkins University, Baltimore, Maryland

Maria Rodriguez-Barradas Departments of Medicine, Microbiology, and Immunology, Baylor College of Medicine, Houston, Texas

Mathuram Santosham Center for American Indian and Alaskan Native Health, Department of International Health, The Johns Hopkins University, Baltimore, Maryland

Mitchell G. Scott Departments of Pathology and Medicine, Washington University School of Medicine, St. Louis, Missouri

Penelope G. Shackelford The Edward Mallinkrodt Department of Pediatrics, Washington University School of Medicine, St. Louis, Missouri

Eugene D. Shapiro Department of Pediatrics, Yale University School of Medicine, New Haven, Connecticut

George R. Siber Massachusetts Public Health Biologic Laboratories and Harvard Medical School, Dana-Farber Cancer Institute, Boston, Massachusetts

Gregg J. Silverman Department of Medicine, University of California—San Diego, La Jolla, California

Aino K. Takala Department of Infectious Disease Epidemiology, National Public Health Institute, Helsinki, Finland

Claudette M. Thompson Department of Infectious Diseases, Dana-Farber Cancer Institute, Boston, Massachusetts

Constance M. Vadheim UCLA Center for Vaccine Research, Harbor-UCLA Medical Center, UCLA School of Medicine, Torrance, California

Loek van Alphen Department of Medical Microbiology, University of Amsterdam, Amsterdam, The Netherlands

Phillip P. Vella* Virus and Cell Biology, Merck Research Laboratories, West Point, Pennsylvania

Jean-Claude Vincent-Falquet Pasteur-Mérieux Serums & Vaccines, Marcy l'Etoile, France

Joel I. Ward UCLA Center for Vaccine Research, Harbor-UCLA Medical Center, UCLA School of Medicine, Torrance, California

*Retired

1

Immunological Basis for PRP Vaccines

Helena Käyhty and P. Helena Mäkelä

National Public Health Institute, Helsinki, Finland

Heikki Peltola

Children's Hospital, University of Helsinki, Helsinki, Finland

I. INTRODUCTION

The history of vaccine development and prevention of serious *Haemophilus influenzae* type b (Hib) infections relates back to the 1930s, when Margaret Pittman discovered that most strains of *H. influenza* that caused serious infections were of one capsular type, type b (1). First evidence of the importance of antibodies in host defense against Hib infection came from Fothergill and Wright, who showed in 1933 that blood of young children lacked bactericidal activity, whereas blood from older children and adults was bactericidal for Hib (2). The specificity of bactericidal antibodies was discussed during the 1930s and 1940s, when intrathecally-given horse antiserum to Hib was tried in experimental animals as a cure for meningitis (3), and later when rabbit hyperimmune serum was used successfully for immunotherapy of Hib infections (4,5). The same investigators showed that absorption with purified type b polysaccharide could remove the protective activity of this rabbit antiserum (6).

The advent of effective antibacterial agents interrupted the interest in Hib vaccine development for decades. It was only in the late 1960s and early 1970s that scientists again became interested in developing a vaccine against Hib. Type b capsular polysaccharide was the object of interest of several groups. The structure of that polysaccharide was discovered to be polyribosylribitol phosphate (7) (usually abbreviated as PRP because of its initially mistaken identification as polyribosyl phosphate). At the beginning of the 1970s, two groups began research on the purification and immunogenicity of PRP (8,9,10). They also developed radioimmunological methods for quantitation of anti-PRP antibodies in human sera (11,12). Basically the same methods are still in use. Later, a pair of curves similar to that of Fothergill and Wright (2) relating incidence of disease at different ages to serum antibodies was drawn on the basis of antibodies to PRP (13,14), indicating their decisive role in protection from invasive disease.

The capsular polysaccharide was fairly easily purified from the culture supernatant, and the product was proven immunogenic first in human adults (8–11). The subsequent immunogenicity studies in infants and children showed that the immune response was clearly age-dependent (11,13–18) and that children under 2 years of age who were at the greatest risk to fall ill with invasive Hib infection responded only poorly to immunization.

At the same time, two clinical efficacy studies were performed. The study in North Carolina by Parke et al. failed to show clinical protection, but the number of cases in the control group was too small for significant conclusions (18). By contrast, the Finnish study gave clear evidence for protective activity of anti-PRP antibodies (19). Largely based on this latter trial the PRP vaccine was licensed in the United States in 1985 for children at least 2 years of age (20). Because the polysaccharide vaccine was not immunogenic or protective among infants and young children, who would have needed it most, research was directed towards an improved PRP-based vaccine. Conjugation of PRP to a protein carrier (21–24) proved successful, and the resulting conjugate vaccines have now proven efficacious in preventing Hib infections even in young infants.

The large amount of research performed in connection with PRP efficacy studies and the subsequent pre- and postlicensure investigations have taught us much about the safety and immunogenicity of PRP. These studies have also provided valuable information about the immune response to polysaccharide antigens in general, and in fact made it clear that this response differs in fundamental ways from the human immune response to proteins.

II. SAFETY OF PRP VACCINE

PRP is one of the safest vaccines. The first experimental lots used in Finland contained impurities and caused local reactions in 51% of the vaccinees (19), but systemic reactions were rare. One serious, but nonfatal, apparently anaphylactic reaction was registered among the 50,000 vaccinees (65,000 doses). The postlicensure lots were purer, and the number of systemic and local reactions decreased significantly after the licensure of the vaccine. Among 4557 vaccinees, only 2.3% had a temperature of

>38°C, 4.8% had local erythema, 2.9% local swelling, and 12.6% local tenderness (25). After administration of several million doses of PRP vaccine, no association between PRP vaccine and serious reactions could be found (26) in a one-year postmarketing surveillance study. During this period 152 spontaneous reports on adverse reactions after vaccination with PRP were received by FDA. Most of the reactions were benign. The more severe ones included convulsions (17 cases), anaphylactoid reactions (2 cases), serum sickness–like reactions (10 cases), erythema multiforme (4 cases), vomiting (16 cases) and one death. However, the causality could not be inferred from any single report.

Some investigators have been worried about an increased risk for Hib infection during the first week following vaccination with PRP (27–30). In the study of Black et al. the risk was 6.4-fold (95% confidence interval, CI, 2.1–19.2) as compared to unvaccinated children (27). The study conducted by the Centers for Disease Control in six areas of the United States revealed an 1.8-fold (CI 95%; 0.3–10.2) increase in the occurrence of invasive Hib disease in the first week after immunization as compared to expectation based on the population at large (28), which did not speak for a significantly increased risk of Hib disease in the week following immunization. In both studies the comparison group is unfair because the vaccinated children were mostly immunized due to an increased risk of Hib infection—a recent exposure to a Hib disease, day-care attendance, or increased susceptibility to Hib disease because of sickle cell disease, Down syndrome, or a history of recurrent Hib infections (29). No cases of Hib disease were seen in the first week after vaccination in the previous, randomized trial (our own unpublished data). Nevertheless, the possibility of a slight increase of Hib susceptibility cannot be excluded, especially since it would have a rational basis in the observation that the anti-PRP antibody concentrations were shown to fall during the first days after vaccination (30). This is believed to reflect neutralization of the small amount of anti-PRP present in children until the antibody response starts 4–7 days after vaccination. However, the practical significance of this theoretically interesting finding is small, as can be deduced from a comparison of an at most 1.8- to 6.4-fold increase of risk over one week with a 90% prevention of cases over the following several years.

III. CLINICAL EFFICACY OF PRP

The PRP vaccine was used in 1974 as a control vaccine in the Finnish group A meningococcal double-blind efficacy trial. The results after a 4-year follow-up were reported in 1984 (19). The vaccine was given to 50,000 infants and children 3–72 months of age. Three- to 17-month-old infants received two doses of vaccine with a 3-month interval. The protective efficacy was clearly age-dependent, since there was no protection before the age of 18 months. Two cases occurred among children immunized at 18–29 months of age but none among older vaccinees, as compared to 20 cases in the control group of same age immunized with group A meningococcal vaccine (19). Thus the overall efficacy was 90% (CI 95%; 55–98) at 18–71 months of age. The exact age at which the efficacy of PRP commenced could not be determined from this study, because there were too few cases in the control group in the critical age group of 18–23 months.

Another study was carried out among 16,000 infants and children in North Carolina (18). In this study half of the 2-month- to 5-year-old children received PRP and the other half group C meningococcal capsular polysaccharide vaccine. No conclusions regarding age-specific efficacy could be drawn, because of the limited number of Hib infections in the study group during the follow-up period of 2 years. The overall protective efficacy was 40% (with probable effectiveness of −10 to 70%). Consistent with the poor protective efficacy, a serum antibody response was only seen in children older than 3 years.

Largely based on the Finnish efficacy trial and the immunogenicity study connected with it, the PRP vaccine was licensed in the United States in 1985 for use among children older than 23 months of age and among those 18–23 months old who are at increased risk to fall ill with Hib infection (20). The United States was the only country to use the polysaccharide vaccine. Five postlicensure case-control studies showed varying results of the efficacy of PRP in the U.S. population (27,28,31–33). In Minnesota the PRP recipients were even reported to have been prone to Hib infections; the vaccine efficacy was −55% (CI 95%; −238 to 29) (31). Four other U.S. studies (27,28,32,33) showed protective efficacy varying between 45% and 88%; so the Minnesota data disagreed sharply with all other data obtained. Overall, the rate of efficacy of PRP in the United States was lower than in Finland, even though the postlicensure lots of PRP proved equally immunogenic than the lot used in the Finnish study (34). Another important reason for the lower postlicensure figures may be that these studies were based on case-control methodology that underestimates vaccine efficacy, especially in diseases like Hib infections in which environmental and socioeconomic risk factors are not easily definable (35). The successful new Hib conjugate vaccines have now decreased the interest in the problems connected with the PRP efficacy.

IV. IMMUNOGENICITY OF PRP

A. Serum Antibody Response to PRP

Pre- and postlicensure immunogenicity studies showed that antibody response to PRP is age-dependent and thus correlates with the age-dependent protective efficacy found in the Finnish study. In the first studies of Smith et al. only 4 out of 18 5- to 12-month-old infants had a significant antibody increase, while the majority of the 123 older children responded after immunization with 0.67- to 67-μg doses of PRP (15). Robbins et al. (11) showed also that 2- to 3-month-old infants responded poorly to PRP and that the response was short lasting. In 1977 Anderson et al. (13) concluded that PRP did not provoke a protective immune response in young infants. In this study only 7 and 17% produced a significant response when immunized at 2–6 or 7–12 months, respectively. Consistent with this, in the Finnish study 9.1–40%, depending on the age group, had a greater than twofold response when immunized during the first year of life. The proportion of responders increased with increasing age, so that almost all (93.3%) responded when immunized at 4–5 years (16). The geometric mean concentration increased correspondingly (Table 1). This and the study of Granoff and Munson showed a great heterogeneity of responses at all ages (36).

The reasons that young infants respond poorly to polysaccharide antigens are not entirely known. An interesting aspect is that all bacterial capsular polysaccharides do not behave similarly. Some, e.g., group A meningococcal or type 3 pneumococcal capsular polysaccharides, are fairly good immunogens even in infancy, while others, such as *E. coli* K1, group B meningococcal, or type 6 pneumococcal capsular polysaccharides are hardly immunogenic even in adults (37).

In mice, the B cells that respond to polysaccharides belong to the $Ly5^+$ subset (38). This subset of lymphocytes develops 7–10 days after birth and reaches adult levels at 3–4 weeks of age. $Ly5^-$ cells, which are responsible for responses to protein antigens (38), are present already at birth (39). The $Ly5^+$ cells are rarer than $Ly5^-$ cells and have a longer half-life. In humans the precise equivalent of murine later-developing B cells has not been described. Barrett et al. (40) showed that human anti–type 4 pneumococcal antibody secreting cells were found in a $CD5^-$ B-cell population ($Ly1^-$ in the murine system). They suggest that acquisition of responsiveness to polysaccharide antigens in humans is associated with the developmental maturation of the $CD5^-$ subset of B cells. Like the $Ly5^+$ subset in mice, the $CD5^-$ cells are relatively rare in infants and young children, and their proportion increases with age throughout childhood (40).

Consistently, isoelectric focusing experiments have shown that only a few B cell clones are triggered by PRP, in contrast to the polyclonal responses induced by protein antigens (41). The oligoclonal nature of the response is in accordance with the limited number of V genes capable of coding for antibody with anti-PRP specificity (42,43).

In mice, the magnitude of the antibody response to the capsular polysaccharides of several bacteria is regulated in a positive and negative manner by thymus-derived lymphocytes. These regulatory T cells are called

Table 1 Antibody Concentrations in Serum Samples of Infants and Children Immunized with *Haemophilus influenzae* Type b Capsular Polysaccharide (PRP) Vaccine

Age (months)	Serum[b]	N	Anti-PRP (μg/ml) GMT[c]	%>0.15[d]	%>1.0[e]
3–5	1	25	0.1 (<0.1–0.23)	0	0
	2	25	0.11 (<0.1–0.19)	8	0
6–11	1	52	0.11 (<0.1–1.73)	12	2
	2	52	0.20 (<0.1–4.69)	59	20
12–17	1	58	0.14 (<0.1–1.18)	21	3
	2	58	0.79 (<0.1–15.0)	81	45
18–23	1	30	0.28 (<0.1–5.16)	63	13
	2	30	3.07 (0.14–>20.0)	97	77
24–35	1	101	0.34 (<0.1–6.77)	66	18
	2	101	5.81 (0.19–>20.0)	100	91
36–37	1	73	0.35 (<0.1–4.25)	66	25
	2	72	6.91 (0.57–>20.0)	100	97
48–71	1	158	0.48 (<0.1–10.04)	81	29
	2	157	10.03 (0.54–>20.0)	100	99

[a]Anti-PRP antibodies in samples taken before and one month after vaccination were measured by radioimmunoassay.
[b]1, serum sample taken before vaccination; 2, serum sample taken one month after vaccination.
[c]Geometric mean and range (in parentheses) of antibody concentrations.
[d]Percent of vaccinees >0.15 μg/ml.
[e]Percent of vaccinees >1.0 μg/ml.
Source: Ref. 19.

amplifier T cells (T_a, $CD4^+CD8^-$) and suppressor T cells (T_s, $CD4^-CD8^+$) (44). T_a cells are not T helper cells (T_h); they represent a separate subset with a different function and different specificity. T_h-cell receptors recognize short peptides bound to a specific groove of the MHC molecules of antigen-presenting cells, and it is indeed unlikely that an oligosaccharide would mimic this activity. By contrast, the T_a and T_s cells are likely to be part of the general immunological regulatory network—directed to the antibodies ("anti-idiotype") formed to PRP (44). In contrast to T_h cells, which act mainly to initiate antibody formation, T_a cells enlarge or expand an ongoing antibody response. In mice, T_s activity is fully developed at 2 weeks of age, when B cells are capable of synthesizing and secreting antipolysaccharide antibodies. By contrast, T_a activity matures much more slowly and is not maximal until 8–10 weeks of age (44).

The persistence of vaccine-induced anti-PRP antibodies is also age-dependent (45–47). This is of importance because the protection after immunization with polysaccharide vaccine is believed to be dependent only on the existence of humoral antibodies; these vaccines do not induce immunological memory (45). In addition to the low antibody responses before the age of 2 years, the antibody concentrations achieved by vaccination at this age decline rapidly to the levels in unimmunized children (45–47). Among older children, the elevated antibody levels persist 1.5–3.5 years after vaccination (45). These data suggest that for children vaccinated at 2–3 years, a revaccination should be considered 1–2 years thereafter.

Varying doses of PRP were tested in the first immunogenicity trials. These studies suggest that a wide range of doses can induce a significant antibody response. The study of Smith et al. (15) compared doses ranging from 0.67 to 67 μg in children of ages between 5 and 59 months. Even though all doses were able to elicit an immune response, doses of 3.3 and 17 μg were superior to 0.67 and 67 μg. In a study by Robbins et al. (11) a 10-μg dose was slightly more immunogenic than a 50-μg dose in children approximately 4 years of age. Anderson et al. (13) compared doses ranging from 0.2 to 50 μg in infants younger than 12 months of age. Probably because of the low overall rate of responsiveness at this age, no difference in the anti-PRP responses could be seen when different doses were used. After licensure of the PRP, 12.5 and 25 μg were found to be equally immunogenic in 24-month-old children (34).

The antibodies induced by vaccine have proven functionally active and protective in several studies. They are complement-activating (48–50), bactericidal (15,49,51,52), and opsonizing (15,51–55). Following either active (56) or passive (52,57,58) immunization, they protect animals from death, bacteremia, or meningitis after experimental challenge with Hib. However, the most important evidence for the functional activity of anti-PRP antibody is the protective immunity induced in older children immunized with purified PRP (19) and the fact that passive administration of bacterial polysaccharide immunoglobulin or anti-PRP–containing antiserum protects infants and agammaglobulinemic patients from Hib infections (59,60).

B. T-Cell–Independent Characteristics of the Antibody Response to PRP

Many bacterial polysaccharide antigens behave in mice as T-cell–independent type 2 (TI-2) antigens (61). These antigens do not recruit T-helper cells, even though T cells can suppress or augment the antibody response, as has been shown for several capsular polysaccharide antigens (44). Typically, the response to TI-2 antigen in mice is restricted to IgM, and no booster-type responses can be seen after repeated immunizations, which means that there is neither a switch from IgM to IgG nor increased antibody response when compared to the response after the first immunization (61). Consistent with this, PRP was not found to induce elevated booster responses or switches from IgM to IgG among Finnish children (62). In contrast to the predominantly IgM responses to polysaccharide antigens in mice, the human response includes IgM, IgA, and IgG (62,63). In some studies, somewhat elevated booster-type responses have been found in both rats and human children when PRP was given together with whole cell pertussis vaccine or with pertussis outer membrane complex (47,64). This finding, which initially caused high hopes of being able to extend the protective activity of PRP to young infants, could not be repeated (62,65–67).

The predominant IgG subclass of human antibodies to polysaccharide TI-2 antigens was previously believed to be IgG2 corresponding to IgG3 in mice (68,69), in contrast to predominantly IgG1 response to proteins, which are typical T-cell–dependent antigens (70,71). However, different bacterial polysaccharides seem to differ in this respect; the IgG antibodies evoked by some of them are mainly IgG2, while in some cases both IgG1 and IgG2 responses are induced (72–75). It should be noted here that children less than 2 years of age are largely unable to produce IgG2, and therefore their IgG response is mainly of IgG1 isotype (75–77). Human adult responses to PRP have been proven to be of three types: in some vaccinees equal amounts of IgG1 and IgG2 are formed, while others show mainly IgG1 or IgG2 responses (72,75). The significance of the IgG isotype distribution in anti-PRP antibody response is not clear. There are indications that anti-PRP antibodies of the IgG2 isotype can have lower functional activity than those of the IgG1 isotype (78).

Typical for TI-2 antigen is also slow maturation of affinity of antibodies (61). Consistently, the intrinsic affinity of anti-PRP antibodies after immunization is low (79). However, the functional affinity (avidity), which is probably biologically more relevant for protective capacity than intrinsic affinity, can increase after immunization (80). On the other hand, some vaccinees can have antibodies of low avidity, which may explain some of the vaccine failures seen in a population whose antibody response measured by routine immunochemical methods (not affected by antibody avidity) is satisfactory (81).

C. Genetic Markers Associated with the Antibody Response to PRP

Several studies have aimed at finding genetic markers associated with poor responses to polysaccharide vaccines. Granoff et al. suggested that genetic factors may play a role in the susceptibility to Hib infection based on their study in which siblings of Hib patients had lower antibody responses to PRP than controls of the same age (82). Certain immunoglobulin allotypes have been connected to a poor antibody response to polysaccharide antigens. However, the results from these studies are conflicting. The Km(1) allotype has in many studies been associated with anti-polysaccharide responses. In one study Km(1)-positive white, but not black, children had lower anti-PRP responses than those lacking this allotype (83). In the second study Km(1)-positive white adults had decreased anti-PRP antibody production compared to Km(1)-negative individuals (84). In a third study (85) Km(1)-positive black children had higher responses than those who were Km(1) negative. This study could not show any association between Km(1) allotype and anti-PRP responses in white populations.

Similarly, conflicting data have been presented for another allotype, G2m(n). Three studies speak for higher [either IgG (86) or IgG2 (87,87a)] anti-PRP responses in adult vaccinees who are positive for this allotype. The study by Granoff et al. (85) in children did not show this connection. Furthermore, infants and children under 2 years of age, a high-risk group for Hib infection, rarely produce the IgG2 isotype, suggesting that any IgG2 allotype would be irrelevant at this age. Accordingly, the presence or absence of this allotype did not influence the risk of invasive Hib disease in Finnish children (88).

D. The Minimal Protective Concentration of Anti-PRP Antibodies

Serum anti-PRP antibody concentrations ranging from 0.05 to 1 μg/ml have been proposed as providing minimal protection (89,90). It is very difficult to determine a minimal protective concentration at an individual level, because the isotype distribution and the functional properties of antibodies can vary greatly. The other factor that makes these estimations difficult is the use of slightly differing methods for anti-PRP antibody determination in different studies (91,92). When evaluating vaccine responses at the population level, several groups have assumed the concentration of 0.15 μg/ml to provide protection at the time of the assay. The antibody concentrations after vaccination fall fairly quickly (45), especially in younger vaccinees. Therefore, for long-lasting protection, higher concentrations than 0.15 μg/ml are needed.

During the Finnish PRP trial a postvaccination concentration of 1 μg/ml (see Table 1) was estimated to predict long-lasting protection after PRP immunization (89,90). This concentration only pertains to antibodies induced by the PRP vaccines. The situation is quite different as regards Hib conjugate vaccines that are able to evoke immunological memory. In this case, protection is not dependent solely on antibody concentrations but also on a quick booster-type antibody response when a vaccinee meets PRP antigen (93,94).

E. Efforts to Make PRP More Immunogenic

The poor immunogenicity and limited protective efficacy of PRP led many groups to try to improve the immunogenicity of PRP or to find other surface components that could induce protective immunity. Feeding of *E. coli* K100 bacteria, which has a capsular polysaccharide cross-reacting with PRP, was an interesting approach to induce both mucosal and humoral immunity (95). Animals colonized by *E. coli* K100 had an anti-PRP response, and accelerated induction of antibody-producing cells was found in spleen, mesenteric lymph nodes, and Peyer's patches after challenge with Hib (95).

Enhancement of immunogenicity by mixing PRP with adjuvants was an obvious possibility, and several approaches were taken: *Bordetella pertussis* cells or outer membrane proteins (64,96), DPT vaccine (62,65), outer cell wall complexes of Hib (97), or proteins, like bovine serum albumin (98), used as carriers in conjugate vaccines. In most studies the adjuvant indeed improved the antibody response, but only slightly in infants and with inconsistent results. Interest in this kind of approach was limited by the apparent success of the development of vaccines based on covalent conjugation of PRP to a carrier protein.

REFERENCES

1. M. Pittman, Variation and type specificity in the bacterial species *H. influenzae*, *J. Exp. Med. 53*:471 (1931).

2. L. D. Fothergill and J. Wright, Influenzal meningitis: the relation of age incidence to the bactericidal power of blood against the causal organism, *J. Immunol.* *24*:273 (1933).
3. M. Pittman, The action of type-specific *H. influenzae* antiserum, *J. Exp. Med.* *58*:683 (1933).
4. H. E. Alexander, C. Ellis, and G. Leidy, Treatment of type-specific *Hemophilus influenzae* infections in infancy and childhood, *J. Ped.* *20*:673 (1942).
5. H. E. Alexander, Experimental basis for treatment of *H. influenzae* infections, *Am. J. Dis. Child.* *66*:160 (1943).
6. H. E. Alexander, M. Heidelberger, and G. Leidy, The protective or curative element in type b *H. influenzae* rabbit serum, *Yale J. Biol. Med.* *16*:425 (1944).
7. R. M. Crisel, R. S. Baker, and D. E. Dorman, Capsular polymer of *Haemophilus influenzae* type b. Structural characterization of the capsular polymer of strain Eagan, *J. Biol. Chem.* *250*:4926 (1975).
8. P. Anderson, G. Peter, R. B. Johnston Jr, L. H. Wetterlow, and D. H. Smith, Immunization of humans with polyribophosphate, the capsular antigen of *Hemophilus influenzae*, type b, *J. Clin. Invest.* *51*:39 (1972).
9. L. P. Rodrigues, R. Schneerson, and J. B. Robbins, Immunity to *Hemophilus influenzae* type b. I. The isolation, and some physicochemical, serological and biological properties of the capsular polysaccharide of *Hemophilus influenzae* type b, *J. Immunol.* *107*:1071 (1971).
10. P. Anderson and D. H. Smith, Isolation of the capsular polysaccharide from culture supernatant of *Haemophilus influenzae* type b, *Infect. Immun.* *15*:472 (1977).
11. J. B. Robbins, J. C. Parke Jr., R. Schneerson, and J. K. Whisnant, Quantitative measurement of "natural" and immunization induced *Haemophilus influenzae* type b capsular polysaccharide antibodies, *Pediatr. Res.* *7*:103 (1973).
12. P. Anderson, Intrinsic tritium labeling of the capsular polysaccharide antigen of *Haemophilus influenzae* type b, *J. Immunol.* *120*:866 (1978).
13. P. Anderson, D. H. Smith, D. L. Ingram, J. Wilkins, P. F. Wehrle, and V. M. Howie, Antibody to polyribophosphate of *Haemophilus influenzae* type b in infants and children: effect of immunization with polyribophosphate, *J. Infect. Dis.* *136* (Suppl):S57 (1977).
14. H. Peltola, H. Käyhty, A. Sivonen, and P. H. Mäkelä, *Haemophilus influenzae* type b capsular polysaccharide vaccine in children: A double-bind field study of 100,000 vaccinees 3 months to 5 years of age in Finland, *Pediatrics* *60*:730 (1977).
15. D. H. Smith, G. Peter, D. L. Ingram, A. L. Harding, and P. Anderson, Responses of children immunized with the capsular polysaccharide of *Hemophilus influenzae* type b, *Pediatrics* *52*:637 (1973).
16. P. H. Mäkelä, H. Peltola, H. Käyhty, H. Jousimies, O. Pettay, E. Ruoslahti, A. Sivonen, and O-V. Renkonen, Polysaccharide vaccines of group A *Neisseria meningitidis* and *Haemophilus influenzae* type b: a field trial in Finland, *J. Infect. Dis.*, *136* (Suppl):S43 (1977).

17. D. J. Pincus, D. Morrison, C. Andrews, E. Lawrence, S. H. Sell, and P. F. Wright, Age-related response to two *Haemophilus influenzae* type b vaccines, *J. Pediatr. 100*:197 (1982).
18. J. C. Parke Jr, R. Schneerson, J. B. Robbins, and J. J. Schlesselman, Interim report of a controlled field trial of immunization with capsular polysaccharides of *Haemophilus influenzae* type b and group C *Neisseria meningitidis* in Mecklenburg County, North Carolina (March 1974–March 1976), *J. Infect. Dis., 136* (Suppl):S51 (1977).
19. H. Peltola, H. Käyhty, M. Virtanen, and P. H. Mäkelä, Prevention of *Hemophilus influenzae* type b bacteremic infections with the capsular polysaccharide vaccine, *N. Engl. J. Med. 310*:1566 (1984).
20. Centers for Disease Control, Polysaccharide vaccine for prevention of *Haemophilus influenzae* type b disease, *MMWR 34*:201 (1985).
21. P. Anderson, M. Pichichero, and R. Insel, Immunization of 2-month-old infants with a protein-coupled oligosaccharides derived from the capsule of *Haemophilus influenzae* type b, *J. Pediatr. 107*:346 (1985).
22. J. Eskola, H. Peltola, P. H. Mäkelä, H. Käyhty, V. Karanko, and J. Samuelson, Antibody levels achieved in infants by course of *Haemophilus influenzae* type b polysaccharide/diphtheria toxoid conjugate vaccine, *Lancet 1*:1184 (1985).
23. M. S. Einhorn, G. A. Weinberg, E. L. Anderson, P. D. Granoff, and D. M. Granoff, Immunogenicity in infants of *Haemophilus influenzae* type b polysaccharide in a conjugate vaccine with *Neisseria meningitidis* outer-membrane protein, *Lancet 2*:299 (1986).
24. B. A. Claesson, R. Schneerson, J. B. Robbins, J. Johansson, T. Lagergard, D. Bryla, L. Levi, T. Cramton, and B. Trollfors, Protective levels of serum antibodies stimulated in infants by two injections of *Haemophilus influenzae* type b capsular polysaccharide-tetanus toxoid conjugate, *J. Pediatr. 114*:97 (1989).
25. S. B. Black, H. R. Shinefield, and the Northern California Permanente Medical Care Program Departments of Pediatrics Study Group, b-CAPSA I *Haemophilus influenzae*, type b, capsular polysaccharide vaccine safety, *Pediatrics 79*:321 (1987).
26. J. B. Milstien, T. B. Gross, and J. N. Kuritsky, Adverse reactions reported following receipt of *Haemophilus influenzae* type b vaccine: an analysis after 1 year of marketing, *Pediatrics 80*:270 (1987).
27. S. B. Black, H. R. Shinefield, R. A. Hiatt, B. H. Fireman, and the Kaiser Permanente Pediatric Vaccine Study Group, Efficacy of *Haemophilus influenzae* type b capsular polysaccharide vaccine, *Pediatr. Infect. Dis. J. 7*:149 (1988).
28. L. H. Harrison, C. V. Broome, A. W. Hightower, C. C. Hoppe, S. Makintubee, S. L. Sitze, J. A. Taylor, S. Gaventa, J. D. Wenger, R. R. Facklam, and The *Haemophilus* Vaccine Efficacy Study Group, A day care-based study of the efficacy of *Haemophilus* b polysaccharide vaccine, *J. Am. Med. Assoc. 260*:1413 (1988).
29. J. I. Ward, C. V. Broome, L. H. Harrison, H. Shinefield, and S. Black, *Haemophilus influenzae* type b vaccines: Lessons for the future, *Pediatrics 81*:886 (1988).

30. S. K. Sood and R. S. Daum, Disease caused by *Haemophilus influenzae* type b in the immediate period after homologous immunization: immunologic investigation, *Pediatrics*, *85* (Suppl.):698 (1990).
31. M. T. Osterholm, J. H. Rambeck, K. E. White, J. L. Jacobs, L. M. Pierson, J. D. Neaton, C. W. Hedberg, K. L. MacDonald, and D. M. Granoff, Lack of efficacy of *Haemophilus* b polysaccharide vaccine in Minnesota, *J. Am. Med. Assoc. 260*:1423 (1988).
32. E. D. Shapiro, T. V. Murphy, E. R. Wald, and C. A. Brady, The protective efficacy of *Haemophilus* b polysaccharide vaccine, *J. Am. Med. Assoc. 260*:1419 (1988).
33. L. H. Harrison, C. V. Broome, A. W. Hightower, and the *Haemophilus* Vaccine Efficacy Study Group, *Haemophilus influenzae* type b polysaccharide vaccine: an efficacy study, *Pediatrics 84*:255 (1989).
34. H. Käyhty, H. Peltola, and J. Eskola, Immunogenicity and reactogenicity of four *Haemophilus influenzae* type b capsular polysaccharide vaccines in Finnish 24-month-old children, *Pediatr. Infect. Dis. J. 7*:574 (1988).
35. A. K. Takala, Epidemiologic characteristics and risk factors for invasive *Haemophilus influenzae* type b disease in a population with high vaccine efficacy, *Pediatr. Infect. Dis. J. 8*:343 (1989).
36. D. M. Granoff and R. S. Munson, Prospects for prevention of *Haemophilus influenzae* type b disease by immunization, *J. Infect. Dis. 153*: 448 (1986).
37. J. B. Robbins, Vaccines for the prevention of encapsulated bacterial diseases: current status, problems and prospects for the future, *Immunochemistry 15*:839 (1978).
38. D. E. Mosier, A. J. Feeney, and P. Scherle, The physiology of B lymphocytes capable of generating anti-polysaccharide antibody responses, *Towards Better Carbohydrate Vaccines* (R. Bell and G. Torrigiani, ed.). John Wiley & Sons Ltd, Chichester, UK, 1987, pp. 243–261.
39. K. E. Stein, Network regulation of the immune response to bacterial polysaccharide antigens. *Curr. Top. Microbiol. Immunol. 119*:57 (1985).
40. D. J. Barrett, J. W. Sleasman, D. A. Schatz, and M. Steinitz, Human antipneumococcal polysaccharide antibodies are secreted by $CD5^-$ B cell lineage, *Cell. Immunol. 143*:66 (1992).
41. R. A. Insel, A. Kittelberger, and P. Anderson, Isoelectric focusing of human antibody to the *Haemophilus influenzae* b capsular polysaccharide: restricted and identical spectrotypes in adults, *J. Immunol. 135*:2810 (1985).
42. E. E. Adderson, P. G. Shackelford, A. Quinn, and W. L. Carroll, Restricted Ig H chain V gene in the human antibody response to *Haemophilus influenzae* type b capsular polysaccharide, *J. Immunol. 147*:1667 (1991).
43. J. J. Tarrand, M. G. Scott, P. A. Takes, and M. H. Nahm, Clonal characterization of the human IgG antibody repertoire to *Haemophilus influenzae* type b polysaccharide. Demonstration of three types of V regions and their association with H and L chain isotypes, *J. Immunol. 142*:2519 (1989).
44. P. J. Baker, Regulation of magnitude of antibody response to bacterial polysaccharide antigens by thymus-derived lymphocytes, *Infect. Immun. 58*:3465 (1990).

45. H. Käyhty, V. Karanko, H. Peltola, and P. H. Mäkelä, Serum antibodies after vaccination with *Haemophilus influenzae* type b capsular polysaccharide and responses to reimmunization: no evidence of immunologic tolerance or memory, *Pediatrics 74*:857 (1984).
46. K. P. Ramsay, L. A. Popejoy, S. W. Jesse, and I. Gonzales-Torres, *Haemophilus* B polysaccharide vaccine, *Am. J. Dis. Child. 143*:28 (1989).
47. M. P. Glode, L. S. Joffe, R. Brogden, and J. Kuo, Reimmunization of children at 18 months of age with *Haemophilus influenzae* type b vaccine, *J. Pediatr. 112*:703 (1988).
48. P. I. Tarr, S. W. Hosea, E. J. Brown, R. Schneerson, A. Sutton, and M. M. Frank, The requirement of specific anticapsular IgG for killing of *Haemophilus influenzae* by the alternative pathway of complement activation, *J. Immunol. 128*:1772 (1982).
49. N. P. Steele, R. S. Munson, D. M. Granoff, J. E. Cummins, and R. P. Levine, Antibody-dependent alternative pathway killing of *Haemophilus influenzae* type b, *Infect. Immun. 44*:452 (1984).
50. S. V. Hetherington and C. C. Patrick, Complement component 3 binding to *Haemophilus influenzae* type b in the presence of anticapsular and anti-outer membrane antibodies, *Infect. Immun. 60*:19 (1992).
51. A. Deveikis, J. Ward, and K. S. Kim, Functional activities of human antibody induced by the capsular polysaccharide or polysaccharide-conjugate vaccines against *Haemophilus influenzae* type b, *Vaccine 6*:14 (1988).
52. J. R. Schreiber, V. Barrus, L. Cates, and G. R. Siber, Functional characterization of human IgG, IgM, and IgA antibody directed to the capsule of *Haemophilus influenzae* type b, *J. Infect. Dis. 153*:8 (1986).
53. G. J. Noel, S. Katz, and P. J. Edelson, Complement-mediated early clearance of *Haemophilus influenzae* type b from blood is independent of serum lytic activity, *J. Infect. Dis. 157*:85 (1988).
54. S. L. Newman, B. Waldo, and R. B. Johnston Jr, Separation of serum bactericidal and opsonizing activities for *Haemophilus influenzae* type b, *Infect. Immun. 8*:488 (1973).
55. K. L. Cates, K. H. Marsh, and D. M. Granoff, Serum opsonic activity after immunization of adults with *Haemophilus influenzae* type b-diphtheria toxoid conjugate vaccine, *Infect. Immun. 48*:183 (1985).
56. N. A. Halsey, T. L. Johansen, L. C. Bowman, and M. P. Glode, Evaluation of the protective efficacy of *Haemophilus influenzae* type b vaccines in an animal model, *Infect. Immun. 39*:1196 (1983).
57. D. Ambrosino, J. R. Schreiber, R. S. Daum, and G. R. Siber, Efficacy of human hyperimmune globulin in prevention of *Haemophilus influenzae* type b disease in infant rats, *Infect. Immun. 39*:709 (1983).
58. P. F. Weller, A. L. Smith, D. H. Smith, and P. Anderson, Role of immunity in the clearance of bacteremia due to *Haemophilus influenzae*, *J. Infect. Dis. 138*:427 (1978).
59. F. S. Rosen and C. A. Janeway, The gamma globulins: III. The antibody deficiency syndromes, *N. Engl. J. Med. 275*:709 (1966).

60. M. Santosham, R. Reid, D. M. Ambrosino, M. C. Wolff, J. Almeido-Hill, C. Priehs, K. M. Aspery, S. Garrett, L. Croll, S. Foster, G. Burge, P. Page, B. Zacher, R. Moxon, B. Chir, and G. R. Siber, Prevention of *Haemophilus influenzae* type b infections in high-risk infants treated with bacterial polysaccharide immune globulin, *N. Engl. J. Med 317*: 923 (1987).
61. K. E. Stein, Thymus-independent and thymus-dependent responses to polysaccharide antigens, *J. Infect. Dis. 165* (Suppl. 1):S49 (1992).
62. H. Käyhty, J. Eskola, H. Peltola, M. Stout, J. S. Samuelson, and L. K. Gordon, Immunogenicity in infants of a vaccine composed of *Haemophilus influenzae* type b capsular polysaccharide mixed with DPT or conjugated to diphtheria toxoid, *J. Infect. Dis. 155*:100 (1987).
63. H. Käyhty, R. Schneerson, and A. Sutton, Class-specific antibody response to *Haemophilus influenzae* type b capsular polysaccharide vaccine, *J. Infect. Dis. 148*:767 (1983).
64. N. Monji, M. R. Stebbins, D. W. McCoy, and J. S.-C. Kuo, Isolation of the outer membrane components of *Bordetella pertussis* which enhance the immunogenicity of *Haemophilus influenzae* type b capsular polysaccharide polyribosyl ribitol phosphate, *Infect. Immun. 51*:865 (1986).
65. E. R. Moxon, A. Anderson, D. H. Smith, B. Adrianzen, G. G. Graham, and R. S. Baker, Antibody response to a combination vaccine against *Haemophilus influenzae* type b, diphtheria, pertussis, and tetanus, *Bull. World Health Organ. 52*:87 (1975).
66. D. M. Ambrosino, M. P. Glode, C. L. Williams, and G. R. Siber, Antibody response of infants to *Haemophilus influenzae* type b capsular polysaccharide combined with *Bordetella pertussis*, *J. Infect. Dis. 151*:1174 (1985).
67. J. I. Ward, G. Brenneman, M. Lepow, M. Lum, K. Burkhart, and C. Y. Chiu, *Haemophilus influenzae* type b anticapsular antibody responses to PRP-pertussis and PRP-D vaccines in Alaska native infants, *J. Infect. Dis. 158*:719 (1988).
68. D. J. Barrett and E. M. Ayoub, IgG2 subclass restriction of antibody to pneumococcal polysaccharides, *Clin. Exp. Immunol. 63*:127 (1986).
69. W. F. Riesen, F. Skvaril, and D. G. Braun, Natural infection of man with group A streptococci. Levels; restriction in class, subclass and type; and clonal appearance of polysaccharide-group-specific antibodies, *Scand. J. Immunol. 5*:383 (1976).
70. I. J. T. Seppälä, N. Rautonen, A. Sarnesto, P. A. Mattila, and O. Mäkelä, The percentages of six immunoglobulin isotypes in human antibodies to tetanus toxoid: standardization of isotype-specific second antibodies in solid phase-assay, *Eur. J. Immunol. 14*:868 (1984).
71. A. Sarnesto, I. Julkunen, and O. Mäkelä, Proportions of Ig classes and subclasses in mumps antibodies. *Scand. J. Immunol. 22*:345 (1985).
72. O. Mäkelä, P. Mattila, N. Rautonen, I. Seppälä, J. Eskola, and H. Käyhty, Isotype concentrations of human antibodies to *Haemophilus influenzae* type b polysaccharide (Hib) in young adults immunized with the polysaccharide as

such or conjugated to a protein (diphtheria toxoid), *J. Immunol. 139*:1999 (1987).

73. N. Rautonen, J. Pelkonen, S. Sipinen, H. Käyhty, and O. Mäkelä, Isotype concentration of humans antibodies to group A meningococcal polysaccharide, *J. Immunol. 137*:2670 (1986).
74. S. Oldfield, S. Jenkins, H. Yeoman, D. Gray, and I. C. M. MacLennan, Class and subclass anti-pneumococcal antibody responses in splenectomized patients, *Clin. Exp. Immunol. 61*:664 (1985).
75. P. G. Shackelford, D. M. Granoff, S. J. Nelson, M. G. Scott, D. S. Smith, and M. H. Nahm, Subclass distribution of human antibodies to *Haemophilus influenzae* type b capsular polysaccharide, *J. Immunol. 138*:587 (1987).
76. V. A. Oxelius, IgG subclass levels in infancy and childhood, *Acta Paediatr. Scand. 68*:23 (1979).
77. H. Käyhty, O. Mäkelä, J. Eskola, L. Saarinen, and I. Seppälä, Isotype distribution and bactericidal activity of antibodies after immunization with *Haemophilus influenzae* type b vaccines at 18–24 months of age, *J. Infect. Dis. 158*:973 (1988).
78. J. Amir, M. G. Scott, M. H. Nahm, and D. M. Granoff, Bactericidal and opsonic activity of IgG1 and IgG2 anticapsular antibodies to *Haemophilus influenzae* type b, *J. Infect. Dis. 162*:163 (1990).
79. S. V. Hetherington, The intrinsic affinity constant (K) of anticapsular antibody to oligosaccharides of *Haemophilus influenzae* type b, *J. Immunol. 140*:3966 (1988).
80. W. R. Griswold, A. H. Lucas, L. F. Bastian, and G. Garcia, Functional affinity of antibody to the *Haemophilus influenzae* type b polysaccharide, *J. Infect. Dis. 159*:1083 (1989).
81. J. Amir, X. Liang, and D. M. Granoff, Variability in the functional activity of vaccine-induced antibody to *Haemophilus influenzae* type b, *Pediatr. Res. 27*:358 (1990).
82. D. M. Granoff, J. E. Squires, R. S. Munson, and B. Suarez, Siblings of patients with *Haemophilus* meningitis have impaired anticapsular antibody responses to Haemophilus vaccine, *J. Pediatr. 103*:185 (1983).
83. J. P. Pandey, H. H. Fudenberberg, G. Virella, C. U. Kyong, C. B. Loadhold, R. M. Galbraith, E. C. Gotschlich, and J. C. Parke Jr., Association between immunoglobulin allotypes and immune responses to *Haemophilus influenzae* and meningococcus polysaccharides. *Lancet 1*:190 (1979).
84. D. M. Ambrosino, V. A. Barrus, G. G. DeLange, and G. R. Siber, Correlation of the Km(1) immunoglobulin allotype with anti-polysaccharide antibodies in Caucasian adults, *J. Clin. Invest. 78*:361 (1986).
85. D. M. Granoff, P. G. Shackelford, J. P. Pandey, and E. G. Boies, Antibody responses to *Haemophilus influenzae* type b polysaccharide vaccine in relation to Km(1) and G2m(23) immunoglobulin allotypes, *J. Infect. Dis. 154*:257 (1986).
86. D. M. Ambrosino, G. Schiffman, E. C. Gotschlich, P. H. Schur, G. A. Rosenberg, G. G. DeLange, E. van Loghem, and G. R. Siber, Correlation

between G2m(n) immunoglobulin allotype and human antibody response and susceptibility to polysaccharide encapsulated bacteria, *J. Clin. Invest. 75*:1935 (1985).

87. H. Sarvas, N. Rautonen, H. Käyhty, M. Kallio, and O. Mäkelä, Effect of Gm allotypes on IgG2 antibody responses and IgG2 concentrations in children and adults, *Intern. Immunol. 2*:317 (1990).

87a. D. M. Granoff, B. K. Suarez, J. P. Pandy, and P. G. Shackelford, Genes associated with the G2m(23) immunoglobulin allotype regulate the IsG subclass response to *Haemophilus influenzae* type b polysaccharide. *J. Infect. Dis. 157*:1142 (1988).

88. A. K. Takala, H. Sarvas, E. Kela, P. R. Rönnberg, and P. H. Mäkelä, Susceptibility to invasive *Haemophilus influenzae* type b disease and the immunoglobulin G2m(n) allotype, *J. Infect. Dis. 163*:637 (1991).

89. H. Käyhty, H. Peltola, V. Karanko, and P. H. Mäkelä, Protective level of serum antibodies to the capsular polysaccharide of *Haemophilus influenzae* type b, *J. Infect. Dis. 147*:1100. (1983).

90. P. Anderson, The protective level of serum antibodies to the capsular polysaccharide of *Haemophilus influenzae* type b, *J. Infect. Dis. 149*:1034 (1984).

91. J. I. Ward, D. P. Greenberg, P. W. Anderson, K. S. Burkart, P. D. Christenson, L. K. Gordon, H. Käyhty, J. S. Kuo, and P. Vella, Variable quantitation of *H. influenzae* type b anticapsular antibody by radioantigen binding assay, *J. Clin. Microbiol. 26*:72 (1988).

92. P. Anderson, R. A. Insel, S. Porcelli, and J. Ward, Immunochemical variables affecting radioantigen-binding assays of antibody to *Haemophilus influenzae* type b capsular polysaccharide in children's sera, *J. Infect. Dis. 156*:582 (1987).

93. M. L. Barbour, R. Booy, D. W. Crook, H. Griffiths, H. Chapel, E. R. Moxon, and R. T. Mayon-White, *Haemophilus influenzae* type b: carriage and immunity four years after conjugate vaccination. *Program and Abstracts of the 32nd ICAAC*, Anaheim, California, 1992, p. 273.

94. H. Käyhty, J. Eskola, H. Peltola, L. Saarinen, and P. H. Mäkelä, High antibody responses to booster doses of either *Haemophilus influenzae* type b capsular polysaccharide or conjugate vaccine after primary immunization with conjugate vaccine, *J. Infect. Dis. 165* (Suppl.):S165 (1992).

95. Z. T. Handzel, M. Argaman, J. C. Parke Jr., and R. Schneerson, Heteroimmunization to the capsular polysaccharide of *Haemophilus influenzae* type b induced by enteric cross-reacting bacteria, *Infect. Immun. 11*:1045 (1975).

96. S. D. King, A. Ramlal, H. Wynter, K. Moodie, D. Castle, J. S. C. Kuo, L. Barnes, and C. L. Williams, Safety and immunogenicity of a new *Haemophilus influenzae* type b vaccine in infants under one year of age, *Lancet 2*: 705 (1981).

97. P. Anderson and R. A. Insel, A polysaccharide-protein complex from *Haemophilus influenzae* type b. I. Activity in weanling rabbits and human T lymphocytes, *J. Infect. Dis. 144*:509 (1981).

98. R. Schneerson, J. E. Robbins, C. Chu, A. Sutton, G. Schiffman, and W. F. Vann, Semi-synthetic vaccines composed of capsular polysaccharides of pathogenic bacteria covalently bound to proteins for the prevention of invasive diseases, *Prog. Allergy 33*:144 (1983).

2

Perspectives on Vaccine Development

Ronald W. Ellis

Merck Research Laboratories, West Point, Pennsylvania

Development is that group of activities that translates a research lead into a commercial product. For vaccines, development encompasses the technical, clinical, regulatory, and associated activities that result in licensure by governmental regulatory agencies. The vaccine development process usually takes at least 4 years and requires very close coordination of the activities of company personnel with clinical investigators in field trials and with regulatory agencies. Scores of individuals in the company work together in an integrated team effort covering the following areas: preclinical, clinical, process, analytical, regulatory, biostatistics, manufacturing, quality assurance, quality control, legal, and marketing. This chapter will provide a general overview of the development process for *Haemophilus* b (Hib) conjugate vaccines. While the development programs for each of the four licensed Hib conjugate vaccines were distinct, most of the points discussed in this review are generally applicable to each of the programs.

As discussed in Chapter 1, vaccines consisting of polyribosylribitol phosphate (PRP) were being licensed in the mid-1980s for use in children at the same time that Hib conjugate vaccines based on the linkage of PRP to various carrier proteins were being developed. The confluence of these development efforts facilitated the ultimate licensure of conjugate vaccines in several ways:

1. Methods for the production, analysis, and quality control of PRP became established for the field in general (Chap. 5), especially by Praxis and Connaught, who had licensed PRP vaccines before their conjugate vaccines.
2. Antibodies to PRP (anti-PRP) were recognized as mediating protection against Hib disease (Chap. 1). The movement toward standardization of the radioimmunoassay (RIA) to measure anti-PRP (Chap. 14) made it readily possible to quantitate anti-PRP levels in the serum of vaccinees in clinical trials, such that the anti-PRP assay became the established method for evaluating the immunogenicity of Hib conjugate vaccines.
3. Investigators in many clinical centers became experienced in evaluating PRP vaccines in routine clinical trials for safety and immunogenicity.
4. Several clinical centers set up extensive networks for the surveillance of Hib disease, which enabled the efficacy of PRP vaccines, then later of Hib conjugate vaccines (Chap. 18), to be evaluated.
5. Regulatory agencies became experienced with the above issues for PRP vaccines, almost all of which became applicable for the eventual licensure of Hib conjugate vaccines (Chap. 24).
6. The awareness of the epidemiology (Chap. 11), morbidity, and mortality of invasive Hib diseases grew in the medical community, such that there became a strong impetus for manufacturers to develop conjugate vaccines.

With the realization that PRP vaccines were neither adequately immunogenic nor efficacious in children less than 18–24 months of age (Chap. 1), the target group with the highest incidence of invasive Hib diseases, several groups turned to conjugate technology for improving the immunogenicity of PRP. It became recognized in the early 1980s that PRP likely would become a licensed vaccine for older children. Therefore, the choice of carrier protein became a significant developmental decision (Chap. 4). Two manufacturers chose licensed vaccine antigens as carrier proteins—diphtheria (D) toxoid for PRP-D (ProHIBit®, Connaught) and tetanus (T) toxoid for PRP-T (ActHIB®, Pasteur-Mérieux)—which are chemically inactivated toxins of *Corynebacterium diphtheriae* and *Clostridium tetani*. Since these antigens had been injected into hundreds of millions of infants as part of the DTP vaccine, their use in conjugate vaccines had not been expected to present any appreciable safety concern. These protein antigens were well characterized. In addition, since Hib conjugate vaccines were expected to be administered to young infants concomitantly with DTP vaccines, it was possible that carrier priming could augment the immunogenicity of the respective Hib conjugate vaccines (Chaps. 4 and 6). Praxis chose a mutant D toxin (CRM_{197}) as carrier protein for its vaccine (HibTITER®, Lederle). Since CRM_{197} has a point mutation which substantially reduces its toxin activity (1), it does not need to be inactivated with formalin as does wild-type D (or T) toxin for DTP vaccine or conjugate carrier. Since formalin treatment chemically alters the toxin, it was hoped that CRM_{197} would have carrier properties superior to those of D and T toxoids by obviating potential chemical alteration of T-cell epitopes in the carrier. Moreover, CRM_{197} also might benefit from carrier priming by D toxoid in DTP vaccine. The fourth manufacturer chose an outer membrane protein complex (OMPC) isolated by detergent extraction of *Neisseria meningitidis* B (NMB) cells as carrier protein for PRP-OMPC (PedvaxHIB®, Merck). Being a large particle, OMPC was expected to afford a superior immunogenic presentation of PRP conjugated onto its surface. OMPC itself has an adjuvant effect as well as a constituent protein with a strong carrier effect (Chap. 4). OMPC vaccines have shown some protective efficacy against NMB diseases. In addition, since meningococcal antigens were not administered as part of other routinely used vaccines, OMPC was not expected to elicit any potential immunological interference.

All the conjugate vaccines utilize PRP derived from fermentations of Hib organisms. Three of the vaccines are conjugates to PRP as a polysaccharide, i.e., generally >50 repeat units of the ribosyl-ribitol-phosphate monomer. The fourth vaccine is a conjugate of CRM_{197} as carrier to oligosaccharides of PRP, i.e., <30 repeat units, and is known as Haemophilus b Oligosaccharide Conjugate or HbOC (HibTITER®). The details of the four chemical strategies used for these vaccines and their rationales are discussed in Chapter 3. Since each of the four vaccines uses different PRP sizes, conjugation chemistries, and carrier proteins, it is not yet possible to state definitively which element of each contributes to its immunogenic properties and is desirable from the perspectives of clinical efficacy, tolerability, and process considerations. Nevertheless, some associations can be drawn regarding certain carrier proteins and their conjugation chemistries with their effect upon immunogenicity (Chap. 6).

Research in conjugate technology as applied to Hib vaccines began at the laboratory scale and was carried out by research chemists. At that time, success typically was judged from some evidence that conjugation of Hib polysaccharide (Ps) to carrier protein had taken place. This evidence included analytical proof of covalent bond formation between Ps and protein, chromatographic or electrophoretic analysis showing an association between Ps and protein, and immune responses in the animal models described below which are qualitatively different from those of the PRP vaccine (Chap. 5). When such evidence had been obtained coupled with process research that showed some reproducibility in the conjugation chemistry and in the preparation of Ps and carrier protein, the decision could be made to initiate product development.

Different development strategies can be followed in a successful program. One strategy, which enables initial clinical data to be obtained rapidly, is to use a laboratory-scale process (hundreds to thousands of doses per batch) to produce vaccine for early clinical trials, a pilot-scale process (thousands to tens of thousands per batch) for later trials including efficacy trials, then the manufacturing-scale process (tens of thousands to over one hundred thousand per batch) for final licensure trials. A second strategy is to use a pilot-scale process for most of the clinical trials including the efficacy studies. A third strategy is to use a pilot-scale process for many clinical studies but the manufacturing-scale process for efficacy and final licensure studies. Yet another strategy is to use a manufacturing scale process for all but the initial clinical studies. It is not possible to state which strategy is most advantageous for the timing and eventual success of development and licensure. Each company has a different "philosophy" for the strategy of developing a vaccine. Each strategy staggers the financial risk and staffing level of development and capital investment in a manufacturing facility in different ways, the first being the most conservative and the last the most risky. There are differences in process risk, since subtle changes may occur during the scale-up process which are not apparent at the time. In this regard, the last strategy is most conservative, while the first two strategies may spawn a manufactured vaccine that is (subtly) different from that used in efficacy studies. Within each company, competition for resources among other non-Hib research, development, and manufacturing projects can dictate the availability of trained staff, facilities, and other resources consistent with only one or two of the above strategies. Nevertheless, each of the different strategies can be and has been executed successfully.

Preclinical biological studies are performed in vitro and in vivo for Hib conjugate vaccines to support development efforts. Mice and infant monkeys have been used as animal models for immunogenicity (Chap. 4). These studies demonstrated that Hib conjugate vaccines were immunogenic in models where the PRP vaccine was nonimmunogenic. These models have been used in development to demonstrate that the vaccine retains the same immunogenic properties as it proceeds through different phases of development. In addition, immunogenicity in inbred mice can be used as a release test for the vaccine. Serological testing is used to measure the immune response to the vaccine in animal models as well as in humans. In the mid-1980s, the Farr-type RIA was standardized according to a single serum standard provided to all laboratories such that a single assay would be used to measure total serum anti-PRP levels in all preclinical and clinical studies (Chap. 14). Other serological assays used to measure anti-PRP have included: (a) enzyme-linked immunoassays to measure IgG, IgG1–4,

IgM and IgA anti-PRP, (b) serum bactericidal assays that measure the ability of serum anti-PRP to mediate in vitro killing of Hib organisms, (c) opsonic assays that measure the capacity for anti-PRP to mediate the ingestion of Hib organisms by neutrophils or macrophages in vitro, and (d) infant rat protection models in which anti-PRP injected into infant rats is shown to prevent Hib-induced bacteremia (Chap. 14).

One of the keys to an effective vaccine development program is the availability of a comprehensive array of analytical techniques. Chapters 3 and 5 describe the major assays used for each of the Hib conjugate vaccines to monitor intermediate steps in the process as well as to analyze the final product. Initially, a wide range of assays is identified, which may provide data relevant to the safety, immunogenicity, consistency, and stability of the product and process. Based upon experience with many lots, select assays eventually are chosen as the key assays for testing each process intermediate and final product lot. Validation assures that each assay is providing accurate results. Ordinarily, the assays used to characterize the process and product should be validated for testing clinical lots. During the several-year period of product development, new assays are introduced as the state of the art advances, which can provide useful new information about the vaccine at the same time that the vaccine proceeds through further clinical trials.

Thorough analytical characterization provides a useful bridge from research lots to clinical lots to manufactured lots in terms of assuring similarity of these lots throughout the development program (2). This is important for both regulatory and financial reasons. When the Hib conjugate vaccine is produced in a manufacturing facility, similarity of its analytical properties to those of the vaccine produced during development provides good assurance that the manufactured vaccine will have a similar safety and immunogenicity profile to that tested during clinical trials. In addition, as a company makes the very large financial commitment to build a manufacturing facility, it must be able to assure through analytical testing that it produces a vaccine equivalent to that tested during clinical trials. This assurance is attained by means of specifications on release assays, which are tests performed on each lot of vaccine produced for clinical trials or commercial distribution (Chap. 5). Each production lot of the four Hib conjugate vaccines undergoes approximately 8–12 release tests. Based upon the range of data for each analytical test on vaccine lots tested clinically and shown to be immunogenic and well tolerated, a limit or specification is established, e.g., phosphate content of PRP as a weight percent of PRP has a release specification of 6.8–9.0%. Any vaccine lot or intermediate which has an analytical test result outside of the release specification is not used further, e.g., a batch of PRP with phosphate as 6.0% of PRP would not be used to make a lot of Hib conjugate vaccine. Unexpected immunogenicity data on a particular clinical lot should be attributable to its analytical characteristics. If a particular lot has an immunogenicity profile higher or lower than others produced by the same process, it may be because of a trend in data from a particular analytical test; the specification then may be reset on the basis of these data. Alternatively, retrospective analysis of such a lot by an assay not routinely used to characterize all previous lots may show a difference or tend in the analytical data. Such an assay then would be established as a release assay for future lots, with the specification set accordingly. Release assays for Hib conjugate vaccines are summarized in Chapter 5.

Once a research-scale process has been established and appropriate analytical tests have been identified and validated, process development begins (3). The goal of this phase of development is to translate a laboratory-scale process into one that can operate at a larger (pilot) scale reproducibly and with high yield for ultimate implementation at the manufacturing scale. It is recognized that the Hib conjugate vaccine is a biological product which, due to its relatively large size and complexity, cannot be completely characterized at the molecular level as can a pharmaceutical product. The pilot-scale process makes use of individual steps; analytical characterization of each of the process intermediates is performed to assure consistency. Since all the Hib conjugate vaccines are the products of numerous chemical reactions, it is important that the process be validated to assure the clearance of all chemicals from the product stream. This validation also relies on extensive analytical testing. Since Hib conjugate vaccines are of high molecular weight relative to chemicals used in the process, a final filtration, chromatography, or ultracentrifugation step can assure the clearance of chemicals from the final product. Another key facet of process development is the identification and testing of all raw materials used in the process, including components of fermentation media, chemical reagents, and chromatography and filtration buffers. Specifications are placed on the testing of all raw materials in order to assure their identity, degree of purity, reproducibility, and effectiveness in the process.

Once the final purified bulk conjugate vaccine has been produced, analytical testing in stability studies becomes the basis for determining a suitable form and temperature of storage. Such testing can be performed initially on research-scale preparations in order to establish storage conditions for the vaccine lots to be used in clinical trials. Further testing of clinical vaccine lots assures that each lot is stable during the course of clinical trials, such that the clinical data on safety and immunogenicity are valid from a regulatory perspective. Probe stability studies can focus upon vaccine in liquid or lyophilized form, stored at either 2–8°C (refrigerated) or −15°C (frozen), which are suitable for conducting clinical trials. From all the analytical assays performed on the final product, several assays considered to be "stability-indicating" are selected. Vaccine is placed at the indicated storage temperatures and tested periodically in the stability-indicating assays at, e.g., 0, 1, 3, 6, 12, 18, and 24 months. Any significant change in analytical data from one of the assays may indicate a time limit for storage at that temperature. Each storage station (refrigerator or freezer) must be validated, i.e., independently certified by temperature recorders to have maintained the indicated temperature during the study. Such studies established that all the Hib conjugate vaccines would be stable at 2–8°C during the course of clinical studies. Two of the vaccines (PRP-D, HbOC) were shown to be stable in liquid storage, while the other two (PRP-OMPC, PRP-T) were shown to be stable in lyophilized form. PRP-OMPC has been developed subsequently into a liquid, aluminum-adsorbed formulation.

The formulation refers to those components of the final vaccine, other than the Hib conjugate itself, that contribute to the appearance, tolerability, immunogenicity, and stability of the vaccine. The formulation should contain a physiological concentration of saline in order to minimize stinging upon injection. The saline solution may be buffered or unbuffered. One of the vaccines contains aluminum hydroxide as adjuvant, to which the Hib conjugate (PRP-OMPC) is adsorbed through ionic bonding. The aluminum adjuvant enhances the immune response to the vaccine. Furthermore, early clinical trials indicated that PRP-OMPC adjuvanted to aluminum was much better tolerated than PRP-OMPC in aqueous solution (Chap. 15); the aluminum formulation has been used henceforth. The Hib conjugate vaccines may also contain thimerosal as preservative. The four Hib conjugate vaccines contain no other significant components as part of their formulation. The lyophilized vaccines (PRP-T, PRP-OMPC) are reconstituted in saline or saline with aluminum, respectively, at the time of administration.

Once the initial process and analytical assays have been developed and the stability of the storage form and the formulation have been assured, an initial clinical lot is prepared, tested, and released. In the United States, an Investigational New Drug (IND) application is prepared and submitted to the Center for Biologics Evaluation and Research (CBER) of the Food and Drug Administration (Chap. 24). The IND application contains detailed technical information (process, analytical, stability, biological, etc.) on the Hib conjugate vaccine, especially on the actual vaccine lot to be evaluated clinically, as well as the details of the plans for the conduct and evaluation of clinical trials. For studies carried out in other countries, an analogous Clinical Study Authorization application is filed with the regulatory agency in the particular country. There is a 30-day waiting period for CBER to review the IND, after which Phase I clinical studies may commence. If

CBER feels that there is a significant unresolved safety issue(s) with regard to the vaccine or plan for clinical trials, it may place the IND on hold, in which case clinical studies would not commence until the sponsor and CBER have resolved the safety issue.

Prelicensure clinical trials are categorized as Phase I, Phase II, or Phase III (Chap. 13). In Phase I trials, the vaccine is studied for safety. Since the primary target group for Hib conjugate vaccines is 2-month-old infants and trials in infants should be approached conservatively, safety is first assessed in adults and then children (e.g., 2–5 years of age) before infants, usually in groups of 10–20 subjects each. Frequently occurring adverse experiences (AEs), such as observed changes at the injection site, fever, crying, and discomfort, are typically tabulated at daily intervals following each injection. Immunogenicity also might be assessed to a limited degree. Vaccine trials are expanded in Phase II to encompass hundreds to 1000 or more infants. These trials include regimens and dose-ranging studies that enable an optimal dosage level and vaccination schedule to be selected for Phase III trials and ultimate licensure. A complete immunogenicity profile for the vaccine is established both in normally responsive populations as well as hyporesponsive groups (Chaps. 15, 16). As discussed above, immunogenicity trials for all Hib conjugate vaccines have made use of the Farr-type RIA for measuring levels of anti-PRP in serum. An expanded database for safety is obtained, where less frequent occurring AEs are observed and tabulated. Other trials include vaccine interaction studies, where the Hib conjugate vaccine is tested by concomitant administration with other pediatric vaccines such as DTP, polio, measles-mumps-rubella, and hepatitis B, to assure that coadministration does not result in clinically significant diminished immune responses to either Hib or to any of the coadministered vaccines. These studies pave the way to enabling the Hib conjugate vaccine to be approved for coadministration with these other required or recommended pediatric vaccines at 2, 4, 6, and 12–15 months as indicated for each product. In this regard, studies also have been performed where Hib conjugate vaccines are mixed with DTP vaccines. HbOC has been blended with DTP and filled into vials at the time of manufacture into a combined quadrivalent vaccine, which has been licensed (4). Additionally, lyophilized PRP-T vaccine has been rehydrated with DTP vaccine for coadministration in a single shot (5).

Once a dosage level has been selected and the tolerability profile of the vaccine established and deemed acceptable, Phase III efficacy trials can be undertaken. Efficacy trials with PRP vaccines had suggested that a serum anti-PRP level of 0.15 μg/ml was generally associated with short-term protection against invasive Hib diseases, while a level of 1.0 μg/ml was associated with long-term protection in children who had received PRP vaccines (Chap.

1). Therefore, it was generally expected that, if Hib conjugate vaccines were able to elicit such anti-PRP levels in infants, these vaccines would be efficacious in preventing invasive Hib diseases in infants less than 6 months of age. Three of the Hib conjugate vaccines (HbOC, PRP-T, PRP-OMPC) elicit $>1.0\ \mu g$ anti-PRP/ml in fully vaccinated infants (post doses 3, 3, 2, respectively), while PRP-D elicits >0.15 but $<1.0\ \mu g$ anti-PRP/ml (post dose 3).

Several different study designs have been used in Phase III efficacy trials (Chap. 18). In double-blind, placebo-controlled trials, the sponsor and clinical investigators are both unaware of whether a subject is receiving vaccine or placebo in order to eliminate bias in trial observations and analysis. Vaccine vials used in the study are filled with either vaccine or with placebo and then together are randomly numbered by code on common labels to assure blinding at the study site. The rate of efficacy is calculated based upon the difference in rates of Hib disease between the two groups. In case-control trials, infants are either vaccinated or unvaccinated, with the sponsor and parents being fully aware of the vaccination status of each infant. Vaccine efficacy is calculated based on a difference in observed disease between groups, which can be adjusted for possible differences in risk factors between the groups. All these studies are designed in collaboration with biostatisticians to ensure that the study groups are of sufficient size to assure adequate statistical significance to their outcome based upon the epidemiology of Hib disease in the target population for the trial (Chap. 11). In open trials, an entire large population is vaccinated, e.g., the annual birth cohort in Finland, and efficacy is calculated based upon the difference in Hib disease incidence in the trial compared to the historical rate of disease (Chap. 23). Each of the Hib conjugate vaccines has been licensed as being effective in preventing invasive Hib infections on the basis of one of these efficacy study designs.

As clinical trials proceed, companies make their plans for establishing a manufacturing facility (6). The major basis for establishing the size of a facility is a marketing projection for the particular Hib conjugate vaccine product. Given the then increasing awareness of the incidence, morbidity, and mortality of invasive Hib diseases, it was anticipated during the time of clinical trials that the Hib conjugate vaccines eventually would be recommended for routine vaccination of infants in developed countries. This defined the eventual annual market size for these vaccines as the birth cohort in the United States, Europe, and other developed countries. Increasing percentages of infants in each country where the vaccine would be licensed were expected to be vaccinated in each subsequent year, with the anticipation that 90% or more of infants eventually would be vaccinated, as is the case with other recommended pediatric vaccines. Each company then forecasts what percentage of the market in each country it thinks it will attain. The forecast is usually for a period of several years, beginning with the year in which the vaccine is expected to receive its first regulatory agency approval in a major market. This forecast becomes the basis for defining the capacity of the manufacturing facility needed to support worldwide demand year by year. It is important to assure flexibility in the operation of the manufacturing facility, whereby the company can smoothly increase or decrease its rate of production in response to higher- or lower-than-anticipated market demand without affecting product quality. It can take 2 or more years from the initial planning of a manufacturing facility until it is actually producing finished vaccine. Furthermore, vaccine produced at scale in the manufacturing facility as consistency lots (see below) is tested clinically for safety and immunogenicity before a license application is filed and approved by a regulatory agency. This means that it is several years before the time of license approval when a marketing projection needs to be made for building a manufacturing facility. The assumptions inherent in such an early marketing forecast may have a relatively low accuracy, especially with regard to dates of licensure of both the subject vaccine as well as its competing vaccines. Estimating these relative timings is critical to the forecast in that, other things being relatively equal, the first product and to some extent the second product licensed usually have the largest shares in a given market.

These uncertainties regarding the marketing forecast make the establishment of a manufacturing facility a very risky and substantial financial commitment, one which can total tens of millions of dollars. If the forecast is too low, then the manufacturing facility will be unable to produce enough doses to satisfy demand, and the company may be unable to launch the Hib conjugate vaccine in all approved markets in a timely fashion. This can allow a competitive vaccine to establish a significantly higher share in the market than it otherwise would have, such that the particular vaccine would have a permanently lowered financial value to its company relative to the situation where it had been able to fully satisfy market demand. If such a shortfall in supply relative to demand is recognized early enough approaching the time of licensure or soon thereafter, the facility and process can be increased in size and capacity but inevitably at a greater cost in time, money, and personnel than if the facility had been appropriately sized originally. Such changes in the process and/or facility entail significant regulatory activities in terms of license amendments, as described below. Another way in which the company can accommodate an unforeseen increase in demand is to design enough flexibility into the operation of the manufacturing facility such that a greater number of lots can be produced each year without changing the process. This means increasing the number of production shifts per week. Conversely, if the original marketing forecast is too high, then the facility will operate below full capacity. Since the overhead costs for operating the facility are spread over fewer doses, the manufacturing cost of the vaccine is higher than it would have been if made in a smaller facility. Furthermore, if demand is low enough, then the company might not even earn back its investment in the facility. These are some of the financial risks inherent in projecting long-term market demand during clinical trials, which nevertheless are necessary risks in launching any new vaccine.

Once sufficient data have accumulated to assure the company that the conjugate vaccine is sufficiently well tolerated and immunogenic and therefore likely to be efficacious in preventing invasive Hib diseases, the company is in the position to make the commitment to building a manufacturing facility (although the company certainly is free to take the risk to build a facility before such clinical data are available). Since licensure for vaccines and biologicals entails the approval by regulatory agencies of the production facility in addition to the actual product, the facility needs to be specially designed to meet extensive regulatory requirements (7) according to the highest expected standards in the industry, which are generally referred to as current Good Manufacturing Practices (cGMP). The cGMP standards include but are not limited to the following provisions:

1. Standard Operating Procedures (SOPs) are used, which systematically describe every process step and analytical procedure in enough detail to enable them to be performed by trained personnel who might not have a scientific background. There is a record of SOPs used for producing and testing each production batch, which are signed by those performing the procedure.
2. There is a complete accounting for all raw materials used in production. Raw materials must meet established quality standards.
3. A purified source of water, e.g., Water for Injection (WFI), must be used for all solutions in the product stream.
4. The facility must be constructed and operated in a way that minimizes the potential for microbial contamination. This includes the use of certain construction designs, building materials, air-pressure patterns, and air-filtration devices.
5. The facility typically is dedicated to the manufacture of a single product. If it is used for a second product, there must be a proven procedure for validating that the facility is thoroughly cleansed of the first product so that there is no possible cross-contamination of products.
6. All raw materials, process intermediates, and final products should be clearly labeled and segregated in a way that assures no cross-contamination or accidental switching of such materials.

7. All processes, analytical procedures, and equipment must be validated, i.e., proven to perform as intended.
8. Personnel working in the facility must be appropriately dressed. In particular, those who come in contact with the process stream should wear gowns, facemasks, shoe covers, and hair covers.
9. Access to the facility, especially where process steps are being performed, should be strictly limited to those who *need* to be there. The routes of access should be controlled in a way that limits the potential for microbial contamination.
10. Samples and final products should be retained for a stipulated period of time after manufacture in case these materials need to be retested for an unforeseen reason.
11. The allowable holding periods for raw materials, solutions, product intermediates, and final products should be established through appropriate stability studies, as described below.

Once the final manufacturing facility is fully operational, it is important to demonstrate that the Hib conjugate vaccine made in this facility is not different from that tested during clinical trials. Unless the vaccine tested in Phase III clinical trials was produced at full scale in the manufacturing facility as consistency lots (see below), the vaccine produced in the facility would be tested in further clinical trials in order to assure similar immunogenicity and tolerability to that used in Phase III. The scale of manufacturing is defined according to marketing projections. Each lot is large enough to assure supplying enough vaccine with an economy of scale to keep direct production costs under control. At the same time, each lot is not so large as to incur excess financial risk in the event that a lot fails a release specification and thus is discarded. In addition, it is important to show that the manufacturing-scale process performs consistently in the final manufacturing facility operated by the production personnel, who are less trained scientifically than the R&D staff. For this purpose, the process is demonstrated by the R&D staff to the manufacturing staff as part of a series of "manufacturing consistency" lots. This is a series of three to five consecutive lots, manufactured by production personnel under cGMP according to SOPs and rigorously analyzed by validated release assays, which affirm that all the lots are produced consistently and are analytically similar. Typically, three of the lots are used to vaccinate the target population (infants) to confirm the "clinical consistency" of tolerability and immunogenicity among these lots. Once the consistency lots have been produced and analytically affirmed for manufacturing consistency and released for evaluation of clinical consistency, the manufacturing facility continues to produce additional lots of vaccine by the same process and tested by the same release assays as inventory for eventual commercial distribution once the vaccine has been licensed. The timing for accumulation of this inventory is important and is another financial risk. Sufficient inventory needs to be accumulated by the time of licensure to be able to support the launch of the product, e.g., a one-year supply of vaccine according to anticipated market demand may be deemed desirable by a manufacturer to minimize the possibility of a stockout should demand be higher than forecast. On the other hand, accumulating an excess inventory in the face of unanticipated slack demand can result in some of the vaccine exceeding its established shelf life and having to be discarded.

There are groups within the manufacturing operation that are responsible for the quality of the production process as well as the final product (7). The Quality Control group is responsible for performing all release testing of process intermediates and final products. Those who perform the tests are ordinarily unaware of the identity of samples they test in order to assure objectivity of the data. The head of the Quality Control group is responsible for reviewing all data from release tests and assuring that the test results all fall within specifications. The group head will release a particular vaccine lot for commercial distribution only if it meets all release specifications. Hence, this individual, whose role is to release only the highest quality product, has a different objective from that of the manufacturing group, which is trying to produce as much vaccine as possible to meet market requirements. The failure of a lot to pass any particular release test is investigated, which can provide valuable feedback to the manufacturing group regarding any unforeseen problems in the process. The Quality Assurance group performs an internal auditing function. It is responsible for reviewing all procedures and data and assuring compliance with SOPs and cGMP. It notes any deviations from proper procedures in order to prevent recurrences. In this way, the group should spot and correct deviations that would have been detected by a regulatory agency in the course of an external audit of the manufacturing operation.

Each of the consistency lots is put into a long-term stability study, as described above. The vaccine may be held at different temperatures, e.g., frozen, refrigerated, and room temperature, for 2 or more years and tested periodically (e.g., 0, 1, 3, 6, 12, 18, 24 months) in stability-indicating assays. By means of such studies on the consistency lots, the shelf life for the vaccine is established. All four Hib conjugate vaccines are indicated for storage at 2–8°C for at least 2 years. The date of expiration is noted on each vial of vaccine. For distribution within the United States, Europe, and other developed countries, given that pediatricians and public health clinics ordinarily have refrigerators in their offices, it is very important that the Hib conjugate vaccine be indicated for storage at refrigerator temperature.

Should Hib conjugate vaccines be utilized in the future in developing countries, which ordinarily lack both a "cold chain" for distribution as well as refrigerators in clinics, then stability at room temperature or higher will become a critical issue for vaccine utilization (Chap. 16). Stability testing also is extended to process intermediates such as PRP, carrier protein, and bulk conjugate vaccine (before filling). To the extent to which stability testing enables such intermediates to be held in storage during a production campaign, the manufacturing facility can operate production in a more flexible fashion.

At the time the consistency lots are prepared, filling of the bulk conjugate vaccine is demonstrated and also must be performed in a consistent fashion. As noted above, two of the vaccines are filled directly as liquid vaccines. The other two are filled as liquid vaccines, then immediately are freeze-dried in a lyophilizer. The vaccine diluent to resuspend the lyophilized vaccine is filled separately, and a vial of diluent is supplied in the field with each vaccine vial. The filling can take place in different types of containers. Single-dose vials, multidose vials, and syringes can all be filled with the vaccine product. Each container must be validated for storage conditions and shelf life according to separate stability studies. Each manufacturer decides upon which containers it should distribute according to marketing surveys. The entire filling operation as well as the vials/syringes also fall under cGMP guidelines.

Once the company has obtained all relevant clinical data and process information and has a manufacturing facility with data on consistency lots, it can apply for licensure of the vaccine (Chap. 24). In the United States, a Product License Application (PLA) and an Establishment License application (ELA), containing all relevant information on the manufacturing facility, are filed with CBER Outside the United States, the same information is filed in a Marketing Authorization Application (MAA) with each regulatory agency. The timing between filing of the PLA/ELA/MAA and granting of a Product License varies among vaccines and among regulatory agencies. Questions from agencies may be answered in writing or at face-to-face meetings. Additional studies may be required before licensure. In order to minimize the possibility that licensure might be delayed by having to perform such additional studies, it is most efficient for the manufacturer to fully discuss the project and anticipated filing needs with key regulatory agencies throughout the development process in order to anticipate all potential issues that might be raised by the agencies and address these *before* it submits the PLA/ELA/MAA There may be formal meetings with individuals outside regulatory agencies where the advice of academic/government scientists and leaders in the fields of Hib, vaccines, and infectious diseases is sought as a recommendation to license the vaccine. During the course of review of the license applications, regulatory agencies may choose to conduct external audits or inspections of the manufacturing facility and its operations in order to assure compliance with cGMP and accuracy of reporting of information. Following licensure, a regulatory agency, typically the one from the country where the product is manufactured, may inspect the facility on a periodic yet unannounced basis in order to assure compliance with the Product and Establishment Licenses.

One of the most critical prelicensure discussions between the manufacturer and regulatory agency is the agreement on the precise wording in the package insert, which contains all key information on the vaccine, especially clinical trial experience, vaccine claims, and trials with competitive products. The wording in the package insert becomes the basis upon which promotional literature is written, i.e., if a property of the vaccine or a perceived competitive advantage is not described in the package insert, then the manufacturer should not be promoting the vaccine on that basis. For this reason, it is important that clinical trials be designed prospectively in a way that enables the results of the trial, in particular competitive trials, to be spelled out in the package insert so that the results can be promoted.

Once a Product License has been granted, development activities can continue for many years. These activities fall into several areas: clinical studies, process improvements, analytical improvements, and facility changes. In order to keep at the state of the art and to be as competitive as possible, a manufacturer ordinarily continues to support the vaccine with these activities.

Postlicensure clinical studies fall into Phases IV and V. A Phase IV trial is an extended safety study conducted in a large number of subjects, typically 10,000 or more, and is designed to detect AEs occurring much less frequently than those detected in the course of prelicensure clinical trials in thousands of subjects. Conducting such a postmarketing surveillance study often is a condition at the time of licensure for granting of the license. A Phase V study is used to seek expanded indications for the vaccine not originally obtained, e.g., vaccination of special populations such as HIV-positive children or concomitant administration with a new vaccine.

Once the process used to make consistency lots has been established, the manufacturer begins to accumulate inventory for launching the vaccine. During this period, there is the opportunity to develop changes in the process which may further improve product purity and consistency, increase yield, assure other sources of raw materials, or accommodate changes in equipment. Some of these changes are minor and can be implemented readily as long as they do not affect the quality or characteristics of the product. Significant changes must be reviewed with regulatory agencies prior to implementation through a formal process of amending the Product License. If such changes are judged to be significant enough based on analytical data that show that the product has changed or if there is presumptive evidence that the product has changed even in lieu of actual analytical data showing a change, then it may be necessary to perform clinical evaluation of the vaccine produced by the new process. The judgment as to the significance of a process change should be a conservative one, given that the Hib conjugate vaccines, being complex biological products, cannot be totally characterized as can pharmaceutical products. In fact, changes in the immunogenic properties of these vaccines have been documented (Chap. 15), even though the vaccines had passed all release tests at the time of manufacture.

Now that the Hib conjugate vaccines have been commercially available for several years, the state of the art with regard to analytical testing has advanced (Chap. 5). While it is not necessarily required that the manufacturer continually update all analytical assays, it may be desirable to apply new assays to the product and to product intermediates. New assays may give valuable information about the product and process not previously available or may give more accurate data than ones already in use. In cases such as these, the manufacturer may implement a new assay as a release assay in addition to those already in use or as a substitution for an available assay. Such changes also are formally documented with and approved by regulatory agencies.

Finally, the manufacturer may wish to make a change in process or scale of operation, as described above, which is so extensive as to require an alteration in the manufacturing facility or operation of the facility or even building a new facility. In such a case, the manufacturer would thoroughly document the changes and formally submit them to regulatory agencies as amendments to the Establishment License, which then proceed through an independent approval process before the vaccine made in the changed/new facility is distributed commercially.

A further phase of development for Hib conjugate vaccines is their combination with other required or recommended pediatric vaccines as a combination product. This involves the formulation of the Hib conjugate vaccine with another vaccine(s). Such a combination product is treated as a new product and is developed according to most of the criteria outlined in this chapter. As described above, the first such combination vaccine developed is a mixture of DTP and HbOC (9). Other combinations being developed include mixtures of Hib conjugate vaccines with DTP, hepatitis B, and inactivated polio vaccines.

It can be seen that the development of a vaccine extends for many years both before and after licensure and requires the commitment of a broad range of expertise. It is clear that rigorous planning, attention to detail, and strong commitment are critical to the successful development of Hib conjugate vaccines, which serve as the prototypes for other conjugate vaccines.

REFERENCES

1. G. Giannini, R. Rapproli, and G. Ratti, *Nucleic Acids Research 12*:4063 (1984).
2. R. L. Garnick, M. J. Ross, and R. A. Baffi, Characterization of proteins from recombinant DNA manufacture, *Drug Biotechnology Regulation* (Y.-Y. H. Chiu and J. L. Gueriguian, eds.), Marcel Dekker, New York, 1991, pp. 263–313.
3. R. G. Werner, H. Langlouis-Gau, F. Walz, H. Allgaier, and H. Hoffmann, Validation of biotechnological production processes, *Drug. Res. 38:* 855 (1988).
4. FDA approval of use of a new Haemophilus b conjugate vaccine and a combined diphtheria-tetanus-pertussis and Haemophilus b conjugate vaccine for infants and children, *MMWR 42*:296 (1993).
5. C. Ferreccio, J. Clemens, A. Avendano, I. Horwitz, C. Flores, L. Avila, M. Cayazzo, B. Fritzell, M. Cadoz, and M. Levine, The clinical and immunologic response of Chilean infants to *Haemophilus influenzae* type b polysaccharide-tetanus protein conjugate vaccine with diphtheria-tetanus toxoids-pertussis vaccine at two, four, and six months of age, *Pediatr. Infect. Dis. J. 10*:764 (1991).
6. D. T. Smith, Recent developments in the design and construction of facilities for the production of human injectables, *Vaccine 5*:5 (1987).
7. D. Hill and M. Beatrice, Facility requirements for biotech plants, *J. Parenter. Sci. Technol. 45*:132 (1991).
8. R. S. Garnick, N. J. Solli, and P. A. Papa, The role of quality control in biotechnology: an analytical perspective, *Anal. Chem. 60*:2546 (1988).
9. D. Hogerman, F. J. Malinoski, D. V. Madore, and P. R. Paradiso, Safety and immunogenicity of DTaP-HbOC in toddlers primed by DTP and HbOC as separate injections or DTP HbOC combination vaccine, *Pediatr. Res. 33*:171A (1993).

3

Conjugation: Design, Chemistry, and Analysis

Peter J. Kniskern

Merck Research Laboratories, West Point, Pennsylvania

Stephen Marburg

Merck Research Laboratories, Rahway, New Jersey

I. INTRODUCTION

Evolution has endowed pathogenic bacteria with various mechanisms designed to avoid evoking strong immune responses in their hosts, thereby enhancing their ability to survive in a hostile environment. Some encapsulate themselves in polysaccharide (Ps), taking advantage of the fact that the immune response to these antigens matures slowly in mammals. These Ps antigens are not able to involve T cells in the immune response of the infant (1) and, therefore, a number of such bacteria pose pathological problems for such individuals. *Haemophilus influenzae* type b (Hib) is such an organism, causing meningitis among other disease states. On the other hand, antigens of a protein (Pr) nature can involve T cells and are immunogenic in infants, as exemplified by efficacious Pr vaccines directed against diphtheria, tetanus, and pertussis. These are used successfully in infants as young as 2 months of age. In the past 15 years research efforts have been directed toward linking the ineffective Ps antigens to fully competent T-cell–involving Pr antigens with the objective of making the former useful as vaccines for these young infants. Such research has its roots in the work of W. F. Goebel and O. T. Avery (2), who showed that small saccharide molecules could be

Table 1 Polysaccharide Treatment and Size of Reaction Partners

Conjugate	Molecular sizing method	PRP m.w.[a]	Protein m.w.	Unbound PRP[b] (%)
PRP-D	hydrolysis @ 100°C	2×10^5–2×10^7	6.2×10^4	<37
HbOC	$NaIO_4$ treatment	3400–11000	6.2×10^4	<10
PRP-OMPC	oxalic acid[c] treatment	$\sim 8 \times 10^4$	3–5×10^7	<15
PRP-T[d]	none	$\sim 1 \times 10^5$	1.5×10^5	<20

[a]From literature reports or estimated from K_d data.
[b]In the final conjugate.
[c]This is not a sizing operation per se but a chemical event during a derivatization step.
[d]Direct published data are unavailable, but see Ref. 13.

transformed to immunologically effective antigens by covalently bonding them to Pr carriers. This research has been fruitful so that in the past few years four conjugate vaccines comprised of the capsular Ps of Hib and various carrier Pr have been developed and licensed. These are PRP-D (Connaught), HbOC (Lederle-Praxis), PRP-OMPC (Merck), and PRP-T (Mérieux).

These vaccines differ from one another in fundamental ways (Table 1); the differences involve the type of carrier Pr, the size of the Ps, the conjugation chemistry, and the details of the manufacturing processes. Although a comprehensive overview dealing with bacterial Ps-Pr conjugates in general appeared recently (3), it is one of the goals of this chapter to provide a description of the synthetic processes for the four commercial Hib vaccines and a critical delineation of their differences. This review also will focus on several critical issues that have emerged during the development of these Hib vaccines in the hope that they can be used as paradigms for future conjugate vaccines.

II. CRITICAL ISSUES

A. Process Control

Since the macromolecular reaction partners in a conjugation of Ps and Pr are polyfunctional and in the case of the Ps also polydisperse, a closely related family of products generally is obtained. Current technology allows neither facile separation of, nor analytical discrimination among the members of the family. Therefore, since immunogenicity may vary across the distribution of products, it is important that the same distribution of products is obtained in each preparation. This requires rigorous control of the process and extensive characterization of the product and the intermediates to ensure reproducibility. In addition, the process is tripartite, involving not only the conjugation but also the isolation and processing of the two macromolecular reactants (i.e., Ps and Pr). In addition, the Ps generally is processed to a material whose molecular weight is lower and less disperse (Table 1). Because of constraints of space we will not discuss the generation and isolation of the raw materials but will touch on their modification (i.e., size reduction of the Ps) as it bears directly on the design of the synthetic scheme. However, it should be emphasized that the ability to produce consistent starting materials bears directly on the ability to control the ensuing chemistry and process; consequently, analytical control of all steps is of paramount importance. The analytical characterization assays for process intermediates and products are summarized in Table 2 and also discussed further below.

Table 2 Analytical Characterization of Intermediates in the Manufacture of PRP Conjuate Vaccines

Vaccine	Intermediate[a]	Assay	Readout	Indication
PRP-D	**2**	not specified (n.s.)	n.s.[b]	n.s.
	4	1,3,5-trinitro benzene-sulfonic acid	OD[c] vs. concentration DT	level of derivatization
PRP-OMPC	**6**	none	—	—
	8	none	—	—
	10	NMR	butane diamine vs. PRP resonances integration	level of derivatization
	11	NMR	"	level of bromoacetylation
	13	Ellman	OD	level of thiolation
	14	amino acid analysis	areas of **16** and **17** vs. lysine	level of covalency and level of capping
PRP-T	**18**	1,3,5-trinitro benzene-sulfonic acid	OD vs. weight of PRP	level of derivatization
HbOC	**20**	alkaline ferricyanide ribose	reducing titer vs. PRP	degree of polymerization
	22	amino acid analysis	n.s.	level of covalency

[a]See text.
[b]n.s. = not specified.
[c]OD = Optical Density.

B. Covalency

The significance of covalency derives from the requirement for two signals required for a T-cell–mediated response. One signal, which provides the antigenic specificity, resides in the Ps, and the other, which is necessary for T-cell involvement, resides in the carrier Pr. If these two components are linked by electrostatic or hydrophobic (i.e., noncovalent) forces, their separation in vivo becomes possible and the efficacy of the conjugate potentially is compromised. Therefore, a stable connection with a covalent bond is required. Since the conjugation products have high molecular weights (m.w.), the conventional physicochemical analyses of structure are not applicable and it is difficult to assess the nature of the chemical changes that have occurred. It is a formidable task for infrared or NMR spectroscopy or elemental analysis (for carbon, hydrogen, nitrogen, etc.) to detect the small changes that a few atoms experience in going from starting material to product when these few atoms exist in a matrix of hundreds or thousands of atoms. Therefore, defining the structural nature of the product(s) becomes problematical, and the crucial issue of the covalency of the bond between the two macromolecules must be addressed in other ways. There are two salient ways of dealing with the covalency issue. One method relies on separation of products and starting materials on the basis of size, using techniques such as size exclusion chromatography (SEC) or filtration through membranes of known molecular weight cut-off (MWCO). The argument can then be made that if Pr and Ps are found in the same solution after separation from their congeneric reactants, then a bond between the two must now exist to allow this observation. However, that observation does not specify what type of interaction, electrostatic or covalent, is present. This form of reasoning also requires that control experiments show that all precursors would not find their way into fractions containing the conjugation product. The other more direct method involves design of the conjugation chemistry to allow detection of a unique molecule, which contains the bond formed in the conjugation of the two macromolecules.

C. Separation of Unconjugated Ps

It is not clear that unconjugated carrier Pr must be removed from the product. However, unconjugated Ps should not be present in appreciable quantities in the vaccine material, because the vaccine dosage is defined as weight of *conjugated* Ps and the analytical methods that define this weight cannot discriminate between conjugated and unconjugated Ps. Moreover, there is evidence that unconjugated Ps has the potential to depress the immune response to conjugates (4). Therefore, the need for removal of unbound Ps must be taken into account when designing a synthesis.

D. Sterility and Safety

Small-molecule injectable drugs are sterilized readily by filtration, but some of the conjugates under consideration have very large m.w., either by design or as a result of polymerization during processing, so that they do not pass through such filters. Therefore, the process design must address this issue either by development of appropriate filtrations or by a totally aseptic manufacturing operation. In addition, the introduction of reactive functional groups during the various stages of the conjugation process introduces a potential safety issue, which requires demonstrating that these are not reactive in the final vaccine; this issue will be discussed in more detail below.

E. Stability

Stability of the formulated vaccine, which is reflected in its shelf life, is of course a major concern. The amide, carbamate, thioether, and amine bonds that are introduced in the PRP-OMPC and HbOC products respectively, are highly stable under the hydrolytic and enzymatic conditions that these products might encounter. Less is known about the iminocarbazate and diacyl hydrazide groups that are features of the respective PRP-D and PRP-T products, but they generally are considered to be stable. However, the effect of these groups in the matrix of a polymeric structure is unknown, and the problem is best addressed empirically. A variety of stability-indicating assays, which track such parameters as antigenicity, immunogenicity, unbound Ps, or phosphate release, must be followed over time under the appropriate conditions of temperature, pH, etc., to establish a stability profile.

III. CHEMISTRY

As mentioned, there are three critical features that a Ps-Pr conjugate material should have to become a successful and immunogenic vaccine. First, the two entities must be joined together by covalent bonds rather than noncovalent interactions. Second, there should not be significant quantities of unconjugated Ps in the final product, and third, the final product must be stable, relatively safe, and sterile. These considerations affect the synthetic design and the details of the preparation. If one regards the conjugation of a Ps to a Pr as an exercise in organic chemistry, then a number of differences become apparent that distinguish this process from one involving small molecules. These differences derive from the nature of the starting materials, which generally:

1. have m.w.s of more than 40,000 daltons;
2. are polyfunctional in that each saccharide molecule has many hydroxyl groups and each Pr molecule has many amino and carboxylate groups;

3. are soluble only in water and not in organic solvents;
4. in the case of the Ps have m.w.s that are polydisperse (i.e., have a distribution of m.w.s that can range easily from twice to one half of a nominal weight);
5. have topological features that cannot be perturbed lest the relevant antigenic quality is lost.

These considerations have implications that must be taken into account when designing the conjugation process. In addition, because of considerations of polyfunctionality and poydispersity, the final material is a mixture of molecular species, and the classical characterization procedures used to define a single compound, such as sodium dodecyl sulfate-polyacrylamide gel electrophoresis (SDS-PAGE), are not always applicable. Therefore, for a conjugate vaccine to be reproducibly manufactured, it is essential that analytical controls be instituted at most, if not all, synthetic steps.

The capsular Ps of Hib, commonly known as PRP (polyribosylribitol phosphate), is a linear polymer consisting of ribose, ribitol, and phosphoric acid, which has the monomeric structure:

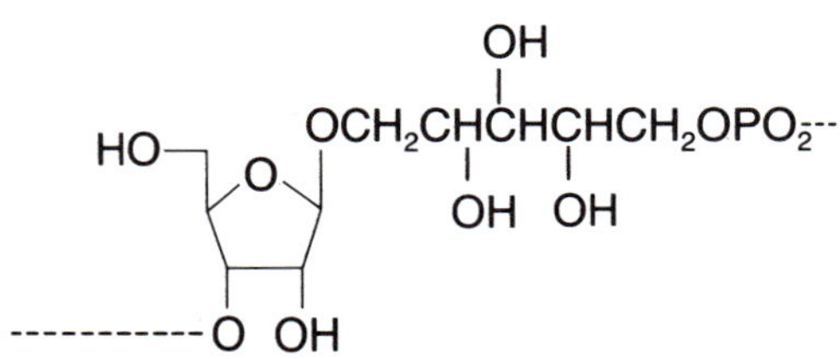

PRP

It should be noted that PRP contains only hydroxyl groups that might be used for generating stable covalent bonds (in the case of the HbOC vaccine, several of these are transformed into aldehyde functions). Conjugation through the acidic hydroxyl on the phosphodiester moiety, which would generate a tri-substituted phosphoric acid derivative, would risk hydrolytic instability in the conjugate. The Pr that have been employed as carriers are different for each of the conjugates under consideration (See Section III.A.), but all have the same functional groups available for conjugation chemistry: the amino groups of lysine, the carboxyl groups of aspartic and glutamic acids, and to a lesser extent the phenolic moiety of tyrosine and the imidazole of histidine. The following is a discussion of how each vaccine manufacturer has used these groups to form covalent bonds to link the two different macromolecules.

A. Outline of the Processes

1. PRP-D

This process (5) involves hydrolyzing and lowering the m.w. of the PRP followed by activation to an electrophilic species with cyanogen bromide, **1**. Although the product of the reaction can assume several structural forms, for the purpose of the discussion it is described as a cyanate ester, **2**. There is no reported assay that quantitates the degree of cyanation. Distortion of the antigenic character of PRP can occur at high levels of derivatization, and the determination of such values would be useful.

$$\text{PRP-}H_2O(100°C) \rightarrow \text{PRP(m.w.} = 2 \times 10^5\text{–}2 \times 10^6) + \underset{\mathbf{1}}{\text{BrCN}} \rightarrow \underset{\mathbf{2}}{\text{PRP-OCN}}$$

In a separate process stream, diphtheria toxoid (DT) is functionalized with adipic acid dihydrazide, **3**, using the water-soluble 1-ethyl-3-(3-dimethylaminopropyl) carbodiimide (EDAC) as the condensing agent and creating the nucleophilic DT derivative, **4**. This reaction utilizes the carboxyl groups of the toxoid and there is an opportunity for crosslinking two or more molecules of DT with **4**.

$$\text{DT} + \underset{\mathbf{3}}{H_2NHNCO(CH_2)_4CONHNH_2} + \text{EDAC} \rightarrow \underset{\mathbf{4}}{\text{DT— }HNNHCO(CH_2)_4CONHNH_2}$$

Compound **4** was evaluated in the early research* by SEC (K_d on Sepharose Cl-4B = 0.75) and found to have a m.w. of 139,000. This m.w., which is about twice the weight of the toxoid, probably reflects a crosslinking reaction. The electrophilic **2** and nucleophilic **4** intermediates then are combined and the conjugate product, **5**, subjected to SEC on Sephacryl S-300. All material of m.w. less than 140,000 daltons is discarded.

$$\mathbf{4} + \mathbf{2} \rightarrow \underset{\mathbf{5}}{\text{DT— }HNNHCO(CH_2)_4CONHNHC(=N)O\text{-PRP}}$$

---

*In routine manufacture the hydrazide 4 is not evaluated by SEC.

The product is characterized by ribose (PRP) and Pr assays (PRP/Pr = 1.12), and SEC on Sepharose Cl-2B and 4B (vide infra). The latter indicates a molecular size of 6.7×10^5. Since other SEC assays indicate that there is no unconjugated Pr in the product, it is inferred that the Pr is covalently bound to the Ps. However, none of these data excludes the presence of unconjugated PRP in the product. This latter fact can have a significant impact on dosage formulation and immunogenicity (vide infra). Because of the polyfunctionality of both Pr and Ps, the product is a mixture of stoichiometries and can be described as the simple lattice type (3) as depicted in schematic form in Figure 1.

2. PRP-OMPC

This process also proceeds in two streams (6,7). One involves derivatization of PRP (which has not been treated to reduce its m.w.) in a non-aqueous system. It was felt that the hydroxyl groups on PRP could not effectively compete as nucleophiles with the hydroxyls of water in an aqueous system. Therefore, PRP was converted to the tetrabutyl ammonium

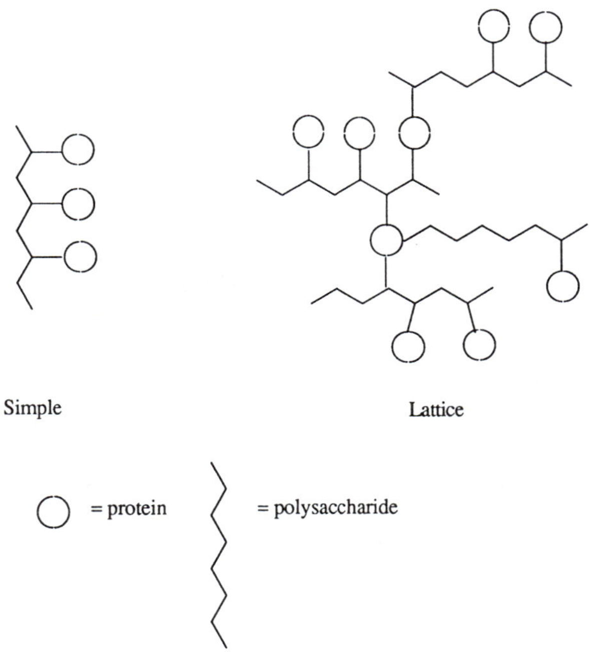

Figure 1 Models of the PRP-T and PRP-D conjugates.

salt, **6**, which is soluble in dimethylformamide (DMF), thus allowing chemistry in a nonaqueous system:

PRP (Ca salt) + oxalic acid

$$\rightarrow \text{PRP } (H^+) + (n\text{-}C_4H_9)_4N^+ \ OH^- \rightarrow \text{PRP}[(n\text{-}C_4H_9)_4N^+]$$

6

The treatment with oxalic acid reduces the m.w. to about 80,000 daltons. This material now is treated in DMF with carbonyl diimidazole, **7**, which converts some of the hydroxyls to electrophilic imidazolyl urethane functions as in the intermediate **8**. There is some NMR evidence that suggests that this activation takes place at the primary C-5 hydroxyl of the ribose (B. Arison, unpublished data):

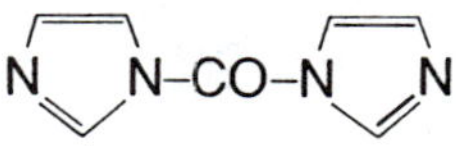

7

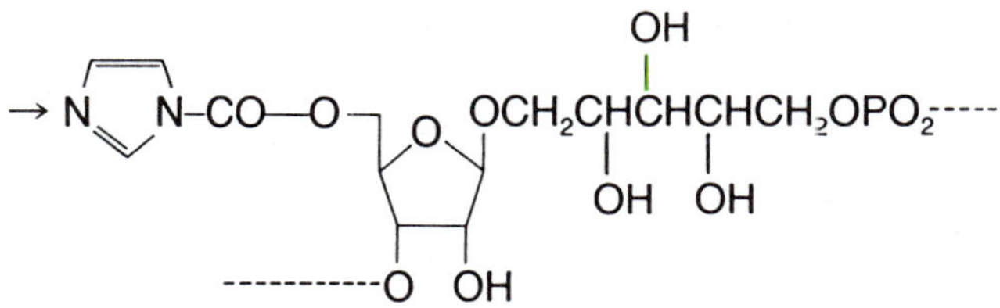

8

The activated PRP, **8**, then is reacted directly with an aqueous solution of 1,4-butane diamine, **9**, transforming the imidazolyl urethane to the urethane of butane diamine, **10**, which has a pendant amine. The use of high concentrations of **9** lessens the probability that crosslinking or cyclization will occur.

$$8 + H_2NCH_2CH_2CH_2CH_2NH_2 \rightarrow$$

9

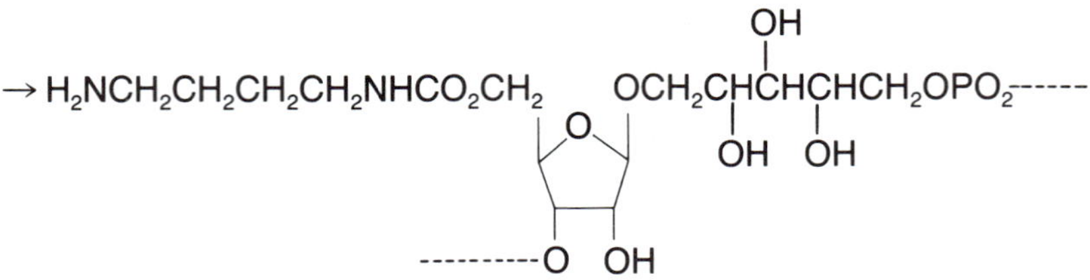

10

After removal of excess **9** by diafiltration, the level of derivatization of **10** can be determined using proton NMR by comparing the integrals of the butane diamine resonances to the integrals of the PRP resonances. The NMR spectrum also indicates that there is little if any crosslinking. The optimal level of butane diamine derivatization is about 20% (that is, one Ps monomeric repeat unit in five contains a butane diamine moiety). This level allows the pendant amine to engage in subsequent chemical steps at reasonable reaction rates and at the same time does not distort the antigenic quality of the PRP to any significant degree. The final step in the PRP derivatization stream involves the bromoacetylation of the pendant amine in **10** by bromoacetyl chloride:

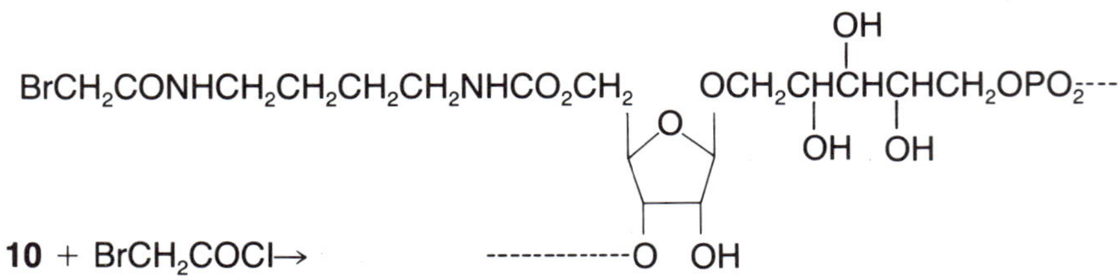

11

After diafiltration, the resultant bromoacetamide **11** is isolated free of all bromoacetic acid species and monitored by NMR for degree of bromoacetylation and derivatization.

The Pr carrier is an outer membrane Pr complex from *Neisseria meningitidis* B designated OMPC. This material is a particle, approximately 100–200 nm in diameter, which is composed of an aggregate of Pr and lipopolysaccharide (LPS) (8). The major Pr, the class 2 Pr, has a m.w. of 42,000 daltons and comprises >60% of the Pr mass. The m.w. of the particle is estimated to be between 3×10^7 and 5×10^7 daltons. This high m.w. confers on OMPC a colloidal nature in aqueous systems and allows the Pr and its conjugates to be ultracentrifuged to a pellet. Moreover, OMPC is retained easily by ultrafiltration membranes through which unconjugated PRP can permeate. OMPC is reacted with *N*-acetylhomocysteine thiolactone, **12**, so that the amino groups of the lysines open the thiolactone forming an amide bond and generating a pendant thiol in the intermediate **13**.

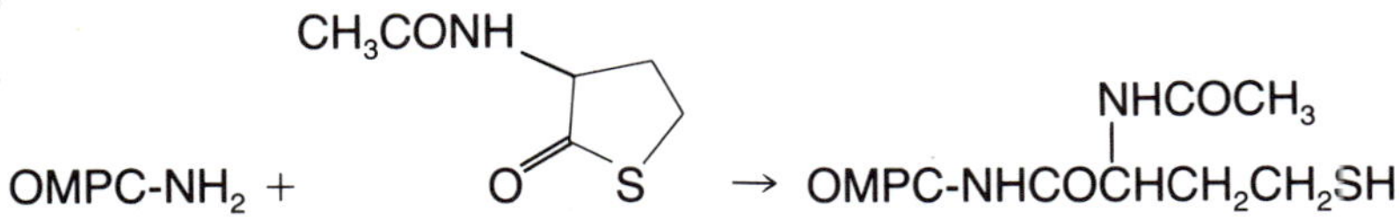

12 **13**

The protein-normalized thiol titer is determined by Ellman (9) and Lowry (10) assays as a control of this step. Then **11** and **13** are reacted resulting in a thioether bond being formed by bromide displacement from **11** with the thiol in **13**. This forms the conjugate, **14**, and the thioether (the encircled atoms) is the relevant covalent bond.

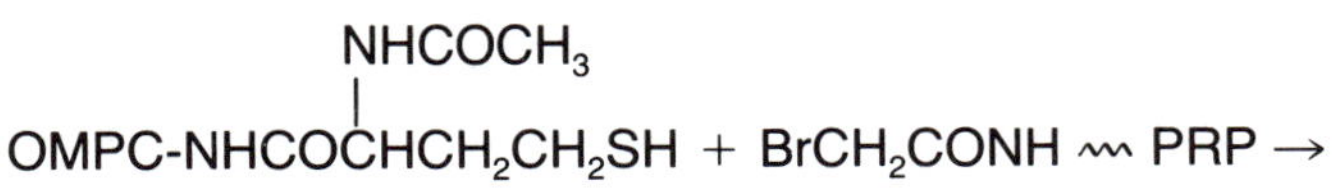

13 **11**

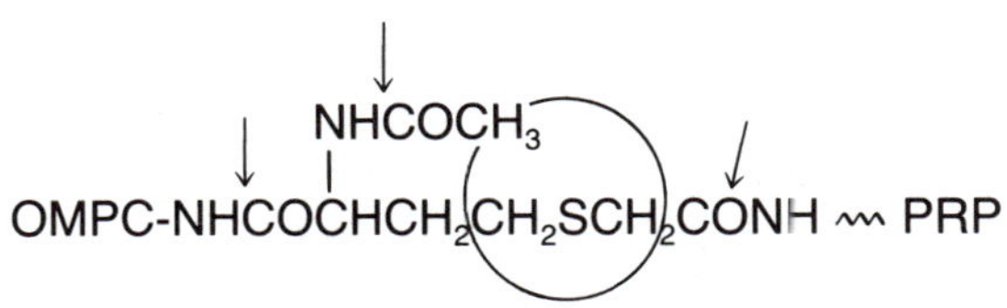

14

Excess bromoacetyl groups in the conjugate **14** that did not react with the OMPC thiols are reacted with *N*-acetylcysteamine, **15**, affording a "capped" conjugate, **14′**.

$CH_3CONHCH_2CH_2SH + BrCH_2CONH_{excess}$ ~ PRP

15

$\rightarrow CH_3CONHCH_2CH_2S{-}CH_2CONH_{excess}$ ~ PRP

capped excess bromoacetyl

14′

The capped conjugate **14′** (m.w. ≈ 5 × 10^7) is then readily separated from unconjugated **11** (m.w. 8 × 10^4) by diafiltration. It is quantitated by PRP (ribose) (11) and Pr (Lowry) (10) assays to give a PRP/Pr value of approximately 0.05–0.10. An aliquot of **14′** is hydrolyzed with HCl to cleave all the peptide bonds in the Pr and the amide bonds indicated by the arrows above. In addition to releasing all the component amino acids of OMPC, two novel amino acids, S-carboxymethylhomocysteine (SCMHC), **16**, and S-carboxymethylcysteamine (SCMC), **17**, are released and are detectable in the amino acid analysis spectrum. Both **16** and **17** are referenced internally to a constituent amino acid of OMPC (in this case lysine is used as an internal standard). Compound **16** is derived from the conjugation step, and each mole represents a mole of covalent bonds that were formed and therefore constitutes a proof of covalency. This approach for defining covalency has been termed the "bigeneric spacer" method (6,7). Compound **17** arises from the capping of excess bromoacetyl groups.

$$HO_2C\overset{\displaystyle NH_2}{\overset{|}{C}}HCH_2CH_2SCH_2CO_2H \qquad\qquad H_2NCH_2CH_2SCH_2CO_2H$$

16 **17**

Knowing the titers of lysine, **16**, **17**, the butane diamine loading and the thiol titer on OMPC affords a significant amount of analytical control over the manufacturing process. This value of extensive analytical monitoring is illustrated clearly for PRP-OMPC, where certain post-licensure lots showed less than expected immunogenicity in the field (Chap. 5). A thorough investigation by the manufacturer revealed that, for some lots manufactured consecutively, a sub-fraction of PRP could become over-derivatized (reduced in antigenicity) and react preferentially with OMPC. This "hyperconjugation," which resulted in reduced immunogenicity, now has been controlled by a process modification. In addition, numerous analytical parameters (Section III.B) were being monitored to provide information about process consistency, and from these additional release specifications have been established for SCMHC/PRP and [SCMHC + SCMC]/PRP; the upper limits of these specifications provide a check of all lots to ensure that the implemented changes continue to control the process and eliminate hyperconjugation. It is unclear whether hyperconjugation can occur with other conjugation chemistries, but the case for PRP-OMPC clearly illustrates the value of extensive analytical monitoring of such complex processes (also see Section IV below).

Figure 2 presents a diagrammatic representation of this conjugate. Essentially there are a number of Ps molecules of varying chain length linked

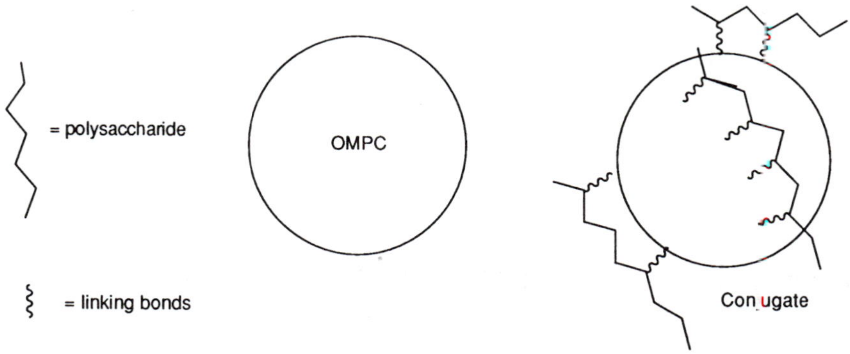

Figure 2 Model of the PRP-OMPC conjugate.

via a variable number of linking moieties to each large OMPC particle. It is unlikely that a significant percentage of Pr is crosslinked, since light scattering analysis indicates little change in particle size distribution (J. Hennessey, private communication). This type of structure differs from the lattice type associated with the PRP-D vaccine in that each Ps molecule is linked to only one Pr molecule. The term "ladder"-type conjugate seems appropriate in describing the OMPC conjugates with the linear Ps taking the part of a rail and the linking molecules the part of the rungs.

3. PRP-T

This vaccine, which is only sparsely described in the literature (12), is prepared by the method of Schneerson et al. (13). PRP is not deliberately size-modified. It then is activated with cyanogen bromide and reacted in situ with adipic acid dihydrazide to form the derivative **18**:

$$\text{PRP} + \mathbf{1} + \mathbf{3} \rightarrow H_2NNHCO(CH_2)_4CONHNHC(=NH)O\text{-PRP}$$

18

The degree of derivatization (i.e., the number of adipic hydrazide units per 100 repeat units of PRP) is defined by a 1,3,5-trinitrobenzenesulfonic acid assay affording a 2% weight loading, which translates to 4 adipic hydrazide units per 100 repeat units of PRP. The carrier protein is tetanus toxoid (TT) obtained by formalin treatment of tetanus toxin. The untoxoided toxin has a m.w. of approximately 150,000 (15). The carboxyl groups of TT are condensed with the hydrazide group of **18**, with 1-ethyl-3(3-dimethylaminopropal) carbodiimide (EDAC) forming the conjugate **19**:

$TT\text{-}CO_2H + EDAC + 18$

$$\rightarrow TT\text{-}CONHNHCO(CH_2)_4CONHNHC(=NH)O\text{–}PRP$$

19

Low m.w. byproducts are removed and then the high m.w. material, contained in the void volume after chromatography on Sepharose Cl-4B, is filter sterilized and affords a PRP/Pr ≈ 0.5. Because of the polyvalency of both TT and **18**, the material can best be described as a lattice-type conjugate (see Fig. 1).

4. HbOC

This methodology involves size reduction of the PRP polymer by cleavage of the glycol functionality in the ribitol moiety. This is accomplished by using sodium metaperiodate (16,17), and cleavage occurs at the sites indicated by the arrows:

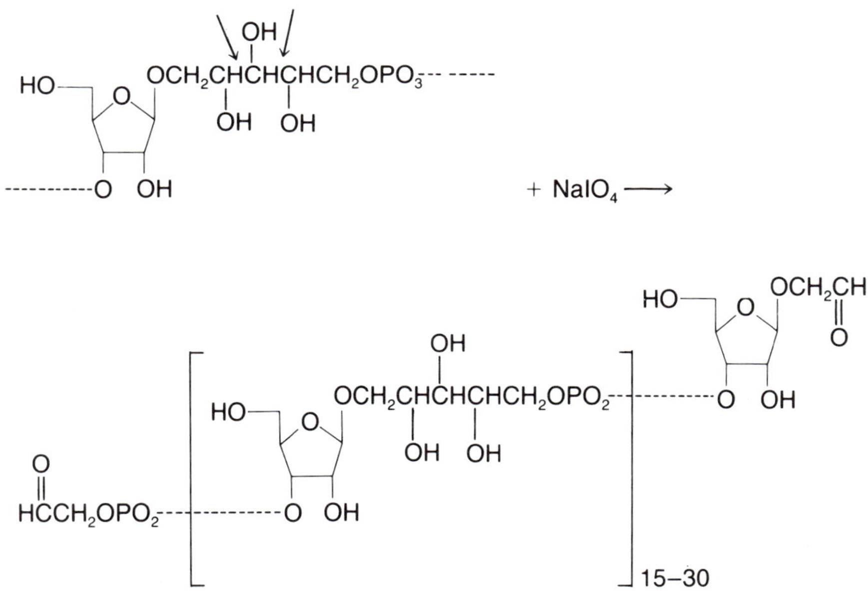

20

The product of the reaction is sized by ultrafiltration through a 30,000 MWCO membrane, rejecting the retentate (i.e., m.w. > 30,000 daltons) and then ultrafiltration through a 10,000 MWCO membrane. At this point the filtrate is rejected and the retentate contains the dialdehyde PRP derivative **20**. This derivative is analyzed for ribose and reducing titer (for aldehydes), and the degree of polymerization (DP, the number of repeat units in a single molecule) is between 15 and 30. The weight average DP is 20.

The Pr carrier used for HbOC is a nontoxic, mutant form of diphtheria toxin known as CRM_{197} (m.w. 58,329). CRMs, or cross-reacting materials, are antigenically equivalent to their cognate Pr and offer two advantages as carriers over their congruent toxoids: there is no potential for reversion to a toxic form, and, since the available lysines were not used in a toxoiding process (i.e., with formaldehyde), there are more nucleophilic nitrogens available to form bonds with electrophilic partners such as the aldehyde groups in **20**. The bond-forming chemistry used for this process is termed reductive amination and involves the reaction of an amine with an aldehyde to form a Schiff base, which is then reduced in situ by sodium cyanoborohydride, **21**, resulting in an alkylated amine:

$$RCH(=O) + H_2NR' \rightarrow RCH{=}NR' + NaBH_3CN \rightarrow RCH_2NHR'$$

21

Compound **21**, which is a less reactive reducing agent than sodium borohydride, does not readily reduce aldehydes (which would simultaneously destroy starting material in the above reaction). Thus **20** and CRM_{197} are reacted to form the conjugate **22** (an example where both reducing ends have been reductively aminated):

20 + H_2N ∿∿ CRM_{197} + **21** →

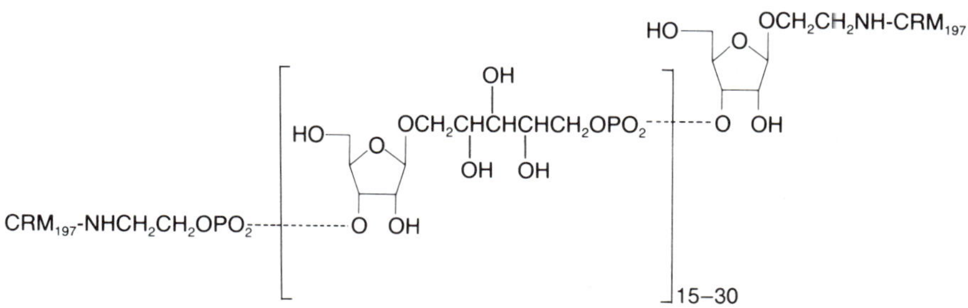

22

The unreacted aldehydes then are reduced with sodium borohydride and the conjugate is ultrafiltered through a 30,000 MWCO membrane to remove small reagents and unconjugated **20**. The retentate contains the conjugate **22**, which is assayed for Ps and Pr (PRP/Pr ≈ 0.4). Since the reactant Ps **20** was sized to pass through a 30,000 MWCO filter, the copresence of Ps and Pr is indirect support for covalency. Subsequently, two other types of analysis provide direct evidence for covalency (19,20). One involves the coincidence of antigenic reactivity to PRP and to CRM_{197} after SDS-PAGE and immunoblotting. The other approach involves the detection of the new amino acid moiety formed when the lysines on the CRM_{197} are reductively aminated with **20**. When the conjugate is hydrolyzed in acid (the arrows show the sites of cleavage) N_ϵ-(2-hydroxyethyl)lysine, **23**, is formed and detected by amino acid analysis (see the PRP-OMPC covalency scheme):

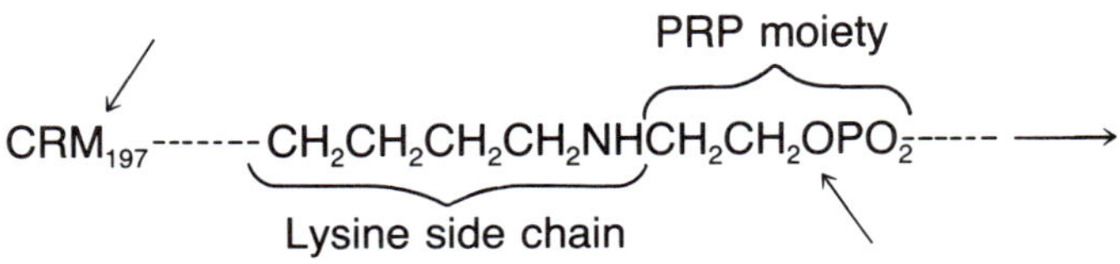

$HO_2CCH(NH_2)CH_2CH_2CH_2CH_2NHCH_2CH_2OH$

23

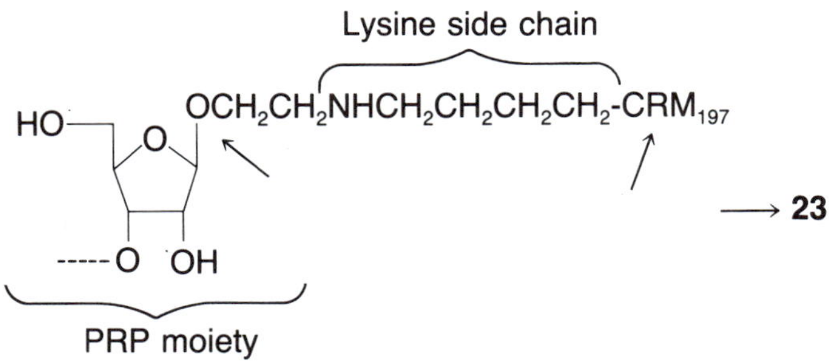

One can depict the HbOC product as a mixture of a neoglycoprotein model (3) and a lattice; the latter is considered modified lattice because **20** is only bi- and not polyfunctional. These models are shown in Figure 3.

B. Quantitative Aspects of Covalency

In both the PRP-OMPC and HbOC conjugates, the amino acid analysis allows one to quantitate the number of covalent bonds per weight of PRP or Pr. What structural inferences can one make from those values, and what immunological consequences follow from those structural features?

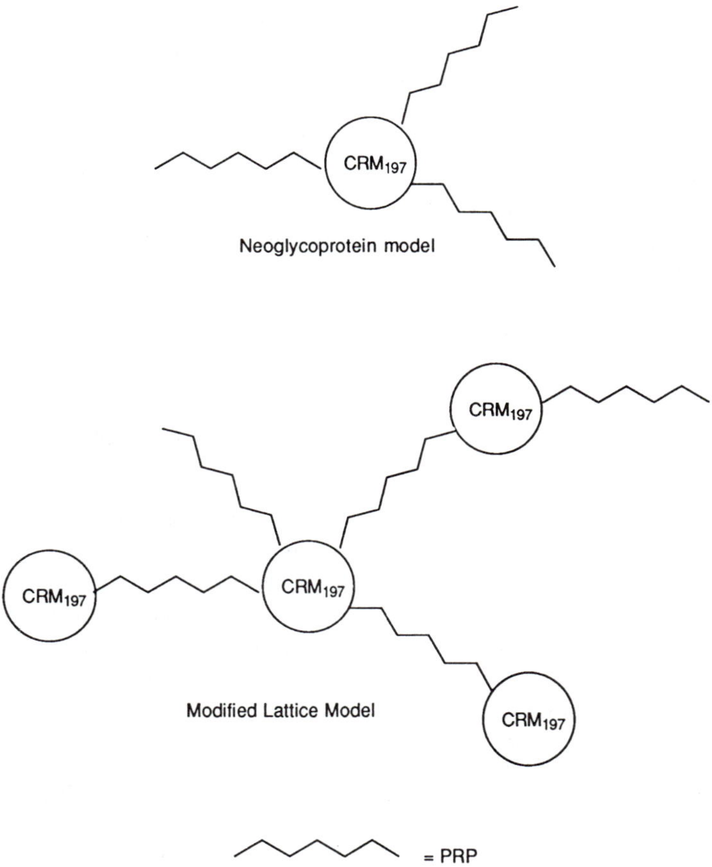

Figure 3 Models for the HbOC conjugate.

In the HbOC case, if one considers a monodisperse Ps or one with a very narrow m.w. distribution, there are two structural cases. If only one end of the PRP is bonded to Pr, this gives rise to a value of 1 hydroxylethyllysine, **23**, per known number of repeat units in a PRP molecule. If both ends of the PRP are bonded, a value of 2 is indicated as an upper limit. For a given value of **23** per weight of PRP, the fractions that are singly and doubly bonded are calculable. If one can vary the fractional value among conjugate preparations, one can correlate it with an immunological consequence. However, if there is a sizable polydispersity of the Ps, the relative fractions no longer are calculable.

In the PRP-OMPC scenario the number of covalent bonds per weight of PRP (titer of **16**/weight PRP) is much more difficult to interpret in a structural sense. Even if the PRP were monodisperse, each molecule is polyderivatized; that is, about 20 sites are functionalized on a molecule of 100 repeat units. In addition, the loci of derivatization on the repeat units are not known. If one now considers that the thiol groups on the OMPC particle are geometrically fixed, it would seem reasonable that there are constraints on which bromoacetyl moieties can form covalent bonds. In addition, the geometry of the available thiols for the second derivatized PRP molecule will be different from that for the first. Therefore, it is almost impossible to extract structural information by knowing the degree of covalency. However, such a value has use as a process control parameter.

C. Safety Considerations as a Consequence of Covalent Chemistry

The fact that these conjugates are the results of reactions involving reactive chemical intermediates raises unique safety concerns, which are added to those generally associated with classical bacterial vaccines (see Sec. IV.B. and Chap. 3). This derives from the fact that functional groups that were created for forming the requisite covalent bonds might also modify host Pr and other host biochemicals (e.g., glutathione) if they remained in reactive form in the final vaccine preparation. To quote the World Health Organization (21):

> Residual unreacted functional groups potentially capable of reacting *in vivo* may be present following the conjugation process. The manufacturing process shall be validated to show that it does not produce bulk vaccines containing such groups; any remaining groups should be made unreactive during manufacture by means of "capping agents."

For HbOC, unreacted aldehydes are reduced with sodium borohydride to unreactive alcohols. The capping of the cyanate ester, which is the reactive form of PRP in the PRP-D and PRP-T products, is not described in the available literature, and thus it is presumed that the manufacturers have validated the absence of such groups. Although not described by the manufacturer, clearly a test utilizing NMR or an assay for reducing groups (22) could be established for HbOC to measure aldehydes following borohydride reduction. For the case of PRP-OMPC, potentially reactive bromoacetyl moieties (i.e., any that did not react with the OMPC thiols) are "capped" with *N*-acetylcysteamine. In addition, analytical verification of the lack of reactive bromoacetyls may be derived by computing the ratio of the sum of the SCMHC plus SCMC determinations to the value determined for butanediamine (all expressed per PRP repeating unit); a value of unity for this ratio indicates indirectly that all potentially reactive bromoacetyls have participated either in conjugation (SCMHC) or capping (SCMC). All the Hib conjugates, however, have an excellent clinical safety record, and these issues are most relevant to future conjugates for which they must be established as they have been for the licensed PRP conjugates.

D. Removal of Unconjugated PRP

Because of the polyfunctional character of the reactants, each of the above preparations consists of a family of conjugates. Since the physicochemical properties of the members of each family of conjugates differ only slightly and as a continuum from the starting material, separations of unconjugated PRP based on these properties are difficult. For instance, separations based on ion exchange chromatography or precipitation with ammonium sulfate would be difficult for a conjugate in which the PRP was the predominant partner. The most general way to make the separation of free (i.e., unconjugated) from conjugated Ps is on the basis of molecular size.* This most often can be accomplished by such techniques as diafiltration or ultracentrifugation. However, when the Pr component dominates the mass of the conjugate, as in the case of the PRP-OMPC conjugate, separations based on the Pr character can be effected. For example, such a conjugate might be precipitated with ammonium sulfate while the free PRP would not.

Although size exclusion media that could be used for most conjugate molecules are available, column separations are cumbersome, expensive, difficult to operate aseptically, and therefore not desirable for manufacturing processes. Ultrafiltration membranes with defined MWCOs are the preferred technology for separations on a manufacturing scale. However, the availability of membranes is limited to sizes with MWCOs below 850,000 (*N.B.*: this is a rapidly changing field and larger MWCOs should be available in the future), and obviously Ps larger than this cannot be separated from their conjugates by this methodology. It should be noted that MWCOs are nominal values, empirically determined with globular Pr, and they may not reflect what is retainable for Ps. In addition, smaller molecules are frequently retained in the presence of high-m.w. species. It is generally acknowledged that for efficient fractionation to take place there should be a 10-fold difference in m.w. (23). It is therefore instructive to consider how this 10-fold ratio might be determined for a conjugate and its congeneric unbound PRP [i.e., if one wants a (m.w. of conjugate)/(m.w.

*At this point it must be mentioned that molecular weights determined by different methods may not be equivalent and that comparisons made in this text may not be valid.

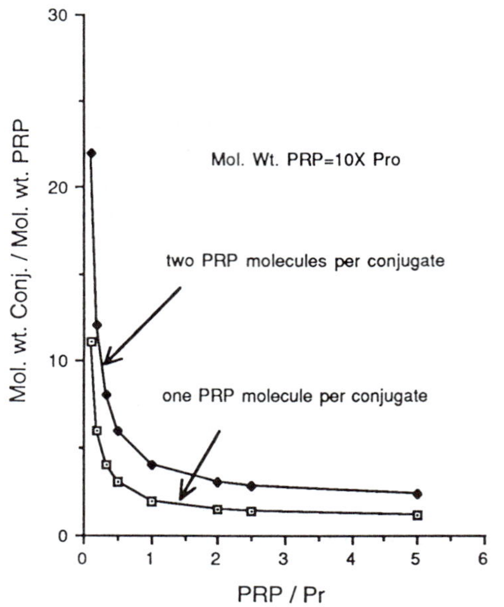

Figure 4 The predicted relationship between the ratio of the m.w. of a conjugate and the m.w. of its congeneric PRP as function of PRP/Pr ratio, calculated for one and two PRP molecules per conjugate and a PRP m.w. 10 times the Pr m.w.

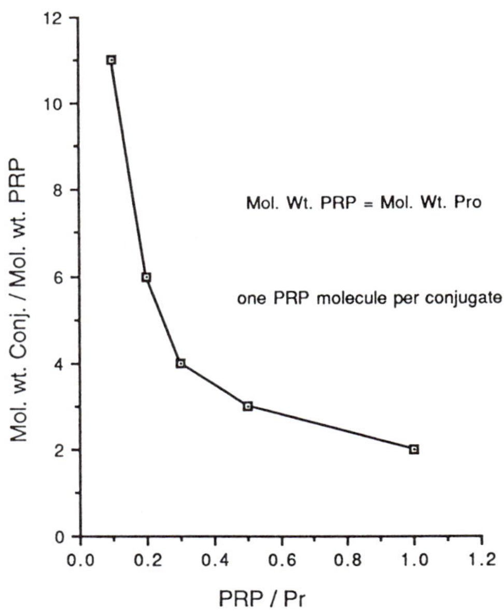

Figure 5 The predicted relationship between the ratio of the m.w. of a conjugate and the m.w. of its congeneric PRP as function of PRP/Pr ratio and involving equal m.w. for PRP and Pro and one molecule of PRP per conjugate.

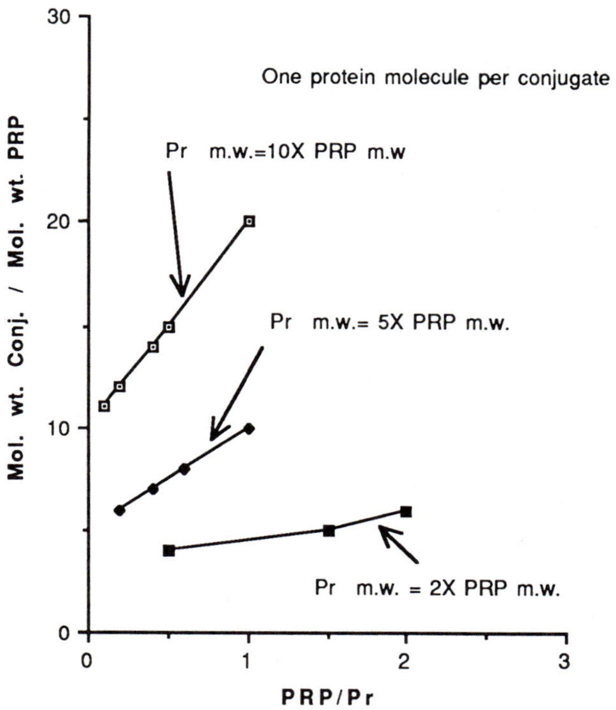

Figure 6 The predicted relationship between the ratio of the m.w. of a conjugate and the m.w. of its congeneric PRP as function of PRP/Pr ratio and describing conjugates whose Pr m.w. is 10 times, 5 times, and 2 times larger than PRP and which are calculated for one Pr molecule per conjugate.

PRP) > 10]. The relevant data, which are available generally, are the m.w. of the Pr, the approximate m.w. of the starting PRP, and the weight ratio, PRP/Pr, of the conjugate. Using these data and assuming certain stoichiometries in the conjugate and certain m.w. ratios for unconjugated Pr and PRP, the relationship between (m.w. conjugate/m.w. PRP) and the PRP/Pr can be defined.

The most demanding case for the desired 10-fold ratio is one in which the macromolecule with the larger m.w. is present in the conjugate with a stoichiometry of one. Using that scenario and others, one can construct a series of graphs that delineate relevant situations and one can estimate the practical limits of a size-based separation. Figures 4 through 7 show the theoretical dependency of those m.w. ratios on the PRP/Pr ratio in which various stoichiometries and m.w.s are considered. Figure 4 is calculated for one and two PRP molecules per conjugate and a PRP m.w. 10 times the Pr m.w. Figure 5 involves equal m.w. for PRP and Pr and one molecule of

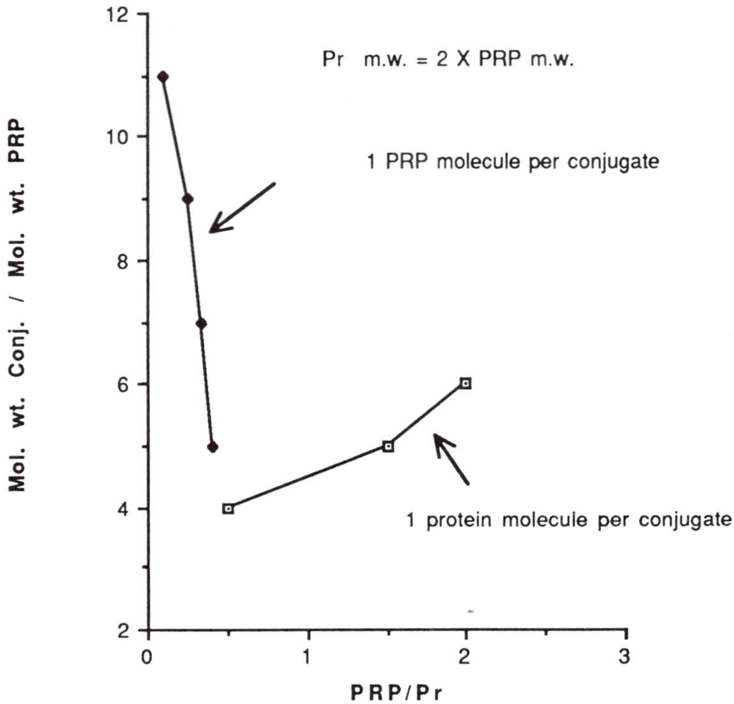

Figure 7 The predicted relationship between the ratio of the m.w. of a conjugate and the m.w. of its congeneric PRP as function of PRP/Pr ratio and describing two different stoichiometries for the situation where the Pr m.w. is twice the PRP m.w.

PRP per conjugate. Figure 6 describes conjugates whose Pr m.w. is 10 times, 5 times, and 2 times larger than PRP and which are calculated for one Pr molecule per conjugate. Figure 7 describes two different stoichiometries for the situation where the Pr m.w. is twice the PRP m.w.

Although the real situation is even more complex, given the fact that the PRP molecules are polydisperse and that multiple stoichiometries are possible, these figures teach that (a) when the Pr is much larger (e.g., 10 times) than the PRP (such as is the case for PRP-OMPC and for HbOC), the 10-fold difference in m.w. needed to separate unconjugated PRP from conjugate is easily reached (Fig. 6) and ultrafiltration can be used to separate the saccharide. As the m.w.s of the two macromolecules approach each other (such as may be the case for PRP-T and to a lesser extent for PRP-D), the 10-fold difference is attainable only at low values of the PRP/Pr ratios (Fig. 5). (b) When different stoichiometries obtain, the relationships change drastically (Fig. 7), (c) when the m.w. of the PRP is the same (Fig. 5) or larger (Fig. 4) than that of the Pr, separations on the basis of size will be difficult except at very low PRP/Pr ratios.

Although it is vital to take these concepts into account in the conjugation design, ultimately the product must be and is assayed for unbound PRP. This usually is done using SEC, ultrafiltration, or hydrophobic chromatography (21). These free PRP assays are reflected in the release specifications, which show major differences for the four conjugates (see Tables 4 and 5). It is interesting to compare two of these, PRP-D and PRP-T, which have specifications of <37%* and <20%, respectively, for their free PRP content. PRP-D is significantly less immunogenic in infants than PRP-T (24,25) despite the fact that both are prepared from formalin-treated Pr by very similar chemistries. One could posit that TT is an inherently more immunogenic carrier than DT. However, CRM_{197}, which has essentially the same amino acid sequence as diphtheria toxin, serves as a highly effective carrier, thus vitiating that argument. It is, therefore, tempting to conclude that for PRP-T, the larger m.w. of TT facilitates more efficient removal of the free PRP relative to PRP-D. (It should be noted that CRM_{197}, which has about the same m.w. as DT, is conjugated to much lower m.w. oligosaccharide fragments, which should allow for efficient removal of those fragments.) Considering this type of argument, there seems to be some validity to the above analysis. However, it also should be noted that the processes for preparation of both of these conjugates do not offer *direct*** proof of covalency and thus the immunogenicity differences might be related to this critical property as well.

IV. PROCESS CHARACTERIZATION AND CONTROL

Process consistency and control are of paramount importance in defining the PRP conjugates. Analytical and biological assays (as summarized in Table 3) are employed not only for process control but also for product characterization. Such characterization assays demonstrate and assure process consistency, define the vaccine (and its dosage), and establish release tests, which ensure that product is well tolerated, immunogenic, and stable. These assays and their development will be discussed in more detail in Chapters 3 and 5 and also will be discussed briefly below as they relate to the manufacturing process. The choice and characterization of the Pr

---

*These values are upper limits for the released vaccines; in routine manufacturing, the values vary between 20 and 30%.

**The covalency of PRP-D has been validly, but indirectly, established by the hydrophobic interaction chromatography method.

Table 3 Characterization Assays

CHEMICAL ASSAYS
Assays on Ps and Intermediates
Molecular weight
Degree of derivatization or functionalization
Antigenicity
Assays on Pr and Intermediates
Degree of derivatization or functionalization
Assays on Conjugate
Percent unconjugated Ps
Assurance of covalency
Degree of crosslinking
Antigenicity
Ps/Pr ratio
BIOLOGICAL ASSAYS
Preclinical Immunogenicity
T-cell dependency
In vivo potency (ED_{50})
Infant primate immunogenicity
Safety
Pyrogen
General safety
STABILITY-INDICATING ASSAYS
Antigenicity (in vitro potency)
In vivo potency
Covalency
% Unconjugated PRP
pH
Completeness of adsorption[a]

[a]At present, only PRP-OMPC is adsorbed to aluminum hydroxide as an adjuvant; future combination vaccines, containing other PRP conjugate vaccines, also probably will be adsorbed.

carriers used in the synthesis of the PRP conjugates are discussed in Chapter 4.

A. Characterization of Starting PRP

1. Chemical

Numerous publications and patents exist describing the purification and characterization of PRP (26,27). Specifications (21) have been established, and these will be discussed in detail in Chapter 5. In terms of the process and its control, the consistency of the PRP starting material is most critical. Chemical assays for PRP constituents (ribose, ribitol, and phosphate) and contaminants (Pr and nucleic acids) are used in conjunction with assays for molecular weight and polydispersity to define PRP as narrowly as possible, thereby better controlling the conjugation reactions and ultimately limiting the variability of the final vaccine.

2. Antigenic

In addition, the PRP starting material must display the protective epitope(s) of the capsule as it exists on the surface of the Hib bacterium in order for the conjugate to provide protective efficacy. These data are determined immunologically by RIA or ELISA or nephelometric methods (see below and Chapter 3).

3. Molecular Weight

PRP is a polymer of a variable number of repeating units, each composed of ribose, ribitol, and phosphate (28), and therefore the starting Ps can vary widely in m.w. A distribution coefficient [K_d] is measured, which can be used to calculate the average m.w. of the molecules in a population comprising the PRP preparation (29). This value is determined by size exclusion chromatography (SEC). In some cases, an index of this m.w. heterogeneity is determined, and this involves more complex methods such as laser light scattering (30). The average size must be capable of assuming the conformation of the protective epitope(s) as displayed on the capsule of Hib bacterium. For PRP-D, PRP-OMPC, and PRP-T, the m.w. of the starting PRP is similar to that of the Ps when it is shed by the Hib bacterium growing in liquid culture. These PRP sizes initially are several hundred repeating units long, but some m.w. degradation does occur as they are processed chemically. For the case of HbOC, the chemistry employed, as described above, results in the partial depolymerization of PRP. By controlling the amount of periodate used for the oxidation reaction, oligosaccharide fragments are obtained that are within the range of sizes empirically determined to result in an immunogenic conjugate (31). Indeed, for all the PRP conjugates, both the oligo- and Ps starting m.w.s result in syntheses of efficacious vaccines. This indicates that at least some of the protective epitopes are displayed on the final conjugates. However, as one seeks to employ the PRP conjugates as prototypes for vaccines against other targets, it must be noted that some Ps [notably those of *Neisseria meningitis* B (32), of *Streptococcus pneumoniae* type 14 (33) and group B Streptococcus type III (34)] have been shown to display conformational (i.e., discontinuous) epitopes which elicit the relevant neutralizing antibodies. Such epitopes are associated with high m.w. molecules (32–34). Although it is not known whether PRP contains such epitopes, for future Ps conjugates it may be critical that synthesis of the conjugate start with Ps with sufficiently large m.w. to ensure efficacy by maintenance of these size-associated conformers in the final conjugate.

B. Assays of the Bulk Conjugate and Final Container Vaccine

1. Chemical Characterization

The results of assays for PRP concentration [generally using the orcinol assay for ribose (11)] and Pr concentration [by the method of Lowry (10)] and their calculated ratio (PRP/Pr) are employed to describe the conjugates and establish that they are synthesized in a consistent and reproducible manner. The PRP/Pr ratios vary considerably among the licensed conjugates, being 0.3–0.6 for HbOC, 1.2–1.7 for PRP-D, 0.05–0.10 for PRP-OMPC, and 0.3–0.6 for PRP-T (Table 4). It is thus probable that the PRP/Pr ratios, in these ranges, have little effect on the immunogenicity of the vaccines but, within a vaccine type, this determination will give an important indication of process consistency.

2. In Vitro Antigenicity Assays

The chemical assays, mentioned in Section IV.B.1., measure total PRP in the conjugate whether or not it retains those topological features that are recognized by the relevant antibodies (this quality is termed antigenicity and is measured by binding experiments using the relevant antibodies). Antigenic quality sometimes can be lost during the processing steps [especially in cases of branched Ps such as *S. pneumoniae* types 18C, 23F etc. (35)] and, in these cases, chemical analyses can be revealing but are not sufficient for characterization.

Table 4 Characteristics of Bulk Conjugates

Vaccine	PRP Kd(CL-4 B)[a]	Proof of covalency	PRP/ Protein ratio	Unconjugated PRP removal	% Free PRP	Ref.
HbOC	0.3–0.6[b]	Direct and indirect	ca. 0.4	Ultrafiltration	<10%	16,17, 22,46
PRP-D	95% < 0.75	Indirect	ca. 1.4[c]	$(NH_4)_2SO_4$ Precipitation	<37%	5,13, 22,46
PRP-OMPC	85%< 0.25	Direct and indirect	ca. 0.06	Ultrafiltration	<15%	6,7, 22,46
PRP-T	60%< 0.20	Indirect	ca. 0.5	Proprietary process	<20%	46

[a]Percentage of starting PRP whose distribution constant (Kd) is below the value specified.
[b]PRP is reduced to an oligosaccharide by periodate oxidation prior to conjugation (see text for detailed description of the process).
[c]Range 1.2–1.7 (P. H. McVerry, personal communication).

The processes should be and are controlled (vide supra) by monitoring PRP antigenicity of intermediates and products; i.e., the reactivity of the vaccine product and its synthetic intermediates are assayed with anti-PRP antibodies to verify that the final conjugates retain the relevant antibody binding activity as compared to the starting PRP. It seems that the next logical step will be to employ quantitative antigenicity assays to determine the conjugate dosage based on a measure of the 'active principal' (i.e., the *antigenic* Ps) in the vaccine. Both the regulatory agencies and the vaccine manufacturers seem to be moving in this direction, although standardization of such assays will require additional development before implementation will be possible.

3. In Vivo Immunogenicity Assays

Because analytical characterization (including determination of antigenicity) per se does not predict an immunological outcome, the determination of the ability of the final vaccine to elicit functional antibodies in an appropriate animal model was an indispensable guide for the development of the various conjugation processes. Such assays also remain useful as qualitative release tests, as a vaccine lot which was not immunogenic in laboratory animals or was incapable of inducing an antibody response in a T-dependent manner might be unlikely to protect human infants. To this end, in vivo assays have been developed which measure the ability of conjugate preparations to actively induce anti-PRP antibodies in experimental species which do not respond to nonconjugated PRP (36–38). The T-cell dependency of the immune response to the conjugates (which provides biological confirmation of covalency) also can be determined by comparing the anti-PRP responses of athymic nude mice, which are congenitally devoid of T cells, with those of their heterozygous littermates, which have a normal complement of T-helper cells (39). These tests, along with assays that verify the functional activity (i.e., its ability to kill Hib) of the conjugate-induced anti-PRP (40–42), will be reviewed in detail in Chapter 5.

4. Assays for Proof and Quantitation of Covalency

As discussed in Section III.B., the synthetic process must result in a stable covalent bond between the PRP and Pr in order to convert the PRP to a T-dependent antigen. Also as discussed in detail above, all conjugate scenarios measure covalency indirectly, and for PRP-OMPC and HbOC determination of a newly created amino acid provides further quantitative and direct proof that a covalent bond has been formed. This degree of covalency must be below a value that would reduce the antigenicity and immunogenicity of the vaccine but not so low as to adversely affect the stability of the vaccine by providing insufficient covalent bonds between each Ps and Pr. The optimal degree of covalency must be determined empirically for each conjugate type, but within a type, assays to verify for each conjugate lot that this value is within the specifications are critical.

5. Assays for Unconjugated PRP

As discussed in detail in Section III. C., determination of the fraction of the Ps in the final vaccine that is unconjugated (this usually is expressed as % free Ps) is important for reasons that derive from the fact that the active form of the immunogen is Ps as the covalent conjugate. Although unconfirmed as yet for PRP conjugates, unconjugated Ps has been reported to decrease the immunogenicity of a conjugate prepared with the type 4 Ps of *Streptococcus pneumoniae* (4). Moreover, the efficacious dosage of the vaccine must be determined as the amount of conjugated Ps (active immunogen) and, if the fraction of unconjugated Ps becomes large, the active dose may be insufficient to induce an effective immune response. For the licensed vaccines, the specifications for % free Ps are generally 10–37% (Table 4).

6. Safety Testing

The PRP conjugate vaccines are indicated for administration to infants as young as 2 months old and, therefore, safety is of primary concern. Special safety considerations, which derive from the fact that these conjugates are the products of chemical reactions that create biologically reactive functional groups during the process, have been discussed in Section III.B. Additionally, because PRP is isolated from a gram-negative bacterium, which contains the pyrogenic lipopolysaccharide (LPS) molecule (OMPC also is derived from an LPS-containing gram-negative bacterium), all the vaccines are release tested for pyrogenicity in rabbits (43) (Table 5). All of the vaccines are also tested for safety in mice and guinea pigs, in which they may not cause loss of weight during a specified observation period (44).

7. Stability-Indicating Assays

In order to study and determine the stability and determine the shelf-life of the vaccines, the assays that measure Ps antigenicity, conjugate immunogenicity, conjugate covalency, and absence of free PRP (vide supra) are followed over time at the recommended storage temperature for the vaccine (other temperatures also may be studied to give additional information). In addition, determination of the pH of the vaccine also may provide useful information regarding stability, as the phosophodiester bonds of PRP are most stable at or near neutrality and a pH drift during storage may provide the earliest indication of a potential for hydrolysis of the antigen.

Table 5 Characteristics of Final Container Vaccines

Vaccine	PRP dose	Protein dose	Pyrogen[a]	Form	Adjuvant	Preservative	Ref.
HbOC	10 μg	ca.25 μg	1 μg/kg	Liquid	None	Thimerosal	22, 46
PRP-D	25 μg	ca.18 μg	1 μg/kg	Liquid	None	Thimerosal	22, 46
PRP-OMPC	15 μg[b]	ca.250 μg[b]	1 μg/kg[c]	Lyo[d,e]	$Al(OH)_3$	Thimerosal	22, 46
PRP-T	10 μg	ca. 24 μg	1 μg/kg	Lyo[d]	None	None	22, 46

[a]Minimum dose not causing a febrile response in rabbits as defined in 21 CFR 610.13; see also footnote (c) below.
[b]Manufacturer is in the process of changing dose to 7.5 μg PRP and ca.125 μg protein based on immunological equivalence.
[c]Administered I.M.; 0.025 μg/kg when administered I.V.
[d]Reconstituted with diluent supplied by the manufacturer at time of use.
[e]A liquid formulation is also being developed.

At the present time all the licensed vaccines are stable for and have expiry dating of at least 2 years (21,45).

V. FUTURE DIRECTIONS

The Hib conjugate vaccines are immunogenic and efficacious in children and infants. HbOC, PRP-OMPC, and PRP-T have been licensed in numerous countries and are recommended for infant immunization by the Advisory Committee on Immunization Practices (ACIP) and the American Academy of Pediatrics (AAP). In areas where usage of the Hib conjugate vaccines has been high, these vaccines have already had a significant impact on disease incidence, perhaps portending eventual eradication of Hib disease. It is thus likely that future work on these vaccines will be confined to the development and refinement of assays controlling their production and release and to formulating and evaluating them in combination with other vaccine components (e.g., diphtheria-tetanus-pertussis [DTP], hepatitis B, hepatitis A, injectable polio, etc.) for universal pediatric administration.

In addition, the successful development of these vaccines, which has involved scores of researchers and years of effort, has at last established several prototype PRP conjugates that can serve to guide the development of other conjugate vaccines in the future. On a long-term research level, some of the lessons learned in the development of these successful PRP conjugates may translate to the successful synthesis of highly immunogenic peptide conjugates which may hold hope as vaccines for viral or parasitic diseases such as AIDS or malaria. In the near future it is, however, a virtual certainty that the PRP conjugates will be excellent prototypes for the development of other Ps conjugates, especially from the capsular Ps of other encapsulated bacteria (such as *S. pneumoniae*, the group B Streptococcus, *N. meningiditis*, *Salmonella typhi*, etc., as well as the opportunistic pathogens such as *Staphylococcus aureus* and *Escherichia coli*). The development of these vaccines already has begun in numerous laboratories, and it is clear that this work owes a debt to the Hib conjugates, which have ushered in an era of vaccine development that should result in a wholly new class of conjugate vaccines during the next decade.

REFERENCES

1. K. E. Stein, Thymus-independent and thymus-dependent responses to polysaccharide antigens, *J. Infect. Dis. 165* (Suppl. 1):S49 (1992).
2. W. F. Goebel and O. T. Avery, Chemo-immunological studies on conjugated carbohydrate-protein, V. The immunological specificity of an antigen prepared by combining one capsular polysaccharide of type 3 pneumococcus with foreign protein. *J. Exptl. Med. 54*:437 (1931).
3. W. E. Dick, Jr. and M. Beurret, Glycoconjugates of bacterial carbohydrate antigens. A survey and consideration of design and preparation factors, *Conjugate Vaccines* (J. M. Cruse and R. E. Lewis, eds.) Karger, Basel, 1989, p. 48.
4. C. C. A. M. Peters, A-M. J. Tenbergen-Meekes, J. T. Poolman, B. J. M. Zegers, and G. T. Rijkers, Immunogenicity of a *Streptococcus pneumoniae* type 4 polysaccharide-protein conjugate is decreased by admixture of high doses of free saccharide, *Vaccine 10*:833 (1992).
5. L. K. Gordon, Polysaccharide endotoxoid conjugate vaccines, U.S. Patent No. 4,619,828 (1986).
6. S. Marburg, D. Jorn, R. L. Tolman, B. Arison, J. McCauley, P. J. Kniskern, A. Hagopian, and P. P. Vella, Bimolecular chemistry of macromolecules—synthesis of bacterial polysaccharide conjugates with *Neisseria meningiditis* membrane protein, *J. Am. Chem. Soc. 108*:5282 (1986).
7. S. Marburg, R. L. Tolman, and P. J. Kniskern, Covalently-modified polyanionic bacterial polysaccharides, stable covalent conjugates of such polysaccharides and immunogenic protein with bigeneric spacers, and methods of preparing such polysaccharides and conjugates and of confirming covalency, U.S., Patent Nos. 4,695,624 (1987) and 4,882,317 (1989).
8. C. E. Frasch, W. D. Zollinger, and J. T. Poolman, Serotype antigens of *Neisseria meningitidis* and a proposed scheme for designation of serotypes, *Rev. Infect. Dis. 7*:504 (1985).

9. G. L. Ellman, Tissue sulfhydryl groups, *Arch. Biochem. Biophys. 82*:70 (1959).
10. O. H. Lowry, N. J. Rosebrough, A. L. Farr, and R. J. Randall, Protein measurement with the folin phenol reagent, *J. Biol. Chem. 193*:265 (1951).
11. Z. Dische and K. Schwarz, Mikromethode zur Bestimmung verschiedener Pentosen nebeneinander bei Gegenwart von Hexosen, *Mikrochem Acta 2*:13 (1937).
12. J. D. Clemens, C. Ferreccio, M. M. Levine, I. Horowitz, M. R. Rao, K. M. Edwards, and B. Fritzell, Impact of *Haemophilus influenzae* type b polysaccharide-tetanus protein conjugate vaccine to concurrently administered diphtheria-tetanus-pertussis vaccine, *JAMA 267*:673 (1992).
13. R. Schneerson, J. B. Robbins, J. C. Parke, C. Bell, J. J. Schlesselman, A. Sutton, Z. Wang, G. Schiffman, A. Karpas, and J. Shiloach, Quantitative and qualitative analysis of serum antibodies elicited in adults by *Haemophilus influenzae* type b and pneumococcus type 6A capsular polysaccharide-tetanus toxoid conjugates, *Infect. Immun. 52*:519 (1986).
14. C. Chu, R. Schneerson, J. B. Robbins, and S. C. Ratogi, Further studies on the immunogenicity of *Haemophilus influenzae* type b and pneumococcal type 6A polysaccharide-protein conjugates, *Infect. Immun. 40*:245 (1983).
15. R. Mangalo, B. Bizzini, A. Turpin, and M. Raynaud, The molecular weight of tetanus toxin, *Biochem. Biophys. Acta 168*:583 (1968).
16. H. J. Jennings and C. Lugowski, Immunogenic polysaccharide-protein conjugates, U.S. Patent No. 4,356,170 (1982).
17. P. W. Anderson and R. Eby, Immunogenic conjugates, U.S. Patent No. 4,902,506 (1990).
18. M. Colombatti, L. Dell'Arciprete, R. Rappuoli, and G. Tridente, Selective immunotoxins prepared with mutant diphtheria toxins coupled to monoclonal antibodies, *Methods Enzymol. 178*:404 (1989).
19. Smith, D. H., Madore, D. V., Eby, R. J., Anderson, P. W., Insel, R. A., and Johnson, C. L., Haemophilus b oligosaccharide-CRM197 and other Haemophilus b conjugate vaccines. A status report, *Immunobiology of Proteins and Peptides V. Vaccines* (M. Z. Atassi, ed.), Plenum Press, New York, 1989, p. 65.
20. R. C. Seid, Jr., R. A. Boykins, D-F. Liu, K. W. Kimbrough, C-L. Hsieh, and R. Eby, Chemical evidence for covalent linkages of a semisynthetic glycoconjugate vaccine for *Haemophilus influenzae* type b disease, *Glycoconjugate J. 6.*:489 (1989).
21. WHO Technical Report, Requirements for *Haemophilus influenzae* type b conjugate vaccines, No. 814, 1991, p. 15.
22. J. T. Park and M. J. Johnson, A submicrodetermination of glucose, *J. Biol. Chem. 181*:149 (1949).
23. S. S. Kulkarni, E. W. Funk, and N. N. Li, Ultrafiltration, *Membrane Handbook*, (W. S. W. Ho and K. K. Sirkar, eds.) Van Nostrand Reinhold, New York, 1989, p. 394.
24. D. M. Granoff, E. L. Anderson, M. T. Osterholm, S. J. Holmes, J. E. McHugh, R. B. Belshe, F. Medley, and T. V. Murphy, Differences in the

immunogenicity of three *Haemophilus influenzae* type b conjugate vaccines in infants, *J. Pediatrics 121*:187 (1992).

25. H. Kayhty, J. Eskola, H. Peltola, P-R. Ronnenberg, E. Kela, V. Karanko, and L. Saarinen, Antibody responses to four *Haemophilus influenzae* type b conjugate vaccines, *AJDC 145*:223 (1991).
26. P. Anderson, J. Pitt, and D. H. Smith, Synthesis and release of polyribophosphate by *Haemophilus influenzae* type b in vitro, *Infect. Immun. 13*:581 (1976).
27. P. J. Kniskern, A. Hagopian, and D. J. Carlo, Meningitis vaccines, U. S. Patent No. 4,307,080 (1981).
28. R. M. Crisel, R. S. Baker, and D. E. Dorman, Capsular polymer of *Haemophilus influenzae* type b I. Structural characterization of the capsular polymer of strain Egan, *J. Biol. Chem. 250*:4926 (1975).
29. W. W. Yau, J. J. Kirkland, and D. D. Bly, *Modern Size-Exclusion Liquid Chromatography*, Wiley, New York, 1979.
30. J. P. Hennessey, B. B. Bednar, and V. Manam, Molecular size analysis of *Haemophilus influenzae* type b capsular polysaccharide, *J. Liquid Chromato.* (in press).
31. P. W. Anderson, M. E. Pichichero, E. C., S. Porcelli, R. F. Betts, D. M. Connuck, D. Korones, R. A. Insel, J. M. Zahradnik, and R. Eby, Effect of oligosaccharide chain length, exposed terminal group and hapten loading on the antibody response of human adults and infants to vaccines consisting of *Haemophilus influenzae* type b capsular antigen uniterminally coupled to the diphtheria Pr CRM_{197}, *J. Immunol. 142*:2464 (1989).
32. M. R. Lifely, C. Moreno, and J. C. Lindon, An integrated molecular and immunological approach towards a meningococcal group b vaccine, *Vaccine 5*:11 (1987).
33. R. Wessels and D. L. Kasper, Antibody recognition of the type 14 pneumococcal capsule. Evidence for a conformational epitope in a neutral polysaccharide, *J. Exp. Med. 169*:2121 (1989).
34. H. J. Jennings, C. Lugowski, and D. L. Kasper, Conformational aspects critical to the immunospecificity of the type III group B streptococcal polysaccharide, *Biochemistry 20*:4511 (1981).
35. J. E. G. van Dam, A. Fleer, and H. Snippe, Immunogenicity and immunochemistry of *Streptococcus pneumoniae* capsular polysaccharides, *Antonie van Leeuwenhoek 58*:1 (1990).
36. C. Y. Chu, R. Schneerson, J. B. Robbins, and S. C. Rastogi, Further studies on the immunogenicity of *Haemophilus influenzae* type b and pneumococcal type 6A polysaccharide-protein conjugates, *Infect. Immun. 40*:245 (1983).
37. P. Anderson and D. H. Smith, Immunogenicity in weanling rabbits of a polyribophosphate complex from *Haemophilus influenzae* type B, *J. Infect. Dis. 136*(Suppl.):S53 (1977).
38. P. P. Vella, J. M. Staub, J. Armstrong, K. T. Dolan, C. M. Rusk, S. Szymanski, W. E. Greer, S. Marburg, P. J. Kniskern, T. L. Schofield, R. L. Tolman, F. Hartner, S-H. Pan, R. J. Gerety, and R. W. Ellis, Immunogenicity

of a new *Haemophilus influenzae* type b conjugate vaccine (meningococcal protein conjugate) (PedvaxHib®), *Pediatrics* (Suppl.):668 (1990).
39. P. J. Baker, Homeostatic control of antibody responses: a model based on recognition of cell-associated antibody by regulatory T cells, *Transplant. Rev. 26*:3 (1975).
40. D. Musher, A. Gorlee, T. Murphy, A. Chapman, J. Zahradnik, M. Apicella, and R. Baughn, Immunity to *Haemophilus influenzae* type b in young adults; correlation of bacteriocidal and opsonizing activity of serum with antibody to polyribosylribitol phosphate and lipopolysaccharide before and after vaccination, *J. Infect. Dis. 154*:935 (1986).
41. A. L. Smith, D. H. Smith, D. R. Averill, J. Marino, and E. R. Moxon, Production of *Haemophilus influenzae* b meningitis in infant rats by intraperitoneal inoculation, *Infect. Immun. 8*:278 (1973).
42. B. M. Gray, Opsonophagocidal activity in sera from infants and children immunized with *Haemophilus influenzae* type b conjugate vaccine (meningococcal protein conjugate), *Pediatrics 85* (Suppl.):694 (1990).
43. *Code of Federal Regulations,* 21CFR 610.13 (1991).
44. *Code of Federal Regulations,* 21CFR 610.11 (1991).
45. *Drug Information for the Health Care Professional*, USP DI, Volume IA, The U.S. Pharmacopeal Convention, Inc., 1992.
46. *Physicians Desk Reference*, 1992.

4

Immunobiology of Protein Carriers

John J. Donnelly and Margaret A. Liu

Merck Research Laboratories, West Point, Pennsylvania

Many potential targets for protective immune responses are peptides or polysaccharides that are not recognized by T lymphocytes and therefore are not highly immunogenic when purified. Coupling such antigens to protein carriers was shown by Avery and Goebel in 1929 (1,2) to increase their immunogenicity. Our level of understanding of the mechanisms by which protein carriers affect immunogenicity has advanced sufficiently over the intervening decades to enable the rational design of conjugate vaccines. The two most important features of this knowledge are the elucidation of the cellular mechanisms of dual-antigen recognition by T and B lymphocytes and the understanding of the role played by the three-dimensional structure of antigens in the activation of B cells. This chapter will focus primarily on the former aspect of protein carriers. The first section will summarize the current understanding of how carrier recognition works. Second, we will discuss the ability of carriers and conjugates to regulate immune responses. Finally, the immunological mechanisms of the *Haemophilus influenzae* type b (Hib) conjugate vaccines currently in use will be described in detail.

I. MECHANISMS OF ACTION OF CARRIER PROTEINS

A. Why Are There T-B Interactions?

The division of lymphocytes into immunoglobulin (Ig)-producing ("B") and regulatory ("T") subpopulations is readily demonstrated in all vertebrates with the exception of sharks, lampreys, and hagfish (3,4). This division is coincident with the ability to make Ig of more than one isotype and suggests that dual control of the Ig isotype produced is highly favorable from an evolutionary standpoint (5–9). In mice, teleost fish, and amphibians, for example, Ig heavy-chain class switching generally requires the cooperation of T and B lymphocytes (10–12). However, polyvalent antigens, such as the Hib capsular polysaccharide polyribosyl ribitol phosphate (PRP), can elicit an IgM antibody response in the absence of T cells (13,14). These antigens are termed type 2 T-independent (TI) antigens and are thought to activate B cells directly by cross-linking surface immunoglobulin molecules (15). Detailed studies of the physical properties of type 2 TI antigens have shown that size and epitope density are key factors in determining their immunogenicity (see Chapter 6). For example, dextrans of less than 70,000 daltons (Da) are minimally immunogenic in humans, while haptenated polymers are most immunogenic in mice when their molecular weights are between 500,000 and 1,000,000 Da (16,17).

B. What Do T Cells "See"?

The T-cell receptor for antigen recognizes antigens that have been "processed" and displayed on the surface of an "antigen-presenting cell" bound to major histocompatibility complex (MHC) molecules (18,19). Processing involves cleavage of polypeptide antigens into peptides 8–20 amino acid residues in length and is thought to occur by partial proteolysis, predominantly in an endosomal compartment (for presentation by MHC Class II molecules) or in the cytosol (for presentation by MHC Class I) (20–22). The interactions of peptides with MHC Class I molecules are well understood (23–28). The relevance of this information to MHC Class II may be inferred from the similarities in amino acid sequence between the peptide-binding regions of the two classes of MHC molecules (29). "Processed" peptides bind in a groove located in the apical portion of the MHC Class I molecule (23–28). Binding results from energetically favorable interaction of amino acid side chains of the peptide with amino acid residues lining the groove of the MHC molecule (25,26). Therefore, selection of peptides for presentation is dependent on the sequences both of the peptide antigen and of the MHC molecule (18–28). Both the peptide and the MHC molecule may undergo conformational changes during binding, and different residues of the peptide may interact with the MHC molecule, thus increasing the diversity of peptides capable of binding to a given MHC molecule (25,26). This model of MHC structure would predict that recognition of this complex by the T-cell receptor occurs when the surface presented by the processed peptide and the flanking portions of the MHC molecule can bind stably to the apical surface of the T-cell receptor (25,28,30). Thus the recognition of antigen by T cells is restricted on two levels: selection of antigen peptides that bind stably to host MHC molecules and selection of T-cell receptors capable of binding with appropriate affinity to MHC molecules (18,30,31). This model provides an explanation for the inability of humans and experimental animals of certain genotypes to respond to particular naturally occurring and synthetic peptides (32). Inability of a given MHC molecule to bind a particular peptide renders an individual unable to present that peptide to T cells. Activation of T cells by recognition of the MHC-peptide complex would be predicted to result from interaction of amino acid side chains of the peptide with complementarity-determining regions of the T-cell receptor (28–32). Thus particular residues of a processed peptide may be involved in binding to MHC ("agretope") or may interact with the T-cell receptor ("epitope") (25–28,30,32).

This understanding of the nature of antigen recognition by T cells leads to two important conclusions relevant to the design of vaccines using protein carriers. First, chemical modifications of protein carriers may influence the ability of T cells to provide "help;" that is, to activate B cells for Ig isotype switching. Large constituents (such as high-molecular weight polysaccharides) or coupling methodologies that render carrier protein molecules resistant to proteolysis may result in conjugates that do not provide efficient T-cell help. Second, putative carrier proteins must contain a sufficiently large diversity of potential T-cell epitopes to ensure that as many members of an outbred population as possible will be capable of recognizing at least one such peptide in association with MHC. Furthermore, the ability of an individual with given MHC molecules to respond to a potential carrier protein in its native state does not necessarily predict his ability to recognize it when conjugated. Modifications of key residues may alter or destroy an agretope or epitope unless the modifications are removed during antigen processing. In some instances chemical modifications of peptides (for example, with TNP) may be recognized by T cells as novel epitopes (33). Partial removal of conjugated polysaccharides during processing might similarly destroy or create new epitopes that could be capable of mediating T-cell help. Thus selection of the optimal protein carrier for a particular conjugate vaccine would require consideration of the ligand of interest, the desired coupling technique, and the planned target population. In practice, most large naturally occurring proteins that might be used as carriers appear to contain a sufficient diversity of potential peptides to function well as carriers in an outbred human population. However, these considerations become of great importance if one attempts to use a limited number of selected peptides to create a synthetic carrier.

C. What Is Antigen Processing?

Antigenic peptides bound to MHC Class I molecules are predominantly recognized by T cells of the CD8+ phenotype, while those bound to MHC Class II molecules are predominantly recognized by T cells of the CD4+ phenotype. Delivery of a nonreplicating antigen, such as a conjugate vaccine, by injection generally predisposes to presentation in association with MHC Class II (22). Both uncomplexed antigen and antigen-antibody complexes may be processed by this pathway (34). MHC Class II–restricted presentation occurs when antigen is endocytosed to an endosomal compartment and undergoes proteolysis in the acidic environment of the early endosome (35,36). Concurrently, both nascent MHC Class II molecules, with their peptide-binding sites occupied by the invariant chain (a nonpolymorphic protein that aids the assembly and intracellular trafficking of MHC Class II) and peptide-bearing MHC Class II molecules recycled from the cell surface are targeted to the same compartment. The invariant chain is proteolytically cleaved, and invariant chain or other preexisting peptides are removed and replaced with newly processed peptides (37–39). The resulting complex is returned to the cell surface via the normal recycling pathway from early endosomes (40). This process can occur in macrophages and B lymphocytes (35,41,42). Small resting B lymphocytes are relatively inefficient at presenting antigen, while activated B lymphocytes present antigen efficiently to primed T cells but not to unprimed T cells (41,42). In lymph nodes, B cells may internalize organelles, containing antigen-antibody complexes, that have been shed by follicular dendritic cells (43). Furthermore, B cells target internalized surface Ig (sIg) to a compartment containing MHC Class II and invariant chains, allowing for processing of internalized complexes of antigen and specific antibody (44). The ability of B cells to process and present antigens, selectively internalized via their sIg molecules, allows for highly efficient cognate interactions of antigen-specific B cells with antigen-specific helper T cells (45).

D. What Do B Cells "See"?

The sIg molecules on B cells serve as surface receptors for antigenic stimulation (46). Signaling from sIg is thought to occur via three membrane proteins associated with the sIg molecules that are phosphorylated following cross-linking of sIg (47,48). Phosphorylation of these membrane proteins results in increased phosphoinositide turnover, leading ultimately to activation of the B cell (49,50). The ability of Ig molecules to bind antigen based on three-dimensional structure is well defined (51). However, two aspects of antibody-antigen interactions are worthy of consideration in the selection of carrier proteins for use in conjugate vaccines. First, B-cell activation requires interaction of antigen with multiple sIg molecules on the B cell surface (17) (see Chapter 6). Thus the density of antibody-binding sites ("epitopes") on the carrier may affect the avidity of antibody obtained by immunization with a conjugate vaccine. Very large carriers, or carriers with a very high density of coupled polysaccharide or small molecular constituent ("hapten"), may interact stably with B cells bearing sIg molecules of relatively low avidity for the desired epitope. If the density of epitopes on the native antigen were much lower than that of the conjugate vaccine, B cells activated by the conjugate may not be activated by the native antigen, leading to a failure of protection. Conversely, too low a density of epitopes in a conjugate vaccine may be so inefficient at activating B cells as to be unable to elicit any antibody response (17) (see Chapter 6). Second, antigen-antibody interactions can be exquisitely stereospecific (51). Conjugation of small haptens may lead to antibody responses with high avidity for the conjugated form and lower avidity for the native epitope present on the pathogen of interest. Conjugation of peptides in particular may alter conformational mobility and lead to an antibody response against conformers absent from the native antigen. Thus selection of carrier proteins must be made to present the optimal epitope density and conformation for eliciting the strongest possible antibody response to the desired pathogen.

E. Effect of Structure on T-Cell Help

Cognate recognition requires that antibody-binding epitopes ("B-cell epitopes") and processed polypeptide complexed to MHC class II ("T-cell epitopes") exist in close proximity, probably on the same antigen-presenting cell. This can be accomplished by linking B- and T-cell epitopes in an immunogen by a variety of methods, including chemical conjugation, tandem expression in a synthetic peptide or fusion protein, or stable noncovalent association (52–58). Expression of B- and T-cell epitopes in tandem in a synthetic peptide has been shown to induce antigastrin antibodies efficiently in guinea pigs (52). A synthetic copolymer consisting of the B-cell epitope Pro-Pro-Pro-Pro-Asn-Pro-Asn-Asp (PPPPNPND) from the circumsporozoite protein (CSP) of *Plasmodium berghei*, in tandem with a T-cell epitope, on a skeleton of polylysine (MAP) induced a protective antibody response to *P. berghei* in mice (53). Expression of the peptide epitope Asn-Ala-Asn-Pro (NANP), derived from the CSP of *Plasmodium falciparum*, in tandem with T-cell epitopes in a fusion protein, elicited antipeptide IgG antibody in strains of mice that were incapable of responding to the NANP peptide alone (54). Stable noncovalent interactions, such as those between the surface (HBsAg) and core (HBcAg) antigens of hepatitis B virus, also may mediate T-cell help. Strains of mice whose MHC molecules are unable to present HBsAg to T cells but do present HBcAg can make IgG antibodies to HBsAg if immunized with a noncovalent complex of the two proteins (55). Weaker noncovalent interactions are not sufficient to produce cognate help. For example, simple mixtures of polysaccharides such as PRP with a carrier, the outer membrane protein complex (OMPC) of *Neisseria meningitidis* serogroup B NMB, do not elicit IgG antibody responses to PRP in mice or infant nonhuman primates, in contrast to conjugates in which the two components are covalently linked by chemical means (56–58). The size and physical form of the covalent conjugates also may significantly affect their ability to mediate T-cell help. Very large aggregates may not be internalized efficiently by B cells and therefore may require processing by macrophages or dendritic cells for presentation to T cells. The clearance rates of such conjugates may be relatively slow. This may be beneficial to secondary responses for both T and B cells, since the persistence of antigen is thought to enhance the persistence of immunological memory (58). Small soluble complexes may be more readily processed by antigen-specific B cells because of their ability to focus and internalize antigen bound to sIg (45). The resulting presentation of processed antigen to T cells might lead to efficient cognate priming of high-affinity B cells, but a shorter persistence of immunological memory due to the more rapid clearance of the antigen (46,58). However, antigen-antibody complexes may be degraded during processing in a slightly different pattern from that of monomeric antigen molecules (59). Binding of antibodies to polypeptides is thought to protect residues in and near the site of antibody attachment from proteolysis (59). Thus, the proximity of hapten constituents to T-cell epitopes on the carrier may significantly affect the immunogenicity of conjugates, particularly upon secondary immunization.

II. IMMUNOREGULATORY MECHANISMS OF CONJUGATE VACCINES

A. Epitopic Suppression

Prior immunization of mice (60) and humans (61) with a carrier protein may result in a decreased antihapten antibody response to subsequent immunization with a hapten coupled to the same carrier. This phenomenon has been termed epitopic suppression (60) and is thought to result from competition between B cells specific for the carrier and those specific for the hapten (62). Prior immunization with the carrier protein can expand the frequency of carrier-specific B cells by as much as 30-fold (62). These cells can then compete with hapten-specific B cells for internalization of the hapten-carrier conjugate and for presentation to carrier-specific helper T cells (62). This would result in a reduced level of cognate help available for the hapten-specific B cells (62). Increasing the density of hapten on the conjugate, increasing the dose of conjugate, or expanding the population of hapten-specific B cells by prior immunization with the hapten conjugated to an unrelated carrier can abrogate epitopic suppression (60–64). Inclusion of adjuvants such as *Bordetella pertussis,* muramyl dipeptide, or lipopolysaccharide (LPS) in the conjugate also can restore the antihapten response to normal levels (63). This phenomenon poses a theoretical consideration for the selection of carrier proteins for clinical use in conjugate vaccines. Where common immunogens are used as carriers, increased substitution with hapten, higher doses of conjugate, or stronger adjuvants may be needed to achieve the desired antihapten antibody response (61–63). When the same carrier is used repeatedly with different haptens, a similar phenomenon may be expected. However, tetanus toxoid (TT) has been used successfully as a carrier protein in both infant humans and nonhuman primates previously immunized with TT, suggesting that, for at least some carriers, epitopic suppression may not pose a significant clinical problem.

B. Mitogens as Carriers

The use of protein carriers that are also mitogens or superantigens may significantly increase the immunogenicity of conjugate vaccines and also may potentially avoid epitopic suppression. Cholera toxin (holotoxin and B subunit), *Pseudomonas aeruginosa* exotoxin A (PE), mycobacterial heat-shock proteins, and outer membrane proteins from gram-negative bacteria such as *N. meningitidis* have been used successfully as protein carriers (64–68). Que et al. compared cholera toxin, PE toxin and TT as carriers for a recombinant polypeptide (R32) from the CSP of *P. falciparum* (64). The resulting IgG antipeptide antibody titers in rabbits were more than twofold greater when cholera toxin or PE was used as carrier rather than TT (64). Immunization of mice with a synthetic peptide from the CSP of *P. falciparum* ($NANP_{40}$) conjugated to the heat-shock proteins hsp65 of *Mycobacterium bovis* or the hsp70 of *M. tuberculosis* yielded IgG antipeptide antibody resposes without the use of additional adjuvants (65). Immunization of humans with *P. aeruginosa* O-polysaccharide coupled to PE or cholera toxin yielded both IgG antibody against the polysaccharide moiety of *P. aeruginosa* LPS and also neutralizing antibody against the toxins (66).

The OMPC of NMB has been used as a carrier for PRP (56,57,67–71).

In adult mice and infant nonhuman primates and humans, this conjugate vaccine induces high titers of serum IgG antibody and protective immunity to Hib infection (56,57,67,68). In addition to possessing T-cell epitopes for carrier recognition, OMPC has been shown to be a mitogen for both T and B cells (69–71). This mitogenicity is independent of the effects of any residual LPS (69–71). The principal protein constituent (class 2) of OMPC, MIEP (major immunoenhancing protein), has been purified and shares the mitogenic activity of OMPC (69–71). MIEP also functions as an effective carrier for PRP in mice and infant rhesus monkeys (69).

C. Carriers and Adjuvants

It is worthwhile to emphasize the distinction between carriers and adjuvants. Carriers act by the specific provision of peptide epitopes which, when presented in association with MHC Class II molecules to T-helper lymphocytes, stimulate the T cells to produce cytokines that affect the B-cell antibody response. Protein carriers should be covalently linked to the polysaccharide or hapten. The carriers are responsible for the T-cell help that induces the B cell to generate the type of antibody response characteristic of T-dependent antigens (i.e., antigens for which the immune response depends upon recognition of the antigen by both T and B cells). These responses include class switching from the production of IgM antibody to high-affinity IgG antibody and the induction of memory or anamnestic responses upon reexposure to the antigen. Adjuvants provide augmentation of the immune response by the more generalized mechanisms of providing a depot effect or by including reactogenic components for various cells of the immune system, rather than by providing T-helper cell–specific epitopes.

The importance of T-cell help becomes clear when devising strategies to induce protective immune responses in young children, particularly those less than 2 years of age who are unable to generate an appropriate immune response against polysaccharides such as PRP (72). Young children respond poorly to PRP when it is presented either as a purified polysaccharide vaccine (73,74) or even following infection with the organism itself. Attempts were made to simply mix PRP with other vaccines (pertussis or DTP) in order to improve the immune response (75–77). However, these did not consistently (76,77) increase the immunogenicity of the PRP. Likewise, infant rhesus monkeys, which have proven to be a useful model for immune responses in humans, do not respond to PRP alone or mixed with (i.e., not conjugated to) carriers (68,78). Thus efforts were turned toward the conjugation of PRP to a carrier protein in order to transform it into a T-dependent antigen.

III. Hib CONJUGATE VACCINES

A. Carrier Effects

Four vaccine conjugates of PRP and carrier proteins have been licensed (see table in preface). These differ in the size of the capsular saccharide used, the protein carrier, and the chemical conjugation technology. These have been extensively described in other reviews (79–86). This article will focus on the differences in immunogenicity and the potential mechanisms related to the various carriers. PRP-D utilizes diphtheria toxoid (DT) covalently linked to sized PRP. HbOC employs a mutant diphtheria toxin, CRM_{197} (*C*ross-*R*eacting *M*utant, a nontoxic single amino acid mutant form of DT) conjugated to an oligosaccharide of PRP of an average length of 20 units. PRP-OMPC conjugates the OMPC of NMB to native PRP polysaccharide. PRP-T utilizes TT as the carrier for native PRP.

All four conjugate vaccines transform the Hib capsular saccharides into T-dependent antigens, although their immunogenicity profiles for infants differ. The immune system, and hence the immune responses, of infants differ from those of older children and adults, revealing varied responses to the four vaccines as a function of age (see Chapter 15). Although the vaccines also differ in the size of saccharide used, it is not clear that this results in any functional in vivo difference in the effect of the anti-PRP antibodies (80,87,88). Thus we will focus on the clear chemical and physical differences among the four carriers.

The size of the carrier may affect the immunogenicity of the conjugate in several ways. Larger proteins are often thought to be more immunogenic and are used routinely as carriers for peptides and haptens for eliciting antibodies in preclinical experiments. One a priori rationale for considering TT a potentially better immunogen and carrier than DT was its larger size. A larger protein, or a carrier with multiple proteins, can potentially provide more MHC Class II epitopes than a smaller protein. In addition, the degree of hapten loading may also be a function of the size of the carrier as well as the chemistry of the conjugation (see Chapters 3 and 6).

B. Carrier Priming

PRP-OMPC elicits antibodies to PRP (anti-PRP) in some strains of adult mice, unlike PRP-D and HbOC (56,57). The latter two vaccines did not generate anti-PRP even following carrier priming or a booster injection. Efficient class switching of antibody class and subclass was seen in mice immunized with PRP-OMPC, such that IgG1, IgG2a, and IgG3 anti-PRP were made in response to PRP-OMPC, but not to PRP-D or HbOC. A memory response was seen when the mice were boosted with a second injection of PRP-OMPC. In order to confirm that these results were due to the ability of the OMPC to act as a carrier, spleen cell transfer experiments were done. These experiments revealed that OMPC did function as a classical carrier, in addition to having adjuvant activities discussed below. These results in mice are reflected in the immunogenicity of these conjugates in infant humans. PRP-OMPC induces titers ≥ 1 μg anti-PRP/ml in the majority of 2- to 6-month-old infants following a single injection (67,89), whereas HbOC and PRP-T do not induce titers of this magnitude until after a second dose in this age group (90,91).

Note that these children are receiving concomitant immunization with DTP (at 2, 4, and 6 months), which may provide increased carrier priming for the latter two vaccines. Indeed, in primate studies, using an earlier PRP-T conjugate, no or low-level anti-PRP were seen (depending upon the dose of PRP-T) unless the monkeys were primed with TT (92). Similarly, three serial immunizations with HbOC ($\pm$TT) were incapable of generating anti-PRP antibody titers in infant rhesus monkeys unless the monkeys were concomitantly given diphtheria (and tetanus) toxoid(s) (68). The monkeys immunized with HbOC did not produce antibodies against DT, unless coimmunized with the DT (and TT), suggesting that the CRM_{197} carrier is not a strong immunogen. As previously suggested (86), this may be due to the lack of formalin inactivation, which is unnecessary for this mutant nontoxic protein (93). The apparent relevance of the infant monkey model to the infant human responses to at least certain PRP conjugates raises theoretical issues about the possible requirement for co-priming with the carrier in the case of HbOC (perhaps reflected in the kinetics of the immune response) or about nonresponders to DT (94).

C. Secondary Responses

As anticipated by the effective T-dependent response, boosts with these vaccines result in a strong anamnestic response of the anti-PRP titers (86,95,96). Interestingly, giving a third dose of PRP-OMPC at 6 months of age does not boost the anti-PRP antibody titer, although a booster dose at 12–15 months does. (In contrast to PRP-OMPC, in a vaccination series with a pneumococcal-OMPC conjugate, a third dose of the conjugate does boost the antibody response.) In certain instances, boosting may be performed with a different conjugate than the one used for the priming series (97), and free polysaccharide alone has also resulted in increased anti-PRP titers (98). This would indicate that once the appropriate help and antibody responses have been generated, induction of memory B cells also occurs, and a TI antigen alone is sufficient to produce the anamnestic response.

D. Adjuvant Effects

OMPC differs from DT, CRM_{197}, and TT in that it is not a single protein, and thus has additional effects to its T-dependent carrier activity. On a macromolecular level, the OMPC carrier is actually a liposome 100–200 nm in diameter. Particulate antigens are thought to be taken up more readily into antigen presenting cells both by being phagocytosed by the antigen presenting cells and by augmented retention of the particles in the reticuloendothelial system. In addition, PRP-OMPC is administered on aluminum, which should provide adjuvant activity by decreasing the dispersal rate of the injected immunogen. The OMPC carrier was also shown to have adjuvant activity, as measured by the ability to increase the immune responses against an antigen mixed with the OMPC (57). The OMPC could augment the antibody response directed against a protein antigen (TT), a polysaccharide conjugated to a protein (PRP-D), or a peptide (when the peptide was precipitated on alum). As expected, this adjuvant activity required the protein to be physically mixed with the OMPC. It is possible that the lipids and LPS present in the OMPC vesicle contributed to this adjuvant activity; however, the adjuvant activity for TT occurred even in LPS-hyporesponsive C3H/HeJ mice. In addition, a single protein component (MIEP), when purified free of detectable LPS, induced proliferation, cytokine production, and immunoglobulin secretion by naive lymphocytes (69–71) thus providing a novel potential explanation for the increased immunogenicity of PRP-OMPC in infants.

E. Antibody Responses in Compromised Hosts

The transformation of TI Hib saccharides into T-dependent conjugates improves the immunogenicity for children with impaired immunity to polysaccharides. This inability or decreased ability to respond to polysaccharides may be as a result of (a) conditions that result in immunocompromise such as sickle cell disease or splenectomy plus therapy for Hodgkin's disease, (b) genetic background (including certain groups of Native Americans and blacks lacking a particular immunoglobulin allotype), or (c) low anti-PRP titers following Hib invasive disease, even following prior vaccination with PRP vaccine. PRP-D, HbOC, and PRP-T were shown to be effective immunogens in infants who had failed to develop protective antibody titers following Hib invasive disease (99–101). Likewise, PRP-OMPC and PRP-D could generate protective anti-PRP titers in children who developed Hib disease following vaccination with the PRP vaccine (102,103). Additionally, vaccination with conjugates has been shown to be effective in certain immunodeficient individuals. Immunization with PRP-T (101),

PRP-D (104), and HbOC (105) resulted in anti-PRP responses in infants or children with sickle cell disease who, prior to immunization, had low antibody titers. Conjugate administration successfully immunized children with the Km(1) Ig allotype who have a higher risk of Hib invasive disease (102). Persons susceptible to recurrent infections or with primary immunodeficiencies (e.g., Wiskott-Aldrich syndrome) developed higher anti-PRP IgG titers following immunization with PRP-T than with the PRP vaccine (106). Men infected with HIV responded to HbOC with higher anti-PRP titers than to the unconjugated PRP (107). PRP-D given to splenectomized patients with Hodgkin's disease who had also received radiation and/or chemotherapy resulted in an increase in anti-PRP titers, although the titers did not boost following a second injection (108). In certain of the cases described above, the antibody titers did not reach levels noted in the control population. Nevertheless, conjugate vaccines clearly induced increases in anti-PRP antibody titers when PRP vaccine, invasive disease, or "natural immunity" was inadequate.

IV. CONCLUSIONS

Conjugation of PRP to a carrier protein has been shown to induce effective anti-PRP levels in infants and immunocompromised children who do not effectively response to PRP alone or PRP presented during invasive infection with Hib organisms. The effectiveness of a carrier in a conjugate varies among carrier proteins, suggesting that in addition to differences in conjugation chemistries, saccharide size, and PRP-protein ratios, factors such as carrier size, adjuvant ability, and particulate nature may affect the immunogenicity in ways beyond the conferring of T-helper cell epitopes.

REFERENCES

1. O. T. Avery and W. F. Goebel, Chemo-immunological studies on conjugated carbohydrate-proteins. II. Immunological specificity of synthetic sugar-protein antigens, *J. Exp. Med. 50*:533 (1929).
2. W. F. Goebel, Studies on antibacterial immunity induced by artificial antigens. I. Immunity to experimental pneumococcal infection with an antigen containing cellobiuronic acid, *J. Exp. Med. 69*:53 (1939).
3. A. Zapata, Phylogeny of the fish immune system, *Bull. Inst. Pasteur. 81*:165 (1983).
4. L. DuPasquier, Phylogenesis of the vertebrate immune system *27. Mosbacher Colloquium* (F. Melchers and K. Rajewsky, eds.), Springer-Verlag, Berlin, 1976, p. 101.
5. G. W. Litman and J. J. Marchalonis, Evolution of antibodies, *Immune Regula-*

tion (L. N. Ruben and H. E. Gershwin, eds.), Marcel Dekker, New York, 1982, p. 29.

6. R. L. Raison, C. J. Hull, and W. H. Hildeman, Characterization of immunoglobulins from the pacific hagfish, a primitive vertebrate. *Proc. Natl. Acad. Sci. USA 75*:5679 (1978).
7. J. C. Atwell and J. J. Marchalonis, Phylogenetic emergence of immunoglobulin classes distinct from IgM. *J. Immunogenet. 1*:367 (1975).
8. E. Hsu and L. DuPasquier, Studies on *Xenopus* immunoglobulins using monoclonal antibodies, *Mol. Immunol. 21*:257 (1984).
9. L. A. Steiner, C. A. Mikyorak, A. D. Lopes, and C. Green, Immunoglobulins in ranid frogs and tadpoles, *Adv. Exp. Biol. Med. 64*:173 (1975).
10. D. H. Katz, T. Hamaoka, and B. Benacerraf, Cell interactions between histocompatible T and B lymphocytes. II. Failure of physiologic cooperative interactions between T and B lymphocytes from allogeneic donor strains in humoral response to hapten-protein conjugates, *J. Exp. Med. 137*:1405 (1973).
11. K. Sailendri and V. R. Muthukkaruppan, The immune response of the teleost, *Tilapia mossambica*, to soluble and cellular antigens, *J. Exp. Zool. 191*:371 (1975).
12. J. Manning and J. D. Horton, RES Structure and function of the amphibia, *The Reticuloendothelial System*, Vol. 3, *Phylogeny and Ontogeny* (N. Cohen and M. M. Sigel, eds.), Plenum Press, New York, 1982, p. 423.
13. B. Andersson and H. Blomgren, Evidence for thymus-independent humoral antibody production in mice against polyvinylpyrrolidone and *E. coli* lipopolysaccharide, *Cell. Immunol. 2*:411 (1971).
14. M. Feldman and A. Basten, The relationship between antigenic structure and the requirement for thymus-derived cells in the immune response, *J. Exp. Med. 134*:103 (1971).
15. H. M. Dintzis, R. L. Dintzis, and B. Vogelstein, Molecular determinants of immunogenicity: the immunon model of the immune response, *Proc. Natl. Acad. Sci. USA 73*:3771 (1976).
16. E. A. Kabat and A. E. Bezer, The effect of variation in molecular weight on the antigenicity of dextran in man, *Arch. Biochem. 78*:306 (1958).
17. R. Z. Dintzis, M. Okajima, M. H. Middleton, G. Greene, and H. M. Dintzis, The immunogenicity of soluble haptenated polymers is determined by molecular mass and hapten valence, *J. Immunol. 143*:1239 (1989).
18. S. Buus, A. Sette, S. M. Colon, C. Miles, and H. M. Grey, The relation between major histocompatibility complex (MHC) restriction and the capacity of Ia to bind immunogenic peptides, *Science 235*:1353 (1987).
19. A. R. Townsend and H. Bodmer, Antigen recognition by Class I MHC-restricted T lymphocytes, *Annu. Rev. Immunol. 7*:601 (1989).
20. D. F. Hunt, H. Michel, T. A. Dickinson, J. Shabanowitz, A. L. Cox, K. Sakaguchi, E. Appella, H. M. Grey, and A. Sette, Peptides presented to the immune system by the murine Class II major histocompatibility complex molecule I-A^d, *Science 256*:1817 (1992).

21. D. F. Hunt, R. A. Henderson, J. Shabanowitz, K. Sakaguchi, H. Michel, N. Sevilir, A. L. Cox, E. Appella, and V. H. Engelhard, Characterization of peptides bound to the Class I MHC molecule HLA-A2.1 by mass spectrometry, *Science 255*:1261 (1992).
22. F. M. Brodsky, Intracellular routes for antigen processing and presentation, *Res. Immunol. 142*: 453 (1991).
23. P. J. Bjorkman, M. A. Saper, B. Samraoui, W. S. Bennett, J. L. Strominger, and D. C. Wiley, The foreign antigen binding site and T cell recognition regions of class I histocompatibility antigens, *Nature 329*:512 (1987).
24. D. R. Madden, J. C. Gorga, J. L. Strominger, and D. C. Wiley, The structure of HLA-B27 reveals nonamer self-peptides bound in an extended conformation, *Nature 353*: 321 (1991).
25. D. H. Fremont, M. Matsumura, E. A. Sture, P. A. Peterson, I. A. Wilson, Crystal structure of two viral peptides in complex with murine MHC Class I H-2K^b, *Science 257*:919 (1992).
26. M. Matsumura, D. H. Fremont, P. A. Peterson, and I. A. Wilson, Emerging principles for the recognition of peptide antigens by MHC Class I molecules, *Science 257*:927 (1992).
27. F. Latron, L. Pazmany, J. Morrison, R. Moots, M. A. Saper, A. McMichael, and J. L. Strominger, A critical role for conserved residues in the cleft of HLA-A2 in presentation of a nonapeptide to T cells, *Science 257*:964 (1992).
28. W. Zhang, A. C. M. Young, M. Imarai, S. G. Nathenson, and J. C. Sacchettini, Crystal structure of the major histocompatibility complex Class I H-2K^b molecule containing a single viral peptide: Implications for peptide binding and T-cell receptor recognition, *Proc. Natl. Acad. Sci. USA 89*:8403 (1992).
29. J. H. Brown, T. Jardetsky, M. A. Saper, B. Samraoui, P. J. Bjorkman, and D. C. Wiley, A hypothetical model of the foreign antigen binding site of Class II histocompatibility molecules, *Nature 332*:845 (1988).
30. M. M. Davis and P. J. Bjorkman, T cell antigen receptor genes and T-cell recognition, *Nature 334*:395 (1988).
31. K. Matsui, J. J. Boniface, P. A. Reay, H. Schild, B. Fazekas de St. Groth, M. M. Davis, Low affinity interaction of peptide-MHC complexes with T cell receptors, *Science 254*:1788 (1991).
32. E. Heber-Katz, D. Hansburg, and R. H. Schwartz, The Ia molecule of the antigen-presenting cell plays a critical role in immune response gene regulation of T cell activation, *J. Mol. Cell. Immunol. 1*:3 (1983).
33. S. Martin, B. Ortmann, U. Pflugfelder, U. Birsner, and H. U. Weltzien, Role of hapten-anchoring peptides in defining hapten-epitopes for MHC-restricted cytotoxic T cells. Cross-reactive TNP-determinants on different peptides, *J. Immunol. 149*:2569 (1992).
34. S. Ozaki and J. A. Berzofsky, Antibody conjugates mimic specific B cell presentation of antigen: Relationship between T and B cell specificity, *J. Immunol. 138*:4133 (1987).
35. K. Ziegler and E. R. Unanue, Decrease in macrophage antigen catabolism by

ammonia and chloroquine is associated with inhibition of antigen presentation to T cells, *Proc. Natl. Acad. Sci. USA 78*:175 (1982).
36. C. V. Harding and E. R. Unanue, Antigen processing and intracellular Ia: Possible roles of endocytosis and protein synthesis in Ia function, *J. Immunol. 142*:12 (1989).
37. P. J. Peters, J. J. Neefjes, V. Oorschot, H. L. Ploegh, and H. J. Geuze, Segregation of MHC Class II molecules from MHC Class I molecules in the Golgi complex for transport to lysosomal compartments, *Nature 349*:669 (1991).
38. C. A. Lamb and P. Cresswell, Assembly and transport of invariant chain trimers and HLA-DR-invariant chain complexes, *J. Immunol. 148*:3478 (1992).
39. C. A. Lamb, J. W. Yewdell, J. R. Bennink, and P. Cresswell, Invariant chain targets HLA class II molecules to acidic endosomes containing internalized influenza virus, *Proc. Natl. Acad. Sci. USA 88*:5998 (1991).
40. Schwartz, A. L., Cell biology of intracellular protein trafficking, *Ann. Rev. Immunol. 8*:195 (1990).
41. E. J. Grosselin, H. P. Tony, and D. C. Parker, Characterization of antigen processing and presentation by resting B lymphocytes, *J. Immunol. 140*:1408 (1988).
42. M. Frohman and C. Cowing, Presentation of antigen by B cells: Functional dependence on radiation dose, interleukins, cellular activation, and differential glycosylation, *J. Immunol. 134*:2269 (1985).
43. A. K. Szakal, M. H. Kosco, and J. G. Tew, A novel in vivo follicular dendritic cell-dependent iccosome-mediated mechanism for delivery of antigen to antigen-processing cells, *J. Immunol. 140*:341 (1988).
44. L. E. Guagliardi, B. Koppelman, J. S. Blum, M. S. Marks, P. Cresswell, and F. M. Brodsky, Co-localization of molecules involved in antigen processing and presentation in an early endocytic compartment, *Nature 343*:133 (1990).
45. A. Lanzavecchia, Antigen-specific interaction between T and B cells, *Nature 314*:537 (1985).
46. T. Kishimoto and K. Ishizaka, Regulation of antibody response *in vitro*. IX. Induction of secondary anti-hapten IgG antibody response by anti-immunoglobulin and enhancing soluble factor, *J. Immunol. 114*:585 (1975).
47. J. Himbach, L. Leclerq, A. Radbruch, K. Rajewsky, and M. Reth, A novel 34-kd protein co-isolated with the IgM molecule in surface IgM-expressing cells, *EMBO J. 7*:3451 (1988).
48. K. S. Campbell and J. C. Cambier, B lymphocyte antigen receptors (mIg) are non-covalently associated with a disulfide-linked, inducibly phosphorylated glycoprotein complex, *EMBO J. 9*:441 (1990).
49. M. M. Harnett and G. G. B. Klaus, G protein coupling of antigen receptor-stimulated polyphosphoinositide hydrolysis in B cells, *J. Immunol. 140*:3139 (1988).
50. J. G. Monroe and S. Haldar, Involvement of a specific guanine nucleotide

binding protein in receptor immunoglobulin stimulated inositol phospholipid hydrolysis, *Biochim. Biophys. Acta 1013*:273 (1989).
51. J. Sharon, E.A. Kabat, and S.L. Morrison, Studies on mouse hybridomas secreting IgM or IgA antibodies for $\alpha(1\rightarrow6)$-linked dextran, *Mol. Immunol. 18*:831 (1981).
52. E. Wunsch, L. Moroder, G. Huebner, H. J. Musiol, R. von Grunigen, W. Gohring, R. Scharf, C. H. Schneider, Fully synthetic immunogens. Part III. Synthesis of hinge peptide/gastrin conjugates and their immunological properties, *Int. J. Pept. Prot. Res. 37*:90 (1991).
53. J. P. Tam, P. Clavijo, Y. Lu, V. Nussenzweig, R. Nussenzweig, and F. Zavala, Incorporation of T and B epitopes of the circumsporozoite protein in a chemically defined vaccine against malaria, *J. Exp. Med. 171*:299 (1990).
54. J. F. Young, W. T. Hockmeyer, M. Gross, W. R. Ballou, R. A. Wirtz, J. H. Tresper, R. L. Beaudoin, M. R. Hollingdale, L. H. Miller, C. L. Diggs, and M. Rosenberg, Expression of *Plasmodium falciparum* circumsporozoite protein in *Escherichia coli* for potential use in a human malaria vaccine, *Science 228*:958 (1985:).
55. D. R. Milich, A. McLachlan, G. B. Thornton, J. L. Hughes, Antibody production to the nucleocapsid and envelope of the hepatitis B virus primed by a single synthetic T cell site, *Nature 329*:547 (1987).
56. Vella, P. P., J. M. Staub, J. Armstrong, K. Dolan, C. M. Rusk, S. Szymanski, W. E. Greer, S. Marburg, P. J. Kniskern, T. L. Schofield, R. L. Tolman, F. Hartner, S.-H. Pan, R. J. Gerety and R. W. Ellis, Immunogenicity of a new *Haemophilus influenzae* conjugate Vaccine (PedvaxHIB®). *Pediatrics 85*: 665 (1990).
57. J. J. Donnelly, R. R. Deck, and M. A. Liu, Immunogenicity of a *Haemophilus influenzae* polysaccharide-*Neisseria meningitidis* outer membrane protein complex conjugate vaccine, *J. Immunol. 145*:3071 (1990).
58. D. Gray and P. Matzinger, T cell memory is short-lived in the absence of antigen, *J. Exp. Med. 174*:969 (1991).
59. F. Manca, D. Fenoglio, A. Kinkl, C. Cambiaggi, M. Sasso, and F. Celada, Differential activation of T cell clones stimulated by macrophages exposed to antigen complexed with monoclonal antibodies. A possible influence of paratope specificity on the mode of antigen processing, *J. Immunol. 140*:2893 (1988).
60. M.-P. Schutze, C. Leclerc, F. R. Vogel, and L. Chedid, Epitopic suppression in synthetic vaccine models: Analysis of the effector mechanisms, *Cell. Immunol. 104*:79 (1987).
61. D. DiJohn, S. S. Wasserman, J. R. Torres, M. J. Cortesia, J. Murillo, G. A. Losonsky, D. A. Herrington, D. Sturcher, and M. M. Levine, Effect of priming with carrier on response to conjugate vaccine, *Lancet 2*:1415 (1989).
62. M.-P. Schutze, E. Deriaud, G. Przewlocki, and C. Leclerc, Carrier-induced epitopic suppression is initiated through clonal dominance, *J. Immunol. 142*:2635 (1989).
63. F. R. Vogel, C. Leclerc, M.-P. Schutze, M. Jolivet, F. Audibert, T. W. Klein,

and L. Chedid, Modulation of carrier-induced epitopic suppression by *Bordetella pertussis* components and muramyl peptide, *Cell. Immunol. 107*:40 (1987).

64. J. U. Que, S. J. Cryz, R. Ballou, E. Furer, M. Gross, J. Young, G. F. Wasserman, L. A. Loomis, and J. C. Sadoff, Effect of carrier selection in immunogenicity of protein conjugate vaccines against *Plasmodium falciparum* circumsporozoites, *Infect. Immun. 56*:2645 (1988).
65. A. R. Lussow, C. Barrios, J. van Embden, R. van der Zee, A. S. Verdini, A. Pessi, J. A. Louis, and G. Del Giudice, Mycobacterial heat shock proteins as carrier molecules, *Eur. J. Immunol. 21*:2297 (1991).
66. S. J. Cryz, A. S. Cross, J. C. Sadoff, A. Wegmann, J. U. Que, and E. Furer, Safety and immunogenicity of *Escherichia coli* O18 O-specific polysaccharide (O-PS)-toxin A and O-PS-cholera toxin conjugate vaccines in humans, *J. Infect. Dis. 163*:1040 (1991).
67. V. I. Ahonkai, L. J. Lukacs, L. C. Jonas, and G. B. Calandra, Clinical experience with PedvaxHIB, a conjugate vaccine of *Haemophilus influenzae* type b polysaccharide-*Neisseria meningitidis* outer membrance protein, *Vaccine 9*:S38 (1991).
68. P. P. Vella and R. W. Ellis, Immunogenicity of *Haemophilus influenzae* type b conjugate vaccines in infant rhesus monkeys, *Pediatr. Res. 29*:10 (1991).
69. M. A. Liu, A. Friedman, A. I. Oliff, J. Tai, D. Martinez, R. R. Deck, J. T.-C. Shieh, T. D. Jenkins, J. J. Donnelly, and L. A. Hawe, Major membrane protein of *N. meningitidis*: A novel lymphocyte mitogen and vaccine carrier protein. *Proc. Natl. Acad. Sci. USA 89*:4633 (1992).
70. L. A. Hawe, J. J. Donnelly, R. R. Deck, A. Friedman, and M. A. Liu, Major Immunoenhancing Protein isolated from *N. meningitidis* is mitogenic for T lymphocytes, *Proceedings of Modern Approaches to New Vaccines,* Cold Spring Harbor Laboratories, Cold Spring Harbor, NY, 1992, p. 353.
71. R. R. Deck, J. J. Donnelly, L. A. Hawe, A. Friedman, M. A. Liu, Class-2 outer membrane protein isolated from *N. meningitidis* induces antibody secretion by murine B lymphocytes, *Proceedings of Modern Approaches to New Vaccines,* Cold Spring Harbor Laboratories, Cold Spring Harbor, NY, 1992, p. 359.
72. D. M. Granoff and R. S. Munson, Prospects for prevention of *Haemophilus influenzae* type b disease by immunization, *J. Infect. Dis. 153*:448 (1986).
73. H. Peltola, H. Kayhty, M. Virtanen, and P.H. Makela, Prevention of *Haemophilus influenzae* type b bacteremic infections with the capsular polysaccharide vaccine, *N. Engl. J. Med. 310*:1561 (1984).
74. H. Kayhty, V. Karanko, H. Peltola, and P. H. Makela, Serum antibodies after vaccination with *Haemophilus influenzae* type b capsular polysaccharide and responses to reimmunization: No evidence of immunologic tolerance or memory, *Pediatrics 74*:857 (1984).
75. M. L. Lepow, G. Peter, M. P. Glode, R. S. Daum. G. Calnen, K. M. Knight, D. Mayer, J. S. C. Kuo, and N. S. T. Lui, Response of infants to *Haemophilus influenzae* type b polysaccharide and diphtheria-tetanus-pertussis vaccines in combination, *J. Infect. Dis. 149*:950 (1984).

76. D. M. Ambrosino, M. P. Glode, C. L. Williams, and G. R. Siber, Antibody response of infants to *Haemophilus influenzae* type b capsular polysaccharide combined with *Bordetella pertussis*, *J. Infect. Dis. 151*:1174 (1985).
77. H. Käyhty, J. Eskola, H. Peltola, M. G. Stout, J. S. Samuelson, and L. K. Gordon, Immunogenicity in infants of a vaccine composed of *Haemophilus influenzae* type b capsular polysaccharide mixed with DPT or conjugated to diphtheria toxoid, *J. Infect. Dis. 155*:100 (1987).
78. J. Y. Tai, P. P. Vella, A. A. McLean, A. F. Woodhour, W. J. McAleer, A. Sha, C. Dennis-Sykes, and M. R. Hilleman, *Haemophilus influenzae* type b polysaccharide-protein conjugate vaccine, *Proc. Soc. Exp. Biol. Med. 184*:154 (1987).
79. S. K. Sood and R. S. Daum, *Haemophilus influenzae* type b conjugate vaccines, *Vaccines and Immunotherapy* (S. J. Cryz, ed.), McGraw-Hill, New York, 1991, pp. 36–58.
80. R. W. Force, R. A. Lugo, and M. C. Nahata, *Haemophilus influenzae* type b conjugate vaccines, *Ann. Pharmacol. 26*:1429 (1992).
81. H. Käyhty, J. Eskola, H. Peltola, P.-R. Rönnberg, E. Kela, V. Karanko, and L. Saarinen. Antibody responses to four *Haemophilus influenzae* type b conjugate vaccines, *AJDC 145*:223 (1991).
82. J. Ward, Prevention of invasive *Haemophilus influenzae* type b disease: Lessons from vaccine efficacy trials, *Vaccine 9*:517 (1991).
83. S. J. Holmes, T. V. Murphy, R. S. Anderson, S. L. Kaplan, E. P. Rothstein, V. N. Gan, and D. M. Granoff, Immunogenicity of four *Haemophilus influenzae* type b conjugate vaccines in 17- to 19-month-old children, *J. Pediat 118*:364 (1991).
84. S. L. Kaplan, *Haemophilus influenzae* type b conjugate vaccines, *Pediatr. Ann. 19*:712 (1990).
85. M. D. Decker, K. M. Edwards, R. Bradley, and P. Palmer, Comparative trial in infants of four conjugate *Haemophilus influenzae* type b vaccines, *J. Pediatr. 120*:184 (1992).
86. P. P. Vella and R. W. Ellis, *Haemophilus* b conjugate vaccines, *Vaccines: New Approaches to Immunological Problems*, Butterworth-Heinemann, Boston, 1992, pp. 1–22.
87. P. W. Anderson, M. E. Pichichero, R. A. Insel, R. Betts, R. Eby, and D. H. Smith, Vaccines consisting of periodate-cleaved oligosaccharides from the capsule of *Haemophilus influenzae* type b coupled to a protein carrier: Structural and temporal requirements for priming in the human infant, *J. Immun. 137*:1181 (1986).
88. S. Pillai, S. Ciciriello, M. Koster, and R. Eby, Distinct pattern of antibody reactivity with oligomeric or polymeric forms of the capsular polysaccharide of *Haemophilus influenzae* type b, *Infect. Immun. 59*:4371 (1991).
89. A. A. Lenoir, P. D. Granoff, and D. M. Granoff, Immunogenicity of *Haemophilus influenzae* type b polysaccharide-*Neisseria meningitidis* outer membrane protein conjugate vaccine in 2- to 6-month-old infants, *Pediatrics 80*:283 (1987).

90. D. M. Granoff, E. L. Anderson, M. T. Osterholm, S. J. Holmes, J. E. McHugh, R. B. Belshe, F. Medley, and T. V. Murphy, Differences in the immunogenicity of three *Haemophilus influenzae* type b conjugate vaccines in infants, *J. Pediatr. 121*:187 (1992).
91. D. V. Madore, C. L. Johnson, D. C. Phipps, L. A. Popejoy, R. Eby, and D. H. Smith, Safety and immunologic response to *Haemophilus influenzae* type b oligosaccharide-CRM_{197} conjugate vaccine in 1- to 6-month-old infants, *Pediatrics 85*:331 (1990).
92. R. Schneerson, J. B. Robbins, C. Chu, A. Sutton, W. Vann, J. C Vickers, W. T. London, B. Curfman, M. C. Hardegree, J. Shiloach, et al., Serum antibody responses of juvenile and infant rhesus monkeys injected with *Haemophilus influenzae* type b and pneumococcus type 6A capsular polysaccharide-protein conjugates, *Infect. Immun. 45*:582 (1984).
93. M. Porro, M. Saletti, L. Nencioni, L. Tagliaferri, and I. Marsili, Immunogenic correlation between cross-reacting material (CRM197) produced by a mutant of *Corynebacterium diphtheriae* and diphtheria toxoid, *J. Infect. Dis. 142*:716 (1980).
94. E. Gold, A. Fevrier, M. H. Hatch, K. L. Herrmann, W. L. Jones, R. D. Krugman, and P. D. Parkman, Immune status of children one to four years of age as determined by history and antibody measurement, *N. Engl. J. Med. 289*:231 (1973).
95. G. A. Weinberg, M. S. Einhorn, A. A. Lenoir, P. D. Granoff, and D. M. Granoff, Immunologic priming to capsular polysaccharide in infants immunized with *Haemophilus influenzae* type be polysaccharide-*Neisseria meningitidis* outer membrane protein conjugate vaccine, *J. Pediatr. 111*:22 (1987).
96. B. Fritzell and S. Plotkin, Efficacy and safety of a *Haemophilus influenzae* type b capsular polysaccharide-tetanus protein conjugate vaccine, *J. Pediatr. 121*:355 (1992).
97. G. Peter, J. G. Easton, N. A. Halsey, et al. Committee on Infectious Diseases, 1990 to 1991, *Haemophilus-influenzae* type-b conjugate vaccines: Recommendations for immunization of infants and children 2 months of age and older: Update, *Pediatrics 88*:169 (1991).
98. P. W. Anderson, M. E. Pichichero, K. Edwards. C. R. Porch, and R. Insel, Priming and induction of *Haemophilus influenzae* type b capsular antibodies in early infancy by Dpo20, an oligosaccharide-protein conjugate vaccine, *J. Pediatr. 111*:644 (1987).
99. S. L. Kaplan, J. M. Zahradnik, E. O. Mason, Jr., et al., Immunogenicity of the *Haemophilus influenzae* type b capsular polysaccharide conjugate vaccine in children after systemic *Haemophilus influenzae* type b infections, *J. Pediatr. 113*:272 (1988).
100. K. M. Edwards, M. D. Decker, C. R. Porch, P. Palmer, and R. Bradley, Immunization after invasive *Haemophilus influenzae* type b disease, *AJDC 143*:31 (1989).
101. S. L. Kaplan, T. Duckett, D. H. Mahoney, Jr., L. L. Kennedy, D. M. Dukes,

D. M. Schaffer, and E. O. Mason, Jr., Immunogenicity of *Haemophilus influenzae* type b polysaccharide-tetanus protein conjugate vaccine in children with sickle hemoglobinopathy or malignancies, and after systemic *Haemophilus influenzae* type b infection, *J. Pediatr. 120*:367 (1992).

102. G. A. Weinberg and D. M. Granoff, Immunogenicity of *Haemophilus influenzae* type b polysaccharide-protein conjugate vaccines in children with conditions associated with impaired antibody responses to type b polysaccharide vaccine, *Pediatrics 85* (Suppl.):654 (1990).

103. G. A. Weinberg, T. V. Murphy, and D. M. Granoff, *Haemophilus influenzae* type b polysaccharide-diphtheria toxoid conjugate vaccine in vaccinated children who developed *Haemophilus* disease, *Pediatrics 86*:617 (1990).

104. J. F. Marcinak, A. L. Frank, R. L. Labotka, S. Rao, L. Drawhorn, C. Damplier, L. R. Frisone, R. Yogev, and P. McVerry, Immunogenicity of *Haemophilus influenzae* type b polysaccharide-diphtheria toxoid conjugate vaccine in 3- to 17-month-old infants with sickle cell disease, *J. Pediatr. 118*:69 (1991).

105. L. G. Rubin, D. Boulalas, and L. Carmody, Immunogenicity of *Haemophilus influenzae* type b conjugate vaccine in children with sickle cell disease, *AJDC 146*:340 (1992).

106. A. Barra, C. Bremard-Oury, A. Bajart, C. Griscelli, B. Fritzell, and J.-L. Preud'homme, Immunogenicity of *Haemophilus influenzae* type b capsular polysaccharide and its tetanus toxoid conjugate in patients with recurrent infections or humoral immunodeficiency, *Int. J. Clin. Lab. Res. 21*:231 (1992).

107. M. C. Steinhoff, B. S. Auerbach, K. E. Nelson, et al. Antibody responses to *Haemophilus influenzae* type b vaccines in men with human immunodeficiency virus infection, *N. Engl. J. Med. 325*:1837 (1991).

108. R. Jakacki, N. Luery, P. McVerry, and B. Lange, *Haemophilus influenzae* diphtheria protein conjugate immunization after therapy in splenectomized patients with Hodgkin's disease, *Ann. Int. Med. 112*:143 (1990).

5

Quality Control

Lallan Giri*

Connaught Laboratories, Inc., Swiftwater, Pennsylvania

Jean-Claude Vincent-Falquet

Pasteur-Mérieux Serums & Vaccines, Marcy l'Etoile, France

I. INTRODUCTION

The control of vaccines is crucial to ensuring safety and efficacy. Every manufactured lot of vaccine must pass general safety, sterility, purity, identity, potency, and level of constituent materials added during manufacturing. The current trend also emphasizes thorough characterization of vaccines.

Out of the six strains of *Haemophilus influenzae*, type b (Hib) is responsible for the cases of serious meningitis. The first Hib vaccine was the purified capsular polysaccharide, polyribosylribitol phosphate (PRP). The PRP vaccine fails to elicit T-cell–dependent immune responses in children. Therefore, to enhance immunogenicity and provide for a booster response, the PRP was covalently linked to a protein carrier (1–4). Thus the conjugate vaccine for this organism is an improved version of the earlier PRP vaccine. As a result of molecular conjugation of a protein carrier to a polysaccharide hapten, the manufacturing, purification, characterization, and quality control testing of the vaccine have become more complex. Both the configuration and size of the polysaccharide and the carrier proteins vary from one manufacturer to the other. However, they all have one common feature, i.e., Hib conjugate vaccines are capable of stimulating

**Present affiliation:* B. W. Manufacturing, Inc., West Greenwich, Rhode Island

the production of specific antibodies in infants or young children at a desired level necessary for protection against disease.

The first Hib conjugate vaccine was licensed in the United States in 1987 by Connaught Laboratories, Inc. Since then, several other companies (Merck, Lederle-Praxis Biologics, and Pasteur-Mérieux) have joined the market. Although the chemical nature of the PRP antigen is identical in vaccines from all four manufacturers, the size of the polymer, chemistry of conjugation, and protein carriers differ (see Chapter 3). Also, there is considerable variability in the procedures used in manufacturing, characterization, and quality control of the conjugate vaccines.

II. REQUIREMENTS AND IN-PROCESS QUALITY CONTROLS OF *HAEMOPHILUS INFLUENZAE* TYPE b CONJUGATE VACCINE

To ensure the quality and safety of Hib conjugate vaccines, guidelines have been set up by the governmental regulatory agency in several countries and at the international level by the World Health Organization (WHO). The WHO guidelines were assembled in concert with experts from the vaccine-producing countries, including U.S. Food and Drug Administration (FDA), and published in 1991 (5). Although each manufacturer is likely to have developed a unique and proprietary procedure to prepare the conjugate, the salient features of the guidelines are as follows.

A detailed operating procedure for the preparation and testing of Hib conjugate vaccines and the facility must be approved by the Center for Biologics Evaluation and Research (CBER), a division of FDA. Any modifications of the manufacturing and/or control methods must also be approved by CBER through an amendment process. Personnel employed in production and quality control of the vaccine should be adequately trained and protected against accidental infection with *H. influenzae* type b.

The Hib strain shall be identified by its source, genotype, and phenotype and by tests to ascertain its characteristics. The strain must have been shown to produce specifically type b polysaccharide. A Master Seed lot of uniform composition is established from a strain processed as a single lot and maintained in the freeze-dried form or frozen at or below −45 to −50°C. A Working Seed lot is prepared through several passages from the Master Seed (5).

The Working Seed lot is inoculated in a liquid medium that does not contain any blood-group substances or other polysaccharides of high relative molecular mass. Consistency of growth of Hib is demonstrated by its growth rate, pH, and yield of PRP. Samples of the culture are taken before killing and tested for any contamination by Gram stain smears and inoculation on appropriate media plates.

The carrier proteins such as diphtheria toxoid, tetanus toxoid, and outer membrane protein complex (OMPC) are derived from *Corynebacterium diphtheriae*, *Clostridium tetani*, and *Neisseria meningitidis* B, respectively. These organisms are maintained and grown following the approved procedures identical to those used for their own vaccine production. The carrier proteins must be characterized and shown to be safe and nontoxic. Prior to conjugation, the diphtheria and tetanus toxins are purified, detoxified, and sterilized by filtration. The protein concentration is estimated by protein nitrogen assay and purity determined by electrophoresis and A^{280}/A^{260} ratio. Appropriate assays are carried out to determine residual phosphorus and formaldehyde. Any toxoid reversal, pyrogenicity, as well as antigenic purity (>1500 Lf/mg protein nitrogen) and sterility of the toxoid must also be determined before conjugation. OMPC is purified and characterized by protein assay, chromatography, and assays to determine residual sialic acid, nucleic acid, and other pyrogenic materials, before conjugation.

Current manufacturing practices (6) are followed using chemicals of an appropriate purity. Each lot of PRP is tested for purity, and all chemical analyses are based on the dry weight of the PRP in its salt form. Any batch of partially purified PRP powder and solution should be stored frozen at or below −20°C. The methods for the analyses of purified PRP, i.e., moisture content, ribose content, phosphorus content, protein content, nucleic acid content, endotoxin content, molecular size, and identity test, are validated and approved by FDA for their suitability, accuracy, and reproducibility.

For in-process control, the moisture content of the dry PRP powder is determined in order to adjust all other assay results to the dry weight of PRP. Ribose content is measured as the active component and should be no less than 32% as estimated by orcinol reaction according to Bial's test procedure (7). Each lot of purified PRP should contain ≤1% nucleic acid and protein contaminants as determined spectrophotometrically and by Lowry's method, respectively. Phosphorus content, which represents the phosphodiester linkage between each repeat unit of the polysaccharide, should be 6.0–9.0% determined as described (8). The endotoxin level should be <10 IU/mg by LAL assay. Also, the purified PRP must pass a pyrogen test in rabbits at 1.0 μg PRP per kg of rabbit weight. The molecular size distribution constant (Kd) is determined by measuring the molecular distribution on Sepharose CL-4B or CL-2B size exclusion chromatography gel and may range from 0.2 to 0.6 depending upon the manufacturing process and the chromatography gel used. The purified PRP is verified for its identity by a serological method or ^{13}C-nuclear magnetic resonance (NMR) spectroscopy (9).

The purified PRP is subjected to chemical modification for conjugation to protein carrier following appropriate validated chemical procedures developed by the manufacturer and approved by the FDA. The chemical conjugation procedure may vary from one product or manufacturer to another. The degree of conjugation must be determined. The conjugate is purified by a proven procedure that has been validated to remove the chemical reagents used for conjugation and capping including the unreacted chemically modified PRP. After the conjugate has been purified, quality control tests must be carried out according to the criteria discussed later in Section IV. Although there may be no limit established, the protein-to-ribose ratio is determined.

III. CHARACTERISTICS OF Hib VACCINES

Before the discussion on conjugate vaccines, it would be useful to review the PRP vaccine that was licensed before conjugate vaccines were developed, since the criteria established for PRP set the analytical basis for the PRP used in the preparation of the conjugates.

A. PRP Vaccine

The first Hib nonconjugate vaccine was a purified PRP and manufactured and licensed by at least three manufacturers, namely, Connaught Laboratories, Inc. (HibVAX®); Lederle Laboratories (Hib-Immune®); and Praxis Biologics (b-Capsa®). Their main release criteria (10) included (a) purity of PRP (>32% ribose), (b) molecular size distribution (Kd = 0.30 on a Sepharose CL-4B column; see Sec. IV.B.6., (c) contamination of nucleic acid and protein (<1% each), (d) low level of endotoxin, and (e) PRP content of 25.0 μg per 0.5-ml dose. The vaccines were stabilized in lactose or sucrose solutions.

B. Conjugate Vaccines

Some of the general properties of the Hib conjugate vaccines produced by various manufacturers are provided in Table 1. The conjugate vaccines exploit the principles of "carrier-hapten" antigen presentation that was successfully demonstrated in bacterial vaccine development (11). In the Hib conjugated vaccine, there are two major components—a polysaccharide, which serves as "hapten," and a carrier-protein molecule. The presence of the conjugated carrier-protein represents a major and basic structural difference from the PRP vaccines. The current criteria require a thorough characterization of the carrier-protein and the polysaccharide at intermediate and final product stages.

Before conjugation, the PRP is isolated from the culture broth of *H. influenzae* type b. It is further purified by precipitation, centrifugation, and phenol extraction. The size distribution of polysaccharide in the vaccines ranges from oligosaccharide (HbOC) to large polymers (PRP-D, PRP-T, and PRP-OMPC).

Table 1 Quality Control Tests for Hib Vaccines at Bulk and Final Product Stages

General Tests[a]	
	General safety
	Sterility
	Identity
	Pyrogenicity
	Limulus amebocyte lysate (LAL) assay for endotoxin
	Osmolality
	Moisture analysis
	Preservative
	Adjuvant (aluminum)
Product-Specific Tests[a]	
	Purity determination
	PRP content
	Free PRP (Ribose)
	Phosphorous analysis
	Protein analysis
	Molecular size distribution
	In vitro antigenicity by ELISA
	Immunogenicity assays
	Mouse immunogenicity
	Monkey immunogenicity

[a]Not all tests are performed on each available vaccine.

There is a considerable degree of variability in the preparation of PRP and conjugate. Some manufacturers prepare their PRP by heat-sizing (PRP-D) whereas others create a comparatively smaller polymer (oligosaccharide) by periodate oxidation (HbOC) (see Chapter 3). The carrier proteins in the conjugate vaccines are diphtheria toxoid (PRP-D), a genetically created mutant diphtheria toxoid CRM_{197} (HbOC), tetanus toxoid (PRP-T) or meningococcal Group B outer membrane protein complex (PRP-OMPC).

The general approach for creating Hib conjugate from PRP and protein has been reviewed in detail in Chapter 3. In PRP-D or PRP-T it involves activation of electrophilic groups on the PRP polymers by cyanogen bromide. For PRP-D conjugate, diphtheria toxoid (D) is derivatized with adipic acid dihydrazide in a separate reaction using carbodiimide chemistry. Thus a nucleophilic diphtheria toxoid derivative is created, which is then conjugated to the electrophilic groups on the activated PRP, thereby creating the PRP-D conjugate (13). For the PRP-T conjugate, a six-carbon spacer molecule is attached to the activated polymer by reaction with adipic acid dihydrazide. Thus the derivatized PRP (called AH-polysaccharide) then is conjugated to 1-ethyl-3-dimethylamino-propyl carbodiimide (EDAC)-activated tetanus toxoid, and the ensuing conjugate is purified. In the HbOC conjugate, a direct covalent coupling between PRP and the mutant diphtheria toxoid CRM_{197} is used without any spacer. The oligosaccharides of approximately 20 repeating units are generated by limited periodate cleavage to create free aldehyde termini. These termini allow efficient coupling to the CRM_{197} protein by reductive amination. In the PRP-OMPC conjugate, a different chemistry and two spacer molecules are used (see Chapter 3). The process involves a multistep procedure to derivatize both PRP and OMPC, each of which is reacted separately with different spacer molecules. The two components (derivatized PRP and protein) with spacers then are covalently linked. This conjugate contains a bigeneric spacer between PRP and the OMPC (4,14). The bigeneric spacer contains S-(carboxylmethyl)-homocysteine, a novel amino acid which can be easily detected and quantitated to determine the degree of linkage (see Chapter 3).

The conjugate vaccines are purified by a combination of physicochemical procedures that involve chemical precipitation and extraction, enzymatic digestion of host nucleic acids and proteins, chemical modifications, ultracentrifugation, and chromatography. The determination of residual contamination by chemicals and reagents added during the processing to ensure the safety of the purified conjugate becomes an important part of vaccine production. Therefore, the quality control tests are carried out at intermediate, bulk, and final product stages. The analyses involve various biological, immunological, analytical, and physicochemical approaches.

IV. VACCINE RELEASE CRITERIA USED BY THE MANUFACTURERS

General and specific guidelines for vaccines are discussed in the WHO guidelines and Code of Federal Regulations (CFR) (5,15). The general requirements for the vaccines are based on those established for other bacterial vaccines. Specifications for the vaccine are developed by manufacturers during the research and clinical studies. These specifications are based on specific immunological, antigenic, and physicochemical properties of the PRP in the Hib vaccine. A reference vaccine that meets all the established specifications is used to monitor the consistency of each manufactured lot of vaccine. For Hib conjugate, a human reference antiserum is available from WHO and is used to determine antigenicity of vaccine.

After the completion of the tests, a release protocol containing all test results is submitted along with vaccine samples to CBER for final release of the vaccine. No vaccine is distributed commercially until a written release has been received by the manufacturer from CBER. Individual laboratories are expected to develop their own test procedures and to validate them for routine application followed by approval by CBER. Similar procedures are required by regulatory authorities in other countries. It is important that test methods are validated for their accuracy, precision, limit of detection, selectivity, range, linearity, and ruggedness (16). Some of the major release criteria are listed in Table 1.

A. General Criteria

The following general tests are required by CFR or European Pharmacopeia (EP) or WHO guidelines. Readers should consult the current CFR Part 21 or EP or WHO technical monograms for detailed guidelines for compliance with the criteria.

1. General Safety

A general safety test on the Hib conjugate vaccine is carried out to detect any toxic contaminants that may be in the vaccine. The test is carried out in mice and guinea pigs. Animals are observed for 7 days for any abnormal clinical manifestation after 1 and 10 human equivalent doses of the vaccine have been injected intraperitoneally in mice and guinea pigs, respectively (15). According to EP and WHO guidelines, 1 human dose in mice and 5 human doses in guinea pigs are administered (5).

2. Sterility

All vaccines are tested for fungal or bacterial contaminants at the bulk and final product stages. The sterility tests are carried out according to the United States Pharmacopeial procedure (16) using membrane filtration and thioglycolate medium. After inoculation, the containers are incubated at 30–35°C for at least 14 days. The medium is tested for its growth-promoting properties using test organisms per CFR (15) before its application in the sterility test.

3. Identity

The CFR regulation requires that the content of final-container vaccine be tested for its antigenic identity after the filled vials have been labeled. The purpose of this test is to distinguish the filled vaccine from any other product being processed in the same laboratory, manufacturing facility, and filling and packaging line. Although the actual procedures vary, the basic principle is based on an antigen-antibody reaction. One of the following procedures is used for the identity test.

a. Rocket Immunoelectrophoresis

Some manufacturers (PRP-D) perform rocket immunoelectrophoresis using specific antibodies against the conjugate vaccine. One of the reactants, usually anti-PRP serum, is incorporated into an agarose gel, and wells cut out in the gel are filled with the second reactant, the vaccine antigen. An electric current is applied so that the antigen migrates into the gel. As a result of the antigen-antibody reaction, rocket-shaped precipitin lines are formed, which become visible after staining with Coomassie blue. The area of the rocket-shaped zone of precipitation is linearly proportional to the concentration of antigen (Fig. 1).

b. Ouchterlony Double-Diffusion

In this method the antigen (PRP-T) and antiserum are initially separated by a gel. Wells are cut out in the gel and filled with antigen and antiserum. The two reactants diffuse toward each other, and, when equivalence is reached, a precipitin line is formed between the two wells.

c. Rate Nephelometry

This procedure is based on the measurement of light scattered by the antigen-antibody immune complexes (16,17). The rate at which light-scattering complexes are formed is proportional to the amount of antigen present, when carried out in the presence of excess antibody. This procedure is used to ensure identity and to measure antigen in the PRP-OMPC conjugate vaccine.

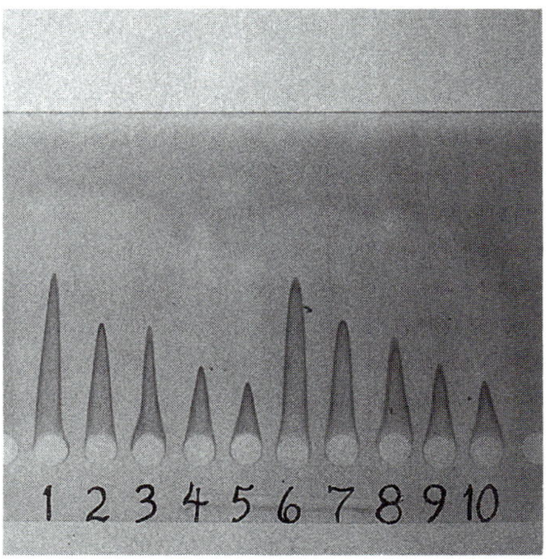

Figure 1 Identity test by rocket immunoelectrophoresis of PRP-D antigen in agarose gel containing anti–PRP-D serum. The antigen was applied in the wells (circles) and electrophoresed at 60 volts for 16 hours. The gel was stained with Coomassie blue. The height of the rocket is proportional to the concentration of the antigen.

Some manufacturers (PRP-T) carry out an identity test also to confirm the specificity of the carrier protein. The procedures for the identity test of the carrier proteins are identical to those used for the PRP antigen. In fact, it is possible to carry out tests for both antigens, PRP and carrier protein, in a single experiment.

4. Pyrogenicity

Pyrogens are fever-causing substances which are high molecular weight endotoxin complexes associated with the outer membrane of gram-negative bacteria. The USP (16) and WHO (5) recommend a rabbit pyrogen test for the final-container Hib vaccine. The rabbit pyrogen test involves measuring the rise in temperature of rabbits following an intravenous injection of 0.025–1.0 μg dose per kilogram of rabbit body weight. Three rabbits are used for the initial test. No individual rabbit should show a rise in temperature of ≥0.6°C over the preinjection temperature. The sum of the three rabbits' individual maximum temperature rises must not exceed 1.4°C according to USP (16) or 1.15 per WHO guidelines (5). If these criteria are not met, the test must be repeated using five additional rabbits (16) or three additional rabbits (5). In the USP assay the temperature rises for all eight rabbits are used in evaluating the final results. The vaccine passes the test for absence of pyrogen if not more than three of the eight rabbits show individual rises in temperature of ≥0.6°C and if the sum of the eight rabbits' maximum temperature rises is ≤3.7°C.

5. Limulus Amebocyte Lysate (LAL) Assay for Endotoxin

LAL is used to determine endotoxin level in vaccine by measuring the protein clotting of the lysate-vaccine mixture. The clotting is an enzyme-catalyzed process which is activated by endotoxin. Thus the clotting is dependent on the concentration of endotoxin (18). Some Hib conjugate vaccine products (PRP-D) are tested for endotoxin level by the LAL assay method in addition to rabbit pyrogen test. The LAL tests are carried out at the purified PRP concentrate and postconjugation stages using the LAL assay described by the USP monograph (16).

6. Osmolality

The osmolality of a vaccine is directly related to the isotonicity of bodily fluid. It is important that the isotonicity of the local fluid is not perturbed after injection to a critical level so as to cause pain and discomfort. Osmolality of some of the final-container vaccine or vaccine diluent for lyophilized vaccines is measured by osmometry according to the procedure described (16,19). The osmometer measures freezing-point depression, which is then converted to osmolality values.

7. Residual Moisture

In lyophilized vaccines such as PRP-T and PRP-OMPC, the residual moisture is determined by thermogravimetric or coulometric method. Thermogravimetry enables continuous recording of the weight of a sample placed in a boat, which is gradually heated. Volatiles given off by the test sample are entrapped by dehydrated helium or nitrogen. When the sample has been totally dried, the weight remains constant. The reduction in weight due to moisture loss is expressed as a percentage of the original sample weight and represents the residual moisture from the sample. The moisture can also be determined by other methods: Karl-Fischer titrimetric or coulometric method (16). The Karl-Fischer titrimetric apparatus consists of a titration cell with compartments. The water is titrated with Karl-Fischer reagent produced by electrolytic generation of iodine in the electrolyte. There is a direct relationship between the electric charge, the quantity of iodine produced and the amount of water, thus allowing a quantitative analysis of moisture. The freeze-dried Hib vaccine is added to the anodic compartment. At the end of the titration, a value of water in micrograms is displayed on the system, which is then converted into percent (%) moisture. The moisture limit in the final lyophilized PRP-T and PRP-OMPC vaccines is $<3\%$.

8. Preservative (Thimerosal) Assay

Thimerosal is a mercury-containing preservative used in liquid Hib conjugate vaccine by some manufacturers. Generally, it is added at the final bulk stage at a final concentration of 0.008–0.012% (80–120 μg/ml). It is assayed in the vaccine by either polarography or colorimetry. The polarographic method involves measurement of *diffusion current* (id) which is proportional to the concentration of electroactive species such as thimerosal. To carry out a quantitative measurement of thimerosal in vaccine, the diffusion current of the vaccine sample and a reference standard (thimerosal standard solution) is measured and the concentration of the sample is calculated from the ratio of the sample to the reference diffusion current. The colorimetric method involves acid hydrolysis and extraction of mercury with either chloroform or carbon tetrachloride in the presence of dithizone, which gives a typical orange color (20). The concentration of thimerosal is determined by interpolation from a standard curve of thimerosal (μg/ml) and A^{480}.

9. Aluminum

The lyophilized PRP-OMPC vaccine is reconstituted with saline containing aluminum hydroxide adjuvant to a concentration of 450 μg aluminum/ml. The concentration of aluminum in a vaccine or diluent can be determined either by spectrophotometric method or by atomic emission spectrometry (16).

B. Product-Specific Criteria

As mentioned earlier, by the time of Phase III clinical studies, the specification of the vaccine is finalized. Typically, three consistency lots of vaccines are produced and tested to ensure that they meet the established specifications. From this point, these specifications become release criteria for every lot of vaccine. The product-specific criteria are related to the immunological or physicochemical properties of Hib conjugates vaccines (21). There is no direct method as yet for measuring the immunological potency of these vaccines that relates directly to protective immunity. Therefore, one has to rely on the tests for purity, content of undegraded ribose, molecular size and composition, and immunogenicity studies in mice and monkeys. These properties confirm the consistency of production and conformity with the specifications of the vaccine used in pivotal clinical trials. Some salient features of Hib conjugate vaccines are discussed in Table 2.

Table 2 Salient Features of *Haemophilus influenzae* Type b Conjugate Vaccines

Properties	PRP-D (ProHIBit®)	HbOC (HibTITER®)	PRP-OMPC (PedvaxHIB®)	PRP-T (Act HIB™)
Polysaccharide characteristics	Heat sized	Oligo-saccharide	High molecular weight polysac-charide	High molecular weight polysac-charide
Molecular size (Kd)[a]	<0.75	0.3–0.6	<0.25	<0.20
Free PRP	<37%	<10%	<15%	<20%
PRP per human dose (μg)	25	10	15	10
Carrier protein	Diphtheria toxoid	Diphtheria CRM 197	Outer membrane protein complex (OMPC) of *Neisseria meningitidis* Group B	Tetanus toxoid
Protein quantity per human dose (μg)	18	25	250	20
Form of vaccine	Liquid	Liquid	Lyophilized[b]	Lyophilized
Preservatives	Thimerosal	Thimerosal	Thimerosal	—

[a]Determined on CL-4B Sepharose.
[b]A liquid version of PedvaxHIB will be available soon.

1. Purity

Several conjugation methods are currently in use. There is always a possibility that some unreacted functional groups or residual reagents capable of reacting in vivo may be present following the conjugation process. Some of the impurities may be pyrogenic. Therefore, it is critical to assay for such residual impurities, which may include residual phenol, unreacted ADH and residual cyanide, residual EDAC, and endotoxins after the activation and derivatization of PRP. Each manufacturer develops assay procedures for these residual contaminants and sets limits based on the reproducibility and sensitivity of the assay procedures. Some of these assays are carried out at the intermediate steps of the manufacturing process (see Chapter 3), whereas others are done at the bulk or final product stages.

2. PRP Content

The amount of PRP is determined through ribose content at the purified liquid PRP concentrate, purified conjugate pool, bulk, and final product stages. The PRP is quantitated by determination of total ribose using a colorimetric procedure. This procedure is based on dehydration of pentose sugars by hydrochloric acid, followed by the condensation of furfural by orcinol reagent, according to Bial's test procedure (7). A blue-green color is developed in the reaction mixture. The optical density is measured at A^{665} in a spectrophotometer at a 665-nm wavelength. The average amount of the polysaccharide per dose of the Hib conjugate vaccine from each manufacturer is given in Table 2. The PRP in the PRP-OMPC conjugate vaccine is determined by rate nephelometry (16,17) at the bulk conjugate and final container stages. A standard curve is prepared using PRP standards of known concentrations. The concentration of the unknown vaccine sample is estimated from the standard curve, interpolated from the plot of scattered light intensity vs the microgram-standard PRP. The PRP content in the PRP-T conjugate is determined by estimating the stiochiometric amount of phosphorus (see Sec. IV.B.4.) and calculating the amount of PRP from the phosphorus values.

3. Free PRP (Ribose)

The free or unbound PRP is determined for the (PRP-D) vaccine by measuring the ribose by a combination of hydrophobic interaction chromatography and colorimetric assays (7,22). Free ribose determination is used to evaluate the stability of the PRP during the manufacturing process. For the hydrophobic interaction chromatography method, the surface hydrophobicity of the carrier-protein conjugated to PRP is exploited. When a sample of Hib conjugate vaccine is applied to the column, the intact conjugate binds on to the column through its carrier protein moiety, whereas the unbound or unconjugated PRP elutes through the column. The unbound PRP is collected and its ribose content is determined colorimetrically (7). A ratio of free ribose to total ribose value is converted to percent free ribose. Other methods also can be used for measuring free PRP.

4. Phosphorus Content

The quantitative analysis of PRP also can be carried out by measuring its phosphate backbone. Phosphorus content is measured in PRP-T using a published procedure (8), which involves acid hydrolysis at high temperature (150–250°C) and reaction with ammonium molybdenum and ascorbic acid. The reaction produces a phosphate-molybdate complex, which, when reduced, gives a blue color that is measured as A^{825}. The phosphorus content in the sample is interpolated from a standard curve. Phosphorus content also is determined in the high molecular weight fraction of the conjugate vaccine by a two-step precipitation with ethanol followed by phosphorus analysis as discussed above (8).

5. Protein Analysis

Protein assays are carried out either to detect any contaminants in the purified PRP or to calculate protein/ribose ratio in the conjugate vaccine. The most commonly used procedures for protein determination are the Lowry (23) or Bradford (24) assays.

6. Molecular Size Distribution

Chromatographic separation of a mixture of macromolecules on a gel-filtration column provides valuable information about molecular size. Most of the manufacturers use this technique to monitor the size distribution of the conjugate during the manufacturing process. The degradation of conjugate in stability studies is monitored by measuring the Kd of the product on a column of Sepharose CL-2B or Sepharose CL-4B gel. When a sample of Hib conjugate vaccine is applied, each molecular species will elute in a different volume, which will vary according to the size of the molecule. Thus, the elution of a particular size of the conjugate will depend on its distribution coefficient, Kd, which is expressed as follows (25):

$$Kd = \frac{(Ve - Vo)}{(Vt - Vo)}$$

where

Vo = void volume
Ve = elution volume of the sample
Vt = total volume of the column

Larger molecules are expected to have a smaller Kd value and would tend to elute earlier than smaller molecules. In the manufacturing process of conjugate vaccines, Kd values are evaluated for both PRP and protein components and range from 0.2 to 0.6 for PRP and 0.5 to 0.7. for protein carriers D, T, and OMPC. As a measure of conjugate stability, some manufacturers (PRP-D) have established a limit where greater than 60% of the conjugate would have a Kd of <0.30, whereas others (HbOC) have a limit where 50% of the conjugate will have a Kd of 0.30–0.60. A direct relationship between the integrity (Kd) of conjugate and immunogenicity in mice has been established for three of the vaccines (PRP-D, PRP-T, and HbOC).

7. In Vitro Antigenicity Determination by Enzyme Linked Immunosorbent Assay (ELISA)

This is one of the most powerful techniques to quantitate either antigen or to demonstrate specificity. The enzymes are usually coupled to antibody specific to PRP or to anti-immunoglobulin. It is essential that both the enzymatic activity and the immunological reactivity of the reagents be preserved (26).

Manufacturers have developed a solid-phase sandwich procedure for the quantitation of PRP in Hib conjugate vaccines. However, this is not yet used as a routine assay but in the near future it will find its application in the quality control testing of Hib conjugate and Hib combination vaccines. First, the PRP is captured on polystyrene beads coated with anti-PRP serum, then a polyclonal rabbit antibody to PRP is bound to the captured PRP, and finally a goat-derived anti-rabbit IgG conjugated to horseradish peroxidase is bound to the rabbit antibody. The amount of peroxidase-enzyme conjugate is determined from the turnover of the peroxidase substrate, which is monitored spectrophotometrically by measuring the A^{492} of the colored reaction mixture. The concentration of reaction product is directly proportional to the bound peroxidase and the captured PRP antigen. A standard curve is prepared in the range of 1–100 ng/ml of the reference Hib conjugate. Both positive and negative controls should be used. A minimum diluted sample volume of 200 μl is required.

8. Mouse Immunogenicity Assay

In the absence of a direct method for potency measurement, mouse immunogenicity is the method of choice to determine the immunogenicity of final filled container of Hib conjugate vaccine. A group of 8–10 adult mice are injected intraperitoneally or subcutaneously with a single dilution of vaccine. For each vaccine there must be a careful selection of the mouse strain and determination of the optimal age for vaccination to ensure consistency of results. The mice are bled 3 weeks after the injection, and the individual sera are tested for antibody response by radioimmunoassay (RIA) (see Chapter 14). The purpose of the assay is to demonstrate that the Hib conjugate vaccine in its final form is a T-cell–dependent immunogen and elicits the production of antibody similar to that present in human serum when injected in humans. For the RIA, each mouse immune serum is then combined with ^{125}I-labeled PRP. The antigen-antibody complex then is precipitated by saturated ammonium sulfate, pelleted by centrifugation and counted directly in a gamma counter (27). There must be at least six mice represented in each control group and each test group for calculations to be valid. At least four responders should show positive results; otherwise the test will be invalid. There should be no statistical difference in immunogenicity between the vaccine lot tested and a reference vaccine that has proven to be immunogenic in human infants. An alternate method for mouse immunogenicity is to determine relative potency. This is determined from the ratio of ED_{50} (effective dose for seroconverting 50% of the mice in the group) of Hib conjugate vaccine with that of a reference vaccine. The ED_{50} values are determined by ELISA.

9. Immunogenicity Study in Monkeys

Infant monkeys have been found to be a model for the immunogenicity of PRP-OMPC in human infants (28). Two- to three-month-old Rhesus monkeys are injected intramuscularly at 0 and 28 days with a total of 0.5 ml dose per injection. They are bled on days 0, 28, and 42. The antibodies (anti-PRP) are measured by a standardized RIA. The responder monkeys are defined as those with ≥ 1.0 μg anti-PRP/ml. The PRP-OMPC is highly immunogenic as compared to a noncovalent conjugate; another Hib conjugate (HbOC) was not immunogenic even after three injections. Thus, for control testing of immunogenicity, the monkey model correlates much more closely with infant humans than mice. However, the limited supply of infant monkeys precludes this test from being used as a routine quality control assay.

V. STABILITY OF *HAEMOPHILUS* TYPE b CONJUGATE VACCINE

The stability of a pharmaceutical product is directly related to its degradation behavior. The degradation of conventional drugs follows zero- or first-order kinetics and is chemical in nature. Thus it is not too difficult to predict stability of the drug product. In contradiction, the stability-limiting factors in many vaccines are most probably domain-related. The instability may be due to chemical degradation or physical (conformational) changes.

Therefore, often it is difficult to imply zero- or first-order kinetics to predict stability of vaccines from short-term data, and therefore shelf life is determined empirically from real-time data.

Stability of vaccines in their final form and container is always a subject of concern. In most vaccines, stability is measured by potency. The potency of a vaccine may be very much dependent on macromolecular complexity, and, unlike pharmaceuticals, it is impossible to fully characterize the structure of polymeric conjugates. Gradual hydrolysis of PRP in the Hib conjugate vaccine can occur, although the rate of hydrolysis may vary with the type of conjugation chemistry. Stability is monitored by subjecting the Hib conjugate vaccine to incubation at various temperatures, including the recommended temperature (5–8°C) of storage in the field. Three major properties—percentage of free ribose, high molecular weight distribution of PRP by gel filtration, and mouse immunogenicity—are measured.

In order to have a highly stable conjugate vaccine, it is crucial to have a conjugate vaccine completely free of residual reagents used during the activation and derivatization process of manufacturing. The measurement of increase in free ribose or Kd in the vaccine may follow zero- or first-order kinetics. A prediction of shelf life by monitoring the stability of the vaccine at elevated temperatures and kinetics of degradation is not generally possible, since the mode of degradation at elevated temperature may be different from that at the actual storage temperature. Therefore, only real-time measurement at the recommended temperature of storage establishes the certified dating period for the product. A shelf life of 18 months to 2 years has been established by real-time data at 5–8°C for Hib conjugate vaccines. This means that after storage at 5–8°C for 2 years, conjugate vaccines have an acceptable relative potency similar to that obtained at the time of final product manufacturing and release.

VI. FUTURE CHALLENGES

The emergence of conjugate Hib vaccines was one of the most significant milestones in the field of vaccinology in terms of its new technology as well as its providing greater protection against the Hib meningitis in infants, and manufacturers have brought excellent licensed vaccines to the market place. Nevertheless, there is still some variability in their elicited immune responses in infants after primary or booster injections.

Although most of the Hib conjugate vaccines share some properties, not all versions are identical. Because of the aforesaid variability in their immunological responses in humans, they have been labeled as extremely T-cell–dependent, moderately T-cell–dependent, or partially T-cell–independent (29). Although some of the variability can be attributed to genetic difference in the target population, the difference in potency measurements among the laboratories also can play a role. Major differences in the quantitation of antibody among laboratories have been reported (30). Thus the challenge lies ahead to understand the cause of immunological variability and to establish a standardized measurement of some properties of the vaccines that correlates with the variability in the quality control laboratories. One should also consider the feasibility of in vitro assays without the use of animals as a possible correlate.

Recently, greater emphasis is being placed by FDA (CBER) on product characterization. In the future, an understanding of molecular heterogenicity and dynamics of conformational changes in a microenvironment before activation and derivatization processes will provide better control of the processes and final product and its efficacy when tested in an appropriate in vivo or in vitro model. A considerable amount of interest is developing among manufacturers and FDA in developing combination vaccines containing Hib conjugates. This poses another challenge to ensure that immunogenicity of each component vaccine is not compromised as a result of mixing and any interaction. This also puts a burden on the quality control laboratories to develop and validate methods so that each component antigen of the combination vaccine is quantitated accurately to assess the quality of the product. Thus, there is greater need for a standardized measurement of antigen, antibody, and immunogenicity to accurately compare the results among laboratories on global basis and to validate methods so that each component antigen of the vaccine is quantitated accurately to assess the quality of the product.

REFERENCES

1. R. Schneerson, O. Barrera, A. Sutton, and J. B. Robbins, Preparation, characterization, and immunogenicity of *Haemophilus influenzae* type b polysaccharide-protein conjugates, *J. Exp. Med. 152*:361 (1980).
2. P. Anderson, Antibody responses to *Haemophilus influenzae* type b and diphtheria toxin induced by conjugates of oligosaccharide of the type b capsule with the nontoxic protein CRM 197, *Infect. Immun. 39*:233 (1983).
3. P. Anderson, M. E. Pichichero, R. A. Insel, et al., Vaccines consisting of periodate cleaved oligosaccharides from the capsule of *Haemophilus influenzae* type b coupled to a protein carrier: structural and temporal requirement for priming in the human infant, *J. Immunol. 137*:1181 (1986).
4. S. Marburg et al., Bimolecular chemistry of macromolecules—synthesis of bacterial polysaccharide conjugates with *Neisseria meningitidis* membrane protein, *J. Am. Chem. Soc. 108*:5282 (1986).
5. WHO, Requirements for Haemophilus type b conjugate vaccines, *WHO Technical Report Series, No. 814,* Geneva (1991).

6. *Code of Federal Regulation* (*CFR*) *21* (211):95 (1990).
7. G. Rendina, Chemical properties of carbohydrate, *Experimental Methods in Modern Biochemistry*, W. B. Saunders Co., Philadelphia, 1971, p. 138.
8. P. S. Chen, Microdetermination of phosphorus, *Anal. Chem. 28*:1756 (1956).
9. R. M. Crisel, et al., Capsular polysaccharide of *Haemophilus influenzae* type b, *J. Biol. Chem. 250*:4926 (1975).
10. J. Ward, and S. Cochi, *Haemophilus influenzae* vaccine, *Vaccines* (S. A. Plotkin and E. A. Mortimer, eds.), W. B. Saunders Publishing Co., Philadelphia, 1988, p. 309.
11. W. F. Goebel and O. T. Avery, Chemoimmunological studies on conjugated carbohydrate proteins. II. Immunological specificity of I. The synthesis of p-aminophenol B-glucoside, p-aminophenol B-galactoside, and their coupling with serum globulin. *J. Exp. Med. 50*:521 (1929).
12. J. Ward and S. Cochi, *Haemophilus influenzae* vaccine, *Vaccines* (S. A. Plotkin and E. A. Mortimer, eds.), W. B. Saunders Publishing Co., Philadelphia, 1988, p. 310.
13. L. K. Gordon, Characterization of a hapten-carrier conjugate vaccine: *H. influenzae*- diphtheria conjugate vaccine, *Modern Approaches to Vaccines* (R. M. Chanock and R. A. Lerner, eds.), Cold Spring Harbor Laboratory, Cold Spring Harbor, NY, 1984.
14. J. Y. Tai, P. Vella, A. A. McLean, et al., *H. influenzae* type b polysaccharide-protein conjugate vaccine (42460), *Proc. Soc. Exp. Biol. Med. 184*:154 (1987).
15. *Code of Federal Regulation* (*CFR*) *21* (600–630):5 (1990).
16. *United States Pharmacopeia,* Rockville, MD, XXII (1991).
17. G. Zografi, H. Scott, and J. Swarbrick, Disperse System, *Remington's Pharmaceutical Sciences* (A. Genaro, ed.), Mac Publishing Co., Easton, PA, 1990, p. 281.
18. F. C. Pearson, LAL assay, *Pyrogens*, Marcel Decker, 1985, pp. 119–147.
19. F. P. Siegel, Tonicity, Osmolality, and Osmolarity, *Remington's Pharmaceutical Sciences* (A. Genaro ed.), Mac Publishing Co., Easton, PA, 1990, p. 1482.
20. W. J. Blaedel and V. W. Meloche, Complexation titrations, Elementary quantitation analysis—theory and principles, Harper and Row Publishers, NY, 1963, p. 525.
21. J. Ward and S. Cochi, *Haemophilus influenzae* vaccine, *Vaccines* (S. A. Plotkin and E. A. Mortimer, eds.), W. B. Saunders Publishing Co., Philadelphia, 1988, pp. 314–320.
22. R. R. Burgess, Protein purification, *Protein Engineering* (D. L. Oxander and C. F. Fox, eds.), Alan R. Liss, Inc., New York, 1987, p. 74.
23. O. H. Lowry, N. J. Rosebrough, A. L. Farr, and R. J. Randall, *J. Biol. Chem. 193*:265 (1951).
24. M. Bradford, A rapid and sensitive method for the quantitation of microgram quantities of protein using the principle of protein-dye binding, *Anal. Biochem. 72*:248 (1976).
25. Characterization of solute behavior, gel filtration theory and practice, Pharmacia Fine Chemicals AB, Uppsala, Sweden, 1981.

26. A. Voller, D. E. Bidwell and A. Bartlet, The enzyme linked immunosorbent assays (ELISA), Microsystems Ltd. Vale Guernsey, Summerfield House, 1979.
27. J. S. Kuo, C. N. Monji, R. S. Schwalbe, and D. W. McCoy, A radioactive antigen-binding assay for measurement of antibody to *Haemophilus influenzae* type b capsular polysaccharide; *J. Immunol. Methods 43*:35 (1981).
28. P. P. Vella, J. M. Staub, and R. W. Ellis, Biological activity of Hib conjugates, *Vaccines 9*:S26 (1991).
29. P. W. Anderson, Jr., New and improved vaccines against *Haemophilus influenzae* type b, *New Generation Vaccines* (G. W. Woodrow and M. M. Levine, eds.), Marcel Dekker, New York, 1990, pp. 349–355.
30. J. I. Ward, D. P. Greenberg, P. W. Anderson, et al., Variable quantitation of *Haemophilus influenzae* type b anticapsular antibody by radioantigen binding assay, *J. Clin. Microbiol. 26*:72 (1988).

6

Structure/Function Relationships in Vaccines

Renee Z. Dintzis

The Johns Hopkins University School of Medicine, Baltimore, Maryland

I. IMMUNOLOGICAL PROPERTIES OF *HAEMOPHILUS INFLUENZAE* BACILLI

Haemophilus influenzae are gram-negative, nonmotile, antigenically heterogeneous bacilli, occurring in both rough (unencapsulated) and smooth (encapsulated) forms. The capsule contributes greatly to the virulence of the smooth form by helping to protect the organism from phagocytosis and offering resistance to the bactericidal action of complement and serum components.

Encapsulated *H. influenzae* fall into six immunological types, designated as a,b,c,d,e, and f. These types refer to specific capsular polysaccharides. Meningitis due to *H. influenzae* is the most common form of septic meningitis, and almost all of these infections are due to type b (Hib). The specific polysaccharide of type b is a linear polymer (1), polyribosylribitol phosphate (PRP), containing ribose, ribitol, and phosphate as the principal constituents (Fig. 1). Antibodies to PRP provide protective immunity. This protective effect is related to the opsonophagocytic and bactericidal properties of the antibody (2–4) and to its ability to activate complement (5).

H. influenzae type b bacilli can be demonstrated to be immunologically related to other microorganisms since antisera to Hib have been shown to cross-react with *Escherichia coli* K100 and pneumococcus types 6 and 29, as

Serotype	Structure
	O
	|
H. influenzae b	→3)βDRib*f*(1→1)D-Ribitol(5-P-O-
	||
	O

Figure 1 Structure of *Haemophilus influenzae* type b polysaccharide.

well as with a variety of gram-positive bacteria that contain polyribitol phosphate in their cell wall teichoic acids (6).

II. BACTERIAL CARBOHYDRATES AS ANTIGENS

A substance is defined as an immunogen if it can induce a detectable specific immune response when injected in vivo. That immune response can be humoral (antibody secretion), or cellular (T-cell activation), or both. In contrast, an antigen is strictly defined as a substance that can react with antibodies, but might not by itself be immunogenic. Thus, all immunogens are antigens, but all antigens are not necessarily immunogens. Low molecular weight compounds including haptens, many drugs, and antibiotics are nonimmunogenic but, when conjugated to proteins, can induce the formation of antibodies against the hapten, drug, or antibiotic. The term "epitope" has been frequently used as synonymous with antigen. However, an epitope refers to that part of an antigen that binds to the antigen-combining site of a specific B-cell receptor (antibody) or T-cell receptor.

The inherent complexity of polysaccharide structures makes them bearers of a great number of possible antigenic epitopes. Whereas in proteins, three amino acids can be assembled into six different peptides, three hexoses can yield more than 600 different oligosaccharides. This is so because hexoses can form linkages with any of five hydroxyl groups on hexose rings, and these may be in either the a or b configuration. Thus, carbohydrates can be the basis for the many varied type-specificities of bacteria.

As noted above, polysaccharides can occur as pure carbohydrates in the bacterial capsule or can be covalently linked to lipid as in the LPS of the cell wall. Although the most potent immunogens are macromolecular proteins, polysaccharides are immunogenic under appropriate conditions. That they can be used as vaccines was early demonstrated by MacLeod et al. in 1945, using pneumococcal polysaccharide to elicit a type-specific protection against pneumococcal infection (7).

III. CHARACTERISTICS OF T-INDEPENDENT ANTIGENS

Bacterial polysaccharides and lipopolysaccharides are classified as T-independent antigens. Unlike most protein antigens, or hapten-protein conjugates, T-independent antigens appear to be immunogenic without the participation of specific T lymphocytes. Characteristically, T-independent antigens are polymeric with multiple repeating identical epitopes, and they typically induce primarily an IgM response, with a variable but small amount of IgG subclasses, depending upon the antigen and the animal. Booster injections will bring falling antibody levels back to original immunization levels, but they will not produce an augmented response, nor will they promote switching to another class of antibody (isotype). Some experimental evidence indicates that many T-independent antigens do require some degree of T-cell help, although much less than that needed by T-dependent antigens (8,9).

At present, vaccination with the T-independent purified capsular polysaccharide immunogens protects adults and older children from infections by *H. influenzae* type b, *Streptococcus pneumoniae*, and *Neisseria meningitidis*, the major bacterial culprits in cases of meningitis and pneumonia. However, unconjugated polysaccharide vaccines have two major drawbacks: (a) children younger than 18 months of age, some elderly and/or immunocompromised people either fail to produce antibodies after vaccination or produce antibodies in levels that are too low to be protective, and (b) a repeat injection fails to elicit a booster (enhanced) response. In contrast to the T-independent antigens, T-dependent antigens utilize the active participation of T lymphocytes in order to produce an antibody response. The immunological responses to T-dependent immunogens are not, in general, characterized by the disadvantages ascribed to T-independent ones.

IV. CHARACTERISTICS OF T-DEPENDENT ANTIGENS

T-dependent antigens are typically proteins that will produce boosted antibody levels upon subsequent injection and promote antibody class switching. This phenomenon is believed to be due chiefly to the participation of T-helper cells, which are activated during the response to the protein. Upon activation, T-helper cells can produce a variety of lymphokines, some of which aid in the stimulation of B cells. This activation of B cells by antigen and T-helper factors can lead, ultimately, to their differentiation into plasma cells, their antibody-producing descendents. The maturation of a T-dependent response with time is characterized by antibody class-switching, as well as an increase in antibody affinity, resulting from somatic mutation in the B-cell immunoglobulin genes.

V. T-CELL DEPENDENCE AND CONJUGATE VACCINES

In contrast to the rather poor response of high-risk groups and children under the age of 18 months to T-independent antigens, the response to T-dependent antigens can be substantial. For this reason, the aim in vaccine development has been to convert T-independent polysaccharides to T-dependent immunogens. Currently, this has been accomplished by covalently bonding carbohydrate antigens to carrier proteins, resulting in the formulation of conjugate vaccines. The efficacy of such conjugate vaccines has been reported in a number of clinical trials in which the production of protective antibody has been induced in response to previously poorly immunogenic T-independent antigens. The conjugate vaccines have been shown to elicit an increased total antipolysaccharide antibody response as well as an enhanced response to booster injection. In general, the induced antibodies also exhibit an increased IgG/IgM ratio, a property that often correlates with enhanced antibody affinity.

The exact mechanism whereby conjugation of polysaccharide to a protein carrier converts the antipolysaccharide response to a T-dependent one is still not completely understood. Experimental evidence supports the concept that in a T-dependent response, B cells (or other antigen-presenting cells) endocytose antigens such as proteins, process them into peptides, and present them on the cell surface as a peptide–class II MHC complex. The presented complex serves to activate T-helper cells with receptors specific for that complex. The activated T-helper cells in turn release soluble mediators that drive clonal expansion and differentiation of antigen-specific B cells into antibody-secreting plasma cells (10). It has been proposed that the enhanced immunogenicity of conjugate vaccines implicates saccharide-specific B cells that process and present antigen to T-helper cells. However, it is not known whether only the protein component or the entire conjugate molecule is processed by the antigen-presenting cells; nor is it known which fragment of the conjugate is presented with the MHC complex. Polysaccharides do not seem to interfere with peptide-MHC interactions, implying that polysaccharides by themselves do not bind to MHC molecules (11).

VI. PROTEIN CARRIERS IN CONJUGATE VACCINES

Of particular importance is the selection of the most appropriate protein to be used as carrier in the formulation of conjugate vaccines. The number of proteins that are acceptable for use in humans as potential carriers is restricted. Diphtheria (12–17) and tetanus (18–22) toxoids have been used as carriers, as has a nontoxic mutant native form of diphtheria toxin, CRM_{197} (23,24). The use of CRM_{197} as a carrier has been thought to be preferable to the use of formalinized diphtheria toxin or diphtheria toxoid, not only because of its inherent nontoxicity but because it has more amino groups available for coupling. The outer membrane protein complex (OMPC) of *N. meningitidis* B has also been used successfully as a carrier (25–27). Some results indicate that the OMPC used as a carrier may have adjuvant properties, inducing a greater response to the conjugate (26,27).

A. Effect of Carrier Priming

Administration of the carrier protein some time before the administration of the conjugate vaccine containing that same protein is termed "carrier priming." There are a number of potential advantages in using protein carriers to which the vaccine recipient has had previous exposure, such as those in the diphtheria-tetanus-pertussis (DTP) vaccine. Most infants will have received their first injection of a DTP vaccine by the age of 3 months; therefore, the use of diphtheria and tetanus toxoids as carriers for conjugate vaccine administrations avoids the introduction of new components into the immunization protocol for infants. Since two Hib conjugate vaccines have been approved for administration to 2-month-old infants, it is possible that these babies will receive simultaneous carrier and conjugate administration. Periodic booster immunizations are indicated for many immunization procedures, so that the presence of these toxoids in conjugate vaccines could serve to boost antibody titers to diphtheria and tetanus.

Vaccine recipients have been reported to respond well to both the protein carrier and its conjugated epitope (19). Immunization with Hib-TT(a tetanus toxoid conjugate) induced boosted antitetanus toxoid antibody production in 18- to 23-month-old infants. Recipients may actually generate independent populations of antibodies that differ not only in antibody specificity, but in antibody isotype (17,20,21). Some studies have indicated that carrier priming will increase the antibody response to the subsequent administration of a carrier-conjugate vaccine (28,29). However, other studies have suggested that carrier priming may actually suppress the subsequent response to an epitope attached to that carrier (30–32).

The immunological consequences of carrier priming may depend upon specific experimental procedures. In a study in humans on the response to a malaria sporozoite dodecapeptide-tetanus toxoid conjugate (33), it was found that carrier priming did produce epitopic suppression, but that the suppression was dose-dependent. Higher vaccine doses overcame the suppression. Other findings have indicated that carrier-induced epitopic suppression may be modulated by the adjuvants administered with the vaccine (34). Studies in mice suggest that both the nature of the carrier and the dose used for priming can affect the response to the saccharide of a saccharide-protein conjugate (35). A recent study in monkeys on the immunogenicity of an Hib-CRM_{197} conjugate vaccine found that there was no response in infant animals unless they were concurrently primed with diphtheria toxoid (36). This would indicate that in certain cases, carrier priming might not only enhance the response to the epitope conjugated to that carrier, but it would be essential to produce an adequate response at all.

Such contradictory findings indicate that additional well-controlled studies must be carried out regarding the dose and time of carrier administration, the dose and time of conjugate administration, and the choice and use of adjuvant. The findings of both immune enhancement and immune suppression related to carrier priming suggest that, currently, it is difficult to predict which of these immunomodulating effects will predominate in any given situation.

B. T-Cell Epitopes as Carriers

Interesting attempts have been made to circumvent the possible suppression mediated by carrier priming by using as carrier a specific peptide of the carrier protein rather than the entire protein molecule. Bixler et al. (37) used a synthetic T-cell peptide identified as the T-cell epitope of CRM_{197} as carrier in a Hib conjugate vaccine. The peptide region containing the T-cell epitope encompassed 14 amino acids (CRM 370–383). When tested in mice, this conjugate elicited both primary and secondary antibody responses. This approach can be carried still further by making a conjugate immunogen containing not only the T-cell epitope of the carrier, but a B-cell epitopic region of a bacterial or viral pathogen. For example, Etlinger et al. (38) identified a specific peptide fragment of tetanus toxoid as a T-cell epitope. When linked to an immunodominant B-cell peptide epitope of the circumsporozoite protein of P. falciparum and injected into tetanus-toxoid primed mice, the conjugate induced an enhanced antibody response to the malarial circumsporozoite protein.

C. T-Cell/B-Cell Chimeras as Immunogens

Immunogenic conjugates have also been made containing T-cell and B-cell epitopes from the same immunogen (39,40). More than one T-cell epitope can be included in a conjugate. A synthetic peptide containing two T-helper-cell epitopes as well as the dominant neutralizing antibody B-cell epitope from the human immunodeficiency virus envelope gp120 has been found to induce neutralizing antibodies in monkeys (41).

There is evidence that the polarity between the B and T peptides may have an effect on the immunogenicity of the conjugate and may also have a profound effect on the antibody specificity and affinity (42–44). However, there is disagreement as to whether linkage of the T-helper epitope to the C- or N-terminus of the adjacent B epitope leads to maximal immunogenicity. Such findings indicate that the amino acid composition of the epitopes as well as the stoichiometry of the chimeras undoubtedly have an important influence on the manner in which these conjugate molecules, are processed and presented to lymphocytes.

D. The Multiple Antigen Peptide (MAP) System as a Vaccine Model

A novel approach in the engineering of epitope-based vaccines has been the multiple antigen peptide (MAP) system. As in the B-cell/T-cell epitope conjugates, no protein carrier is used. However, instead of a linear arrangement of B-cell and T-cell epitopes, the MAP system builds chemically defined structures obtained directly from the solid-phase synthesis of antigenic peptide epitopes onto an oligomeric branching lysine core (45,46). A number of MAP models have been constructed, but an especially immunogenic arrangement of epitopes has been reported to consist of four B-cell and four T-cell epitopes arranged in tandem on a lysine core matrix (47,48). The conjugate is a macromolecule with multiple clusters of antigenic epitopes at the surface; thus it has the appearance and molecular weight of a small protein.

E. Immunogenicity of Co-Injected B-Cell and T-Cell Epitopes

There is evidence that in some immunization protocols, covalent linkage between the B-cell and T-cell epitope may not even be necessary (49). This was supported by the findings of Partidos et al. (50), who induced antibody to a B-cell epitope by simply co-immunizing mice with synthetic B-cell and T-helper-cell epitopes from glycoproteins of the measles virus. Notable was the fact that the mice used were genetically nonresponsive to the B-cell epitope when it was administered by itself in complete Freund's adjuvant, but were capable of responding to the B-cell epitope when it was injected with adjuvant at the same time and in the same site as the immunogenic T-cell epitope. Possibly, comparable maneuverings with polysaccharide epitopes may lead to novel vaccine designs.

VII. STRUCTURAL REQUIREMENTS FOR IMMUNOGENICITY OF UNCONJUGATED POLYSACCHARIDES

Priming with Hib conjugate vaccines has been reported to lead to higher responses to subsequent unconjugated PRP administration (51). Anderson et al. have noted that after initial immunization with conjugate vaccines, infants respond at an earlier age to unconjugated PRP vaccine than they would if they had not been primed with the conjugate (24,52,53). It has been suggested that, for maintenance of high antibody levels, the unconjugated capsular PRP could be used as an economical booster after an initial priming with the conjugate (54). If unconjugated polysaccharides are to be utilized in vaccination booster protocols, more information as to the structural requirements for the optimal immunogenicity of these types of T-independent antigens will be needed.

The importance of the molecular size and state of aggregation of polysaccharide antigens was early demonstrated in studies on the immunogenicity of dextran, a polysaccharide made by *Leuconostoc mesenteroides*. Molecules with a molecular weight below 70,000 daltons (D) were not immunogenic, while those of greater molecular weight were substantial immunogens (55).

More recently, Dintzis and colleagues have attempted to identify the molecular parameters most relevant to the immunogenicity of T-independent antigens. Their findings also indicated that the molecular weight of the antigen greatly affects its immunogenicity. The antigens studied included a series of carefully size-fractionated pneumococcal polysaccharides (56) and haptenated polymers (57,58). In the haptenated polymer studies, a variety of polymer carriers were used, some of them polysaccharides such as dextran, Ficoll, and carboxymethyl cellulose. These haptenated polysaccharides became immunogenic only when their molecular weights approached roughly 100,000 D. In addition, the number of haptens or epitopes on the carrier polymer had to exceed 20 to stimulate antihapten or antiepitope antibody production. If the mass of the carrier were sufficient, high-density haptens or epitopes yielded the best responses. The optimal molecular weight for immunogenicity in the molecules studied was about 500,000 D. With molecular weights greater than 1 million D, the response began to fall off. Importantly, it was found that smaller molecules of less than 100,000 D were not only nonimmunogenic, but when administered with larger, immunogenic molecules, they proved to inhibit the response to the larger molecules.

Similar results were obtained using nonhaptenated pneumococcal polysaccharides as antigens, indicating that these findings as to optimal molecular weight were not unique to haptenated polysaccharides (56). The pneumococcal polysaccharide studies were carried out on different molecular weight fractions of type 3 (PP3), which is a linear structure of alternating glucose and glucoronic acid subunits. Several PP3 preparations used in human vaccines were size-fractionated and found to be quite heterogeneous, ranging from 70,000 to 620,000 D in size. These fractions were refractionated twice, and their immunogenicity was tested in mice.

As in the case of the haptenated polymers, it was found that preparations of molecular weight less than 100,000 D were not immunogenic. In order to preclude the possibility that the nonimmunogenicity of the smaller fractions was due to an unexpected difference in chemical composition between the material smaller than 100,000 D and the larger material, a center, immunogenic fraction of 250,000 D was ultrasonicated to yield smaller fractions ranging from 20,000 to 50,000 D. Not only were the smaller molecules of PP3 completely nonimmunogenic, but when administered with a comparable (and stimulatory) dose of the larger molecules, they strongly inhibited the immune response to the larger molecules from which they had been fragmented by ultrasonication.

These findings may have important implications when polysaccharides are used in vaccine protocols. They indicate that there is an optimal size for optimal immunogenicity of such materials. Importantly, contamination with smaller molecular fractions is deleterious. Such fractions are not only inactive immunologically, but can actually inhibit the response to the larger fractions. In general, bacterial polysaccharides are obtained from the large molecular complexes of the bacterial capsule or cell envelope or from supernatant fluids in which the bacilli have been cultured. The saccharides to be used as vaccines are derived from chemical degradations of the isolated macromolecular complexes. Such procedures are likely to produce an assortment of saccharides of unequal sizes. The aforementioned studies indicate that careful fractionation to eliminate the smaller sizes is critical for optimal immunogenicity.

VIII. STRUCTURAL REQUIREMENTS FOR OPTIMAL GLYCOCONJUGATE VACCINES

The optimal size for immunogenicity of the saccharide component of a conjugate vaccine may be quite different from the optimal size of the polysaccharide to be used in an unconjugated vaccine. A number of findings have indicated that conjugates made with smaller fractions of polysaccharides (oligosaccharides of varing lengths) could be effective in inducing antibody responses to the polysaccharide from which they were derived. Snippe et al. (59) conjugated pneumococcal hexasaccharide from *Streptococcus pneumoniae* to three different protein carriers and found this conjugated oligosaccharide to be immunogenic and protective against *S. pneumoniae* infection in mice.

Although studies comparing human antibody responses to two conjugate vaccines of Hib-diphtheria toxoid found that differences in response to a polysaccharide vs. an oligosaccharide conjugate were not statistically different (60), it has been noted that conjugate vaccines using oligosaccharides of different sizes and loading density may vary as to their immunogenicity. In a 1983 study, Anderson (61) obtained three sizes of oligosaccharides (designated small, medium, and large) after acid hydrolysis of PRP and conjugated them to the CRM_{197} protein. The three oligosaccharide sizes proved to be approximately equally immunogenic in weanling rabbits. Anderson et al. subsequently conducted more extensive investigations in humans and reported that different sizes of PRP oligomers conjugated to diphtheria toxoid varied in their immunogenicity. Oligomers of 20 repeat units of PRP were more immunogenic than oligomers of smaller repeat units (62). However, further studies revealed that the extent of hapten loading (ribose/protein ratio) was more important for immunogenicity than the size of the oligomer (23).

Studies on the immunogenicity of a dextran-chicken serum albumin conjugate in mice yielded results somewhat contradictory to the above findings (63,64). They indicated that protein conjugates made with low molecular weight dextran oligomers (1000–4000 Da) were more immunogenic than conjugates made with dextrans of higher molecular weight. Increasing the size of the saccharide to 40,000 Da or permitting multiple attachments of the saccharide to the protein reduced its immunogenicity.

From reports such as these, it would seem that comparisons as to the immunogenicity of oligo- and polysaccharide conjugates are difficult to make, since these studies vary in types of antigens, doses, character and age of subjects, methods of conjugation, and characterization of the oligosaccharide as well as of the final conjugate product.

Four *H. influenzae* type b conjugate vaccines have been developed for use in human infants (Table 1) (23,65–68). Each uses a different protein carrier. They also vary in the size of the saccharide epitope. One of the vaccines (HbOC) uses a PRP oligosaccharide rather than the larger polysaccharide for conjugation. The vaccines also vary in the ratio of saccharide to protein. The diphtheria toxoid conjugate (PRP-D) consists, on average of nine toxoid molecules covalently linked to each polysaccharide molecule, with a final molecular weight of 2.1×10^6 D. Preparations of the *N. meningitidis* B outer membrane protein complex conjugate (PRP-OMPC) and the tetanus toxoid conjugates (Hib-TT or PRP-T) have varied in their polysaccharide content (69,70). In general, doses containing 15 μg polysaccharide generate good responses in infants. The one oligosac-

Table 1 *Haemophilus influenzae* Type b Conjugate Vaccines

Abbreviation	Trade name	Carrier protein	Licensed use
PRP-D	ProHIBit	Diphtheria toxoid	for children ≥15 mo of age
HbOC	HibTITER	CRM_{197}	for infants & children ≥2 mo of age
PRP-OMP	PedvaxHIB	OMP	for infants & children ≥2 mo of age
PRP-T	—	Tetanus toxoid	not yet licensed

charide conjugate (HbOC) uses CRM_{197} as the protein carrier with an oligosaccharide averaging 20 repeat saccharide units. In addition, the vaccines vary in the type and method of linkage of the saccharide to the carrier.

It is evident that despite substantial variations in the construction of glycoconjugate vaccines, it has been possible to achieve great improvements in prophylactic immunization. In contrast to the native macromolecular polysaccharide vaccines, which are T-independent, the T-dependent glycoconjugate vaccines are immunogenic in infants and elicit antibody titers which can be boosted with subsequent immunization.

Despite these advances, some confusion still exists as to the optimal molecular characteristics for immunogenicity. Optimal molecular parameters such as saccharide size and substitution density, conjugation procedure, and size of final conjugate are yet to be elucidated. Studies with human subjects are understandably difficult and expensive. Unfortunately, findings using laboratory animals do not always reliably reflect what the human responses will be. Nevertheless, important research continues, using a variety of animal models, some of whose responses yield significant clues as to which molecular structures are likely to lead to efficacious vaccines. More polysaccharides in bacterial cell envelopes are being subjected to conversion into conjugates from organisms such as *Pseudomonas aeruginosa*, *Neisseria gonorrhoeae*, *Neisseria meningitidis*, *Streptococcus pneumoniae*, *Salmonella typhi*, *Escherichia coli*, *Klebsiella*, and *Vibrio cholerae*. Such studies hold much promise for effective vaccines of lasting efficacy against a large variety of serious human infectious diseases.

REFERENCES

1. P. Anderson and D. H. Smith, Isolation of the capsular polysaccharide from culture supernatant of Haemophilus influenzae type b, *Infect. Immun. 15*:472 (1977).

2. P. Anderson, R. B. Johnson, and D. H. Smith, Human serum activities against *H. influenzae* type b, *J. Clin. Invest. 51*:31 (1972).
3. R. Schneerson, L. P. Rodrigues, J. C. Parker, and J. B. Robbins, Immunity to disease caused by *H. influenzae* type b: II. Specificity and some biological characteristics of "natural", infection acquired, and immunization induced antibody to capsular polysaccharide, *J. Immunol. 107*:1081 (1971).
4. S. L. Newman, B. Waldo, and R. B. Johnston, Separation of serum bactericidal and opsonizing activities for *Haemophilus influenzae* type b, *Infect. Immun. 8*:488 (1973).
5. J. A. Winkelstein and E. R. Moxon, Role of complement in the host's defense against *Haemophilus influenzae*, Haemophilus influenzae *Epidemiology, Immunology and Prevention of Disease* (S. H. Sell and P. F. Wright, eds.), Elsevier Biomedical, New York, 1982, pp. 135–144.
6. M. Argaman, T. Y. Liu, and J. B. Robbins, Polyribitol-phosphate: an antigen of four gram-positive bacteria cross-reactive with the capsular polysaccharide of *Haemophilus influenzae* type b, *J. Immunol. 112*:649 (1974).
7. C. M. MacLeod, R. G. Hodges, M. Heidelberger, and W. G. Bernhard, Prevention of pneumococcal pneumonia by immunization with specific capsular polysaccharides, *J. Exp. Med. 82*:445 (1945).
8. B. L. Pike and G. J. V. Nossal, A reappraisal of "T-independent" antigens. I. Effect of lymphokines on the response of single adult hapten-specific lymphocytes, *J. Immunol. 132*:1687 (1984).
9. R. O. Endres, E. Kushnir, J. W. Kappler, P. Marrack, and S. C. Knisky, A requirement for non-specific T cell factors in antibody responses to "T cell independent" antigens, *J. Immunol. 130*:781 (1983).
10. E. C. Snow and R. J. Noelle, Thymus-dependent antigenic stimulation of hapten-specific B lymphocytes, *Immunol. Rev. 99*:173 (1987).
11. F. Leyva-Cobian and E. R. Unanue, Intracellular interference with antigen presentation, *J. Immunol. 141*:1445 (1988).
12. C. Lue, S. J. Prince, A. Fattom, R. Schneerson, J. B. Robbins, and J. Mestecky, Antibody-secreting peripheral blood lymphocytes induced by immunization with a conjugate consisting of *Streptococcus pneumoniae* type 12F polysaccharide and diphtheria toxoid, *Infect. Immun. 58*:2547 (1990).
13. J. Eskola, H. Kayhty, H. Peltola, V. Karanko, J. Samuelson, and L. Gordon, Antibody levels achieved in infants by course of *Haemophilus influenzae* type b polysaccharide/diphtheria toxoid conjugate vaccine, *Lancet 1*:1184 (1985).
14. A. Fattom, C. Lue, S. C. Szu, J. Mestecky, G. Schiffman, D. Bryla, W. F. Vann, D. Watson, L. M. Kimzey, J. B. Robbins, and R. Schneerson, Serum antibody response in adult volunteers elicited by injection of *Streptococcus pneumoniae* type 12F polysaccharide alone or conjugated to diphtheria toxoid, *Infect. Immun. 58*:2309 (1990).
15. D. M. Granoff, E. G. Boies, and R. S. Munson Immunogenicity of *Haemophilus influenzae* type b polysaccharide-diphtheria toxoid conjugate vaccine in adults. *J. Pediatr. 105*:22 (1984).
16. W. L. Nelson and D. M. Granoff, Protective efficacy of *Haemophilus influ-*

enzae type b polysaccharide -diphtheria toxoid-conjugate vaccine, *Am. J. Dis. Child 144*:292 (1990).
17. O. Makela, P. Mattila, N. Rautonen, I. Seppala, J. Eskola, and H. Kayhty, Isotype concentrations of human antibodies to *Haemophilus influenzae* type b polysaccharide (Hib) in young adults immunized with the polysaccharide as such or conjugated to a protein (diphtheria toxoid), *J. Immunol. 139*:1999 (1987).
18. B. A. Claesson, R. Schneerson, B. Trollfors, T. Lagergard, J. Taranger, and J. B. Robbins, Duration of serum antibodies elicited by *Haemophilus influenzae* type b capsular polysaccharide alone or conjugated to tetanus toxoid in 18- to 23-month-old-children, *J. Pediatr. 116*:929 (1990).
19. B. A. Claesson, B. Trollfors, T. Lagergard, J. Taranger, D. Bryla, G. Otterman, T. Cramton, Y. Yang, C. R. Reimer, J. B. Robbins and R. Schneerson, Clinical and immunologic responses to the capsular polysaccharide of *Haemophilus influenzae* type b alone or conjugated to tetanus toxoid in 18- to 23-month old children, *J. Pediatr. 112*:695 (1988).
20. R. Schneerson, J. B. Robbins, J. C. Parke, A. Sutton, Z. Wang, J. J. Schlesselman, G. Schiffman, C. Bell, A. Karpas, and M. C. Hardegree, Quantitative and qualitative analyses of serum *Hemophilus influenzae* type b, pneumococcus type 6A and tetanus toxin antibodies elicited by polysaccharide-protein conjugates in adult volunteers, *Infect. Immun. 52*:501 (1986).
21. T. Legergard, J. Shiloach, J. B. Robbins, and R. Schneerson, Synthesis and immunological properties of conjugates composed of group B streptococcus type III capsular polysaccharide covalently bound to tetanus toxoid, *Infect. Immun. 58*:687 (1990).
22. S. J. Crys, J. C. Sadoff, E. Furer, and R. Germanier, *Pseudomonas aeruginosa* polysaccharide-tetanus toxoid conjugate vaccine: safety and immuneogenicity in humans, *J. Infect. Dis 154*:682 (1986).
23. P. W. Anderson, M. E. Pichichero, E. C. Stein, S. Porcelli, R. F. Betts, D. M. Connuck, D. Korones, R. A. Insel, J. M. Zahradnik, and R. Eby, Effect of oligosaccharide chain length, exposed terminal group, and hapten loading on the antibody response of human adults and infants to vaccines consisting of *Haemophilus influenzae* type b capsular antigen uniterminally coupled to the diphtheria protein CRM197, *J. Immunol. 142*:2464 (1989).
24. P. Anderson, M. E. Pichichero, and R. A. Insel, Immunization of two-month old infants with protein oligosaccharides derived from the capsule of *Haemophilus influenzae* type b, *J. Pediatr. 107*:346 (1985).
25. D. M. Granoff, A. Chacko, K. R. Lottenbach, and K. E. Sheetz, Immunogenicity of Haemophilus influenzae type b polysaccharide-outer membrane protein conjugate vaccine in patients who acquired *Haemophilus* disease despite previous vaccination with type b polysaccharide vaccine, *J. Pediatr. 114*:925 (1989).
26. M. S. Einhorn, G. A. Weinberg, E. L. Anderson, P. D. Granoff, and D. M. Granoff, Immunogenicity in infants of *Haemophilus influenzae* type b polysaccharide in a conjugate vaccine with *Neisseria meningitidis* outer-membrane protein, *Lancet 2*:299 (1986).

27. J. J. Donnelly, R. R. Deck, and M. A. Liu, Immunogenicity of a *Haemophilus influenzae* polysaccharide-*Neisseria meningitidis* outer membrane protein complex conjugate vaccine, *J. Immunol. 145*:3071 (1990).
28. L. K. Gordon, Characterization of a hapten-carrier conjugate vaccine: H. influenzae-diphtheria conjugate vaccine, *Modern Approaches to Vaccines* (R. M. Chanock and R. A. Lerner, eds), Cold Spring Harbor Laboratory, Cold Spring Harbor, NY, 1984, pp. 393–396.
29. L. D. Lise, D. Mazier, M. Jolivet, F. Audibert, L. Chedid, and D. Schlesinger, Enhanced epitopic response to a synthetic human malarial peptide by preimmunization with tetanus toxoid carrier, *Infect. Immun. 55*:2658 (1987).
30. L. A. Herzenberg, T. Tokuhisa, and L. A. Herzenberg, Carrier priming leads to hapten-specific suppression, *Nature 285*:665 (1980).
31. M. P. Schutze, C. Leclerc, M. Jolivet, F. Audibert, and L. Chedid, Carrier-induced epitopic suppression, a major issue for synthetic vaccines, *J. Immunol. 135*:2319 (1985).
32. M. P. Schutze, E. Deriaud, G. Przewlocki, and C. LeClerk, Carrier-induced epitopic suppression is initiated through clonal dominance, *J. Immunol. 142*:2635 (1989).
33. D. DiJohn, J. R. Torres, J. Murillo, D. A. Herrington, S. S. Wasserman, M. J. Cortesia, G. A. Losonsky, D. Sturcher, and M. M. Levine, Effect of priming with carrier on response to conjugate vaccine, *Lancet* (*Dec. 16*):1415 (1989).
34. F. R. Vogel, C. LeClerc, M. P. Schutze, M. Jolivet, F. Audibert, T. W. Klein, and L. Chedid, Modulation of carrier-induced epitopic suppression by *Bordetella pertussis* components and muramyl peptide, *Cell. Immunol. 107*:40 (1987).
35. C. A. M. Peeters, A.-M. Tenberger-Meekes, J. T. Poolman, M. Beurret, B. J. M. Zegers, and G. Rijkers, Effect of carrier priming on immunogenicity of saccharide-protein conjugate vaccines, *Infect. Immun. 59*:3504 (1991).
36. P. P. Vella and R. W. Ellis, Immunogenicity of *Haemophilus influenzae* type b conjugate vaccines in infant rhesus monkeys, *Ped. Res. 29*:10 (1991).
37. G. S. Bixler, R. Eby, K. M. Dermody, R. M. Woods, R. C. Seid, and S. Pillai, Synthetic peptide representing a T-cell epitope of CRM197 substitutes as carrier molecule in a *Haemophilus influenzae* type b (Hib) conjugate vaccine, *Adv. Exp. Med. Biol. 251*:175 (1989).
38. H. M. Etlinger, D. Gillessen, H.-W. Lahm, H. Matile, H.-J. Schonfeld, and A. Trzeciak, Use of prior vaccinations for the development of new vaccines, *Science 249*:423 (1990).
39. M. F. Good, W. L. Maloy, M. N. Lunde, H. Margalit, J. L. Cornette, G. L. Smith, B. Moss, L. H. Miller, and J. A. Berzofsky, Construction of synthetic immunogen: use of new T-helper epitope on malaria circumsporozoite protein, *Science 235*:1059 (1987).
40. C. Leclerc, G. Przewlocki, M.-P. Schutze, and L. Chedid. A synthetic vaccine constructed by copolymerization of B and T cell determinants, *Eur. J. Immunol. 17*:269 (1987).
41. M. K. Hart, T. J. Palker, T. J. Matthews, A. J. Langlois, N. W. Lerche, M. E.

Martin, R. M. Scearce, C. McDanal, D. P. Bolognesi, and B. F. Haynes, Synthetic peptides containing T and B cell epitopes from human immunodeficiency virus envelope gp120 induce anti-HIV proliferative responses and high titers of neutralizing antibodies in rhesus monkeys, *J. Immunol. 145*:2677 (1990).

42. J. H. Cox, J. Ivanyi, D. B. Young, J. R. Lamb, A. D. Syred, and M. J. Francis, Orientation of epitopes influences immunogenicity of synthetic peptide dimers, *Eur. J. Immunol. 18*:2015 (1988).
43. M. E. Levely, M. A. Mitchell, and J. A. Nicholas, Synthetic immunogens constructed from T-cell and B-cell stimulating peptides (T:B chimeras): preferential stimulation of unique T- and B- cell specificities is influenced by immunogen configuration, *Cell Immunol. 125*:65 (1990).
44. C. D. Partidos, C. Stanley, and M. W. Steward, The effect of orientation of epitopes on the immunogenicity of chimeric peptides representing measles virus protein sequences, *Mol. Immunol. 29*:651 (1992).
45. J. P. Tam, High-density multiple antigen-peptide system for preparation of antipeptide antibodies. *Methods Enzymol. 168*:7 (1989).
46. J. P. Tam, Synthetic peptide vaccine design: synthesis and properties of a high-density multiple antigenic peptide system, *Proc. Natl. Acad. Sci. 85*:5409 (1988).
47. J. P. Tam, P. Clavijo, Y. Lu, V. Nussenzweig, R. Nussenzweig, and F. Zavala, Incorporation of T- and B-epitopes of the circumsporozoite protein in a chemically defined vaccine against malaria, *J. Exp. Med. 171*:299 (1990).
48. B. Nardelli, Y.-A. Lu, D. R. Shiu, C. Delpierre-Defoort, A. T. Profy, and J. P. Tam, A chemically defined synthetic vaccine model for HIV-1, *J. Immunol. 148*:914 (1992).
49. P. Sarobe, J. J. LaSatre, J. Golvano, A. Gullo, M. P. Civeira, J. Prieto, and F. Borras-Guesta, Induction of antibodies against a peptide hapten does not require covalent linkage between the hapten and a class II presentable T helper peptide, *Eur. J. Immunol. 21*:1555 (1991).
50. C. D. Partidos, O. E. Obeid, and M. W. Steward, Antibody responses to non-immunogenic synthetic peptides induced by co-immunization with immunogenic peptides, *Immunology 77*:262 (1992).
51. G. A. Weinberg, S. Menachem, S. Einhorn, A. A. Lenoir, P. D. Granoff, and D. M. Granoff, Immunologic priming to capsular polysaccharide in infants immunized with *Haemophilus influenzae* type b polysaccharide—*Neisseria meningitidis* outer membrane protein conjugate vaccine, *J. Pediatr. 111*:22 (1987).
52. P. Anderson, M. Pichichero, K. Edwards, C. R. Porch, and R. Insel, Priming and induction of Haemophilus influenzae type b capsular antibodies in early infancy by Dpo20, an oligosaccharide-protein conjugate vaccine, *J. Pediatr. 111*:644 (1987).
53. R. A. Insel and P. W. Anderson, Oligosaccharide-protein conjugate vaccines induce and prime for oligoclonal IgG antibody responses to the *Haemophilus influenzae* b capsular polysaccharide in human infants, *J. Exp. Med. 163*:262 (1986).

54. P. W. Anderson, New and improved vaccines against *Haemophilus influenzae* type b infections, *New Generation Vaccines* (G. C. Woodrow and M. M. Levine, eds.). Marcel Dekker, Inc., New York, 1990, pp. 349–355.
55. E. A. Kabat and A. E. Bezer, The effect of variation in molecular weight on the antigenicity of dextran in man, *Arch. Biochem. 78*:306 (1958).
56. H. M. Dintzis and R. Z. Dintzis, A molecular basis for immune regulation: the immunon hypothesis, *Theoretical Immunology*, *Part One* (A. S. Perelson, ed.), Addison-Wesley, Redwood City, CA, 1988, pp. 83–103.
57. R. Z. Dintzis, M. H. Middleton, and H. M. Dintzis, Studies on the immunogenicity and tolerogenicity of T-independent antigens, *J. Immunol. 131*:2196 (1983).
58. R. Z. Dintzis, M. Okajima, M. H. Middleton, G. Greene, and H. M. Dintzis, The immunogenicity of soluble haptenated polymers is determined by molecular mass and hapten valence, *J. Immunol. 143*:1239 (1989).
59. H. Snippe, A.-J. Van Houte, J. E. G. Van Dam, M. J. DeReuver, M. Jansze, and J. M. N. Willers, Immunogenic properties in mice of hexasaccharide from the capsular polysacharide of *Streptococcus pneumoniae* type 3, *Infect. Immun. 40*:856 (1983).
60. I. Seppala, H. Sarvas, O. Makela, J. Eskola, and H. Kayhty, Human antibody responses to two conjugate vaccines of *Haemophilus influenzae* type b saccharides and diphtheria toxoid, *Scand. J. Immunol. 28*:471 (1988).
61. P. Anderson, Antibody responses to *Haemophilus influenzae* type b and diphtheria toxin induced by conjugates of oligosaccharides of the type b capsule with the nontoxic protein CRM_{197}, *Infect. Immun. 39*:233 (1983).
62. P. Anderson, M. E. Pichichero, R. A. Insel, R. Betts, R. Eby, and D. H. Smith, Vaccines consisting of periodate-cleaved oligosaccharides from the capsule of *Haemophilus influenzae* type b coupled to a protein carrier: Structural and temporal requirements for priming in the human infant, *J. Immunol. 137*:1181 (1986).
63. O. Makela, F. Peterfy, I. G.Outschoorn, A. W. Richter, and I. Seppala, Immunogenic properties of a(1–6) dextran, its protein conjugates, and conjugates of its breakdown products in mice, *Scand. J. Immunol. 19*:541 (1984).
64. I. Seppala and O. Makela, Antigenicity of Dextran-protein conjugates in mice. Effect of molecular weight of the carbohydrate and comparison of two modes of coupling, *J. Immunol. 143*:1259 (1989).
65. D. H. Smith, D. V. Madore, R. Eby, P. W. Anderson, R. A. Insel, and C. L. Johnson, Haemophilus b oligosaccharide-CRM_{197} and other *Haemophilus* b conjugate vaccines: a status report, *Adv. Exp. Med. Biol. 251*:65 (1989).
66. D. V. Madore, C. L. Johnson, D. C. Phipps, Pennridge pediatric associates, L. A. Popejoy, R. Eby and D. H. Smith, Safety and immunologic response to Haemophilus influenzae type b oligosaccharide CRM_{197} conjugate vaccine in 1-to-6-month old infants, *Pediatrics 85*:331 (1990).
67. P. P. Vella, J. M. Staub, J. Armstrong et al., Immunogenicity of a new

Haemophilus influenzae type b conjugate vaccine (meningococcal protein conjugate), (Pedvax HIB®). *Pediatrics 85*:668 (1990).
68. G. Tudor-Williams, J. Frankland, D. Issacs, et al., *Haemophilus influenzae* type b conjugate vaccine trial in Oxford: implications for the United Kingdom, *Arch. Disease Child. 64*:520 (1989).
69. R. Yogev, M. Arditi, E. G. Chadwick, M. D. Amer, and P. A. Sroka, *Haemophilus influenzae* type b conjugate vaccine (meningococcal protein conjugate) immungenicity and safety at various doses, *Pediatr. 85*:690 (1990).
70. B. A. Claesson, R. Schneerson, J. B. Robbins, J. Johansson, T. Lagergard, J. Taranget, D. Bryla, L. Levi, T. Cramton, and B. Trollfors, Protective levels of serum antibodies stimulated in infants by two injections of Haemophilus influenzae type b capsular polysaccharide (PRP) tetanus antigen (T) conjugate, *J. Pediatr. 114*:97 (1989).

7

Molecular Epidemiology of Hib Strains

Loek van Alphen

University of Amsterdam, Amsterdam, The Netherlands

I. INTRODUCTION

Haemophilus influenzae type b (Hib) causes systemic disease worldwide, although the disease incidence and the disease pattern differ largely among individual populations. In general, the incidence is high (more than 100/100,000 children under 5) in developing countries and among special populations such as Alaskan Eskimos and low in industrialized areas (20–100/100,000 under five). A high incidence coincides with a maximum age-specific incidence below 7 months of age (reviewed in ref. 1). Meningitis is the major Hib disease worldwide. Epiglottitis is common in countries like Finland, but is rare in other populations, such as the Alaskan Eskimos (2,3). In developing countries acute respiratory tract infections (ARI) are frequently caused by Hib (4). These observations have prompted many investigators to study the epidemiology of Hib disease by comparing Hib isolates from different sources in various parts of the world. Presently, these epidemiological studies are based on the analysis of not only general properties of the bacterium but also of virulence factors and other disease-associated markers. Differences in DNA sequences of the chromosome and in the electrophoretic mobility of metabolic enzymes are general epidemiological tools. Analysis of components exposed on the surface of the bacterium, like outer membrane proteins (OMPs) and lipopolysaccharides (LPSs), reveals information about the antigenic composition and diversity of Hib. Identification of specific virulence factors (fimbriae, IgA protease) is important for our understanding of their role in the pathogenesis of Hib disease.

In this chapter I shall summarize the data on the molecular analysis of the epidemiological markers of Hib and their occurrence among disease and carrier isolates of Hib. The molecular epidemiology of Hib is based on the geographical distribution of these markers among Hib isolates and the change in distribution in time and due to vaccination.

II. GENERAL METHODS FOR THE TYPING OF Hib

A. Biotyping

Biotyping was the first method to discriminate between individual *H. influenzae* isolates of a particular type and is based on the presence or absence of urease and ornithine decarboxylase activity and the production of indole (5). All eight theoretical combinations (biotypes) have been described (5–8). Despite an enormous number of studies describing biotypes of *H. influenzae*, this method is of limited value to study the epidemiology of *H. influenzae*, since only four biotypes are frequently found. Invasive disease isolates are mainly biotype I. The expression of the three enzymatic reactions does not seem to be a prerequisite for invasive disease since one fifth of Finnish Hib isolates is biotype II (9).

B. Electrophoretic Typing

With multilocus enzyme gel electrophoresis, genetically controlled variants of enzymes (alloenzymes) are separated in a starch gel due to their differences in charge. The alloenzymes are identified by histochemical staining with specific substrates. The relative mobilities of the enzyme variants are recorded. The electrophoretic type (ET) of an isolate is defined by the combination of electromorphs for the enzymes tested. Using a relatively large number of enzymes (up to 32 for bacteria), differences in mobility reflect differences in genetic structure of the strains, as is described in detail in Chapter 9. Although the number of ETs among Hib isolates is much less than among nontypeable ones, ETing has a high discriminatory power.

C. DNA Restriction Length Polymorphism

Restriction endonuclease analysis of chromosomal DNA has been used by several groups to compare nonencapsulated *H. influenzae* (10,11). Strains that were different by restriction endonuclease analysis appeared in most cases also different by rRNA gene restriction patterns. The interpretation of the rRNA restriction patterns is easier, since the number of bands to be compared is limited (11). Restriction endonuclease analysis of chromosomal DNA is not suitable for *H. influenzae* type b strains, since their relationship is too close to see differences of any significance for the epidemiological analysis of Hib (unpublished observations).

III. METHODS FOR THE ANALYSIS OF SURFACE EXPOSED COMPONENTS OF Hib

Capsular polysaccharides, OMPs, and LPSs of *H. influenzae* have been analyzed extensively, since they are exposed at the surface of the bacteria and are therefore possible candidates for a vaccine to prevent *H. influenzae* disease. Antibodies specific for these surface exposed components may promote antibody-dependent killing by complement and enhance opsonophagocytosis.

A. Capsular Polysaccharides

The typing of the capsular polysaccharides of *H. influenzae* is performed with protein A coagglutination or latex agglutination with polyclonal antisera specific for types a–f. Both techniques give similar results (5).

B. Outer Membrane Proteins

Two systems are used for the nomenclature of the major outer membrane proteins. A numerical numbering (P1–P6) has been described by Granoff and Munson (13). Loeb and Smith (14) and we (15) used an alphabetical numbering. These OMPs include OMP a [or P1, molecular weight 43–50 kilodaltons (kD)] b,c (or P2, 39–42 kD), and d (or P5, 37–39 kD, eCP4, 30 kD) and OMP P6 (16.6 kD). Proteins a (P1) and d (P5) can easily be identified by their heat-modifiability in SDS (15). Protein c is probably a minor protein which is enriched after purification of outer and cytoplasmic membranes of *H. influenzae* by sucrose gradient centrifugation after spheroplast formation (15). Only one gene copy has been found for protein b,c (P2) (16). The protein coded by this gene is a porin, facilitating the diffusion of nutrients and some antibiotics through the outer membrane (17). OMP e (P4) is a conserved nonimmunogenic protein (13–15,18). Protein P6 is a lipoprotein that binds to its DNA, thereby regulating its expression (19). A 15 kD lipoprotein (20) has a restricted homology with OMP P6. The protein patterns are stable in patients and experimental models (21,22).

OMP subtyping of Hib strains is based on differences in the mobility of the major OMPs a (P1), b,c (P2), and d (P5), which show diversity in molecular weight (Fig. 1). A gradient (23,24) and a normal (14,15) SDS-polyacrylamide gel electrophoresis system are in use for the analysis of the

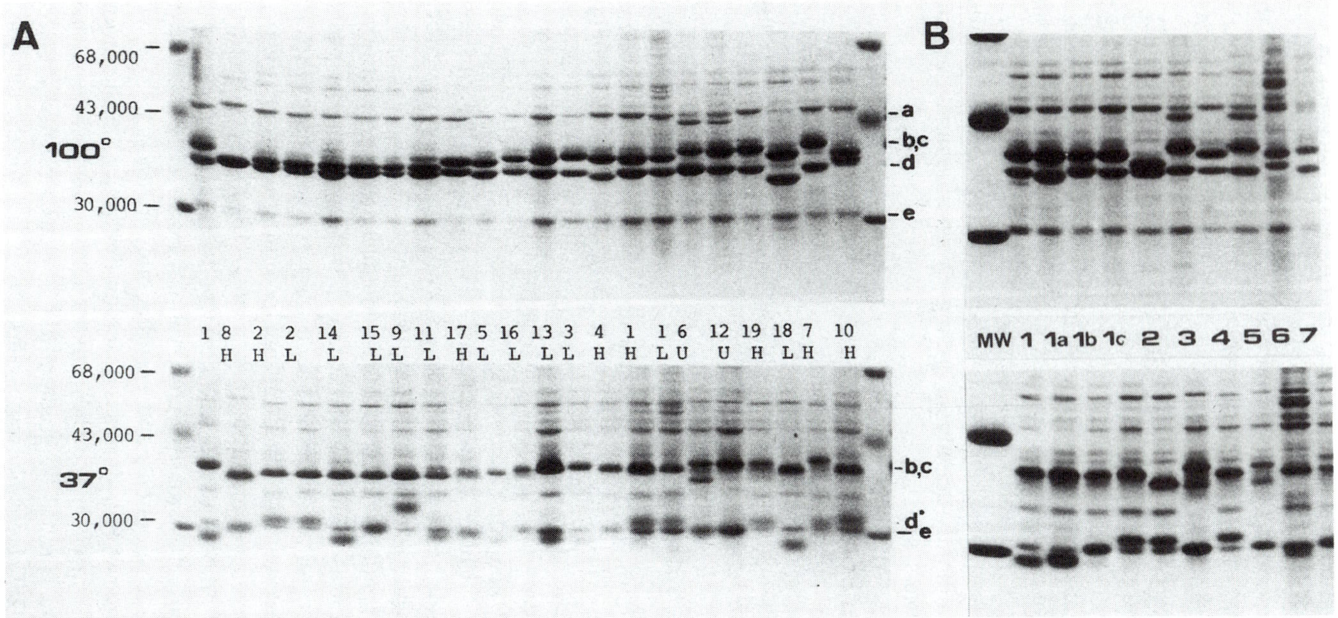

Figure 1 OMP subtypes as analyzed by SDS-polyacrylamide gelelectrophoresis. Only the relevant part of the gel is shown. A, subtypes described by Barenkamp et al. (23); B, by Van Alphen et al. (1).

proteins. The results depend on pretreatment of the samples before they are applied on the gel, since proteins a (P1) and d (P5) are heat-modifiable and since protein b,c (P2) sometimes appears as multiple bands when unheated. Maximum resolution is obtained by analyzing samples boiled in SDS as well as samples treated at 37°C. About 30 different OMP patterns have been recognized among Hib strains. These include 21 different subtypes described by Barenkamp et al. for Hib isolates from patients with invasive disease in the United States (23–25). We have described nine different subtypes, which are partly identical to the subtypes described by Barenkamp (1). In Table 1 these subtyping systems are compared. The two subtyping systems are mutually exchangeable.

The H(eavy or high position in gel), L(ight or low position in gel), or U(nclassified or intermediate position in gel) in the system described by Barenkamp et al. indicates the position of protein a (P1) (23). The small differences in the genes for the H, L, and U forms of OMP a (P1) are located in three regions (26). All L-type strains react with monoclonal antibody 5HA5 (27). Numerical analysis of these protein patterns now adds to our knowledge of the relationship between the various subtypes (28).

C. Lipopolysaccharides

Diversity has been found in LPSs of *H. influenzae* with respect to sugar composition, electrophoretic mobility in SDS-polyacrylamide gels, and

Table 1 Characteristic Features of the Major Outer Membrane Protein Subtypes of *Haemophilus influenzae* Type b

OMP subtype[a]	Major ET[b]	*capb*[c] RFLP	BT	LPS
1L (1c)	1.9	G	I	ND
	12.8, 21.8	G	I	1
1H	1.9	G	I	ND
2L (2)	1.9		I	2
3L (1)	12.5, 12.8	S	I,II	1
6U (3)	25.6	S	II	10
8H	235	O	I	ND
13L	21.6	S	I	ND

[a]Nomenclature according to the system described by Barenkamp et al. (23,24). The figures between brackets indicate the subtypes in the system described by van Alphen et al. (1).
[b]Electrophoretic typing (ET) data from Musser et al. (35)
[c]Restriction fragment length polymorphism (RFLP) of the *capb* locus from Ref. 34. ND, not determined.

antigenic properties. The gel profiles are not epidemiologically stable markers (29). This is caused by variation in the transcription of genes involved in the biosynthesis of LPS (30) and by phenotypic variation depending on the presence of some metabolites in the medium (31). Despite these variations, Hib isolates express under standard laboratory conditions stable epitopes which appeared to be useful epidemiological markers. All different LPSs contain the same sugars, namely *N*-acetyl-glucosamine, galactose, glucose, and L-glycero-D-mannoheptose, although in varying ratios. These epitopes are recognized by a set of serotype specific polyclonal and monoclonal antibodies. Ten serotypes have been described, but a considerable number of Hib strains are nontypeable (32).

IV. METHODS FOR THE ANALYSIS OF VIRULENCE PROPERTIES

Epidemiological data are available on virulence factors that enable Hib to colonize the mucosa and survive in the blood. These suggest that the capsular polysaccharide contributes strongly to the survival of the bacterium in the tissues and the circulation in the absence of specific antibodies. Other factors seem also to be important. These include LPS, IgA protease, and fimbriae (33). Galactose is an important sugar in LPS, since Hib with galactoseless LPS has reduced virulence in the infant rat model. In addition, LPS is an important immunomodulator. Fimbriae promote bacterial colonization in the nasopharynx and may play a role in tissue tropism of Hib. *H. influenzae* IgA protease degrades immunoglobulin IgA1, that is, the predominant immunoglobulin subclass on the mucosa of the respiratory tract.

A number of factors have been described in relation to virulence of *H. influenzae* that have not been analyzed epidemiologically. They include a mucinase, a ciliotoxin, iron-repressible proteins, and heat shock proteins.

A. Restriction Fragment Length Polymorphism of *Capb* Genes

The genetic relationship between encapsulated *H. influenzae* was studied with RFLP analysis of the *H. influenzae* chromosome after restriction endonuclease digestion followed by DNA hybridization with a probe containing the *capb* genes (34). These genes are involved in the synthesis of the type b capsule. The genes for other capsule types of *H. influenzae* cross-hybridize with this probe. Fourteen distinct but closely related chromosomal restriction fragment length polymorphism (RFLP) patterns were identified (34,35). All RFLPs are serotype specific. Allen et al. (34) showed that three RLFPs cover 96% of *H. influenzae* type b strains from all over the world. Each RFLP was associated with its own distinctive set of OMP subtypes and ETs, indicating that they are closely related, thereby strongly supporting the clonal hypothesis (35).

It has now become clear that nontypable *H. influenzae* strains do not produce capsules, since their DNA does not hybridize with genes required for capsule production (34,35). Encapsulated strains sometimes become nonencapsulated by deletions in the *capb* region of their chromosome (36). These "nontypable" strains represent a minority in each pure culture of *H. influenzae* type b, but are rare in nature.

B. Immunoglobulin IgA_1 Protease

Clinial isolates lacking an IgA_1 protease are rare. Since all *H. influenzae* type b strains share the same enzyme, this method is not suitable for typing (38). Nonencapsulated strains have 15 different proteins (37).

C. Fimbriae

Fimbriae on the surface of *H. influenzae* facilitate the interaction of the bacteria with the mucosa of the upper respiratory tract and protect the bacteria against mucociliary clearance. Brinton's group has identified four families of fimbriae with different morphologies (38). LKP fimbriae have been analyzed in great detail. They mediate adherence to oropharyngeal epithelial cells and to those cells in tissue sections that are affected by *H. influenzae* during colonization and infection. Bacteria not expressing these fimbriae have an impaired ability to colonize the nasopharynx of monkeys (39). The gene cluster coding for LKP-4 fimbriae has been cloned and partially sequenced (40). More than 14 different LKP serotypes have been recognized, indicating the presence of type-specific epitopes. These antigenic differences may become the basis of a classification system (38).

V. WORLDWIDE DISTRIBUTION OF Hib STRAINS

The most discriminatory methods for the molecular epidemiological analysis of Hib are OMP subtyping and ETyping. The number of OMP subtypes of Hib is larger than the number of ETs, indicating that strains of a particular ET may have different OMP subtypes. Since ETs are markers for clones (see Chapter 9), a particular clone of Hib may express different OMPs. The reverse is also true, since all major OMP subtypes occur among various clones. Most of the OMP subtypes were in one or two groups of ETs, thereby indicating their clonal structure (35). These clones share many of the characteristics described above (Table 1). The observation that strains belonging to one ET have various OMP subtypes indicates that horizontal exchange of DNA between the clones during evolution contributed to genetic diversity of Hib. Therefore, typing based on OMPs and ETs is in general sufficient to our understanding of the epidemiology of Hib disease. However, these additional typing characteristics may help to discriminate between closely related strains (clones). OMP 2L strains isolated in Iceland were differentiated, for instance, from OMP 2L strains in Finland by LPS serotyping (41).

The most frequently occurring subtypes and the other characteristics of the strains of the subtypes are summarized in Table 1 and the worldwide distribution of the subtypes in Table 2. Five of the 21 OMP subtypes occurring in the United States account for 87% of all Hib isolates (25). The common subtypes [1H, 2L (2), and 3L (1)] appeared more or less randomly distributed over the country in contrast to some of the less common subtypes (24). Subtype 4H strains comprised 24% of isolates from patients in Denver, Colorado, but were rare in the rest of the United States (24). In metropolitan Atlanta, Georgia, 90% of all isolates belonged to one subtype (42). Outside the United States the number of subtypes causing disease in a country is very limited. In The Netherlands more than 80% of all Hib isolates obtained from patients with meningitis were of one subtype (subtype 1, identical to 3L) (43). Subtype 1 (3L) strains are responsible for 15% of the disease isolates in the United States (25). It is the common subtype in Western Europe, except in Iceland (41).

Table 2 Distribution of the Most Predominantly OMP Subtypes on the Continents

OMP subtype	North America	South America	Europe	Asia	Africa	Australia
1H	74	—	2	—	—	—
1L	15	—	48	17	2	19
2H	8	—	1	—	—	—
2L	64	2	44[a]	4	13	—
3L	75	1	238	28	5	19
6U	11	1	3	11	4	1
8H	7	—	—	—	—	—
13L	30	—	—	2	—	1
Total	284	4	336	62	24	40

Data derived from data listed in Ref. 35, supplemented with data for The Netherlands (43) and Finland (9). It is important to note that strong differences exist in the distribution between countries (see text).

[a]Including 11 strains from Iceland, which represent a special clone (41).

Subtype 1 strains comprise not only the great majority of the European Hib isolates, but 80% of the isolates in Australia. A minor difference between the protein mobility of OMP P2 of subtype 1 strains from Europe and from the United States (subtype 3L) was noted by Clements et al. (44). The Australian isolates were identical to the European reference strain. Since the other typing characterictics of the subtype 1 and 3L strains were previously shown to be identical, these subtypes are strongly related, if not identical (35). Although subtype 1 (3L) strains are distributed worldwide, they are absent in Africa (The Gambia, Kenya, Nigeria) with the exception of South Africa, and in defined areas like Iceland (41,45).

In Iceland 84% of all isolates are subtype 2 (2L), a subtype found worldwide. However, subtype 2 (2L) strains in Iceland are LPS-9, while isolates elsewhere are mainly LPS-2. The Icelandic subtype was also isolated in the Canadian Maritime provinces (35). The Icelandic and the Canadian Maritime population are distinct in origin from other Europeans. They probably share Celtic ancestry, suggesting that the subtype 2 (2L), LPS-9 subtype has established in populations of Celtic origin. Since until recently these populations were hardly intermingled by immigration, the subtype 2 (2L), LPS-9 strains probably have stabilized in that area. In Finland 21% of the isolates are subtype 1c (1L), which is a common subtype in the United States. Genetically these subtype 1c and 1 strains in Finland are closely related (ET 21.8 and 12.5) They differ in *capb* locus RFLP (G for subtype 1c and S for subtype 1), but they have the same biotype (I) and LPS serotype (1) (9,46).

The H-subtype strains (1H, 2H, and 8H) are mainly restricted to the United States. Since the H-subtype strains were absent among Hib isolates in the United States before 1954 (47), apparently the H-type OMP P1 (a) was introduced recently. This shows that the distribution of Hib subtypes can change strongly in a few decades. These H subtypes may be more virulent than the L subtypes. This change in the distribution of OMP subtypes is probably not caused by the mobility of the population, since the mobility of people between Europe and the United States has increased over recent decades without causing dramatic shifts in the distribution of the various clones. The clone with OMP subtype 1H is still rare in Europe. This may be because *H. influenzae* type b strains are exchanged primarily by children in a relatively narrow age range (4–7 years), and this age group has relatively low mobility compared to other age groups hardly carrying these bacteria. In this respect it is also intriguing that Iceland still has its own subtype (clone); tourism causes strong increases in the population during the summer, and many Icelanders stay on the mainland of Europe for months. Here, also, the exchange may be restricted to children of a narrow age range. Alternatively, host factors affecting colonization are important for the subtype distribution.

Isolates with the OMP subtype 6U (subtype 3) are rarely observed in Europe, Australia, and the United States, but predominate in Papua New Guinea (48% of isolates) and were also observed among the isolates from Thailand, Nigeria, and Kenya (45). This subtype seems to be distributed locally, since it was not found in the Gambia (27).

It can be concluded that in most countries one or a few subtypes are predominant. Strains with certain OMP subtypes do not spread easily across extended natural borders, like seas. The reason for this phenomenon may be that each population has its own stable reservoir of Hib strains (as in Iceland), that strains are genetically linked to certain populations, or that spread is low due to absence of close contacts between carriers.

VI. SUBTYPES OF Hib AS DISEASE MARKERS

Subtype 1c strains cause proportionally more meningitis and less epiglottitis than subtype 1 strains. Children with subtype 1c disease were mainly between 6 months and 2 years. These two characteristics associated with subtype 1c strains appeared to be statistically independent (46). Although these strains have minor differences in OMPs they are genetically more different as determined by electrophoretic typing. 83% of the subtype 1c (1L) strains are ET 21.8 and subtype 1 (3L) strains are ET 12.5 and ET 12.8 (9). The clone with OMP 13L and ET 21.8 represents a clone that is predominantly isolated from healthy carriers (48). Age dependent differences in subtype distribution have not been found when comparing patients below 5 years with patients older than 7 years. Patients with severe predisposing factors are infected significantly less by the common subtype of Hib. These patients are usually infected at greater than 7 years of age (49).

Subtype 6U strains have been reported to be associated significantly with cases among black children who attended day care (50). Edmonson et al. (51) found that recurrent infections are sometimes caused by the same subtype of Hib, indicating that these patients did not develop protective immunity.

Secondary cases in day care centers were caused by strains with the same subtype. Subtype 1H strains cause significantly more often secondary cases than others (51).

Hampton et al. (48) found similar subtypes in patients and in healthy carriers. Interestingly, Hib strains from carriers in an open population were significantly more often of subtype 13L than those from patients, suggesting that subtype 13L strains are less virulent than others (48). In a carrier study in Amsterdam it appeared that "rare" subtypes were isolated significantly more frequently among carriers than among patients (52) (Table 3). In the Gambia subtypes 5 and 9 were isolated from carriers more fre-

Table 3 Subtyping of Case and Carrier Strains of *H influenzae* b in Amsterdam and The Netherlands

Source of strains	Year of isolation	N	OMP subtype						
			1	1a	1b	1c	2	3	o[a]
Carriers (Amsterdam)	1987	24	12	3	3	1	2	1	2
Patients (Amsterdam)	1975–87	97	80	2	—	4	1	5	5
Patients (Netherlands)	1975–80	80	67	6	2	—	4	1	—
Patients (Netherlands)	1987	96	85	6	1	1	—	—	3

[a]o, other.

Source: Ref. 52.

quently than from patients (27). These results clearly indicate differences between disease and carrier isolates, although the subtypes causing disease are regularly found in the throat of healthy individuals. Since *H. influenzae* is a strictly human pathogen, such carriers can be regarded as the reservoir for the bacteria. Eradication of carriership will most likely prevent Hib disease. Therefore, data from vaccination trials in Finland yielding a decrease of the rate of carriership among vaccinees are exciting (53).

VII. SUBTYPE DISTRIBUTION OF ANTIBIOTIC RESISTANT Hib STRAINS

Comparison of the OMP subtypes of antibiotic resistant strains and of sensitive strains revealed a similar subtype distribution, indicating that *H. influenzae* type b randomly acquires plasmids coding for antibiotic resistance (54,55).

VIII. DISTRIBUTION OF Hib TYPES DURING VACCINATION

Isolates from Finnish Hib patients with systemic disease were collected prior to and during large-scale vaccinations with Hib conjugate vaccines (56). These strains were analyzed by OMP subtyping, LPS serotyping, and BT. Strains with OMP-BT-LPS combinations (clones) 1-I-1 and 1c-I-1 disappeared at the same rate as the disease they were associated with (Fig. 2). A preferential decrease in the number of isolates of a clone with OMP-BT-LPS 1-II-1 was recorded, whereas the reduction in disease caused by strains of OMP-BT-LPS 1-II-9 occurred at a lower rate than expected. The latter clone occurred mainly in the most densely populated area of Finland. Strains belonging to all the common Hib clones were isolated from the 16

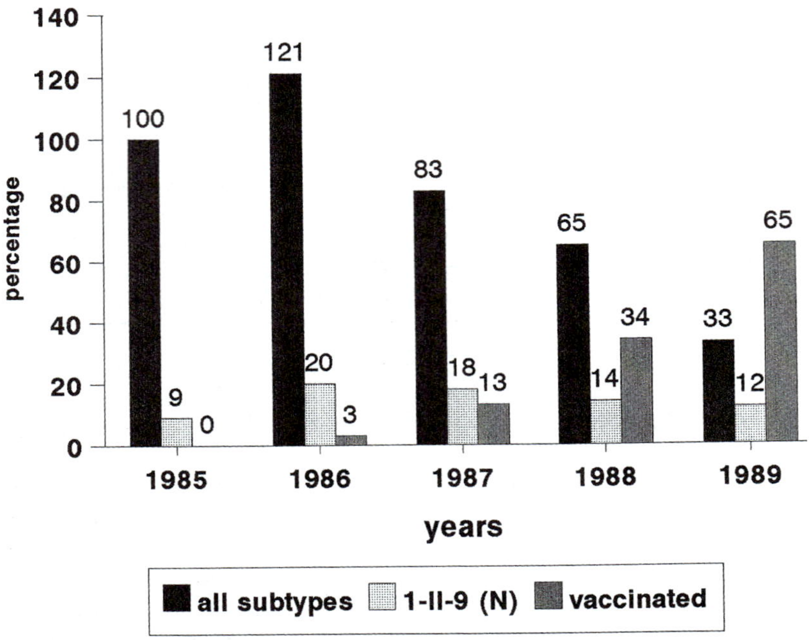

Figure 2 Effect of vaccination on the subtype distribution in Finland during vaccination. Data are derived from Re. 56.

infants who acquired Hib disease despite being (partially) vaccinated. Thus, Hib clones disappeared during mass vaccination with conjugate vaccines, although with different rates. Temporal changes in the distribution of some clones were also observed in the United States (57). The practical conclusion of the present study is that Hib conjugate vaccines were able to prevent invasive Hib disease in children in Finland, irrespective of the subtype (clone) of the Hib bacteria that causes the infection.

IX. CONCLUDING REMARKS

The characteristics of *H. influenzae* type b analyzed include general characteristics like outer membrane protein composition, biotypes, DNA restriction fragments, and also virulence determinants, such as fimbriae, IgA1-protease, capsular polysaccharides, and lipopolysaccharide. Strains that cause spontaneous invasive disease belong to a limited number of clones. These clones have distinct OMP patterns and ETs. These clones probably share all the requirements for full virulence. Clones of less common ETs and OMP subtypes are more probably less virulent and are thereby isolated more often from carriers than from patients. Among the more virulent clones differences were observed in disease specificity and epidemiological characteristics. These observations hint us to the bacterial components that influence the disease process. This is a challenge for the future research on the pathogenesis of *H. influenzae* type b disease.

REFERENCES

1. L. van Alphen and H. Bijlmer, Molecular epidemiology of *Haemophilus influenzae* type b, *Paediatrics 85*(Suppl.):S636 (1990).
2. J. I. Ward, M. K. Lum, D. B. Hall, et al., Invasive *Haemophilus influenzae* type b disease in Alaska: background epidemiology for a vaccine efficacy trial, *J. Infect. Dis. 153*:17 (1986).
3. A. K. Takala, J. Eskola, H. Peltola, and P. H. Mäkelä, Epidemiology of invasive *Haemophilus influenzae* type b disease among children in Finland before vaccination with *Haemophilus influenzae* type b conjugate vaccine, *Pediatr. Infect. Dis. 8*:297 (1989).
4. B. Greenwood, Epidemiology of acute lower respiratory tract infections, especially those due to *Haemophilus influenzae* type b, in The Gambia, West Africa, *J. Infect. Dis. 165*(Suppl.):S26 (1992).
5. M. Kilian, A taxonomic study on the genus *Haemophilus*, with the proposal of a new species, *J. Gen. Microbiol. 93*:9 (1976).
6. T. R. Oberhofer and A. E. Back, Biotypes of *Haemophilus* encountered in clinical laboratories, *J. Clin. Microbiol. 10*:168 (1979).
7. M. Gratten, *Haemophilus influenzae* biotype VII, *J. Clin. Microbiol 18*:1015 (1983).
8. F. O. Sottnek, and W. L. Albritton, *Haemophilus influenzae* biotype VIII, *J. Clin. Microbiol. 20*:815 (1984).
9. A. K. Takala, L. van Alphen, J. M. Musser, L. Geelen, R. Selander, J. Eskola, and P. H. Mäkelä, Bacteriological epidemiology of *Haemophilus influenzae* type b strains causing invasive disease in Finland, *J. Infect. Dis. 160*:237 (1989).
10. K. Groeneveld, L. van Alphen, P. P. Eijk, H. M. Jansen, and H. C. Zanen, Changes in outer membrane proteins of nontypable *Haemophilus influenzae* in patients with chronic obstructive pulmonary disease, *J. Infect. Dis. 158*:360 (1988).
11. K. D. Bruce and J. Z. Jordens, Characterization of noncapsulate *Haemophilus influenzae* by whole-cell polypeptide profiles, restriction endonuclease analysis, and rRNA gene restriction patterns, *J. Clin. Microbiol. 29*:291 (1991).
13. D. M. Granoff and R. S. Munson, Prospects for prevention of *Haemophilus influenzae* type b disease by immunization, *J. Infect. Dis. 153*:448 (1986).
14. M. R. Loeb and D. H. Smith, Outer membrane protein composition in disease isolates of *Haemophilus influenzae*: pathogenic and epidemiological implications, *Infect. Immun. 30*:709 (1980).

15. L. van Alphen, T. Riemens, J. Poolman, and H. C. Zanen, Characteristics of major outer membrane proteins of *Haemophilus influenzae*, *J. Bacteriol. 155*:878 (1983).
16. R. Munson, Jr. and R. W. Tolan, Jr. Molecular cloning, expression, and primary sequence of outer membrane protein P2 of *Haemophilus influenzae* type b, *Infect. Immun. 57*:88 (1989).
17. V. Vachon, D. J. Lyew, and J. W. Coulton, Transmembrane permeability channels across the outer membrane of *Haemophilus influenzae* type b, *J. Bacteriol. 162*:918 (1985).
18. L. van Alphen, T. Riemens, and H. C. Zanen, Antibody response against outer membrane components of *Haemophilus influenzae* type b strains in patients with meningitis, *FEMS Microbiol. Lett. 18*:189 (1983).
19. D. J. Sikkema, M. B. Nelson, M. A. Apicella, and T. F. Murphy, Outer membrane protein P6 of *Haemophilus influenzae* binds to its own gene, *Molecul. Microbiol. 6*:547 (1992).
20. B. A. Green, T. Guinn-Dey, and G. W. Zlotnick, Biological activities of antibody to a peptidoglycan-associated lipoprotein of *Haemophilus influenzae* against multiple clinical isolates of *H. influenzae* type b, *Infect. Immun. 55*:2878 (1987).
21. L. van Alphen, L. Geelen-van den Broek, and M. van Ham, *In vivo* and *in vitro* expression of outer membrane components of *Haemophilus influenzae*, *Mol. Pathogen. 8*:279 (1990).
22. E. J. Hansen, C. F. Frisch, and K. H. Johnston, Detection of antibody-accessible proteins on the cell surface of *Haemophilus influenzae* type b, *Infect. Immun. 33*:950 (1981).
23. S. J. Barenkamp, R. S. Munson, and D. M. Granoff, Subtyping isolates of *Haemophilus influenzae* type b by outer-membrane protein profiles, *J. Infect. Dis. 143*:668 (1981).
24. D. M. Granoff, S. J. Barenkamp, and R. S. Munson, Outer membrane protein subtypes for investigation of *Haemophilus influenzae* type b disease, *Haemophilus influenzae* (S. H. Sell and P. F. Wright, eds.), Elsevier Science Publishing Co., Inc., New York, 1982), p. 43.
25. S. J. Barenkamp, R. S. Munson, and D. M. Granoff, Comparison of outer-membrane protein subtypes and biotypes of isolates of *Haemophilus influenzae* type b, *J. Infect. Dis. 144*:480 (1981).
26. R. S. Munson, B. Brodeur, P. Chong, S. Grass, D. Martin, and C. Proulx, Outer membrane proteins P1 and P2 of *Haemophilus influenzae* type b: structure and identification of surface-exposed epitopes, *J. Infect. Dis. 165* (Suppl.):S86 (1992).
27. H. A. Bijlmer, L. van Alphen, L. Geelen-van den Broek, B. M. Greenwood, H. A. Vakenburg, and J. Dankert, Molecular epidemiology of *Haemophilus influenzae* type b in the Gambia, *J. Clin. Microbiol. 30*:386 (1992).
28. J. A. Elliott, G. S. Bosley, G. M. Carlone, B. D. Plikaitis, and R. R. Facklam, Separation of *Haemophilus influenzae* type b subtypes by numerical analysis, *J. Clin. Microbiol. 25*:1476 (1987).
29. R. W. Tolan, R. S. Munson, and D. M. Granoff, Lipopolysaccharide gel

profiles of *Haemophilus influenzae* type b are not stable epidemiological markers, *J. Clin. Microbiol. 24*:223 (1986).
30. J. N. Weiser, J. M. Love, and E. R. Moxon, The molecular mechanism of phase variation of *H. influenzae* lipopolysaccharide, *Cell 59*:657 (1989).
31. M. R. Loeb, M. Kuratana, and P. Anderson, Cell surface changes in *Haemophilus influenzae* type b associated with a phenotypic increase in resistance to bactericidal antibody, *J. Infect. Dis. 165* (Suppl.):S110 (1992).
32. L. van Alphen, M. Klein, L. Geelen-van den Broek, T. Riemens, P. Eijk, and H. Kamerlingh. Biochemical characterization and worldwide distribution of serologically distinct lipopolysaccharides of *Haemophilus influenzae* type b, *J. Infect. Dis. 162*:659 (1990).
33. E. R. Moxon, Molecular basis of invasive *Haemophilus influenzae* type b disease, *J. Infect. Dis.* 165 (Suppl.):S77 (1992).
34. I. Allen, M. R. Loeb, and E. R. Moxon, Limited genetic diversity of *Haemophilus influenzae* (type b), *Microbiol. Pathogen. 2*:139 (1987).
35. J. M. Musser, J. S. Kroll, D. M. Granoff, E. R. Moxon, B. R. Brodeur, J. Campos, et al., Global genetic structure and molecular epidemiology of encapsulated *Haemophilus influenzae*, *Rev. Infect. Dis. 12*:75 (1990).
36. S. K. Hoiseth and J. R. Gilsdorf, The relationship between type b and nontypable *Haemophilus influenzae* isolated from the same patient, *J. Infect. Dis.* 158:643 (1988).
37. M. Kilian, J. Mestecky, and M. W. Russell, Defense mechanisms involving Fc-dependent functions of immunoglogulin A and their subversion by bacterial immunoglobulin A proteases, *Microbiol. Rev. 52*:296 (1988).
38. C. C. Brinton, M. J. Carter, D. B. Derber, S. Kar, J. A. Kramarik, C-C Agenes, and S. W. Wood, Design and development of pilus vaccines for *Haemophilus influenzae* disease, *Pediatr. Infect. Dis. 8*:S54 (1989).
39. A. Weber, K. Harris, S. Lohrke, L. Forney, and A. L. Smith, Inability to express fimbriae results in impaired ability of *Haemophilus influenzae* b to colonize the nasopharynx, *Infect. Immun. 59*:4724 (1991).
40. S. M. van Ham, L. van Alphen, and F. R. Mooi, Fimbria-mediated adherence and hemagglutination of *Haemophilus influenzae*, *J. Infect. Dis. 165* (Suppl.):S97 (1992).
41. L. van Alphen, L. Geelen, K. Jónsdóttir, A. K. Takala, H. Kayhty, and H. C. Zanen, Distinct geographical distribution of subtypes of *Haemophilus influenzae* type b in western Europe, *J. Infect. Dis. 156*:216 (1987).
42. J. A. Elliott, N. Pigott, S. L. Cochi, and R. R. Facklam, Major subtypes of invasive *Haemophilus influenzae* from 1983 to 1985 in Atlanta, Ga, *J. Clin. Microbiol. 28*:833 (1990).
43. L. van Alphen, T. Riemens, J, Poolman, C. Hopman, and H. C. Zanen, Homogeneity of cell envelope protein subtypes, lipopolysaccharide serotypes, and biotypes among *Haemophilus influenzae* type b from patients with meningitis in The Netherlands, *J. Infect. Dis. 148*:75 (1983).
44. D. A. Clements, S. J. MacInnes, and G. L. Gilbert, Outer membrane protein subtypes of *Haemophilus influenzae* type b isolates causing invasive disease in Victoria, Australia, from 1988 to 1990, *J. Clin. Microbiol. 30*:1879 (1992).

45. R. S. Munson, M. H. Kabeer, A. A. Lenoir, and D. M. Granoff, Epidemiology and prospects for prevention of disease due to *Haemophilus influenzae* in developing countries, *Rev. Infect. Dis. 11*(Suppl.):S588 (1989).
46. A. K. Takala, L. van Alphen, J. Eskola, J. Palmgren, P. Bol, and P. H. Mäkelä, *Haemophilus influenzae* type b strains of outer membrane subtype 1 and 1c cause different types of disease, *Lancet ii*:647 (1987).
47. S. J. Barenkamp, D. M. Granoff, and M. Pittman, Outer membrane protein subtypes and biotypes of *Haemophilus influenzae* type b: relation between strains isolated in 1934–1954 and 1977–1980, *J. Infect. Dis. 148*:1127 (1983).
48. C. M. Hampton, S. J. Barenkamp, and D. M. Granoff, Comparion of outer membrane protein subtypes of *Haemophilus influenzae* type b isolates from healthy children in the general population and from diseased patients, *J. Clin. Microbiol. 18*:596 (1983).
49. L. van Alphen, A. van Dam, P. Bol, L. Spanjaard, and H. C. Zanen, Types and subtypes of 73 strains of *Haemophilus influenzae* isolated from patients more than 6 years of age with meningitis in The Netherlands, *J. Infect. 15*:95 (1987).
50. T. V. Murphy, M. T. Osterholm, L. M. Pierson, K. E. White, J. A. Breedlove, G. B. Seibert, J. N. Kuritsky, and D. M. Granoff, Prospective surveillance of *Haemophilus influenzae* type b disease in Dallas County, Texas and in Minnesota, *Pediatrics 79*:173 (1987).
51. M. B. Edmonson, D. M. Granoff, S. J. Barenkamp, and P. J. Chesney, Outer membrane protein subtypes and investigation of recurrent *Haemophilus influenzae* type b disease, *J. Pediatrics. 100*:202 (1982).
52. L. van Alphen, P. Bol, M. L. K. Kok, and L. Geelen-van den Broek, Differences in subtype distribution of *Haemophilus influenzae* type b from carriers in the general population and patients with meningitis, *J. Med. Microbiol. 34*:313 (1991).
53. A. K. Takala, J. Eskola, M. Leinonen, H. Käyhty, A. Nissinen, E. Pekkanen, and P. H. Mäkelä, Reduction of oropharyngeal carriage of *Haemophilus influenzae* type b (Hib) in children immunized with an Hib conjugate vaccine, *J. Infect. Dis. 164*:982 (1991).
54. J. Campos, S. Garcia-Tornel, J. M. Musser, et al., Molecular epidemiology of multiple resistant *Haemophilus influenzae* type b in day care centers, *J. Infect. Dis. 156*:483 (1987).
55. L. van Alphen, L. A. Arends, T. Riemens, and L. Geelen, Comparison of antibiotic-resistant and -sensitive strains of *Haemophilus influenzae* type b by outer membrane protein subtyping, *Eur. J. Clin. Microbiol. 7*:309 (1988).
56. L. van Alphen, A. K. Takala, L. Geelen-van den Broek, J. Dankert, and J. Eskola, Changes in the distribution of *Haemophilus influenzae* type b clones associated with widespread infant vaccination in Finland, *J. Infect. Dis. 166*:1340 (1992).
57. D. M. Granoff, K. Sheetz, J. P. Pandey, M. H. Nahm, J. H. Rambeck, et al., Host and bacterial factors associated with *Haemophilus influenzae* type b disease in Minnesota children vaccinated with type b polysaccharide vaccine, *J. Infect. Dis. 159*:908 (1989).

8

Molecular Aspects of the Pathogenesis of Invasive *Haemophilus influenzae* Type b Infections

John Simon Kroll and Paul Richard Langford

St. Mary's Hospital Medical School, London, England

I. INVASIVE *HAEMOPHILUS INFLUENZAE* TYPE b INFECTION: THE PATHOGENETIC SEQUENCE

Haemophilus influenzae type b is a normal colonist of the human upper respiratory tract, where it is found in 3–5% of the healthy population (1). Its clinical significance rests almost entirely in its capacity to cause problems in other locations. Infections, at times life-threatening, may arise through superficial spread of organisms to a contiguous site, a possible mode of infection in epiglottitis and bacterial pneumonia, or by invasion of the bloodstream and bacteremic dissemination to distant sites, as occurs in septic arthritis and meningitis.

In order to survive in the relatively hostile environment of the ciliated, mucus-covered, immunoglobulin-coated, phagocyte-endowed human upper respiratory tract and in the desiccating void it must traverse to spread to a new host, the organism possesses characteristics that, viewed from a human perspective, are defined as determinants of virulence when their action leads to spread from the nasopharynx and/or disease (Table 1). Such bacterial factors may interfere with the successful clearance of organisms from the mucosal surface, increase the risk that they penetrate that surface to enter the bloodstream, enhance microbial survival within that compartment, facilitate infection of further normally sterile sites such as the meninges, or lead in any location to release of host factors damaging to the

Table 1 Established and Putative Determinants of Virulence of *H. influenzae* Type b

Capsular polysaccharide
Lipooligosaccharide (LOS)
Fimbriae
IgA-protease
Peptidoglycan
Outer-membrane proteins
Iron-acquisition proteins
Hemocin

tissues. In this chapter we describe the pathogenetic sequence of natural human invasive infection with *H. influenzae* type b, recently reviewed by Stephens and Farley (2), identifying microbial determinants with established or supposed parts to play in the process of infection, and then go on to consider the molecular nature of individual bacterial components in greater detail.

Organisms of *H. influenzae* type b are spread between individuals in respiratory secretions, transmitted as airborne droplets or by direct contact (1). In the case of *Neisseria meningitidis*, the risk that infection will arise in a susceptible individual is related to inoculum size (3). Experimental infection of infant rats and of human nasopharyngeal tissue in organ culture suggests the same to be true of *H. influenzae* type b (4–6). Microbial components that enhance environmental survival, and undefined factors that may increase the intensity of bacterial multiplication in the nasopharynx, are therefore determinants of virulence at this stage.

On arrival on the mucosal surface of the upper respiratory tract, the first host defense that bacteria encounter is mucus. This forms a viscoelastic gel 2–5 μm-thick (7), which protects the underlying epithelium from microbial contact and is kept in continuous cephalad motion by the action of underlying ciliated cells (the mucociliary escalator), tending to clear bacteria out of the system. Nonetheless, organisms of *H. influenzae* type b associate avidly with mucus (2). Mucus consists of a complex hydrated mixture of glycoproteins, immunoglobulins IgG and IgA, and further uncharacterized components; the factor(s) responsible for association with *Haemophilus* have not been identified. Neither microbial fimbriae nor capsule appear critical for this interaction in the nasopharyngeal organ culture system. The part played by mucosal IgA in the balance between microbial clearance and persistent infection appears to be complex. *H. influenzae* type b organisms, in common with the other potentially invasive respiratory tract pathogens *N. meningitidis* and *Streptococcus pneumoniae*, secretes a protein with

IgA_1-protease activity (8), and this enzyme may be a factor facilitating colonization. The enzyme cleaves human IgA_1 in the hinge region of the α chain to yield separate Fab and Fc portions (9). Fab fragments retain their antigen-binding capacity, and it has been proposed that, through their production, bacterial IgA_1 protease may subvert host defenses dependent on recognition of IgA-Fc attached to organisms (10). Experiments to demonstrate the importance of such a mechanism in the pathogenic behavior of *Haemophilus* have so far been frustrated by the specificity of the enzyme for the antibody of humans and higher primates.

As well as associating with mucus, *H. influenzae* type b interferes with the effective action of the mucociliary escalator by disrupting the function of the ciliated columnar epithelium. Shortly after nasopharyngeal tissue explants are exposed to organisms in vitro, there is a slowing and disorganization of ciliary activity, and ciliated cells are later extruded from the surface. These events are not mediated by attachment of bacteria to the epithelial surface or directly to cilia (4,5). A low molecular weight, heat-stable bacterial component of uncertain identity has been implicated (11). There are conflicting data on the importance of lipooligosaccharide (LOS) in this process, whether acting directly on the epithelium or indirectly by stimulating the release of tissue-damaging cytokines. A suggestion that peptidoglycan fragments released from the *Haemophilus* cell wall may be the main cause of ciliary slowing awaits experimental confirmation (12).

Having negotiated the mucociliary escalator, *H. influenzae* type b attaches to the mucosal epithelial surface, associating selectively with nonciliated cells (4,5). Fimbriated and nonfimbriated organisms show a different pattern of association with the surface (5,13). Fimbriated bacteria adhere in substantial clusters all over the surface of the cell, while nonfimbriated organisms, which may have arisen from fimbriated isoforms elsewhere on the surface by phase variation (see below) or may have arrived independently at the surface, are seen in small numbers close to intercellular junctions (5). These different patterns of adherence may be of pathogenic significance, for invasion of *H. influenzae* type b occurs principally between separated tight junctions, and the invading organisms are nonfimbriated (14). This process of nasopharyngeal epithelial invasion appears to be the principal route by which *H. influenzae* type b strains reach the circulation (14). The mechanism by which organisms in the subepithelial space subsequently penetrate the pharyngeal capillary plexus is not known, but once in the bloodstream, bacterial polysaccharide capsule and LOS (discussed in detail below) appear to play a critical role in perpetuating bacteremia (15). These bacterial components endow organisms with antiphagocytic properties, and the result is a higher level of sustained bacteremia, which appears to be the critical factor determining whether the blood-brain barrier (BBB) is penetrated (16). There is no evidence for specific bacterial tropism for cerebral capillary endothelium or for structures in the vascular bed of the choroid plexus, where initial central nervous sytem infection is thought to occur (17). The means by which bacteria extravasate through capillary endothelium is an area of active research. An interaction resembling coiling phagocytosis of *Haemophilus* by an endothelial cell has been observed electron-micrographically in vitro (18), but its importance relative to the nonspecific action of LOS (discussed below) in increasing BBB permeability, or to other so far undefined processes, is uncertain.

From this discussion it should be apparent that the final outcome following the arrival of organisms of *H. influenzae* type b in the human nasopharynx is highly unpredictable. The possession by organisms of an array of factors that can modulate the effect of host defenses may under different circumstances lead to colonization or to invasive infection. It is still not known whether the first is a necessary precursor of the second. The dynamics of experimental infection indicate that organisms with an invasive phenotype can arise within a colonizing population during an incubation phase (see Sec. II.), but it remains possible that natural invasive infection may result from the arrival of small numbers of organisms already expressing an invasive phenotype. It is a striking observation that invasive infection in experimental animals may arise as the result of survival of a single organism from the infecting inoculum (19). The concatenation of events required to lead to invasive infection from the nasopharynx is clearly highly unlikely.

II. FIMBRIAE

Many clinical isolates of *H. influenzae* type b possess surface fimbriae (pili) which, by analogy with other gram-negative organisms, are candidate structures for mediating adherence to host cells. Of four families distinguished on morphological and functional criteria by Brinton et al. (20), the most extensively studied are α fimbriae: nonflagellar filamentous protein appendages 450 nm or more in length and $\approx$5 nm broad, composed of an array of identical $\approx$24 kilodaltons (kD) subunits (pilin molecules) arranged with helical symmetry and speculatively associated with various minor protein components (see Sec. III.C.). Considerable antigenic variation occurs. More than 14 serotypes are known, and immunological studies with intact fimbriae and denatured pilin molecules have demonstrated both type-specific epitopes and others relatively conserved between strains (20,21). While epitopes that are highly conserved between strains are immunodominant when denatured fimbrial subunits are studied, these are not generally accessible to antibody when assembled in fimbriae. Moderately conserved epitopes found on assembled fimbriae of different strains appear to be conformationally dependent, composed of separated tracts of amino acids brought together in the tertiary/quaternary structure of fimbriae (21). In addition to this antigenic variation, α fimbriae are inconstantly expressed, showing phase variation in vitro and in vivo at a frequency of 10^{-4} (5,22).

A. Fimbriae in Host-Parasite Interactions

The relevance of fimbriae to adhesion is demonstrated by the fact that fimbriated *Haemophilus* can be enriched from a phase-varied mixture of fimbriated and nonfimbriated organisms by their capacity to bind to various host cells, including erythrocytes to which they attach via the AnWj antigen (23). The epithelial cell receptor for *Haemophilus* α fimbriae has been partially characterized as containing a sialyl-lactosyl-ceramide structure (24). It is distinct from, though related to, the AnWj blood group antigen, and the two receptors appear to have a common genetic origin (25).

Fimbriae-specific and tissue-specific interactions have been demonstrated between *H. influenzae* type b organisms and human cells, supporting the hypothesis that tissue tropism during colonization and infection might be mediated by fimbriae. Fimbriated variants show increased binding to human oropharyngeal cells in vitro compared to their nonfimbriated counterparts (26,27). Fimbriated organisms bind densely in vitro to upper respiratory tract epithelium and to pulmonary epithelial cells, but only sparsely to kidney or liver cells, and these interactions are inhibited by a fimbriae-specific monoclonal antibody (mAb) (28). A further specific interaction has been suggested between α fimbriae and respiratory mucus (28a).

While fimbriae seem to be involved in the colonization process, it is not clear that they play a part in the pathogenesis of invasive infection. Studies using the infant rat model have the major drawback that the specific interaction between α-fimbriated bacteria and pharyngeal epithelium found in humans is not present. A highly unusual type b strain, genetically divergent from the main bacterial population (29), does, however, show specific binding to infant rat oropharyngeal cells, and with this strain more efficient nasal colonization was found after challenge with the fimbriated variant (30). In nasal washings from colonized animals, however, nonfimbriated organisms greatly predominated. Nasopharyngeal epithelial cells of Rhesus monkeys are bound specifically by α-fimbriated type b strains, allowing studies of experimental infections that more closely resemble human disease. In a recent study, intranasal infection with 10^3 fimbriated organisms was followed after several days by bacteraemia and meningitis (A. Smith, personal communication). However, in the "incubation" period, sampling of the nasopharyngeal flora revealed a gradual switch of the population from α-fimbriated to non–α-fimbriated, and only the latter organisms were isolated from blood or cerebrospinal fluid (CSF). This result parallels the consistent and striking observation in humans that organisms isolated from blood or CSF are devoid of α fimbriae. Such observations have led to the hypothesis that type b strains with α fimbriae may have a survival advantage in initial colonization through their specific adhesive properties, but derive later benefit from losing their fimbriae, perhaps as the result of phase variation. Such an advantage might be a heightened ability to avoid phagocytosis by neutrophils or cells of the reticulo-endothelial system (31).

Studies in which a non–α-fimbriated mutant of *H. influenzae* type b strain Eagan, constructed by interruption of the pilin gene (see Sec. II.B.), has been compared with its wild-type parent, showed that specific adherence to human epithelial cells was reduced 10- to 100-fold and that there was a 10-fold reduction in nasopharyngeal colonization density in Rhesus monkeys (22). Experiments are in progress to determine whether this mutation impairs the capacity of organisms to cause invasive infection (A. Smith, personal communication).

Very little is known of the recently described β fimbriae (32). In contrast to α fimbriae, they are also found on bloodstream and CSF isolates, though simultaneous expression of the two types has not been observed. Further studies are awaited to establish whether this second type of pilus is important in colonization or disease, and what role other fimbriae and nonfimbrial adhesins (13,33) play in *Haemophilus* pathogenicity.

B. Genetics of Fimbriation

Several groups have cloned and sequenced the gene for the major α-fimbrial subunit (*hifA*) from different type b strains of *H. influenzae* (34–37). The genes from strains Eagan and M43 both encode a prepilin with identical 20-amino-acid leader peptides, but show 16% nucleotide sequence divergence (35). Consistent with the antigenic diversity of fimbriae demonstrated by immunological methods, the deduced protein sequences of the mature pilins show 22% divergence, though there is overall biochemical similarity over 95% of the sequence when "conservative" substitutions are taken into account.

Van Ham et al. (34) expressed *H. influenzae* type b fimbrial genes in *Escherichia coli* from a large segment of DNA cloned on a cosmid and showed that the resulting strain expressed *Haemophilus* fimbriae and adhered to human oropharyngeal epithelial cells. Further analysis of the cloned DNA has shown that the pilin structural gene, *hifA*, is expressed divergently from a cluster of at least four other genes, *hifBCDE* (L. van Alphen, personal communication). The *hifB* protein has substantial similarity to *E. coli* PapD, the molecular chaperone mediating transfer of pilin subunits from the inner to the outer membrane (38), and *E. coli* PapD expressed in *H. influenzae* type b restores piliation to a *hifB* mutant, a result that strongly suggests that these genes are homologous (A. Smith, personal communication). Other *hif* genes are thought to encode the fimbrial anchor and minor pilins including the putative adhesin. The divergent promoter regions of *hifA* and *hifB* overlap and are remarkable for a run of repeats of the dinucleotide TA between the respective −35 and −10 motifs. This repeat appears to form the molecular substrate for phase variation in the expression of α fimbriae. Amplification of the region by the polymerase chain reaction from cells of different phases of fimbriation has shown heavily fimbriated cells to have $(TA)_{10}$ in the promoter region and nonfimbriated variants $(TA)_9$ (38a). Thus the TA-copy number varies, through a presumed slip-strand mispairing mechanism, so as to alter the separation of these motifs and thus alter the efficiency with which the region can bind RNA polymerase and so lead to pilin synthesis.

III. LIPOOLIGOSACCHARIDE

The LOS of *H. influenzae* type b contains lipid A linked via 2-keto-3-deoxy-*manno*-octulosonic acid (KDO) to a short antennated oligosaccharide, analogous to the core oligosaccharide of lipopolysaccharide (LPS) in Enterobacteriaceae. This oligosaccharide, containing heptose, glucose, and galactose (39), terminates the structure, which thus lacks the repeating 'O' side chain typical of LPS (40) and, as a consequence, is referred to as LOS. The lipid A domain is responsible for the classic endotoxic properties of the molecule, while the part played by the oligosaccharide side chain in the interactive biology of the organism with its host is the subject of much current interest and speculation.

A. LOS in Host-Parasite Interactions

Experiments in vivo and in vitro have delineated interactions between *H. influenzae* type b LOS and host tissues that seem relevant to *Haemophilus* pathogenicity. Purified *Haemophilus* LOS is cytotoxic in vitro to ciliated epithelium from the upper respiratory tracts of experimental animals (41), and human nasopharyngeal epithelium in tissue culture suffers comparable damage on exposure to washed organisms (4). Intranasal instillation of purified LOS prior to intranasal challenge of infant rats with live organisms has been found to lead to an increased level of bacteremia compared to controls not pretreated with LOS (42). This finding suggests that LOS blebbing from living organisms in outer membrane vesicles (which may act essentially as delivery vehicles of LOS in vivo), or released from dead ones, may have a role in facilitating passage of *Haemophilus* from the nasal cavity to the bloodstream.

Haemophilus LOS has been implicated as a mediator of increased BBB permeability. An early and sustained increase in formation of pinocytotic vesicles and a progressive increase in the separation of tight junctions, indicated experimentally by increased permeability to albumin, occurs after intra-cisternal (i-c) inoculation of *H. influenzae* type b organisms into rats (43). I-c inoculation of purified *H. influenzae* type b LOS leads to a similar effect (44) as does instillation of outer membrane vesicles (45). In experiments using rat brain capillary endothelium in tissue culture, Tunkel et al. (46) showed that purified LOS caused an increase in the permeability to albumin without evidence of cell death and that this effect was observed in the absence of host inflammatory cells. Purified LOS from *H. influenzae* type b has also been shown to be cytotoxic for bovine aortal endothelial cells (47), and addition of live or heat-killed *H. influenzae* type b organisms, or purified LOS, to monolayers of bovine brain microvessel endothelial cells also results in cytotoxicity (48). Patrick et al. (48) found that this cytotoxicity was abrogated by anti-CD14 monoclonal antibody, which is known to block a monocyte receptor involved in mediating the effect of LPS (49).

Recent evidence suggests that the potent effect of LOS on BBB permeability is mediated by the cytokines tumour necrosis factor (TNF) and interleukin-1 (IL-1). These molecules are released primarily by monocytes and macrophages (50), but IL-1 is also produced by "nonprofessional" phagocytic cells, including endothelial cells (51). Both cytokines have been found in the CSF of neonates and older children with meningitis (52) and in rats after i-c inoculation of *H. influenzae* type b LOS (53). I-c inoculation of recombinant human IL-1 into rats causes an increase in BBB permeability prior to the peak response seen after i-c inoculation of *H. influenzae* type b LOS (53). This effect was not observed after i-c inoculation of human recombinant TNF, but when TNF and IL-1 were administered together at a concentration of the latter that produced no change, an enhanced increase in BBB permeability was observed. As TNF can induce production of IL-1 by noncerebral capillary endothelium in vitro, leading to increased permeability, analogous effects occurring in cerebral capillary endothelium could contribute to BBB breakdown in meningitis.

B. LOS Structure-Function Relationships Bearing on Bacterial Virulence

Two distinct mechanisms have been identified by which *H. influenzae* type b LOS may protect the organism from host anti-microbial defenses.

1. Serum Resistance

Strains of *H. influenzae* type b grown in nutrient broth are more susceptible to the complement-mediated bactericidal activity of anti-LOS antibodies than are organisms harvested directly from the nasopharynx (54) or from the blood (55) of infected rats (56,57). These phenotypes have been referred to as serum-sensitive (Sen) and resistant (Res). Broth-grown Sen strains can be converted to the Res phenotype by incubation in filtrates of rat or human serum (55,58), or in a mixture of glucose, lactate, urea, and bicarbonate (59). Res strains have been found to elaborate a three- to fourfold greater quantity of LOS compared to the Sen cells from which they were derived, though this LOS is of unaltered electrophoretic mobility in SDS-PAGE gels (57). The mechanism by which having a greater amount of LOS makes organisms more serum-resistant is unknown, but the observation illustrates the importance of recognizing the effect of environment on bacterial composition and in particular the caution that should be exercised in extrapolating results obtained in vitro to the situation in vivo.

2. LOS Antigenic Variation

Haemophilus LOS shows considerable structural variation, both between strains and within a single strain (phase variation), as evidenced by variable mobility in SDS-PAGE gels and a variable pattern of reactivity with mAbs (60,61). This variability has until now precluded complete structural studies, but it is known that the lipid A backbone consists of phosphorylated diglucosamine substituted with fatty acid residues (62), in particular tetradecanoic acid and its 3-hydroxylated derivative (39), and in the mutant strain I-69 (see Sec. III.C.), which contains the minimum LOS structure known for any viable bacterium, a single unsubstituted KDO moiety is linked to this backbone (62). Wild-type strains show phase variation of epitopes on the oligosaccharide side chain. The potential biological relevance of this variation was first demonstrated by Kimura and Hansen (61), who studied two strains, which on primary screening were unable to bind the mAbs 4C4 and 5G8, but which showed spontaneous and reversible acquisition of these binding characteristics at a frequency of 0.2–16.7%. (4C4/5G8)-deficient strains were of low virulence in infant rats, while variants capable of binding both mAbs were found to produce a greater incidence of bacteremia in infant rats after challenge by the intranasal route (both strains) and in the one strain that was tested by the intraperitoneal route. A (4C4/5G8)-positive variant synthesized an LOS of higher molecular weight than its parent strain. The phase-variable structure recognized by mAb 4C4 has been identified as Galα(1→4)Galβ (63), while another, recognized by mAb 3F11, has been shown to be Galβ(1→4)GlcNAc (64,65). Such structures are present on the surface of glycosylated mammalian cells, and it has been suggested that this molecular mimicry by *Haemophilus* may enhance the organism's ability to evade the immune system (63,65). Evidence that *Haemophilus* LOS phase variation occurs in vivo has been presented by Weiser et al. (66) and Mertsola et al. (67). Weiser et al. showed that while epitopes recognized by mAbs 4C4 and 12D9 were almost universally present on bacteria freshly isolated from the CSF of patients with meningitis, these epitopes were lost on growth in vitro. Mertsola et al. also found that bacteria isolated from the CSF of children with meningitis showed mAb-binding characteristics that were partially lost after passage. One interpretation of these results is that selection of organisms bearing particular oligosaccharide structures from an initially heterogenous population may play an important part in pathogenesis. Such selection could occur at any of several stages in infection from initial nasopharyngeal colonization to invasion of the BBB. This hypothesis is supported by the observation that organisms recovered from the CSF of infant rats after intranasal infection no longer display some LOS antigenic characteristics found in the challenge organisms (67) and is also consistent with the results of experiments with LOS mutants that show a reduced repertoire of antigenic variation (see Sec. III.C.).

C. LOS Genetics

The intriguing proposition that molecular mimicry, exhibited through LOS variation, may contribute to the pathogenicity of *H. influenzae* type b has focused recent attention on the genetics of its synthesis. The complexity of the LOS molecule and the responsiveness of its expression, in both qualitative and quantitative terms, to regulatory stimuli make it likely that multiple, complex, genetic loci will be involved in its expression. A comprehensive review has recently been published (68).

Rd is a nonencapsulated *H. influenzae* strain derived originally from a type d background. Early experiments directed at understanding the genetic basis of type b polysaccharide capsulation resulted fortuitously in the construction of a pair of type b transformants of Rd with different LOS phenotypes (69). These strains, designated Rd^-/b^+:01 and Rd^-/b^+:02, differed in the quantity of galactose in their LOS. Rd^-/b^+:02, with less galactose, was more virulent than Rd^-/b^+:01 in infant rats as judged by the incidence and level of sustained bacteremia following intraperitoneal or intranasal infection. However, further analysis revealed that Rd^-/b^+:02 had a single-copy *cap* locus in contrast to the duplication in Rd^-/b^+:01 (see Sec. IV.B.), and the precise contribution of its LOS phenotype to virulence is still unclear. Nevertheless, Rd^-/b^+:02 has proved useful in establishing a fundamental role for the LOS side chain in *Haemophilus* virulence. Transformation of Rd^{-}/b^{+}:02 with an *H. influenzae* type b gene bank resulted in a mutant termed I-69 (70). This transformant has been shown to have the deeply truncated LOS structure described above, was susceptible in vitro to serum killing and was avirulent in the infant rat model of infection despite possessing a type b capsule. The mutation in the locus responsible for this phenotype is currently unknown.

The capacity of cloned *Haemophilus* gene products to modify the core oligosaccharide of *E. coli* LPS has led to the identification of a complex LOS locus in *H. influenzae* type b containing at least three genes or gene clusters (*lsg1*, *lsg2*, *lsg3*) (71). *E. coli* transformed with the clone pGEMLOS-5 produced an LPS containing an extra 1.4 kD oligosaccharide portion compared to the host strain, and the LPS developed reactivity to a mAb specific for Galβ(1→4)GlcNAc. This mAb failed to bind when further subcloned *Haemophilus* DNA was present (leading to production of a larger recombinant LOS in the *E. coli* recipient), a result suggesting epitope masking by additional sugar residues (72). The part this locus plays in *Haemophilus* LOS synthesis remains to be elucidated.

Three further chromosomal loci (*lic1*, *lic2*, *lic3*) have been identified that are involved in the phenomenon of LOS phase variation (73). *lic1* was identified by screening a genomic library of *H. influenzae* type b for DNA capable of transforming a non–phase-variable strain to express phase-variable LOS epitopes as defined by reactivity to mAbs 6A2 and 12D9 (74). The locus was found to contain four open reading frames (ORFs) *lic1ABCD* with no resemblance to previously known genes. The initiation codons of *lic1B* and *lic1C* each overlapped the extreme 3′ end of the preceding gene, a result suggesting that with *lic1A* these genes formed a single transcriptional unit. Site-directed mutagenesis of *lic1A* resulted in low constitutive expression of previously phase-variable epitopes. At the 5′ end of *lic1A*, a variable number (≈30) of tandem repeats of the tetranucleotide CAAT was found immediately downstream of three ATG codons. Depending on the number of CAAT repeats, one, two, or no initiation codons would be in frame with the rest of the *lic1A* ORF downstream (Fig. 1) and variation in the number of CAAT repeats was indeed found to accompany phase variation in reactivity to mAb 6A2. Conceivably, slip-strand mispairing in this region of *lic1A* could be the molecular event underlying phase variation (75). The loci *lic2* and *lic3* were cloned from the same *H. influenzae* type b gene bank through their hybridization to the oligonucleotide $(CAAT)_5$ (73). *lic2* [probably identical to *lex-1* (76)] consists of a single gene containing tandem repeats of CAAT at its 5′ end. Evidence that *lic2* is involved in LOS expression comes from the observation that mutations in *lic2* abolish reactivity to mAb 4C4 and other undefined structures identifed by further mAbs (76). *lic3* consists of 4 ORFs

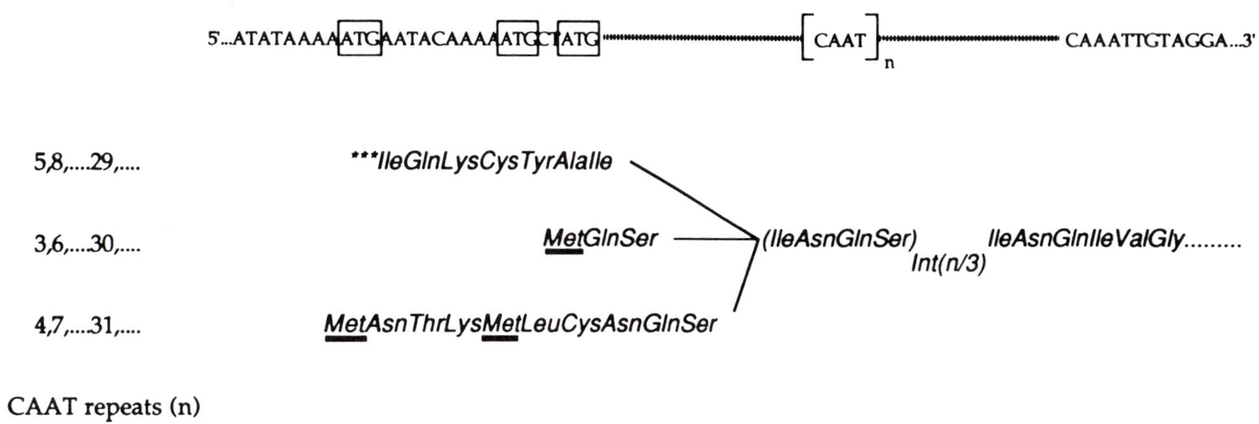

Figure 1 5′ end of *lic1*. The nucleotide sequence shows three possible ATG start codons (boxes), followed by n repeats of the tetranucleotide CAAT and the next 12 nucleotides of the *lic1A* ORF. A translation is shown below the sequence, with different possible N-terminal ends linked via repeats of the tetrapeptide Ile-Asn-Gln-Ser to the rest of the protein. Possible N-terminal methionines corresponding to the different ATG codons are underlined. Which N-terminal end will be linked to the body of the protein depends on the number(n) of CAAT repeats; the number of tetrapeptide repeats found in a particular example is Int(n/3), the largest whole number $\leq n/3$. For $n = 5,8, \ldots$ there is no possible N-terminal methionine linked to the body of the protein.

(77). While *lic3A*, the "CAAT gene," and *lic3C* do not resemble any genes yet described, the deduced *lic3D* product is closely similar in sequence to adenylate kinase, essential for maintaining cell energy balance. No other homolog to the adenylate kinase gene has been identified in *Haemophilus*, and it may be that co-expression of this crucial metabolic enzyme with the products of LOS genes reflects the need for growing cells to coordinate formation of a satisfactory cell envelope. *lic3B* has been shown by complementation studies to encode galactose-4-epimerase (galE) (77). Further *gal* genes, encoding other enzymes of the Leloir pathway for catabolism of exogenous galactose (78), have been located elsewhere in the *Haemophilus* chromosome (79).

Analysis of the effect of LOS gene mutations on bacterial virulence is still at a preliminary stage, which reflects the complexity of the loci under consideration. A *lic1/lic2* mutant of strain RM7004 showed a normal capacity to cause sustained, high-level bacteremia following intraperitoneal inoculation of infant rats and caused a normal incidence and level of prolonged nasopharyngeal colonization after intranasal infection (80). In contrast, the mutant demonstrated decreased capacity to cause bacteremia following intranasal infection, which suggested that this LOS mutant was compromised in its ability to invade from the nasopharynx to the vascular compartment. The involvement of *lex-1* (*lic2*) in virulence has been demonstrated by Cope et al. (76), who compared the type b strain DL42 with a mutant containing a linker insertion in *lex-1* that rendered it incapable of binding the mAb 4C4. The mutant was less virulent, causing only 67% of infant rats challenged intranasally to have bacteremia compared to 90% of those infected with the wild-type. A *lic3* deletion mutant of RM7004, lacking the 3′ end of *lic3A*, *galE* and the 5′ end of *lic3C*, was impaired in its ability to cause bacteremia following either intraperitoneal or intranasal challenge (77). However, the complexity of the phenotype produced by this deletion makes interpretation of these data difficult. In particular, the reactivity of the mutant strain in vitro to the mAb 4C4 (recognizing a galactose-containing epitope) was only manifest when grown in defined medium with no galactose present, so the role of the *galE* mutation could not be interpreted without knowledge of the galactose environment of the organism during infection. To resolve this question, Maskell et al. cloned the remaining *gal* genes (*galR*, *galT*, *galK*, and *galM*) from *H. influenzae* type b (79). A series of single and double mutants (*galE*, *galK*, *galEgalK*) were tested for virulence on intraperitoneal challenge in the infant rat model of infection. With mutants of one strain (Eagan), the incidence of bacteremia was markedly reduced with *galE* and combined *galEgalK* mutations, but not with *galK* mutations alone. However, in another *H. influenzae* type b strain, the reduction in the incidence of bacteremia caused by *galE* and *galEgalK* mutants was considerably less (79). The importance of these interstrain differences in the pathogenic process remains to be evaluated.

IV. CAPSULE

A. Capsule in Host-Parasite Interactions

Both capsulate and noncapsulate *H. influenzae* are responsible for significant human disease. However, whereas organisms responsible for superficial mucosal infections such as otitis media are most often noncapsulate, those that invade the bloodstream to cause serious infections such as meningitis are virtually always capsulate. Polysaccharide and teichoic acid capsules are well-established determinants of virulence in many species of bacteria, as recently reviewed elsewhere (16). These materials endow organisms with a hydrophilic, negatively charged surface that is intrinsically antiphagocytic. Opsonization with complement or antibody increases susceptibility to phagocytosis. However, the presence of capsular polysaccharide may promote inactivation of C3b (81), act as a barrier between the site of deposition of C3b and other necessary factors on the phagocytic cell, or, by continuously being shed from the bacterial surface, nullify the role of capsule-directed host defenses. Of particular clinical significance, capsular polysaccharides interact with the human immune system as relative T-independent antigens that elicit a very poor antibody response in human infants. The result is to delay the clearance of organisms from a naive host by an antibody-mediated process. While these are features of capsules that interest physicians, capsular structures may reasonably be assumed to have a wider function beyond the interactive biology of microbe and host. In upper respiratory colonists such as *Haemophilus*, capsule may well provide a hydrophilic microenvironment that improves the changes of bacterial survival in the environment between hosts as well as on an epithelial surface, let alone in the bloodstream.

A question of enduring interest in relation to *Haemophilus* capsulation is why serotype b strains should apparently have so much greater pathogenic potential than strains of the other five serotypes (a,c–f). Strains causing bacteremia and meningitis outside the neonatal period are almost always found to be type b. Widely differing interpretations can be placed on this intriguing observation. At one extreme, the primacy of type b strains in causing disease might reflect the fact that type b capsule (a linear polymer of the subunit ribose-[1-1]-ribitol-5-phosphate-[3-) in and of itself endows strains with greatly enhanced virulence. At the opposite extreme, the possession of type b capsule might simply be a prominent phenotypic marker in strong linkage disequilibrium with other, as yet undefined, microbial characteristics actually responsible for the virulent behavior. A major goal of research into the molecular basis of pathogenicity of *H. influenzae* has been to explain this striking prominence of type b strains, and both population and molecular genetic studies have made important contributions.

Musser and colleagues (see Chapter 9) have established by multilocus enzyme electrophoretic typing that the bacterial population of capsulate *H. influenzae* responsible for human infection is diverse but has a clonal structure, dividing into two major phylogenetic divisions. A striking observation is that capsular type is in marked linkage disequilibrium with electrotype, although type a and type b strains stand out in being represented in both major phylogenetic divisions (Fig. 2). This result suggests that possession

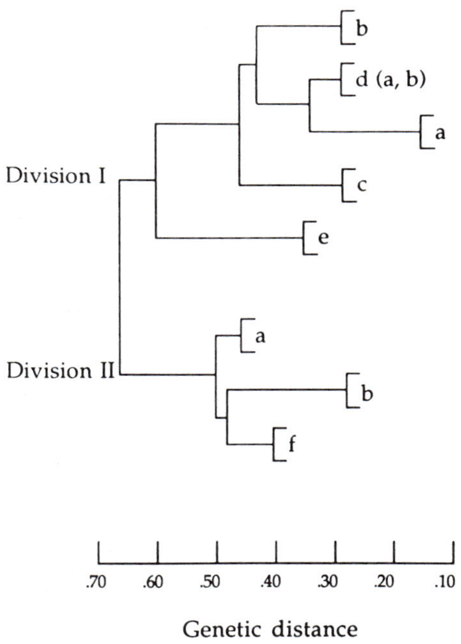

Figure 2 Dendrogram showing serotypes for eight numerically predominant clusters of encapsulated *H. influenzae*. The dendrogram was generated as described, based on electrophoretic typing of 2209 isolates at 17 enzyme loci. Genetic distance (dimensionless) reflecting relatedness between strains is shown at the bottom. Clusters are defined as groups of strains related to each other at, or more closely than, the genetic distance corresponding to the end of each branch. Each cluster contains strains of the serotype(s) indicated. The population divides into two primary phylogenetic divisions (I,II) at a genetic distance of 0.66. (From Ref. 111.)

of type b capsule may not alone be sufficient to explain the virulence of type b strains. Not only do type b strains fall into two clonal groups different in many ways other than capsule from strains of any other serotype but, with the insight that this detailed typing system provides, it has been possible to select strains from each division and compare their virulence in the infant rat model of systemic infection (82). Compared to Division I strains, Division II strains have been found to have a greatly reduced capacity to cause sustained bacteraemia, despite having biochemically identical capsule to division I strains (83–85). Further, a naturally occurring, capsulate example of a division I type b strain has been identified with negligible capacity to cause disease (85). Genetically defined strains are essential to clarify the situation. Zwahlen *et al.* (15) constructed isogenic mutants of a division I strain identical but for capsular type and compared these in the infant rat model. Intranasal or intraperitoneal inoculation of the type b mutant Rd^-/b^+:02 consistently gave higher levels of sustained bacteraemia and a higher frequency of meningitis than did constructs of the other five serotypes. The non-b mutants in general, however, were more virulent in this model system than the natural isolates from which their *cap* genes were derived. Further experiments showed that the higher virulence of type b strains resulted from type b capsule giving organisms a greater resistance to phagocytosis in the spleen. Thus type b capsule has been shown independently to enhance virulence, but other, noncapsular, characteristics are also important in pathogenicity.

B. Genetics of Capsulation

Studies of the genetic basis of capsulation have brought further insights into the virulence of capsulate *H. influenzae*. Genes involved in *Haemophilus* capsulation are clustered at the chromosomal *cap* locus (Fig. 3). In the prototypic type b strain Eagan (86), *cap* contains a direct repeat of two segments of approximately 17 kilobase pairs (kbp) of DNA, an organization anticipated to be highly unstable in a recombination-proficient background (87). In the earliest descriptions of type b capsulation in *H. influenzae*, the phenotype was indeed identified as unstable (88) with slow-growing, pleomorphic capsule-deficient (b-) mutants occurring at high frequency (up to 0.5% of colonies derived from a mid-exponential culture), continuing to produce polysaccharide but failing to export it to the bacterial surface (89,90). More recent studies have shown that export-defective mutants arise at very high frequency but that most die before multiplying to form visible colonies (91). Southern hybridization analysis of strain Eagan and its capsule-deficient mutants using *cap* DNA probes confirms that the duplication is reduced to a single copy in b– mutants (87,90), but shows

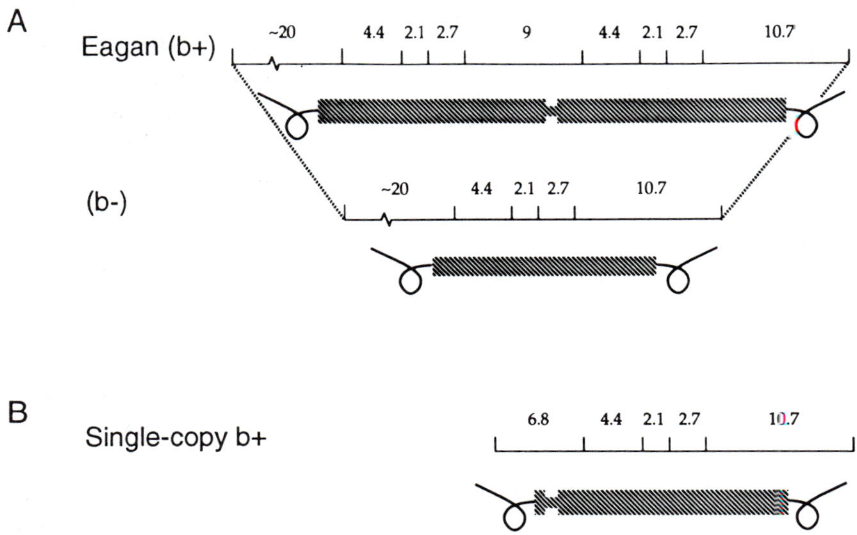

Figure 3 Physical maps of *cap* loci. (A) *cap* in type b strain Eagan (b+) and a spontaneous capsule-deficient mutant (b−). *Eco*RI sites (unmarked vertical lines above the line of the chromosome) divide the locus into fragments of the sizes shown in kilobases. The location and extent of the *cap* gene cluster is shown below the line of the chromosome (hatched bars). In Eagan, direct repeats of ≈17 kbp are separated by the unique bridge region indicated by a constriction between the repeats. In the reduced locus of the capsule-deficient (b−) mutant, generated by recombination between the two sides of the repeat, a single copy without a bridge region is found. (B) The rare single-copy type b capsulation locus, shown aligned with the Eagan *cap* locus to emphasize the presence of the bridge region and small terminal DNA repeat.

further that in the process a "bridge region" of unduplicated DNA lying between the *cap* direct repeats is lost (Fig. 3A). This bridge region contains the gene *bexA*, and site-directed mutagenesis reproduces the polysaccharide export-defective capsule-deficient phenotype (92). Sequence analysis of *bexA* has shown its product to have peptide domains characteristically conserved in ATP-binding proteins found energizing diverse membrane transport systems (93). This result suggests that an analogous transporter, of the "ABC superfamily" type, may be responsible for export of capsule polysaccharide. *bexA* is the fourth gene in the *bex* cluster. The three more 5′ genes—*bexDCB*—are thought to encode other components of the polysaccharide export apparatus (94). BexB has the periodic hydrophobicity of an integral membrane protein characteristically found in such transporters, while Tn*phoA* mutagenesis has established that BexC is a candidate periplasmic component (94). Polysaccharide exporters encoded by genes homologous to members of the *bex* cluster have recently been described at the capsulation loci of *Escherichia coli* and *Neisseria meningitidis* (95,96), and detailed studies in *N. meningitidis* (97) suggest a possible role in capsulation for *H. influenzae* BexD. The *ctrA* gene product of the *N. meningitidis* capsulation locus—a protein sharing 51% sequence identity with BexD—appears to be the outer membrane component of the meningococcal capsule polysaccharide exporter. The same role might be served by BexD in *H. influenzae*, perhaps as part of a pore structure through which capsular material reaches the surface (98).

Surveys of clinical type b isolates have shown showed that although the direct repeat configuration at *cap* is found in more than 99%, there are a few exceptions in which the locus contains only one complete copy of the ≈17 kbp segment, terminating with *bexA* (Fig. 3B). Strains with this single-copy locus make about half as much capsular polysaccharide as those with the usual duplication and give rise to a lower level of sustained bacteraemia in the infant rat model of experimental infection (99). In contrast, *cap* loci from type a, type c, and type d strains all have the single copy pattern: a direct-repeat arrangement is not found (15,100,101). Alignment of restriction endonuclease maps of single-copy *cap* loci demonstrated that they all had the same segmental organization, with serotype-specific DNA (region 2) sandwiched between DNA common to all (regions 1 and 3) (100–102) (Fig. 4). This pattern conforms to the pattern established for the other major gram-negative capsulate pathogens *E. coli* and *N. meningitidis* (103–105).

In the *Haemophilus cap* locus, the whole of region 1 is occupied by the *bex* gene cluster (94). The ORF of *bexA* is followed by a inverted repeats of a degenerate version of the *Haemophilus* 11-base-pair DNA uptake sequence (106). Such a motif has been suggested to act as a transcriptional terminator in *Neisseria gonorrhoeae* (107) and, more recently, in *H. influenzae* (108,109). At the other end of the *bex* cluster, another close match to the uptake sequence is found at the 5′-end of *bexD*. Nucleotide sequences diverge upstream of the *bex* promoter in the different serotypes, where region 2 genes are serotype specific, presumably encoding enzymes necessary for biosynthesis of the type-specific sugar heterodimers. In type b strains a further six ORFS are found in the *cap* locus, four of these (ORF 1 to ORF 4) being unique to type b strains and comprising region 2. A pair of uptake sequences lies between ORF 4 and the next gene (ORF 5) (L. N. Brophy, personal communication). Beyond these, ORF 5 and ORF 6 (encoding unknown functions but containing DNA common to all serotypes) make up region 3. Thus the segmentation of *cap* defined by cross-serotype

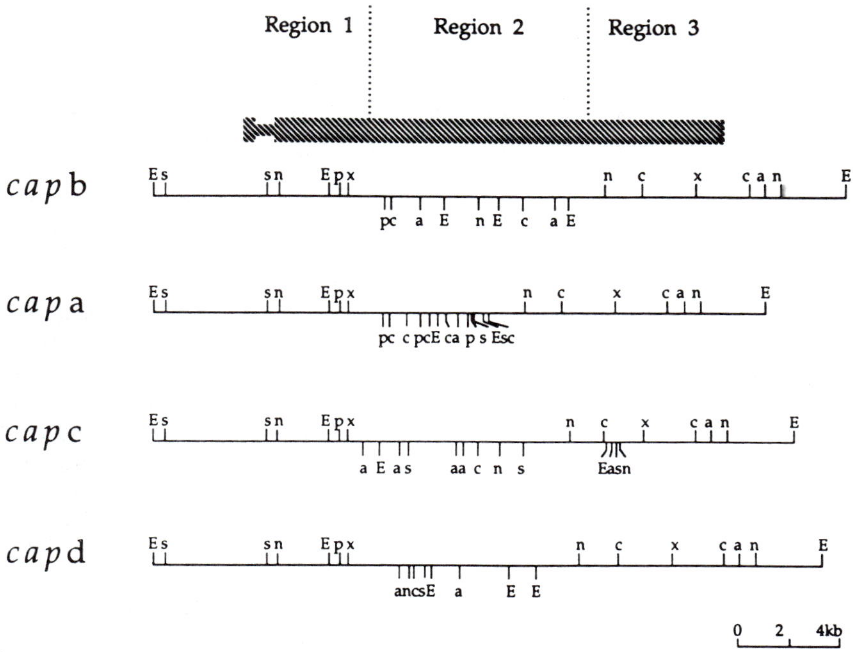

Figure 4 Fine structure maps of type a, type c, and type d *cap* loci aligned at the left-hand end with the single-copy type b locus. The extent of the single-copy type b *cap* locus is depicted as a hatched bar as in Figure 3, with regions 1, 2, and 3 indicated above. Sites shown are cleaved by restriction endonucleases *Eco*RI (E), *Sca*I (s), *Nco*I (n), *Pst*I (p), *Xho*I (x), *Cla*I (c), *Xba*I (a). Regions of map similarity are indicated by upward orientation of the labeling of restriction sites, and regions of map divergence by downward orientation, so delineating region 2 sandwiched between regions 1 and 3.

DNA hybridization apparently reflects the organization of genes into functional groups: an export gene cluster, a biosynthesis gene cluster, and a third, as yet uncharacterized, pair of genes common to all serotypes. This organization, with a "cassette" of biosynthesis genes flanked by uptake sequences and slotted between common regions 1 and 3, is tailor-made for genetic exchange. Such cassette exchange is readily achieved in vitro (15,110), and there is clear evidence that occasional transformation and recombinational integration of heterologous *cap* DNA has occurred in vivo (29). Though such events have clearly been rare (29,111,112), they cannot be concluded to have been of negligible importance in the evolution of *H. influenzae* virulence. The biological success of a single mutant type b clone as described below is a reminder that rare recombinational events in the bacterial chromosome may have major consequences for human disease.

Recent characterization of DNA beyond the ends of regions 1 and 3 has shown that the division I *cap* locus is flanked by directly repeated copies of IS*1016*—a 713bp IS-like element of the Tn*3* family—making it in effect a compound transposon (113) (Fig. 5A). In strain Eagan, representative of type b strains in which *cap* is duplicated, DNA sequencing revealed a truncated second copy of *bexA* running on to a residual part of IS*1016* at the end of *cap* (Fig. 5B). The presence of this truncated second copy strongly suggests that the Eagan *cap* locus arose through a two-stage process (Fig. 6). First, an initial recombination between the small direct repeats of IS*1016* would have generated a perfect duplication. Such duplications have been found at the *cap* loci of serotype a strains (113,114). In type b strains, this recombination was apparently followed by a deletion leaving the centrally located copy of *bex*A unique and type b capsule production absolutely dependent on maintenance of the duplication. To address the question of how the

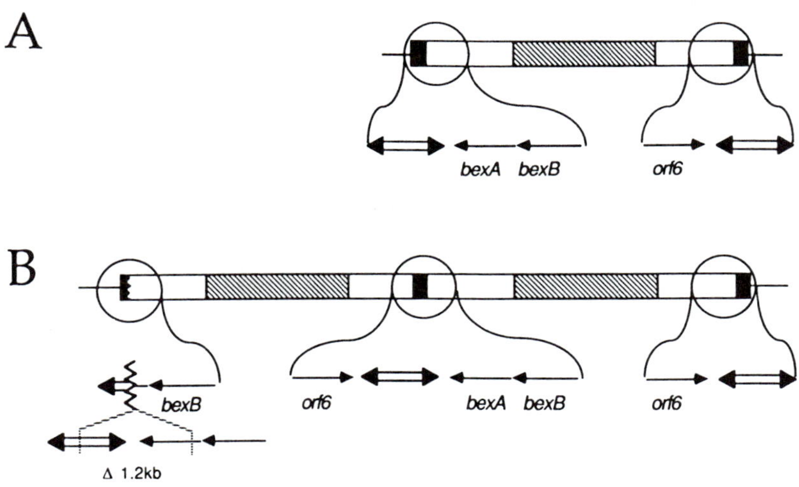

Figure 5 Diagrammatic representations of the type b *cap* locus, with expansions of certain regions to indicate genes of interest. (A) The single-copy locus. The *cap gene cluster is flanked by copies of* IS*1016* (filled rectangles in the diagram, double-headed arrows in the expansion). Region 1 (unshaded) contains the *bex* genes (*bexA* and *bexB* shown as arrows in the expansion), followed by type b–specific region 2 (shaded). In region 3, *orf6* precedes the second copy of IS*1016* (expansion). (B) The Eagan *cap* locus. Shading and symbols are as in A. The locus falls short of being a perfect repeat of the single copy by virtue of the 1.2-kbp deletion (zig-zag line). The extent of DNA deleted is indicated at the bottom.

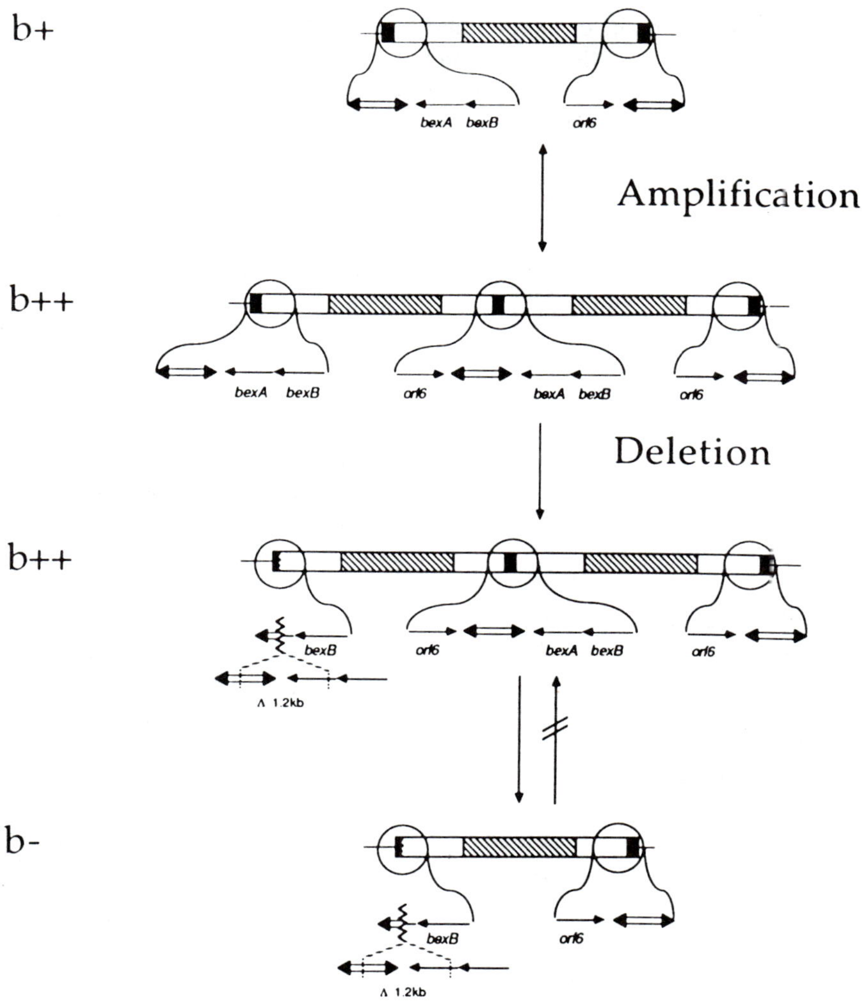

Figure 6 Duplication-deletion mechanism generating the Eagan *cap* locus. Shading and symbols are as in Figure 5. b+ and b++ signify capsule polysaccharide production corresponding to the single- and double-copy loci. b- signifies the capsule-deficient (export-defective) state consequent on lacking *bexA*. The Eagan *cap* locus corresponds to the b++ state following the deletion. Single- and double-headed arrows linking different degrees of *cap* gene amplification signify the possibility of genetic reorganization/mutation leading to one state being converted to the other.

duplicated locus might be maintained in other type b strains, 18 strains, selected from all over the world, have now been examined for terminal deletions in *cap*. These strains, of known diverse electrophoretic types (Fig. 7), all showed an identical deletion to that found in Eagan. DNA sequencing confirmed that the same *bex*A-IS*1016* fusion was present at the end of their

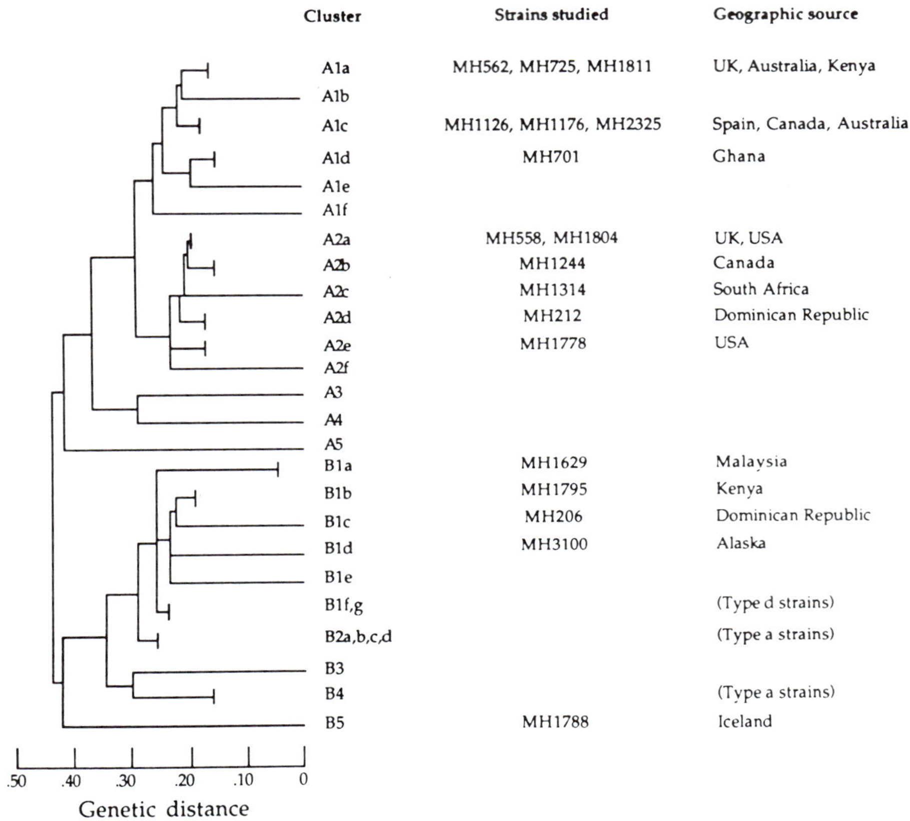

Figure 7 Dendrogram indicating genetic relationships between selected type b strains segregating to phylogenetic division I of the population of capsulate *Haemophilus*. Relationships are displayed as in Figure 2 in terms of the dimensionless quantity genetic distance. Strains segregate into ET clusters, a cluster containing strains related to each other at a maximum of the genetic distance indicated by the vertical line at the end of a "branch." Clusters representing a unique strain thus lie at a genetic distance of zero. Relationships between clusters are indicated by the lines joining them. The major lineages A and B are related at a genetic distance of 0.42, corresponding to differences, on average, at 7/17 enzyme loci assayed. Eighteen strains examined in detail lie in the clusters shown and were isolated from the countries indicated. (Adapted from Ref. 112, where a fuller description of each strain is given.)

cap loci (115). As genetic exchange between capsulate *Haemophilus* strains is very rare (111,112), this result strongly suggests that all type b strains currently responsible for invasive disease are the descendants of an ancestral strain in which a duplication-deletion scenario occurred as depicted in Figure 6. The data imply biological advantage in having a duplicated *cap* locus, as the clonal extinction of single-copy type b strains has not occurred. The larger quantity of capsular polysaccharide made by strains with a duplication at *cap* (99) does not entirely satisfactorily explain their greater propensity to cause disease, as mutants with a *cap* duplication but with a single region 2 deletion retain full virulence despite having half the capsule (116). The biological advantage of having a *cap* duplication may arise from the capacity of such strains to undergo gene amplification readily (Fig. 8). This process, anticipated to be less likely in single-copy strains as the targets for amplification (the two copies of IS*1016* in such a case) are small, can be expected to generate a family of strains with 3-, 4-, and higher multimers of the basic set of *cap* genes, from which a phenotype of amplified polysaccharide may be selected in certain circumstances. This selection has been found to occur in invasive *H. influenzae* type b disease: fresh unpassaged isolates from blood and CSF have been shown to be heavily capsulated and to have *cap* amplified up to five copies, a genetic configuration that degrades rapidly to the two-

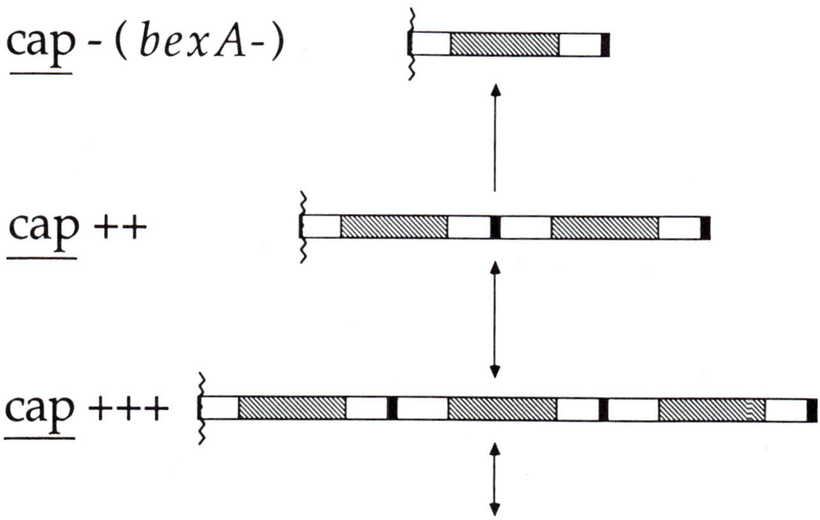

Figure 8 Amplification/reduction of *cap* gene copy number. Double- and single-headed arrows between states signify the possibility of reversibility of the transition. A potential for amplification beyond a triplication is implied by the lowermost double-headed arrow.

copy ground state on cultivation in vitro (117). While a transient high level of capsulation may promote bacterial survival in the bloodstream, leading to meningitis, it remains to be shown what the advantage might be to the organism under normal circumstances in the nasopharynx. Capsule production appears irrelevant to bacterial adhesion (118), and an attractive hypothesis—yet to be established as fact—is that heavily capsulated strains might be implicated in transmission, more readily surviving the desiccating environment between hosts.

V. CONCLUDING REMARKS

Molecular studies of the pathogenicity of *H. influenzae* have established unequivocally that in naturally occurring type b strains, the polysaccharide capsule is a critical determinant of virulence. The particular pathogenicity of type b strains compared to other serotypes appears, at least in isogenic constructions, to derive from the nature of the polysaccharide itself, which may confer particularly antiphagocytic properties. Type b polysaccharide is thus uncompromisingly validated as a component of any vaccine to protect against invasive type b disease. Further conclusions can, however, be drawn.

First, noncapsular determinants make an important contribution to *Haemophilus* pathogenicity (15). LOS and fimbriae are prominent bacterial characteristics with a reputation firmly established in other gram-negative pathogens for critical involvement in bacterial virulence, but while they might reasonably be supposed to make an important contribution to the pathogenicity of *Haemophilus*, the precise part that they play remains open to debate. Current studies appear set to define a part for LOS, but it is still uncertain whether fimbriae contribute to the pathogenetic sequence of invasive disease. Many less well-characterized bacterial features—for example, minor outer membrane proteins (119), iron-acquisition proteins (120), hemocin (121)—are likely also to contribute to the totality of *Haemophilus* virulence, but the roles they play will probably remain unappreciated until molecular genetic techniques are brought to bear. The stimulus to clarify *Haemophilus* pathogenicity further comes in part from consideration of future developments in the vaccine field. Outer membrane proteins in particular are favored candidates for inclusion in vaccines that may protect against a wider spectrum of *H. influenzae* infections than those caused by type b strains alone (see Chapter 7). Immunodominant surface proteins of unknown function possess the minimal credentials necessary for consideration as vaccine components if they can be shown to be antigenically conserved across the bacterial population. However, null mutants need to be generated—which in practice usually means that the gene needs to be cloned—in order to establish that expression is necessarily linked with bacterial virulence. A satisfactory understanding of the more subtle interactions between host and microorganism will require clarification of the genetic basis for expression and a systematic evaluation of isogenic mutants by studies such as those described for fimbriae, LOS, and capsule.

Second, the primacy of type b strains as pathogens is thrown in a somewhat different light by the discovery of the DNA deletion that lies behind the stabilization of the duplicated *cap* locus (115). *cap* duplication is associated entirely with type b capsulation, and any contribution to virulence that may derive from this genetic configuration cannot be distinguished from a contribution of the type b polysaccharide. Nevertheless, as the mutation lies outside DNA specific to type b strains, it is possible that non-b serotypes may acquire it. The prospect, though remote, of non-b serotypes acquiring enhanced virulence in this way is an added incentive to continue molecular genetic studies to define additional bacterial determinants for inclusion in a polyvalent, extended spectrum vaccine against all *Haemophilus* disease.

REFERENCES

1. E. R. Moxon, *Haemophilus influenzae*, *Principles and Practice of Infectious Diseases* (G. Mandell, R. Douglas, and J. Bennett, eds.), Wiley Medical Publications, New York, 1989, p. 1722.
2. D. S. Stephens and M. M. Farley, Pathogenic events during infection of the human nasopharynx with *Neisseria meningitidis* and *Haemophilus influenzae*, *Rev. Infect. Dis. 13*:22 (1991).
3. B. Schwartz, P. S. Moore, and C. V. Broome, Global epidemiology of meningococcal disease, *Clin. Microbiol. Rev. 2*:S118 (1989).
4. M. M. Farley, D. S. Stephens, M. H. Mulks, M. D. Cooper, J. V. Bricker, S. S. Mirra, and A. Wright, Pathogenesis of IgA1 protease-producing and -nonproducing *Haemophilus influenzae* in human nasopharyngeal organ cultures, *J. Infect. Dis. 154*:752 (1986).
5. M. M. Farley, D. S. Stephens, S. L. Kaplan, and E. O. Mason Jr., Pilus- and non-pilus-mediated interactions of *Haemophilus influenzae* type b with human erythrocytes and human nasopharyngeal mucosa, *J. Infect. Dis. 161*:274 (1990).
6. E. R. Moxon, A. L. Smith, D. R. Averill, and D. H. Smith, *Haemophilus influenzae* meningitis in infant rats after intranasal inoculation, *J. Infect. Dis. 129*:154 (1974).
7. I. Carlstedt and J. K. Sheehan, Structure and macro-molecular properties of mucus glycoproteins, *Monogr. Allergy 24*:16 (1988).
8. A. G. Plaut, The IgA1 proteases of pathogenic bacteria, *Annu. Rev. Microbiol. 37*:603 (1983).

9. M. Kilian, B. Thomsen, T. E. Petersen, and H. Bleeg, Molecular biology of *Haemophilus influenzae* IgA1 proteases, *Mol. Immunol. 20*:1051 (1983).
10. M. Kilian, J. Mestecky, and M. W. Russell, Defence mechanisms involving Fc-dependent functions of immunoglobulin A and their subversion by bacterial immunoglobulin A proteases, *Microbiol. Rev. 52*:296 (1988).
11. R. Wilson, D. Robert, and P. Cole, Effects of bacterial products on human ciliary function *in vitro*. *Thorax 40*:125 (1985).
12. R. Wilson and E. R. Moxon, Molecular mechanisms of *Haemophilus influenzae* pathogenicity in the respiratory tract, *Bacterial Infections of Respiratory and Gastrointestinal Mucosae* (W. Donachie, E. Griffiths, and J. Stephen, eds.), IRL Press, Washington, DC, 1988, p. 29.
13. M. R. Loeb, E. Connor, and D. Penney, A comparison of the adherence of fimbriated and non-fimbriated *Haemophilus influenzae* type b to human adenoids in organ culture, *Infect. Immun. 56*:484 (1988).
14. L. G. Rubin and E. R. Moxon, Pathogenesis of bloodstream invasion with *Haemophilus influenzae* type b, *Infect. Immun. 41*:280 (1983).
15. A. Zwahlen, J. S. Kroll, L. G. Rubin, and E. R. Moxon, The molecular basis of pathogenicity in *Haemophilus influenzae*: comparative virulence of genetically-related capsular transformants and correlation with changes at the capsulation locus *cap*, *Microb. Pathogen. 7*:225 (1989).
16. E. R. Moxon and J. S. Kroll, The role of bacterial polysaccharide capsules as virulence factors, *Current Topics in Microbiology and Immunology, Vol. 150, Bacterial Capsules* (K. Jann and B. Jann, eds.), Springer, Berlin, 1990, p. 65.
17. A. L. Smith, M. C. Roberts, J. E. Haas, and P. M. Mendelman, Mechanisms of *Haemophilus influenzae* type b meningitis, *Bacterial Meningitis* (M. A. Sande, A. L. Smith, and R. K. Root, eds.), Churchill Livingstone, Edinburgh, 1985, p. 11.
18. M. Virji, H. Kayhty, D. J. P. Ferguson, C. Alexandrescu, and E. R. Moxon, Interactions of *Haemophilus influenzae* with cultured human endothelial cells, *Microb. Pathogen. 10*:231 (1991).
19. E. R. Moxon and P. A. Murphy, *Haemophilus influenzae* bacteremia and meningitis resulting from survival of a single organism, *Proc. Natl. Acad. Sci. USA 75*:1534 (1978).
20. C. C. Brinton, M. J. Carter, D. B. Derber, S. Kar, J. A. Kramarik, A. C. C. To, S. C. M. To, and S. W. Wood, Design and development of pilus vaccines for *Haemophilus influenzae* diseases, *Pediatr. Infect. Dis. J. 8*:S54 (1989).
21. J. R. Gilsdorf, K. McCrea, and L. Forney, Conserved and nonconserved epitopes among *Haemophilus influenzae* type b pili, *Infect. Immun. 58*:2252 (1990).
22. A. Weber, K. Harris, S. Lohrke, L. Forney, and A. L. Smith, Inability to express fimbriae results in impaired ability of *Haemophilus influenzae* type b to colonize the naso-pharynx, *Infect. Immun. 59*:4724 (1991).
23. L. van Alphen, J. Poole, and M. Overbeeke, The Anton blood group antigen is the erythrocyte receptor for Haemophilus influenzae, *FEMS Microbiol. Lett. 37*:69 (1986).

24. L. van Alphen, L. Geelen-van den Broek, L. Blaas, M. van Ham, and J. Dankert, Blocking of fimbria-mediated adherence of *Haemophilus influenzae* by sialyl gangliosides, *Infect. Immun. 59*:4473 (1991).
25. L. van Alphen, C. Levene, L. Geelen-van den Broek, J. Poole, M. Bennett, and J. Dankert, Combined inheritance of the epithelial cell and erythrocyte receptors for *Haemophilus influenzae*, *Infect. Immun. 58*:3807 (1990).
26. N. G. Guerina, S. Langermann, H. W. Clegg, T. W. Kessler, D. A. Goldmann, and J. R. Gilsdorf, Adherence of piliated *Haemophilus influenzae* type b to human oropharyngeal cells, *J. Infect. Dis. 146*:564 (1982).
27. C. C. Patrick, G. S. Patrick, S. L. Kaplan, J. Barrish, and E. O. Mason, Jr., Adherence kinetics of *Haemophilus influenzae* type b to eukaryotic cells, *Pediatr. Res. 26*:500 (1989).
28. L. M. T. Sterk, L. van Alphen, L. Geelen-van den Broek, H. J. Houthoff, and J. Dankert, Differential binding of *Haemophilus influenzae* to human tissues by fimbriae, *J. Med. Microbiol. 35*:129 (1991).
28a. W. Barsum, R. Wilson, R. C. Read, A. Rutman, P. Webb, H. C. Todd, P. Cole, Interaction of fimbriate (F+) and non-fimbriated (F−) clinical isolates of nontypeable *H. influenzae* (NTHi) with human respiratory tract mucus *in vitro*, *Thorax*, *47*:859 (1992).
29. J. S. Kroll and E. R. Moxon, Capsulation in distantly related strains of *Haemophilus influenzae* type b: genetic drift and gene transfer at the capsulation locus, *J. Bacteriol. 172*:1374 (1990).
30. P. W. Anderson, M. E. Pichichero, and E. M. Connor, Enhanced nasopharyngeal colonization of rats by piliated *Haemophilus influenzae* type b, *Infect. Immun. 48*:565 (1985).
31. M. F. Tosi, D. C. Anderson, J. Barrish, E. O. Mason, Jr., and S. L. Kaplan, Effect of piliation on interactions of *Haemophilus influenzae* type b with human polymorphonuclear leucocytes, *Infect. Immun. 47*:780 (1985).
32. L. J. Forney, T. Giddings, J. Gilsdorf, T. Hoepf, and L. Bakaletz, Expression of pili by systemic isolates of *Haemophilus influenzae* type b, *Proceedings of the 90th annual meeting of the American Society for Microbiology*, Anaheim, CA, 1990.
33. N. S. Sable, E. M. Conner, C. B. Hall, and M. R. Loeb, Variable adherence of fimbriated *Haemophilus influenzae* type b to human cells, *Infect. Immun. 48*:119 (1985).
34. S. M. Van Ham, F. R. Mooi, M. G. Sindhunata, W. R. Maris, and L. Van Alphen, Cloning and expression in *Escherichia coli* of *Haemophilus influenzae* fimbrial genes establishes adherence to oropharyngeal epithelial cells, *EMBO J. 8*:3535 (1989).
35. J. R. Gilsdorf, C. F. Marrs, K. W. McCrea, and L. J. Forney, Cloning, expression and sequence analysis of the *Haemophilus influenzae* type b strain M43p+ pilin gene, *Infect. Immun. 58*:1065 (1990).
36. S. Langermann and A. Wright, Molecular analysis of the *Haemophilus influenzae* type b pilin gene, *Mol. Microbiol. 4*:221 (1990).
37. L. J. Forney, C. F. Marrs, S. Bektesh, and J. R. Gilsdorf, Comparison and

analysis of the nucleotide sequences of pilin genes from *Haemophilus influenzae* type b strains Eagan and M43, *Infect. Immun. 59*:1991 (1991).
38. A. Holmgren, M. J. Kuehn, C-I. Branden, and S. J. Hultgren, Conserved immunoglobulin-like features in a family of periplasmic pilus chaperones in bacteria, *EMBO J. 11*:1617 (1992).
38a. S. M. van Ham, L. van Alphen, F. R. Mooi, J. P. van Putten, Phase variation of *H. influenzae fimbriae*: transcriptional control of two divergent genes through a variable combined promoter region, *Cell 73*:1187 (1993).
39. S. E. Zamze and E. R. Moxon, Composition of the lipopolysaccharide from different capsular serotype strains of *Haemophilus influenzae*, *J. Gen. Microbiol. 133*:1443 (1987).
40. T. J. Inzana, Electrophoretic heterogeneity and interstrain variation of the lipopolysaccharide of *Haemophilus influenzae*, *J. Infect. Dis. 148*:499 (1983).
41. A. P. Johnson and T. J. Inzana, Loss of ciliary activity in organ cultures of rat trachea treated with lipooligosaccharide isolated from *Haemophilus influenzae*, *J. Med. Microbiol. 22*:265 (1986).
42. S. L. Kaplan, E. P. Hawkins, T. J. Inzana, C. C. Patrick, and E. O. Mason, Contribution of *Haemophilus influenzae* type b lipopolysaccharide to pathogenesis of infection, *Microb. Pathogen. 5*:55 (1988).
43. V. J. Quagliarello, W. J. Long, and W. N. M. Scheld, Morphologic alterations of the blood-brain barrier with experimental meningitis in the rat. Temporal sequence and role of encapsulation, *J. Clin. Invest. 77*:1084 (1986).
44. B. Wispelwey, A. J. Lesse, E. J. Hansen, and W. N. M. Scheld, *Haemophilus influenzae* lipopolysaccharide-induced blood brain barrier permeability during experimental meningitis in the rat, *J. Clin. Invest. 82*:1339 (1988).
45. B. Wispelwey, E. J. Hansen, and W. N. M. Scheld, *Haemophilus influenzae* outer membrane vesicle-induced blood brain barrier permeability during experimental meningitis, *Infect. Immun. 57*:2559 (1989).
46. A. R. Tunkel, W. Rosser, E. J. Hansen, and W. N. M. Scheld, Blood-brain barrier alterations in bacterial meningitis: development of an *in vitro* model and observations on the effects of lipopolysaccharide, *In Vitro Cell Dev. Biol. 27A*: 113 (1991).
47. P. R. Langford, M. Szabo, and E. R. Moxon, *In vitro* cytotoxicity of *Haemophilus influenzae* lipopolysaccharides for bovine aortal endothelial cells, *FEMS Microbiol. Lett. 81*:161 (1991).
48. D. Patrick, J. Betts, E. A. Frey, R. Prameya, K. Dorovini-Zis, and B. B. Finlay, *Haemophilus influenzae* lipopolysaccharide disrupts confluent monolayers of bovine brain endothelial cells *via* a serum-dependent cytotoxic pathway, *J. Infect. Dis. 165*:865 (1992).
49. S. D. Wright, R. A. Ramos, P. S. Tobias, R. J. Ulevitch, and J. C. Mathison, CD14, a receptor for complexes of lipopolysaccharide (LPS) and LPS binding protein, *Science 249*:1431 (1990).
50. A. R. Tunkel, B. Wispelwey, and W. N. M. Scheld, Bacterial meningitis: recent advances in pathophysiology and treatment, *Ann. Intern. Med. 112*:610 (1990).
51. P. Libby, J. M. Ordovas, K. R. Auger, A. H. Roblins, L. K. Birinyi, and C.

A. Dinarello, Endotoxin and tumor necrosis factor induce interleukin-1 gene expression in adult vascular endothelial cells, *Am. J. Pathol. 124*:179 (1986).
52. M. M. Mustafa, O. Ramilo, X. Saez-Liorens, J. Mertsola, R. R. Magness, and G. H. McCracken, Prostaglandin E_2 and I_2, interleukin-1β, and tumor necrosis factor in cerebrospinal fluid of infants and children with bacterial meningitis, *Pediatr. Infect. Dis. J. 8*:921 (1989).
53. V. J. Quagliarello, B. Wispelwey, W. J. Long, and W. N. M. Scheld, Recombinant human interleukin-1 induces meningitis and blood-brain barrier injury in the rat: characterization and comparison with tumor necrosis factor, *J. Clin. Invest. 87*:1360 (1991).
54. L. G. Rubin and E. R. Moxon, The effect of serum-factor induced resistance to somatic antibodies on the virulence of *Haemophilus influenzae* type b, *J. Gen. Microbiol. 131*:515 (1985).
55. S. Shaw, A. L. Smith, P. Anderson, and D. H. Smith, The paradox of *Haemophilus influenzae* type b bacteremia in the presence of serum bactericidal activity, *J. Clin. Invest. 58*:1019 (1976).
56. T. J. Inzana and P. Anderson, Serum-factor dependent resistance of *Haemophilus influenzae* type b to antibody to lipopolysaccharide, *J. Infect. Dis. 151*:869 (1985).
57. M. Kuratana, E. J. Hansen, and P. Anderson, Multiple mechanisms in serum-factor induced resistance of *Haemophilus influenzae* type b to antibody, *Infect. Immun. 58*:914 (1990).
58. P. Anderson, A. Flesher, S. Shaw, and A. L. Harding, Phenotypic and genetic variation in the susceptibility of *Haemophilus influenzae* type b to antibodies to somatic antigens, *J. Clin. Invest. 65*:885 (1980).
59. M. Kuratana and P. Anderson, Host metabolites that phenotypically increase the resistance of *Haemophilus influenzae* type b to clearance mechanisms, *J. Infect. Dis. 163*:1073 (1991).
60. R. W. Tolan, R. S. Munson, Jr., and D. M. Granoff, Lipopolysaccharide gel profiles of *Haemophilus influenzae* type b are not stable epidemiologic markers, *J. Clin. Microbiol. 24*:223 (1986).
61. A. Kimura and E. J. Hansen, Antigenic and phenotypic variations of *Haemophilus influenzae* type b lipopolysaccharide and their relationship to virulence, *Infect. Immun. 51*:69 (1986).
62. I. M. Helander, B. Lindner, H. Brade, K. Altmann, A. A. Lindberg, E. T. Rietschel, and U. Zahringer, Chemical structure of the lipopolysaccharide of *Haemophilus influenzae* strain I-69 Rd^-/b^+: a description of a novel deep-rough chemotype, *Eur. J. Biochem. 177*:483 (1988).
63. M. Virji, J. N. Weiser, A. A. Lindberg, and E. R. Moxon, Antigenic similarities in lipopolysaccharides of *Haemophilus* and *Neisseria* and expression of a digalactose structure also present on human cells, *Microb. Pathogen. 9*:441 (1990).
64. A. A. Campagnari, S. M. Spinola, A. J. Lesse, Y. A. Kwaik, R. E. Mandrell, and M. A. Apicella, Lipooligosaccharide epitopes shared among gram-negative non-enteric mucosal pathogens, *Microb. Pathogen. 8*:353 (1990).
65. R. E. Mandrell, R. McLaughlin, Y. A. Kwaik, A. Lesse, R. Yamasaki, B.

Gibson, S. M. Spinola, and M. A. Apicella, Lipooligosaccharides of some *Haemophilus* species mimic human glycosphingolipids and are sialylated, *Infect. Immun. 60*:1322 (1992).
66. J. N. Weiser, A. A. Lindberg, E. J. Manning, E. J. Hansen, and E. R. Moxon, Identification of a chromosomal locus for expression of lipopolysaccharide epitopes in *Haemophilus influenzae*, *Infect. Immun. 57*:3045 (1989).
67. J. Mertsola, L. D. Cope, X. Saez-Llorens, O. Ramilo, W. Kennedy, G. H. McCracken, and E. J. Hansen, *In vivo* and *in vitro* expression of *Haemophilus influenzae* type b lipo-oligosaccharide epitopes, *J. Infect. Dis. 164*:555 (1991).
68. E. R. Moxon and D. Maskell, *Haemophilus influenzae* lipopolysaccharide: the biochemistry and biology of a virulence factor, *Molecular Biology of Bacterial Infection: Current Status and Future Perspectives* (C. E. Hormaeche, C. W. Penn, and C. J. Smyth, eds.), Cambridge University Press, Cambridge, 1992).
69. A. Zwahlen, L. G. Rubin, and E. R. Moxon, Contribution of lipopolysaccharide to pathogenicity of *Haemophilus influenzae*: comparative virulence of genetically-related strains in rats, *Microb. Pathogen. 1*:465 (1986).
70. A. Zwahlen, L. G. Rubin, C. J. Connelly, T. J. Inzana, and E. R. Moxon, Alteration of the cell wall of *Haemophilus influenzae* type b by transformation with cloned DNA: association with attenuated virulence, *J. Infect. Dis. 152*:485 (1985).
71. S. M. Spinola, Y. Abu Kwaik, A. J. Lesse, A. A. Campagnari, and M. A. Apicella, Cloning and expression in *Escherichia coli* of a *Haemophilus influenzae* type b lipooligosaccharide synthesis gene(s) that encodes a 2-keto-3-deoxyoctulosonic acid epitope, *Infect. Immun. 58*:1558 (1990).
72. Y. Abu Kwaik, R. E. McLaughlin, M. A. Apicella, and S. M. Spinola, Analysis of *Haemophilus influenzae* type b lipooligosaccharide-synthesis genes that assemble or expose a 2-keto-3-deoxyoctulosonic acid epitope, *Mol. Microbiol. 5*:2475 (1991).
73. J. N. Weiser, D. J. Maskell, P. D. Butler, A. A. Lindberg, and E. R. Moxon, Characterization of repetitive sequences controlling phase variation of *Haemophilus influenzae* lipopolysaccharide, *J. Bacteriol. 172*:3304 (1990).
74. J. N. Weiser, A. A. Lindberg, E. J. Manning, E. J. Hansen, and E. R. Moxon, Identification of a chromosomal locus for expression of lipopolysaccharide epitopes in *Haemophilus influenzae*, *Infect. Immun. 57*:3045 (1989).
75. J. N. Weiser, J. M. Love, and E. R. Moxon, The molecular mechanism of phase variation of *Haemophilus influenzae* lipopolysaccharide, *Cell 59*:657 (1989).
76. L. D. Cope, R. Yogev, J. Mertsola, J. L. Latimer, M. S. Hanson, G. H. McCracken, Jr., and M. S. Hansen, Molecular cloning of a gene involved in lipooligosaccharide biosynthesis and virulence expression in *Haemophilus influenzae* type b, *Mol. Microbiol. 5*:1113 (1991).
77. D. J. Maskell, M. J. Szabo, P. D. Butler, A. E. Williams, and E. R. Moxon, Molecular analysis of a complex locus from *Haemophilus influenzae* involved in phase-variable lipopolysaccharide biosynthesis, *Mol. Microbiol. 5*:1013 (1991).

78. S. Adhya, The galactose operon, *Escherichia coli* and *Salmonella typhimurium*: cellular and molecular biology (F. C. Neidhart, J. L. Ingraham, K. B. Low, B. Magasanik, M. Schaechter, and H. E. Umbarger, eds.) American Society for Microbiology, Washington, DC, 1988, p. 1503.
79. D. J. Maskell, M. J. Szabo, M. E. Deadman, and E. R. Moxon, The *gal* locus from *Haemophilus influenzae*: cloning, sequencing and the use of *gal* mutants to study lipopolysaccharide, *Mol. Microbiol. 6*:3051 (1992).
80. J. N. Weiser, A. Williams, and E. R. Moxon, Phase-variable lipopolysaccharide structures enhance the invasive capacity of *Haemophilus influenzae*, *Infect. Immun. 58*:3455 (1990).
81. M. K. Pangburn, R. D. Schreiber, and H. J. Müller-Eberhard, Human complement C3b inactivator. Isolation, characterization and demonstration of an absolute requirement for serum protein β1H for cleavage of C3b and C4b in solution, *J. Exp. Med. 146*:257 (1977).
82. A. L. Smith, D. H. Smith, D. R. Averill, Jr, J. Marino, and E. R. Moxon, Production of *Haemophilus influenzae* b meningitis in infant rats by intraperitoneal inoculation, *Infect. Immun. 8*:278 (1973).
83. R. M. Crisel, R. S. Baker, and D. E. Dorman, Capsular polymer of *Haemophilus influenzae* type b. 1. Structural characterization of the capsular polymer of strain Eagan, *J. Biol. Chem. 250*:4926 (1975).
84. P. Branefors-Helander, C. Erbing, L. Kenne, and B. Lindberg, Structural studies of the capsular antigen of *Haemophilus influenzae* type b, *Acta Chem. Scand. Ser. B. 30*:276 (1976).
85. J. S. Kroll and E. R. Moxon, Genetic and phenotypic variation in the capsulation and virulence of Culture Collection strains of *Haemophilus influenzae* type b, *Microb. Pathogen. 7*:449 (1989).
86. P. W. Anderson, R. B. Johnston, Jr., and D. H. Smith, Human serum activities against *Haemophilus influenzae* type b, *J. Clin. Invest. 51*:31 (1972).
87. S. K. Hoiseth, E. R. Moxon, and R. P. Silver, Genes involved in *Haemophilus influenzae* type b capsule expression are part of an 18-kb tandem duplication, *Proc. Natl. Acad. Sci. USA 83*:1106 (1986).
88. L. D. Fothergill and C. A. Chandler, Observations on the dissociation of meningitic strains of *Haemophilus influenzae*, *J. Immunol. 31*:401 (1936).
89. B. W. Catlin and V. R. Tartagni, Delayed multiplication of newly capsulated transformants of *Haemophilus influenzae* detected by immunofluorescence, *J. Gen. Microbiol. 56*:387 (1969).
90. S. K. Hoiseth, C. J. Connelly, and E. R. Moxon, Genetics of spontaneous, high-frequency loss of b-capsule expression in *Haemophilus influenzae*, *Infect. Immun. 49*:389 (1985).
91. L. N. Brophy, J. S. Kroll, D. J. P. Ferguson, and E. R. Moxon, Capsulation gene loss and "rescue" mutations during the Cap+ to Cap− transition in *Haemophilus influenzae* type b, *J. Gen. Microbiol. 137*:2571 (1991).
92. J. S. Kroll, I. Hopkins, and E. R. Moxon, Capsule loss in *H. influenzae* type b occurs by recombination-mediated disruption of a gene essential for polysaccharide export. *Cell 53*:347 (1988).

93. C. F. Higgins, I. D. Hiles, G. P. C. Salmond, D. R. Gill, J. A. Downie, I. J. Evans, I. B. Holland, L. Gray, S. D. Buckel, A. W. Bell, and M. A. Hermodson, A family of related ATP-binding proteins coupled to many distinct biological processes in bacteria, *Nature 323*:448 (1986).
94. J. S. Kroll, B. Loynds, L. N. Brophy, and E. R. Moxon, The *bex* locus in encapsulated *Haemophilus influenzae*: a chromosomal region involved in capsule polysaccharide export, *Mol. Microbiol. 4*:1853 (1990).
95. A. N. Smith, G. J. Boulnois, and I. S. Roberts, Molecular analysis of the *Escherichia coli* K5 *kps* locus: identification and characterization of an inner-membrane capsular polysaccharide transport system, *Mol. Microbiol. 4*:1863 (1990).
96. M. Frösch, U. Edwards, K. Bousset, B. Krause, and C. Weisgerber, Evidence for a common molecular origin of the capsule gene loci in Gram-negative bacteria expressing group II capsular polysaccharides, *Mol. Microbiol. 5*:1251 (1991).
97. M. Frösch, D. Muller, K. Bousset, and A. Muller, Conserved outer membrane protein of *Neisseria meningitidis* involved in capsule expression, *Infect. Immun. 60*:793(1992).
98. M. E. Bayer, Areas of adhesion between wall and membrane of *Escherichia coli*, *J. Gen. Microbiol. 53*:395 (1968).
99. J. S. Kroll and E. R. Moxon, Capsulation and gene copy number at the *cap* locus of *Haemophilus influenzae* type b, *J. Bacteriol. 170*:859 (1988).
100. A. Dhir, Molecular studies on the contribution of capsular polysaccharide to the virulence of *Haemophilus influenzae*, dissertation, Oxford University, Oxford, 1988.
101. J. S. Kroll, S.Zamze, B. Loynds, and E. R. Moxon, Common organization of chromosomal loci for the production of different capsular polysaccharides in *Haemophilus influenzae*, *J. Bacteriol. 171*:3343 (1989).
102. S. Ely, J. Tippett, and E. R. Moxon, Identification and characterization of a serotype b-specific segment of the *Haemophilus influenzae* genome, *Infect. Immun. 57*:2926 (1989).
103. G. J. Boulnois, I. S. Roberts, R. Hodge, K. R. Hardy, K. B. Jann, and K. N. Timmis, Analysis of the K1 capsule biosynthesis genes of *Escherichia coli*: definition of three functional regions for capsule production, *Molec. Gen. Genet. 208*:242 (1987).
104. E. R. Vimr, W. Aaronson, and R. P. Silver, Genetic analysis of chromosomal mutations in the polysialic acid gene cluster of *Escherichia coli* K1, *J. Bacteriol. 171*:1106 (1989).
105. M. Frösch, C. Weisgerber, and T. F. Meyer, Molecular characterization and expression in *Escherichia coli* of the gene complex encoding the polysaccharide capsule of *Neisseria meningitidis* group B, *Proc. Natl. Acad. Sci. USA 86*:1669 (1989).
106. D. B. Danner, R. A. Deich, K. L. Sisco, and H. O. Smith, An 11-base-pair sequence determines the specificity of DNA uptake in *Haemophilus* transformation, *Gene 11*:311 (1980).

107. S. D. Goodman and J. J. Scocca, Identification and arrangement of the DNA sequence recognised in specific transformation of *Neisseria gonorrhoeae*, *Proc. Natl. Acad. Sci. USA 85*:6982 (1988).
108. S. Goodgal and M. A. Mitchell, Sequence and uptake specificity of cloned sonicated fragments of *Haemophilus influenzae* DNA, *J. Bacteriol. 172*:5924 (1990).
109. J. S. Kroll, B. M. Loynds, and P. R. Langford, Palindromic *Haemophilus* DNA uptake sequences in presumed transcriptional terminators in *Haemophilus influenzae* and *H. parainfluenzae*, *Gene 114*:1512 (1992).
110. E. R. Moxon and K. A. Vaughn, The type b capsular polysaccharide as a virulence determinant of *Haemophilus influenzae*: studies using clinical isolates and laboratory transformants, *J. Infect. Dis. 143*:517 (1981).
111. J. M. Musser, J. S. Kroll, E. R. Moxon, and R. K. Selander, Evolutionary genetics of the encapsulated strains of *Haemophilus influenzae*, *Proc. Natl. Acad. Sci. USA 85*:7758 (1988).
112. J. M. Musser, J. S. Kroll, D. M. Granoff, et al., Global genetic structure and molecular epidemiology of encapsulated *Haemophilus influenzae*, *Rev. Infect. Dis. 12*:75 (1990).
113. J. S. Kroll, B. M. Loynds, and E. R. Moxon, The *Haemophilus influenzae* capsulation gene cluster: a compound transposon, *Mol. Microbiol. 5*:1549 (1991).
114. I. Allan, J. S. Kroll, A. Dhir, and E. R. Moxon, *Haemophilus influenzae* serotype a: outer membrane protein classification and correlation with DNA polymorphism at the *cap* locus, *Infect. Immun. 56*:529 (1988).
115. J. S. Kroll, E. R. Moxon, and B.M. Loynds, An ancestral mutation enhancing the fitness and increasing the virulence of *Haemophilus influenzae* type b, *J. Infect. Dis. 168*:172 (1993).
116. S. Ely, J. Tippett, J. S. Kroll, and E. R. Moxon, Mutations affecting expression and maintenance of genes encoding the serotype b capsule of *Haemophilus influenzae*, *J. Bacteriol. 167*:44 (1986).
117. P. G. Corn, J. Anders, A. K. Takala, H. Kayhty, and S. K. Hoiseth, Genes involved in *Haemophilus influenzae* type b capsule expression are frequently amplified, *J. Infect. Dis. 167*:356 (1993).
118. J. J. LiPuma and J. R. Gilsdorf, Role of capsule in adherence of *Haemophilus influenzae* type b to human buccal epithelial cells, *Infect. Immun. 55*:2308 (1987).
119. M. Chanyangam, A. L. Smith, S. L. Moseley, M. Kuehn, and P. Jenny, Contribution of a 28-kilodalton membrane protein to the virulence of *Haemophilus influenzae*, *Infect. Immun. 59*:600 (1991).
120. J. Holland, P. R. Langford, K. J. Towner, and P. Williams, Evidence for *in vivo* expression of transferrin-binding proteins in *Haemophilus influenzae* type b, *Infect. Immun. 60*:2968 (1992).
121. J. J. LiPuma, H. Richman, and T. L. Stull, Haemocin, a bacteriocin produced by *Haemophilus influenzae* type b: species distribution and role in colonization, *Infect. Immun. 58*:1600 (1990).

9

Molecular Population Genetics of *Haemophilus influenzae*

James M. Musser and Vivek Kapur

Baylor College of Medicine, Houston, Texas

I. INTRODUCTION

Population genetic research has a rich history of scientific contributions that is virtually unknown to most medical scientists interested in microbial infectious diseases. In the 1970s, investigators began to exploit the techniques and theory of contemporary molecular population genetic analysis to study natural samples of bacteria recovered from human infections and other sources (1). In addition, scientists whose training and interests were predominantly in the area of evolutionary biology recognized that for several reasons bacteria may be ideal organisms to address certain questions of longstanding interest (2). Initially almost all research examining the population genetics of bacteria focussed on *Escherichia coli* (1–3) or other Enterobacteriaceae (3) because samples of these organisms were easy to obtain and could be grown readily by individuals who, in general, had not handled unicellular haploid pathogens with unfamiliar names and nutritional requirements.

Haemophilus influenzae was one of the first nonenteric bacterial species to be examined in detail by researchers interested in the molecular population genetics of pathogenic organisms (4). The goal of this chapter is to summarize studies addressing the global molecular population structure of the pathogen and to demonstrate how an understanding of the population genetics and evolution of this organism has enriched molecular pathogenesis research and provided an important model for similar studies with other human and veterinary pathogens. In addition, we present data describing serotype b Hib clone frequencies in 17 countries not previously sampled, and molecular phylogenetic analysis of allelic variants of several genes whose products are of potential medical interest. A more extensive description of some of the results summarized in this chapter is presented elsewhere (5).

II. MULTILOCUS ENZYME ELECTROPHORESIS—THE PRIMARY TOOL

A. Theory and Background

Examination of the population genetics of bacteria and other organisms requires a technique that rapidly indexes allelic variation at many chromosomal loci and can easily be applied to large samples—many hundreds to thousands of individual isolates—required to obtain statistically robust results. Notwithstanding the availability of techniques of directly assessing diversity at the gene level by restriction fragment analysis or nucleotide sequencing, in the mid-1980s, the only feasible way to measure allelic variation at large numbers of chromosomal loci on a very large scale in natural populations was by analysis of randomly selected sets of metabolic enzymes for electrophoretically demonstrable mobility variants (6). This statement remains generally true today, although the techniques of arbitrarily primed polymerase chain reaction (PCR) (7) and chromosomal profiling with other approaches based on the PCR (8), and large-scale comparative automated DNA sequence analysis promise to provide viable alternatives.

The multilocus enzyme electrophoresis approach employs starch gel electrophoresis to resolve allelic variants of metabolic "housekeeping" enzymes (6,9,10). Variation in enzyme mobility can be directly related to allelic variation at the genes encoding the proteins. Stated another way, enzyme electromorphs are equated with alleles at the corresponding structural gene locus. Unique combinations of electromorphs over all loci examined can then be equated with distinctive multilocus chromosomal genotypes, which in practice are referred to as electrophoretic types, or ETs. Electrophoresis of proteins detects a large percentage of nucleotide substitutions creating variation in the primary amino acid sequence (11–14). Although the amount of allelic variation detected by multilocus enzyme electrophoresis may underestimate the total nucleotide variation occurring at a locus as a consequence of failure to reveal silent nucleotide substitutions and amino acid replacements, in practice this technique provides ample—and sometimes abundant—polymorphism for indexing overall genomic divergence among isolates and for distinguishing among closely related strains. Through application of the statistics of contemporary molecular population genetic research, estimates of chromosomal relationships and differentiation of phylogenetic lineages are generated for all isolates examined. The relationships are usually graphically represented as a phylogenetic tree in two-dimensional dendrogram form. Importantly, the genomic differentiation revealed by this technique is strongly correlated for many pathogens (10), including *H. influenzae* (15,16), with estimates of nucleotide sequence divergence obtained from DNA hybridization studies. Because the electromorph variation identified by multilocus enzyme electrophoresis is interpretable in terms of allelic variation, access is gained to the extensive statistical methods and theoretical models of molecular population genetics (17). For example, statistical tests (18,18a) permit inferences to be drawn regarding levels of genetic recombination between cell lines in populations.

B. Initial Population Genetic Framework

Study of the population genetics and molecular epidemiology of *H. influenzae* by multilocus enzyme electrophoresis began in earnest in the mid-1980s with an analysis of 177 serotype b strains recovered mainly from patients with invasive disease episodes in the United States (4). Thirty-two distinctive multilocus enzyme genotypes (ETs) were identified, and it was found that 73% of invasive disease episodes were caused by strains of only three ETs. The investigation also showed that serotype b capsular polysaccharide in strains belonging to four rather distinct phylogenetic lineages of the species, each of which is associated with a characteristic set of outer membrane protein (OMP) electrophoretic profiles (OMP subtypes). To explain the occurrence of strong nonrandom associations of multilocus enzyme genotype and OMP subtype, and the repeated recovery of isolates with identical properties in widely separated geographic regions over a 40-year period, it was hypothesized that the structure of natural populations of serotype b *H. influenzae* is basically clonal as a consequence of infrequent recombination of chromosomal genes.

C. Samples Recovered from Global Sources

To study the genetic structure and molecular epidemiology of *H. influenzae* on a global scale, we assembled a collection of 2209 isolates of six polysaccharide capsule types, including 1975 serotype b isolates recovered in 30 countries (5). This sample was characterized for electrophoretically demonstrable allele profiles at 17 metabolic enzyme loci. Two hundred and eighty distinct multilocus genotypes were distinguished, and cluster analysis revealed two primary phylogenetic divisions, summarized by the dendrogram shown in Figure 1. Strains producing serotype c, e, and f capsules belong to single divisions and have no close genetic relationships to strains of other serotypes. Serotype a and b strains occur in both primary phylogenetic divisions. Interestingly, a close genetic relatedness between serotype d iso-

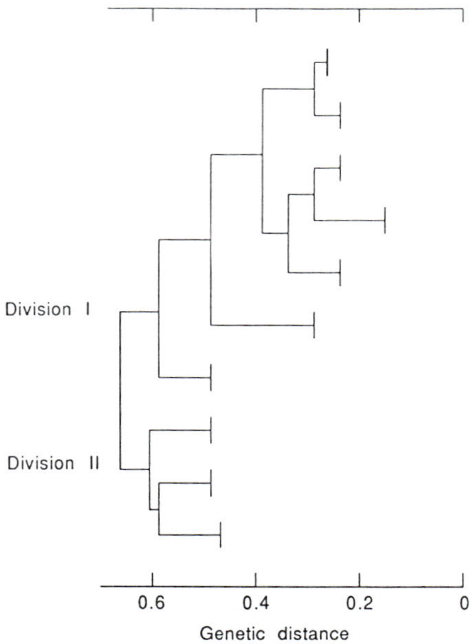

Cluster	Serotype	*cap* RFLP	Common OMP types
A1	b	S, V, G	1H, 1L, 2L
A2	b	S	1L, 2L, 3L
B1	b, d	S	6U
B2	a	T	1U
B4	a, b	N, T	1U, 5L
D	c		
F2	e		
H	a	M	2H, 4H, 6H
J	b	O	8H
K	f		

Figure 1 Dendrogram showing estimates of genetic relationships of 280 ETs of encapsulated *H. influenzae* and serotypes, *cap* region RFLP patterns, and common OMP types. The dendrogram was generated by the average-linkage method of clustering from a matrix of coefficients of pairwise genetic distance, based on 17 enzyme loci. There are two primary divisions: I and II. Groups represented by multiple ETs diverging from one another at a genetic distance of 0.20 or less were truncated; the point of truncation indicates the deepest level of divergence of families of ETs within the cluster. Note that serotype a and b strains with the same OMP subtype designation may not be identical in actual OMP electrophoretic pattern. The dendrogram is modified from data presented in Ref. 5.

lates and some strains of serotypes a and b was identified. This sample of isolates from global sources has served as a convenient source of genetically well-characterized strains useful for several types of investigations summarized in this review.

III. COMMON THEMES

Four common themes have emerged from studies of the global genetic population structure of encapsulated *H. influenzae* strains.

A. Clonal Population Structure

The population structure of encapsulated *H. influenzae* is predominantly clonal (19) as indicated by several lines of evidence (5,19,20), including the repeated recovery of isolates of identical multilocus enzyme genotype over large geographic areas (even globally) and long time periods and by the occurrence of linkage disequilibrium (nonrandom association) between enzyme loci (unpublished data). Because evolutionary convergence through independent mutation to the same multilocus enzyme genotype is highly unlikely (2), ETs are considered to mark clones. A combination of ET and OMP subtype or other traits has also been used to identify clones and subclones. Significant new evidence favoring the interpretation of a clonal structure for encapsulated organisms, derived from comparative gene sequencing studies, is discussed beyond. A basically clonal structure implies that rates of recombination of chromosomal genes between different cell lines are low, perhaps not in excess of the mutation rate.

B. Most Disease Episodes Caused by Few Clones

The number of encapsulated clones in natural populations is relatively small. Given the relatively high average level of allelic diversity at enzyme loci in encapsulated and other strains, a very large number of distinctive multilocus genotypes potentially could occur in natural populations (2). However, the actual number of clones sufficiently common to be recovered in our global sampling program involving thousands of isolates is only on the order of a few hundred. In addition, because the majority of cases of serious invasive infections (meningitis, sepsis, cellulitis, epiglottitis, etc.) is caused by small proportions of the total number of extant clones, the variance in pathogenicity among clones must be very large. Among a sample of 1975 serotype b strains examined, 1609 (81%) were assigned to one of the following nine ETs, each of which was represented by 20 or more isolates: ETs 1.9, 4, 12.5, 12.7, 12.8, 12.9, 21.6, 21.8, and 25.6 (5).

C. Geographic Variation in Clonal Structure

The analysis of the global strain sample identified strong patterns of geographic variation, on an intercontinental scale, in both the extent of genetic diversity and clonal composition of populations (5). For example, in Europe, the clone of *H. influenzae* marked by ET 12.5/3L OMP subtype is the major cause of invasive disease, and clonal diversity in most countries is rather low relative to that in the United States, where ET 1.9/OMP1H subtype is predominant. The analysis also suggested that the present distribution of clones is, in part, related to patterns of racial or ethnic differentiation and historical demographic movements of the human host populations. Patterns of geographic variation in serotype b population structure are described more fully in Section IV.

D. Subspecific Structure and Disease Specificity

Construction of a phylogenetic framework by molecular population genetic techniques permits one to study the manner in which the total genotypic diversity is apportioned with respect to several variables, including disease character. For both encapsulated and serologically nontypable *H. influenzae*, sufficient genetic data are now available to permit the conclusion to be reached that significant ecological, epidemiological, and other natural history correlates occur along clonal lineages (20). These correlates are most striking when the phylogenetic branches are deep, or ancient. For example, there are two deep phylogenetic divisions of encapsulated *H. influenzae*. Serotype b strains represent clones belonging to four distinct phylogenetic lineages, three occurring in primary division I and a fourth in division II (5,19,20). Serotype a strains also belong to divergent lineages in the two primary divisions. For both serotype a and serotype b, there is evidence of difference in virulence between clones in the two divisions. Serotype b clones in division I are responsible for more than 99% of invasive disease worldwide, and clones of serotype a in division I are more frequently recovered from serious disease episodes than are clones of serotype a in division II (5). Another example of the occurrence of nonrandom disease apportionment along phylogenetic lineages is the observation (21) that in Finland, strains of OMP subtype 1 and 1c cause different types of disease. (OMP subtype 1 strains are usually ET 12.5 or ET 12.8, and OMP subtype 1c organisms are mainly ET 21.8.) The observation that a clone marked by ET 21.6 is preferentially associated with the carrier state in several populations (5) and the finding that differences in OMP subtype distribution occur in carriers and patients with invasive disease episodes, (5,22,23) are compatible with the nonrandom apportionment of virulence character along phylogenetic lineages.

IV. OVERVIEW OF GLOBAL DISTRIBUTION OF SEROTYPE b CLONE DISTRIBUTION

The data summarized below were obtained from studies of strains recovered prior to introduction and widespread use of serotype b vaccines in several localities (5). Although in theory it is possible that vaccination has had a preferential detrimental effect on certain clones or subclones, a recent data from Finland suggests that this is not the case (24,24a).

A. United States and Canada

Virtually all cases of invasive serotype b disease in the United States are caused by isolates of two clones marked by ET 1.9/OMP 1H and ET 12/OMP 3L. A small proportion of disease (<5%) is also attributable to the ET 25.6/OMP 6U clone. Barenkamp et al. (25) presented evidence that the frequency of serotype b isolates of the OMP 1H type increased dramatically in the continental United States between the periods 1934–1954 and 1977–1980. In light of the nonrandom association of ET and OMP, this means an increase in the frequency of the ET 1.9/OMP 1H subclone. The virtual absence of variation in biotype (biotype I) among isolates of this subclone is consistent with this thesis. The simplest hypothesis accounting for the apparent temporal change in the composition of the population in the United States postulates an episode of periodic selection (26) involving a fitness mutation in a cell line representing ET 1.9/OMP 1H. An alternative hypothesis is that temporal variation in frequency of this subclone occurred as a consequence of modifications in demographic or other features of the host population, such that the fitness of the already existing ET 1.9/OMP 1H genotype increased relative to that of the other cell lines. For example, there was a marked increase in the frequency of child care outside the home in this period, and, in this regard, isolates of OMP 1H have been shown in certain studies to be associated with an increased risk of primary disease in children attending daycare centers. (27) and an increased risk of secondary transmission (28).

Despite geographic affinity and extensive sharing of ethnic background and cultural history, there are significant differences in the frequency of recovery of serotype b clones in Canada and the United States (5). One striking example was the occurrence of ET 100 throughout Canada (Ontario, Manitoba, Alberta, and British Columbia) but its absence in samples from the United States. We hypothesize that the ET 100 genotype may have its origin in the Ukraine or allied geographic area. Similarly, 17% of Canadian isolates, but only 4% of isolates from the United States, were ET 12.5.

B. Other Countries in the Western Hemisphere

We have recently examined samples from patients in Mexico, Chile (29), Brazil, and Uruguay (Table 1). Virtually all isolates from these countries were assigned to the ET 12 clone family, and most were ET 12.8, and therefore probably characterized by OMP subtype 3L. Uruguay was unusual in that 65% of cases were ET 12.5.

C. Europe

In striking contrast to the situation in the United States, most disease episodes in northern and western Europe are caused by strains of ET 12.5 with OMP subtype 3L (type 1 in the van Alphen system; see Chapter 7).

Recent study of additional strains from several European countries, including Poland, Italy, Germany, Iceland, Ireland, Wales (30), England (30a), Austria, and Belgium (Table 1), extend the general principle that with the exception of Iceland, most disease episodes in western and northern Europe are caused by isolates of ET 12.5. A sample from Greece was notably more heterogeneous in clonal composition and showed that a significant proportion of disease was caused by ET 12.5 (46%) and ET 12.8 (23%).

Examination of relatively large samples of invasive serotype b isolates recovered in Iceland in the 1980s and 1990s demonstrated that in contrast to other European countries, including those in Scandinavia, virtually all serotype b invasive disease occurring in that country is caused not by ET 12.5/OMP 3L, but by ET 1.9/OMP 2L. For several reasons described in detail elsewhere (5), the hypothesis was formulated that strains of ET 1.9/

Table 1 Distribution by Country of *H. influenzae* Serotype b ETs

Source	*n*	1.9	8	12.5	12.6	12.7	12.8	25.6	Other
Mexico	9	2					7		
Brazil	30			5	1	1	21		2
Chile	20					2	12	5	1
Uruguay	20			13		3	3	1	
Iceland	42	23		13				2	4
England	14	12		1			1		
Wales	128	3		100	1	7	7	2	8
Ireland	51			42		3		1	5
Belgium	8			8					
Germany	8			7			1		
Austria	17	1		11			3		2
Poland	4			2	1			1	
Italy	17			17					
Greece	39	1	3	18		3	10		4
Israel	64			10			37	13	4
Lebanon	4							1	3
Jordan	3		1				1		1
Morocco	34						19	5	10
Pakistan	61						3		58[a]
Taiwan	32						24	8	

[a]57 isolates of ET 141 and 1 isolate of ET 140. These ETs are closely allied with ET 25.6

OMP 2L are "old" in Iceland and those of ET 12.5/OMP 3L are relatively newly introduced. Because human population genetic studies demonstrate significant admixture of Celtic ethnicity among Icelanders (31), it was reasoned that the ET 1.9/OMP 2L clone should occur in relatively high frequency among other human populations of Celtic ancestry that have lived in relative geographic isolation. We tested this hypothesis by an analysis of strains recovered from patients living in several maritime provinces of Canada. The discovery of the ET 1.9/OMP 2L clone in relatively high frequency among those Canadian patients strongly supports our hypothesis and provides an explanation for the curiously different population structure of Icelandic serotype b strains. Van Alphen et al. (32) also noted that most strains in Iceland are unusual compared to other areas of Europe.

D. Africa

Serotype b strains recovered from predominantly black populations in Africa represent a heterogeneous array of genotypes (5,33). The ET 1.9/1H clone is notably lacking among samples recovered from several countries on the continent. We favor the notion that the relatively large amount of ET, OMP, and ET/OMP diversity present in African samples is due in large part to relatively longstanding association of serotype b organisms with populations that probably represent an ancestral human group (34).

A recent study by Biljmer et al. (35) of OMP subtypes in samples obtained from The Gambia confirmed several results of our earlier study showing significant diversity among African samples, including those from Gambian patients. However, although Biljmer et al. (35) claimed that most isolates were of OMP subtypes not previously described, those results are surprising inasmuch as a relatively large proportion of strains in the earlier study were subtype 2L (5).

E. Near East

Analysis of samples of strains obtained recently from Israel, Morocco, Lebanon, and Jordan show that most disease episodes are caused by isolates of ET 12.5, 12.8, or 25.6. No isolates of ET 1.9 were identified in these samples.

F. Asia and Australia

Most isolates examined from Asian or Oceania sources were ET 12.8, ET 25.6, or closely related clones (5). Papua New Guinea and Pakistan (36) were notable in that most isolates were of ETs very closely allied with ET 25.6. An extension of our studies to include organisms recovered from

Chinese patients in Taiwan demonstrated that isolates of ET 12.8 and ET 25.6 caused virtually all disease episodes caused by serotype b organisms (Table 1). A recent analysis (37) of 187 strains taken from largely Caucasian Australian patients with invasive disease found that virtually all (87%) organisms were of a single subtype identical to 3L, a result that confirms our previous findings (5) showing a marked predominance of the ET 12.5/3L clone. These data imply that ET 12.5/3L organisms were abundant in the United Kingdom prior to the large-scale colonization of Australia in the nineteenth century. Interestingly, two recent studies (37a,b) found that strains from aboriginal populations are more diverse in OMP subtype and have a higher proportion of OMP 2L one of the two main types recovered in Papua, New Guinea (5).

G. Clonal Turnover

The observation that ET 1.9 causes most invasive disease in Iceland, where ET 12.5 has only rarely been recorded, is compatible with the hypothesis that the European population of *H. influenzae* is experiencing clonal turnover, with ET 12.5 displacing other clones in an episode of periodic selection (26). Additional evidence of clonal turnover has been identified in studies of strains recovered in Minnesota (38) and Finland (39).

H. Global Gaps

The population structure and clonal diversity of serotype b strains circulating in several countries of significant interest, such as the former Soviet Union, India, and mainland China, has not yet been conducted. In addition, more extensive sampling of countries in eastern Europe and the Near East is needed. The senior author (J.M.M.) is very interested in analyzing samples of isolates recovered from these localities, and especially from patients of known ethnicity.

I. Implications for Immunoprophylaxis Research

If future vaccines are formulated to include serotype b OMP alleles that demonstrate significant geographic variation in frequency (such as P1 and P2; see below), it may be appropriate to employ knowledge of local bacterial population structure to tailor the composition of the vaccine. Allelic variants commonly associated with invasive disease in the target population should be employed. With the introduction and relatively widespread use of automated DNA sequencing instruments, it is now possible to define OMP gene allelic variants of large samples of strains in a matter of weeks.

V. COMPARATIVE CHROMOSOMAL ORGANIZATION STUDIES

Several groups have published the results of studies aimed at mapping the chromosomal location of virulence and other genes with pulsed-field gel electrophoresis and Southern blot hybridization techniques (40–42). Lee et al. (41) employed a derivative of a serotype d isolate and identified a chromosome of about 1900 kilobases, a value similar to those published by Kauc et al. (40) and Butler and Moxon (42). Interestingly, study of an epidemiologically unrelated serotype d strain identified a chromosomal pulsed-field restriction pattern indistinguishable from strain Rd, a result consistent with the hypothesis of recent evolutionary origin for serotype d strains (5,20).

Butler and Moxon (42) used contour-clamped homogeneous electric field pulsed-field gel electrophoresis to characterize the chromosomal maps of 11 distinct serotype b strains, selected to represent several divergent phylogenetic lineages, as indexed by multilocus enzyme electrophoresis. Four strains assigned to cluster A1 had similar restriction fragment polymorphism patterns generated by digestion with *Sma*I. Three strains in cluster A2 also had patterns similar to one another, but were clearly distinct from those in cluster A1. In addition, more heterogeneity was observed among the patterns of A2 strains than the A1 strains, a result consistent with the multilocus enzyme electrophoretic data demonstrating that there is substantial metabolic enzyme allelic diversity among isolates in cluster A2. Single *H. influenzae* strains assigned to clusters B1, J1, and J3 had unique *Sma*I cleavage patterns that were quite distinct from strains in major lineage A. Taken together, the pulsed-field gel electrophoretic data are consistent with the overall chromosomal relationships estimated by multilocus enzyme electrophoresis.

VI. ALLELIC VARIATION IN GENES ENCODING PUTATIVE VIRULENCE FACTORS

Knowledge of the global population structure of encapsulated organisms has proven of significant utility in formulating several studies examining allelic variation in genes encoding outer membrane proteins and other putative virulence factors (see Chapter 7). The pertinent results of these investigations are discussed below.

A. Outer Membrane Protein P1 Gene (*omp1*)

Protein P1 is one of the major molecules comprising the *H. influenzae* outer membrane (43). Two electrophoretic forms of this protein have been identified among strains commonly recovered from natural populations and are designated H and L. A relatively small number of strains has a P1 electrophoretic variant that is not H or L, and these organisms are given the "U" OMP1 designation (for "unclassified"). The gene encoding OMP P1 has been sequenced in strains representing three of the major serotype b *H. influenzae* clone families (44). Compared with the gene found in strain MinnA (ET 1.9/OMP subtype 1H), the gene in an ET 12/OMP subtype 3L organism was 94% identical and encoded a predicted protein that was 9% divergent. An ET 25.6/OMP 6U strain had an *ompl* gene that was 90% identical with the MinnA gene and encoded a protein that was 14% divergent. These relationships are shown in Figure 2. Sequence divergence of the 1H and 3L P1 genes was largely localized to two regions (nucleotides 307 to 360 and 646 to 744). The 6U P1 gene also displayed allelic variation in these two regions, and, in addition, had a third variant area encoded by nucleotides 1327 to 1365. Twenty-five *H. influenzae* serotype b strains recovered from global sources were also examined for restriction fragment length polymorphism with an *ompl* gene probe. All 10 strains assigned to OMP subtype 1H, which are a distinct clone as assessed by multilocus enzyme electrophoresis, had a single hybridization band of 6 kilobases. Similarly, all strains of OMP subtypes 3L and 13L, which are found in strains closely related in overall chromosomal character, were characterized by a single band of 8.8 kb. Five isolates of OMP subtype 6U assigned to a third major *H. influenzae* clone family were also identical in *ompl* RFLP pattern. One strain ("Rab") assigned to a very divergent serotype b chromosomal phylogenetic lineage gave a unique hybridization pattern. Taken together, allelic differentiation in *ompl* is cognate with chromosomal divergence assessed by multilocus enzyme electrophoesis.

Proulx et al. (45) developed a panel of eight murine monoclonal antibodies against OMP P1 purified from an ET 12/3L strain. These monoclonal antibodies were used to characterize a sample of 140 encapsulated *H. influenzae* strains recovered worldwide and representative of the major clone families identified among serotype a, b, and d strains. An epitope was identified that reacted with seven monoclonal antibodies and was expressed by all type b strains assigned to lineages A1 and A2. Serotype b strains assigned to cluster B1 (mainly 6U strains) failed to react with these seven antibodies, but did react with antibody P1.8. Interestingly, serotype a strains assigned to cluster B1 were recognized by all monoclonals except P1.8. None of the serotype a and b strains assigned to major phylogenetic division II were recognized by the panel of monoclonal antibodies. Taken together, these results demonstrate that the patterns of P1 surface epitope exposure, like that for OMP P2 (see below), are strongly cognate with genetic lineages of encapsulated *H. influenzae* strains and, therefore, support the hypothesis that the population structure of encapsulated *H. influenzae* is predominantly clonal.

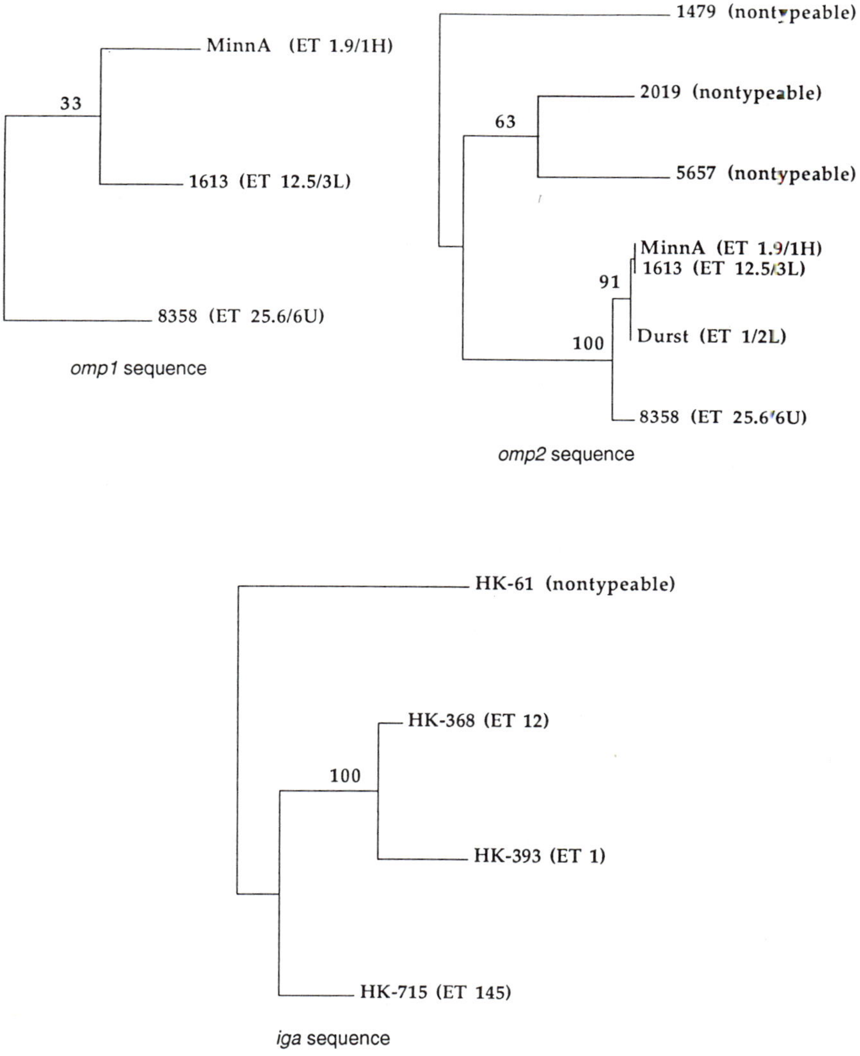

Figure 2 Phylogenetic analysis of putative virulence gene alleles of *Haemophilus influenzae*. The amino acid sequences of alleles of outer membrane protein 1, outer membrane protein 2, and immunoglobulin IgA1 protease were derived from the coding regions of the nucleotide sequences deposited in GenBank [*omp1*, J03381 (MinnA), M63151 (1613), and M73494 (8358); *omp2*, J03359 (MinnA), M93268 (1479), M93269 (2019), and M93270 (5657); and *iga*, M87489 (HK715), M87490 (HK393), M87491 (HK61), and M87492 (HK368)] and aligned with the program Clustal (103). The tree was generated with the computer program PAUP 3.0q (104), and the bootstrap method (105). The numbers adjacent to a node represent the proportion of 2000 trees that contained the variants to the right as a monophyletic group.

A more recent epitope analysis of an immunodominant domain on P1 using synthetic peptides and anti-idiotype antibodies extended these findings (46)

B. Outer Membrane Protein P2 Gene (*omp2*)

1. Serotype b Strains

The observation (47) that polyclonal antibody directed against OMP P2 is protective in an infant rat model of bacteremia led Munson and colleagues to study diversity among the *omp2* gene found in strains selected to represent the major serotype b OMP subtypes recovered from patients with invasive disease in the United States (48). The sequence of the P2 gene from strain MinnA (ET 1.9/1H OMP subtype) was compared with the gene found in organisms assigned to OMP subtype 2L (strain Durst, ET 1), OMP subtype 3L (strains 1613 and 3175 and, ET 12.5), and subtype 6U (strain 8358, ET 25.6). The OMP2 gene found in the ET 12.5/OMP 3L organism was identical to the MinnA sequence and differed from the gene in strain Durst by a single nonsynonymous change (Arg → Gln) at position 186. In constrast, the OMP2 gene in the ET 25.6/OMP 6U organism was characterized by 13 nucleotide changes resulting in 10 amino acid alterations. Interestingly, many of the nonsynonymous changes are clustered in a region (amino acids 181 to 190) that apparently contains an immunodominant epitope (48). An analysis of phylogenetic relationships among the three *omp2* alleles demonstrates that, in general, the phylogeny of the *omp2* alleles is cognate with the overall chromosomal relationships, as indexed by multilocus enzyme electrophoresis.

We note that the *omp2* gene found in MinnA is also identical to the sequence for a strain (DL42) published by Hansen et al. (49). Munson et al. (48) also stated that a second 3L strain had the identical *omp2* gene.

2. Serological Diversity in OMP P2 Occurs Along Clonal Lineages of Encapsulated Strains

Several groups of investigators have developed panels of monoclonal antibodies against OMP P2 (50–52). A set of 16 monoclonal antibodies was used to characterize a sample of 119 encapsulated *H. influenzae* strains recovered worldwide and representative of the major clone families identified among serotype a, b, and d strains. Two antibodies (mAb P2-4 and P2-6) recognized only serotype b strains assigned to primary phylogenetic division I. Three other monoclonal antibodies (P2-3, P2-8, and P2-11) reacted with division I serotype b isolates and also identified all genetically allied strains expressing serotype a and d polysaccharide capsules. In contrast, none of the 16 antibodies reacted with genetically divergent serotype a or b strains assigned to primary phylogentic division II (Fig. 1). The results demonstrate that the patterns of P2 surface epitope exposure are strongly cognate with genetic lineages of encapsulated *H. influenzae* strains and, therefore, support the hypothesis that the population structure of encapsulated *H. influenzae* is predominantly clonal. Recently knowledge of the clonal reactivity pattern of this panel of monoclonal antibodies was exploited to map B-cell epitopes on OMP P2 with recombinant proteins and synthetic peptides (53,54)

3. Unencapsulated Strains

Analysis of several samples of unencapsulated *H. influenzae* recovered from diverse geographic sources and infection types by multilocus enzyme electrophoresis (55,56) and other techniques (57–59) has identified substantial levels of genotypic diversity among these organisms. Forbes et al. (60) studied allelic variation in the structural gene for OMP P2 in a sample of 16 unencapsulated strains by PCR amplification and identified substantial levels of size variation in *omp2*. For example, the size of the amplified gene ranged from 970 to 1090 nucleotides, a length variation of about 15%. A restriction endonuclease map was also generated for the *omp2* gene in 10 strains by cleavage with seven enzymes. All 10 strains had distinct restriction maps and these differed from the map of the single serotype b strains studied.

Recently, Sikkema and Murphy (61) sequenced *omp2* in three unrelated strains of serologically nontypable *H. influenzae*. Four major "hypervariable" regions, each 12–35 amino acids long, and several smaller islands of variation of two to seven amino acids each were identified. Much of the variation was clustered in regions coding for amino acids with high antigenic index and surface exposure probability as shown by computer model analysis. The investigators also confirmed by restriction fragment length polymorphism analysis that substantial levels of heterogeneity exist at the *omp2* locus of natural isolates of serologically nontypable *H. influenzae*.

C. Outer Membrane Protein P6 Gene (*omp6*)

OMP P6 is a 16,000-dalton outer membrane protein that constitutes 1–5% of the protein content of the *H. influenzae* outer membrane (62). Several lines of evidence suggest that antibodies directed against OMP P6 are protective (63,64). Inasmuch as OMP P6 potentially could be incorporated into a *H. influenzae* vaccine, the gene (*omp6*) encoding this molecule was studied for allelic variation by comparative sequencing techniques. The sequence found in MinnA (ET 1.9) differed from that in strain Eagan (ET 6) by two synonymous nucleotides, and the gene in a serologically nontypable strain designated 1479 was found to differ from strain MinnA at 13 nucleotides, all of which were silent substitutions.

Diversity in the *omp6* gene was then studied in a sample of 40 strains (20 expressing serotype b polysaccharide and representing the breadth of diversity, as indexed by OMP subtyping and multilocus enzyme electrophoresis and 20 serologically "nontypable" for capsule) recovered from diverse sources with five oligonucleotide probes in Southern hybridization experiments (65). Thirty-one strains had the identical hybridization pattern for all probes tested, and five strains differed only by the occurrence of a less intense signal for one of the five probes. Taken together, the data indicate that allelic variation at the *omp6* locus is relatively restricted among natural populations of *H. influenzae*. It was hypothesized that allelic diversity is restricted as a consequence of strong selective pressure, presumbly due to functional constraints.

Recently, Murphy et al. (66) characterized the *omp6* gene harbored by strains of unencapsulated biotype IV *H. influenzae* recovered from neonatal sources. These strains are genetically highly divergent from other *H. influenzae* organisms and represent a previously undescribed cryptic genospecies of *Haemophilus* (see beyond). The DNA sequence of *omp6* in two strains (1595 and 1610) previously studied by multilocus enzyme electrophoresis were identical and encoded a predicted protein that differed from previously published sequences at 5 of 153 amino acids. (The number of nucleotide alterations was not given.) Two of the changes occur at positions 59 and 61 and apparently are located in a region that includes an antigenic site. Taken together, the comparative sequencing data are consistent with the population genetic results demonstrating that certain biotype IV strains are actually a previously unrecognized *Haemophilus* species incorrectly classified as *H. influenzae* (55).

D. Immunoglobulin A1 Protease Gene (*iga*)

Strains of *H. influenzae* synthesize an extracellular protease that specifically cleaves human immunoglobulin A1 in the hinge region of the heavy chain (67). Proteolysis results in production of intact Fc and Fab fragments, and the Fab moiety retains antigen-binding capacity. The specific cleavage of human IgA1, the resulting loss of IgA-dependent cell-mediated effector functions (67a), and the strong correlation between protease production and recovery from invasive disease episodes have led to the hypothesis that the enzyme is an important virulence factor.

Poulsen et al. (68) studied restriction fragment length polymorphisms in the *iga* gene region in a sample of 60 serotype b *H. influenzae* strains recovered in the United States and European countries and previously characterized for clonal lineage. Four RFLP classes were identified, and these patterns were strongly cognate with the clonal lineage of the strains.

For example, virtually all strains assigned to ET 1 and closely allied clones of lineage A1 had *iga* RFLP pattern II, ET 12 and related organisms had *iga* RFLP type I, and ET 25.6 and similar multilocus enzyme genotypes had the type III *iga* pattern. Highly divergent serotype b organisms assigned to major phylogenetic division II were *iga* type IV.

Recently, Poulsen et al. (69) studied allelic variation in the *iga* gene by comparative sequencing of the gene from four strains, including three serotype b organisms of known clonal lineage and one serologically non-typable strain that has not been studied by multilocus enzyme electrophoresis. The data demonstrate that the overall phylogeny of the *iga* gene in the three serotype b clones is cognate with the chromosomal relationships identified by multilocus enzyme electrophoresis, despite the occurrence of patterns of variation in the gene consistent with a mosaic structure that are probably due to rare horizontal transfer and recombination events.

E. Pilin Gene (*pil*)

The pilin gene has been studied by several groups of investigators mainly because of the observation that *H. influenzae* pili mediate bacterial adherence to several cell types (70,71). The pilin gene in three serotype b strains (M47, MinnA, and 770235), all of which are ET 1 organisms (unpublished data), are identical (71–73). Forney et al. (74) reported that the pilin gene in strain Eagan, a relatively rare ET 6/OMP 1L isolate, was 16% divergent from the ET 1 isolates, a value that is unusually large for strains that are of relatively related clones. Coleman et al. (72) showed that the pilin gene in an unencapsulated strain is 23% divergent from published serotype b pilin gene sequences.

F. Molecular Variation at the Capsulation Locus

The capsulation locus in *H. influenzae* has been studied extensively in the last decade (75,76,76a). It is now known that this locus in type a, b, c, and d strains is organized in an identical fashion, with a central DNA segment encoding serotype-specific information and flanking sequences common to all encapsulated strains (75). The occurrence of serotype a and serotype b expression in association with chromosomal genotypes that are highly divergent in overall character led to the hypothesis that horizontal transfer and recombination of capsulation genes occurs occasionally in natural populations (20). This hypothesis was subsequently confirmed by comparative gene-sequencing studies (76). Genes clustered in one of the non–serotype-specific *cap* segments (region 1) have diverged to an extent (12% nucleotide dissimilarity) that is essentially equivalent to the expected level of differentiation of the genomes assigned to the two major phylogenetic divisions. In striking contrast, genes in region 2 conferring serotype b–specific expression were identical in a stretch of 230 bp studied and were also identical by restriction endonuclease mapping with 13 enzymes. Taken together, the data strongly support the hypothesis of a recent horizontal transfer event involving region 2 DNA.

G. Superoxide Dismutase Gene (*sod*)

Superoxide dismutases (SOD) are metalloenzymes that detoxify superoxide radicals and therefore protect cells against oxygen damage. It is thought that SOD may be a virulence factor for certain pathogenic bacteria by contributing to resistance to oxygen radicals generated by host cell phagolysomes (77). Recently the gene encoding a copper-zinc superoxide dismutase was cloned and characterized from a *H. influenzae* strain assigned to major phylogenetic division II (78). Interestingly, it was discovered that the *sod* gene occurs only among clones comprising division II and is not found among division I isolates which together account for virtually all invasive disease episodes. In addition, the *sod* gene in division II isolates contains a single base pair change resulting in an inactive enzyme as a consequence of a histidine ↔ tyrosine replacement. An *sod* allele encoding an active enzyme was found in isolates of *Haemophilus parainfluenzae*. Kroll et al. (78) speculated that SOD production might contribute to escape from host mucociliary clearance mechanisms.

VII. OTHER CONTRIBUTIONS MADE BY THE MOLECULAR POPULATION GENETIC APPROACH

A. The Brazilian Purpuric Fever Clone

Brazilian purpuric fever is a serious invasive disease of children that was first characterized in 1984, when an outbreak in Promissao, Sao Paulo State, Brazil, resulted in 10 cases, all of which were fatal (79). Intensive epidemiological investigations demonstrated that *Haemophilus influenzae* biogroup aegyptius (formerly *H. aegyptius*) can be recovered from most patients with BPF (80). Analysis by multilocus enzyme electrophoresis revealed that in all cases isolates were a single clone (81). Subsequent studies demonstrated that biogroup aegyptius isolates form three distinct evolutionary lineages of the species *H. influenzae* and isolates of the case clone are genetically not closely related to other isolates classified as biogroup ageyptius (82). The Brazilian purpuric fever case clone was found to be genetically allied with *H. influenzae* isolates producing serotype c polysaccharide capsule. It has been hypothesized based on the population genetic evidence that biogroup ageyptius isolates may represent cell lineages occasionally transmitted from nonhuman hosts or spawned from a much larger base population consisting of genetically diverse nonpathogenic precursor clones.

The finding that the BPF strains are highly divergent in overall chromosomal genotype from other strains assigned to biogroup ageyptius provides a ready explanation for the results of studies demonstrating that strains of the BPF clone differ from other biogroup ageyptius strains in virtually every characteristic examined (83–91).

B. A New *Haemophilus* Species

In the course of population genetic analysis of a sample of 65 serologically nontypable isolates recovered largely from children with invasive and noninvasive disease in the United States, four closely related biotype IV ETs associated with obstetrical or neonatal bacteremia were found to be highly divergent from all others examined (55). Because estimates of genetic relatedness based on multilocus enzyme electrophoresis for strains of *Legionella* spp. (92) and other species had been shown to be positively correlated with measures of similarity in total nucleotide sequences derived from DNA hybridization experiments, we hypothesized that these isolates were specifically distinct. Subsequently, Quentin et al. (15) examined genetic relationships among a sample of 112 unencapsulated *H. influenzae* strains recovered from genital, obstetric, and neonatal sources in the United States and France by multilocus enzyme electrophoresis and demonstrated that strains of the divergent *Haemophilus* organisms hybridized at well below the 70% level conventionally taken as the criterion of species level differentiation in many groups of bacteria. More recently, the hybridization studies were expanded and definitive evidence was presented that this unusual group of urogenital organisms is a newly recognized *Haemophilus* species (16). Isolates of this species have never been identified in settings other than neonatal, obstetrical, or urogenital disease, an observation that strongly suggests the organism is a urogenital specialist. Consistent with this hypothesis is the discovery that isolates of this species readily adhere to cells of urogenital epithelial, but not cells of respiratory tract origin (93).

VIII. CONCLUDING REMARKS

Global sampling of encapsulated strains of *H. influenzae* has led to definition of the genetic structure of populations and construction of evolutionary frameworks reflecting overall genomic relatedness of strains and clones. This framework has been exploited by several groups of investigators to advance our understanding of pathogenesis and the distribution of virulence characters. With the advent of automated DNA sequencing, one potentially fruitful area for future research is large-scale characterization of allelic variation in virulence genes, in strains selected to represent several distinct clonal lineages. This approach has already proved successful in studies addressing the clonal distribution of alleles of virulence gene, the molecular evolutionary genetics of virulence gene variation, and the molecular basis of temporal variation in disease frequency and severity of another human bacterial pathogen, *Streptococcus pyogenes* (94–102). It would also be useful to more fully understand the forces responsible for subspecific structure in *H. influenzae.* For example, do barriers exist to recombination among the major phylogenetic lineages? Finally, there has been surprisingly little interest in the molecular study of clone marked by ET 21.6/OMP 13L, a line that is frequently found in the carrier state but seldom recovered from invasive infections.

ACKNOWLEDGMENTS

The unflagging support of Professor R. K. Selander is gratefully acknowledged. We thank all our colleagues who generously supplied strains and preprints of unpublished manuscripts.

REFERENCES

1. R. Milkman, Electrophoretic variation in *Escherichia coli* from natural sources, *Science 182*:1024 (1973).
2. R. K. Selander and B. R. Levin, Genetic diversity and structure in *Escherichia coli* populations, *Science 210*:545 (1980).
3. H. Ochman, T. S. Whittam, D. Caugant, and R. K. Selander, Enzyme polymorphism and genetic population structure in *Escherichia coli* and *Shigella*, *J. Gen. Microbiol. 129*:2715 (1983).
4. J. M. Musser, D. M. Granoff, P. E. Pattison, and R. K. Selander, A population genetic framework for the study of invasive diseases caused by serotype b strains of *Haemophilus influenzae*, *Proc. Natl. Acad. Sci. USA 82*:5078 (1985).
5. J. M. Musser, J. S. Kroll, D. M. Granoff, E. R. Moxon, B. R. Brodeur, J. Campos, H. Dabernat, W. Frederiksen, J. Hamel, G. Hammond, E. A. Hoiby, K. E. Jonsdottir, M. Kabeer, I. Kallings, W. N. Khan, M. Kilian, K. Knowles, H. J. Koornhof, B. Law, K. I. Li, J. Montgomery, P. E. Pattison, J.-C. Piffaretti, A. K. Takala, M. L. Thong, R. A. Wall, J. I. Ward, and R. K. Selander, Global genetic structure and molecular epidemiology of encapsulated *Haemophilus influenzae*, *Rev. Infect. Dis. 12*:75 (1990).
6. R. K. Selander, D. A. Caugant, H. Ochman, J. M. Musser, M. N. Gilmour, and T. S. Whittam, Methods of multilocus enzyme electrophoresis for bacte-

rial population genetics and systematics, *Appl. Environ. Microbiol. 51*:873 (1986).
7. J. Welsh and M. McClelland, Fingerprinting genomes using PCR with arbitrary primers, *Nucleic Acids Res. 18*:7213 (1990).
8. J. Versalovic, V. Kapur, E. O. Mason, Jr., U. Shah, T. Koeuth, J. R. Lupski, and J. M. Musser, Penicillin-resistant *Streptococcus pneumoniae* strains recovered in Houston, Texas: Identification and molecular characterization of multiple clones, *J. Infect. Dis., 167*:850 (1993).
9. R. C. Lewontin, *The Genetic Basis of Evolutionary Change*, Columbia University Press, New York, 1974.
10. R. K. Selander and J. M. Musser, The population genetics of bacterial pathogenesis, *Molecular Basis of Bacterial Pathogenesis* (B. H. Iglewski, and V. L. Clark, ed.), Academic Press, Orlando, FL, 1990, p. 11.
11. M. Kreitman, Nucleotide polymorphism at the alcohol dehydrogenase locus of *Drosophila melanogaster*, *Nature 304*:412 (1983).
12. P. H. Cooke and J. G. Oakeshott, Amino acid polymorphisms for the esterase-6 in *Drosophila melanogaster*, *Proc. Natl. Acad. Sci. USA 86*:1426 (1989).
13. K. Nelson, T. S. Whittam, and R. K. Selander, Nucleotide polymorphism and evolution in the glyceraldehyde-3-phosphate dehydrogenase gene (*gapA*) in natural populations of *Salmonella* and *Escherichia coli*, *Proc. Natl. Acad. Sci. USA 88*:6667 (1991).
14. S. W. Schaeffer and E. L. Miller, Molecular population genetics of an electrophoretically monomorphic protein in the alcohol dehydrogenase region of *Drosophila pseudoobscura*, *Genetics 132*:163 (1992).
15. R. Quentin, A. Goudeau, R. J. Wallace, Jr., A. L. Smith, R. K. Selander, and J. M. Musser, Urogenital, maternal, and neonatal isolates of *Haemophilus influenzae*: identification of unusually virulent serologically non-typable clone families and evidence for a new *Haemophilus* species, *J. Gen. Microbiol. 136*:1203 (1990).
16. R. Quentin, C. Martin, J. M. Musser, N. Pasquier-Picard, and A. Goudeau, Genetic characterization of a cryptic genospecies of *Haemophilus* causing urogenital and neonatal infections, *J. Clin. Microbiol. 31*:1111 (1993).
17. M. Nei, *Molecular Evolutionary Genetics*, Columbia University Press, New York, 1987.
18. S. Sawyer, Statistical tests for detecting gene conversion, *Mol. Biol. Evol. 6*:526 (1989).
18a. T. S. Whittaun, H. Ochman, and R. K. Selander, Multilocus genetic structure in natural populations of *Escherichia coli*, *Proc. Natl. Acad. Sci. USA*, *80*:1751 (1983).
19. J. M. Musser, J. S. Kroll, E. R. Moxon, and R. K. Selander, Clonal population structure of encapsulated *Haemophilus influenzae*, *Infect. Immun. 56*:1837 (1988).
20. J. M. Musser, J. S. Kroll, E. R. Moxon, and R. K. Selander, Evolutionary genetics of the encapsulated strains of *Haemophilus influenzae*, *Proc. Natl. Acad. Sci. USA 85*:7758 (1988).

21. A. K. Takala, L. van Alphen, J. Eskola, J. Palmgren, P. Bol, and P. H. Makela, *Haemophilus influenzae* type b strains of outer membrane subtypes 1 and 1c cause different types of invasive disease, *Lancet ii*:647 (1987).
22. C. M. Hampton, S. J. Barenkamp, and D. M. Granoff, Comparison of outer membrane protein subtypes of *Haemophilus influenzae* type b isolates from healthy children in the general population and from diseased patients, *J. Clin. Microbiol. 18*:596 (1983).
23. L. van Alphen, P. Bol, M. L. J. Kok, and L. Geelen-van den Broek, Difference in subtype distribution of *Haemophilus influenzae* type b from carriers in the general population and patients with meningitis, *J. Med. Microbiol. 34*:313 (1991).
24. A. K. Takala, J. Eskola, M. Leinonen, H. Kayhty, A. Nissinen, E. Pekkanen, and P. H. Makela, Reduction of oropharyngeal carriage of *Haemophilus influenzae* type b (Hib) in children immunized with an Hib conjugate vaccine. *J. Infect. Dis. 164*:982 (1991).
24a. L. van Alphen, A. K. Takala, L. Geelen-van den Broek, J. Dankert, and J. Eskola, Changes in the distribution of *Haemophilus influenzae* type b clones associated with widespread infant vaccination in Finland, *J. Infect. Dis. 166*:1340 (1992).
25. S. J. Barenkamp, D. M. Granoff, and M. Pittman, Outer membrane protein subtypes and biotypes of *Haemophilus influenzae* type b: relation between strains isolated in 1934–1954 and 1977–1980, *J. Infect. Dis. 148*:1127 (1982).
26. A. L. Koch, The pertinence of the periodic selection phenomenon to prokaryotic evolution, *Genetics 77*:127 (1974).
27. M. T. Osterholm, J. N. Kuritsky, L. N. Pierson, T.A. Libby, R. A. Kaslow, and D. M. Granoff, Risk of secondary *Haemophilus influenzae* type b (Hib) disease in day care, *Pediatr. Res. 18* (Suppl.): 282A (#1121) (abstr.) (1984).
28. S. J. Barenkamp, D. M. Granoff, and R. S. Munson, Jr., Outer-membrane protein subtypes of *Haemophilus influenzae* type b and spread of disease in day-care centers, *J. Infect. Dis. 144*:210 (1981).
29. R. Lagos, A. Avendano, I. Horwitz, J. M. Musser, S. K. Hoiseth, D. R. Maneval, Jr., M. J. Jones, M. M. Levine, J. P. Dattas, I. Prenzel, N. Enriquez, S. Topelberg, F. Olivari, and J. G. Morris, Jr., Molecular epidemiology of *Haemophilus influenzae* within families in Santiago, Chile, *J. Infect. Dis. 164*:1149 (1991).
30. A. J. Howard, K. T. Dunkin, J. M. Musser, and S. R. Palmer, Epidemiology of *Haemophilus influenzae* type b invasive disease in Wales, *Br. Med. J. 303*:441. (1991).
30a. G. Urwin, J. M. Musser, and M. F. Yuan, Clonal analysis of *Haemophilus influenzae* type b isolates from meningitic and nonmeningitic disease in the United Kingdom, *J. Med. Microbiol.* (in press).
31. E. A. Thompson, The Icelandic admixture problem, *Ann. Hum. Genet. 36*:425 (1973).
32. L. van Alphen, L. Geelen, K. Jonsdottir, A. K. Takala, H. Kayhty, and H. C.

Zanen, Distinct geographic distribution of subtypes of *Haemophilus influenzae* type b in western Europe, *J. Infect. Dis. 156*:216 (1987).
33. R. S. Munson, Jr., M. H. Kabeer, A. A. Lenoir, and D. M. Granoff, Epidemiology and prospects for prevention of disease due to *Haemophilus influenzae* in developing countries, *Rev. Infect. Dis. 11*:S588 (1989).
34. L. Vigilant, M. Stoneking, H. Harpending, K. Hawkes, and A. C. Wilson, African populations and the evolution of human mitochondrial DNA, *Science 253*:1503 (1991).
35. H. A. Bijlmer, L. van Alphen, L. Geelen-van den Broek, B. M. Greenwood, H. A. Valkenburg, and J. Dankert, Molecular epidemiology of *Haemophilus influenzae* type b in The Gambia, *J. Clin. Microbiol. 30*:386 (1992).
36. G. A. Weinberg, A. Ghafoor, Z. Ishaq, N. K. Nomani, M. Kabeer, F. Anwar, M. I. Burney, A. W. Qureshi, J. M. Musser, R. K. Selander, and D. M. Granoff, Clonal analysis of *Haemophilus influenzae* isolated from children from Pakistan with lower respiratory tract infections, *J. Infect. Dis. 160*:634 (1989).
37. D. A. Clements, S. J. MacInnes, and G. L. Gilbert, Outer membrane protein subtypes of *Haemophilus influenzae* type b isolates causing invasive disease in Victoria, Australia, from 1988 to 1990, *J. Clin. Microbiol. 30*:1879 (1992).
37a. G. L. Gilbert, and D. A. Clements, Distribution of *Haemophilus influenzae* type b outer membrane protein subtypes in different ethnic groups in Australia, *J. Infect. Dis. 168*:255 (1993).
37b. D. Hansman, and A. Lawrence, Outer-membrane protein and immunoblot analysis of Australian isolates of *Haemophilus influenza, J. Med. Microbiol. 38*:378 (1993).
38. D. M. Granoff, K. Sheetz, J. P. Pandey, M. H. Nahm, J. H. Rambeck, J. L. Jacobs, J. Musser, R. K. Selander, M. Kabeer, T. V. Murphy, and M. T. Osterholm, Host and bacterial factors associated with *Haemophilus influenzae* type b disease in Minnesota children vaccinated with type b polysaccharide, *J. Infect. Dis. 159*:908 (1989).
39. A. K. Takala, L. van Alphen, J. M. Musser, L. Geelen, R. K. Selander, J. Eskola, and P. H. Makela, Bacteriologic epidemiology of *Haemophilus influenzae* type b strains causing invasive infections in Finland, *J. Infect. Dis. 160*:237 (1989).
40. L. Kauc, M. Mitchell, and S. H. Goodgal, Size and physical map of the chromosome of *Haemophilus influenzae*, *J. Bacteriol. 171*:2474 (1989).
41. J. J. Lee, H. O. Smith, and R. J. Redfield. Organization of the *Haemophilus influenzae* Rd genome, *J. Bacteriol. 171*:3016 (1989).
42. P. D. Butler, and E. R. Moxon. A physical map of the genome of *Haemophilus influenzae* type b, *J. Gen. Microbiol. 136*:2333 (1990).
43. S. J. Barenkamp, R. S. Munson, Jr., and D. M. Granoff, Subtyping isolates of *Haemophilus influenzae* type b by outer-membrane protein profiles, *J. Infect. Dis. 143*:668 (1981).
44. R. Munson, Jr., S. Grass, M. Einhorn, C. Bailey, and C. Newell. Comparative analysis of the structures of the outer membrane protein P1 genes from

major clones of *Haemophilus influenzae* type b, *Infect. Immun.* *57*:3300 (1989).

45. C. Proulx, R. S. Munson, Jr., S. Grass, J. Hamel, D. Martin, and B. R. Brodeur, Identification of a surface-exposed immunodominant epitope on outer membrane protein P1 of *Haemophilus influenzae* type b, *Infect. Immun.* *59*:963 (1991).
46. C. Proulx, J. Hamel, P. Chong, D. Martin, and B. R. Brodeur, Epitope analysis of an immunodominant domain on the P1 protein of *Haemophilus influenzae* type b using synthetic peptides and anti-idiotypic antibodies, *Microb. Pathog.* *12*:433 (1992).
47. R. S. Munson, Jr., J. L. Shenep, S. J. Barenkamp, and D. M. Granoff, Purification and comparison of outer membrane protein P2 from *Haemophilus influenzae* type b isolates, *J. Clin. Invest.* *72*:677 (1983).
48. R. Munson, Jr., C. Bailey, and S. Grass, Diversity of the outer membrane protein P2 gene from major clones of *Haemophilus influenzae* type b, *Mol. Microbiol.* *3*:1797 (1989).
49. E. J. Hansen, C. Hasemann, A. Clausell, J. D. Capra, K. Orth, C. R. Moomaw, C. A. Slaughter, J. L. Latimer, and E. E. Miller, Primary structure of the porin protein of *Haemophilus influenzae* type b determined by nucleotide sequence analysis, *Infect. Immun.* *57*:1100 (1989).
50. D. Martin, J. Hamel, B. R. Brodeur, and J. M. Musser, Antigenic relationships among the porin proteins of encapsulated *Haemophilus influenzae* clones, *J. Clin. Microbiol.* *28*:1720 (1990).
51. E. M. Haase, A. A. Campagnari, J. Sarwar, M. Shero, M. Wirth, C. U. Cumming, and T. F. Murphy, Strain-specific and immunodominant surface epitopes of the P2 porin protein of nontypeable *Haemophilus influenzae*, *Infect. Immun.* *59*:1278 (1991).
52. L. van Alphen, P. Eijk, L. Geelen-van den Broek, and J. Dankert, Immunochemical characterization of variable epitopes of outer membrane protein P2 of nontypeable *Haemophilus influenzae*, *Infect. Immun.* *59*:247 (1991).
53. D. Martin, R. Munson, Jr., S. Grass, P. Chong, J. Hamel, G. Zobrist, M. Klein, and B. R. Brodeur, Mapping of B-cell epitopes on the outer membrane P2 porin protein of *Haemophilus influenzae* by using recombinant proteins and synthetic peptides, *Infect. Immun.* *59*:1457 (1991).
54. J. Hamel, D. Dugourd, D. Martin, C. Proulx, P. Chong, and B. R. Brodeur, Localization of conserved B-cell epitopes among encapsulated and non-encapsulated *Haemophilus influenzae* P2 porin proteins using synthetic peptides, *J. Gen. Microbiol.* *138*:161 (1992).
55. J. M. Musser, S. J. Barenkamp, D. M. Granoff, and R. K. Selander, Genetic relationships of serologically nontypeable and serotype b strains of *Haemophilus influenzae*, *Infect. Immun.* *52*:183 (1986).
56. O. Porras, D. A. Caugant, B. Gray, T. Lagergard, B. R. Levin, and C. Svanborg-Eden, Difference in structure between type b and nontypable *Haemophilus influenzae* populations, *Infect. Immun.* *53*:79 (1986).

57. S. J. Barenkamp, R. S. Munson, Jr., and D. M. Granoff, Outer membrane protein and biotype analysis of pathogenic nontypable *Haemophilus influenzae*, *Infect. Immun. 36*:535 (1982).
58. K. D. Bruce and J. Z. Jordens, Characterisation of non-capsulate *Haemophilus influenzae* by whole-cell polypeptide profiles, restriction endonuclease analysis, and rRNA gene restriction patterns, *J. Clin. Microbiol 29*:291 (1991).
59. K. D. Bruce and T. H. Pennington, Clonal analysis of non-typable *Haemophilus influenzae* by sodium dodecyl sulphate-polyacrylamide gel electrophoresis of whole cell polypeptides, *J. Med. Microbiol. 34*:277 (1991).
60. K. J. Forbes, K. D. Bruce, A. Ball, and T. H. Pennington, Variation in length and sequence of porin (*ompP2*) alleles of non-capsulate *Haemophilus influenzae*, *Molec. Microbiol. 6*:2017 (1992).
61. D. J. Sikkema and T. F. Murphy, Molecular analysis of the P2 porin protein of nontypeable *Haemophilus influenzae*, *Infect. Immun. 60*:5204 (1992).
62. R. S. Munson, Jr., and D. M. Granoff, Purification and partial characterization of outer membrane proteins P5 and P6 from *Haemophilus influenzae* type b, *Infect. Immun. 49*:544 (1985).
63. B. A Green, B. J. Metcalf, T. Quinn-Dey, D. H. Kirkley, S. A. Quataert, and R. A. Deich, A recombinant non-fatty acylated form of the Hi-PAL (P6) protein of *Haemophilus influenzae* elicits biologically active antibody against both non-typeable and type b *H. influenzae*, *Infect. Immun. 58*:3272 (1990).
64. T. F. Murphy, L. C. Bartos, A. A. Campagnari, M. B. Nelson, and M. A. Apicella, Antigenic characterization of the P6 protein of nontypeable *Haemophilus influenzae*, *Infect. Immun. 54*:774 (1986).
65. M. B. Nelson, R. S. Munson, Jr., M. A. Apicella, D. J. Sikkema, J. P. Molleston, and T. F. Murphy, Molecular conservation of the P6 outer membrane protein among strains of *Haemophilus influenzae*: analysis of antigenic determinants, gene sequences, and restriction fragment length polymorphisms, *Infect. Immun. 59*:2658 (1991).
66. T. F. Murphy, C. Kirkham, and D. J. Sikkema, Neonatal, urogenital isolates of biotype 4 nontypeable *Haemophilus influenzae* express a variant P6 outer membrane protein molecule, *Infect. Immun. 60*:2016 (1992).
67. M. Kilian, B. Thomsen, T. E. Petersen, and H. Bleeg, Molecular biology of *Haemophilus influenzae* IgA1 proteases, *Mol. Immunol. 20*:1051 (1983).
67a. M. Kilian, J. Mestecky, and M. W. Russell, Defense mechanisms involving Fc-dependent functions of immunoglobulin A and their subversion by bacterial immunoglobulin A proteases, *Microbiol. Rev. 52*:296 (1988).
68. K. Poulsen, J. P. Hjorth, and M. Kilian, Limited diversity of the immunoglobulin A1 protease gene (*iga*) among *Haemophilus influenzae* serotype b strains, *Infect. Immun. 56*:987 (1988).
69. K. Poulsen, J. Reinholdt, and M. Kilian, A comparative genetic study of serologically distinct *Haemophilus influenzae* type 1 immunoglobulin A1 proteases, *J. Bacteriol. 174*:2913 (1992).

70. M. R. Loeb, E. Connor, and D. Penney, A comparison of the adherence of fimbriated and nonfimbriated *Haemophilus influenzae* type b to human adenoids in organ culture, *Infect. Immun. 56*:484 (1988).
71. S. M. van Ham, F. R. Mooi, M. G. Sindhunata, W. R. Maris, and L. van Alphen, Cloning and expression in *Escherichia coli* of *Haemophilus influenzae* fimbrial genes establishes adherence to oropharyngeal epithelial cells, *EMBO J. 8*:3535 (1989).
72. T. Coleman, S. Grass, and R. Munson, Jr., Molecular cloning, expression, and sequence of the pilin gene from nontypeable *Haemophilus influenzae* M37, *Infect. Immun. 59*:1716 (1991).
73. J. R. Gilsdorf, C. F. Marrs, K. W. McCrea, and L. J. Forney, Cloning, expression, and sequence analysis of the *Haemophilus influenzae* type b strain M43p+ pilin gene, *Infect. Immun. 58*:1065 (1990).
74. L. J. Forney, C. F. Marrs, S. L. Bektesh, and J. R. Gilsdorf, Comparison and analysis of the nucleotide sequences of pilin genes from *Haemophilus influenzae* type b strains Eagan and M43, *Infect. Immun. 59*:1991 (1991).
75. J. S. Kroll, S. Zamze, B. Loynds, and E. R. Moxon, Common organization of chromosomal loci for production of different capsular polysaccharides in *Haemophilus influenzae*, *J. Bacteriol. 171*:3343 (1989).
76. J. S. Kroll and E. R. Moxon, Capsulation in distantly related strains of *Haemophilus influenzae* type b: genetic drift and gene transfer at the capulation locus, *J. Bacteriol. 172*:1374 (1991).
76a. J. S. Kroll, E. R. Moxon, and B. M. Loynds, An ancestral mutation enhancing the fitness and increasing the virulence of *Haemophilus influenza* type b, *J. Infect. Dis. 168*:172 (1993).
77. B. L. Beck, L. B. Tabatabai, and J. E. Mayfield, A protein isolated from *Brucella abortus* is a [Cu,Zn] superoxide dismutase, *Biochemistry 29*:372 (1990).
78. J. S. Kroll, P. R. Langford, and E. R. Moxon, Copper-zinc superoxide dismutase of *Haemophilus influenzae* and *H. parainfluenzae*, *J. Bacteriol. 173*:7449 (1991).
79. Centers for Disease Control, Preliminary report: epidemic fatal purpuric fever among children—Brazil, *MMWR 34*:217 (1985).
80. Brazilian Purpuric Fever Study Group, Brazilian purpuric fever: epidemic purpura fulminans associated with antecedent purulent conjunctivitis, *Lancet ii*:757 (1987).
81. D. J. Brenner, L. W. Mayer, G. M. Carlone, L. H. Harrison, W. F. Bibb, M. C. Brandileone, F. O. Sottnek, K. Irino, M. W. Reeves, J. M. Swenson, K. A. Birkness, R. S. Weyant, S. F. Berkley, T. C. Woods, A. G. Steigerwalt, P. A. D. Grimont, R. M. McKinney, D. W. Fleming, L. L. Gheesling, R. C. Cooksey, R. J. Arko, C. V. Broome, and the Brazilian Purpuric Fever Study Group, Biochemical, genetic, and epidemiologic characterization of *Haemophilus influenzae* biogroup aegyptius (*Haemophilus aegyptius*) strains associated with Brazilian purpuric fever, *J. Clin. Microbiol. 26*:1524 (1988).
82. J. M. Musser and R. K. Selander, Brazilian purpuric fever: evolutionary genetic relationships of the case clone of *Haemophilus influenzae* biogroup

aegyptius to encapsulated strains of *Haemophilus influenzae*, *J. Infect. Dis. 161*:130 (1990).

83. L. W. Mayer, W. F. Bibb, K. A. Birkness, K. Irino, R. S. Weyant, M. W. Reeves, J. M. Swenson, and the Brazilian Purpuric Fever Study Group, Distinguishing clonal characteristics of the Brazilian purpuric fever-producing strain, *Pediatr. Infect. Dis. J. 8*:241 (1989).
84. A. J. Lesse, L. L. Gheesling, W. E. Bittner, S. D. Myers, and G. M. Carlone, Stable, conserved outer membrane epitope of strains of *Haemophilus influenzae* biogroup aegyptius associated with Brazilian purpuric fever, *Infect. Immun. 60*:1351 (1992).
85. M. H. O. Porto, G. J. Noel, P. J. Edelson, and the Brazilian Purpuric Fever Study Group, Resistance to serum bactericidal activity distinguishes Brazilian purpuric fever (BPF) case strains of *Haemophilus influenzae* biogroup aegyptius (*H. aegyptius*) from non-BPF strains, *J. Clin. Microbiol. 27*:792 (1989).
86. L. G. Rubin, E. S. Gloster, G. M. Carlone, and the BPF Study Group, An infant rat model of bacteremia with Brazilian purpuric fever isolates of *Haemophilus influenzae* biogroup aegyptius (*H. aegyptius*), *J. Infect. Dis. 160*:476 (1989).
87. B. Swaminathan, L. W. Mayer, W. F. Bibb, G. W. Ajello, K. Irino, K. A. Birkness, C. F. Garon, M. W. Reeves, M. C. Brandileone, F. O. Sottnek, D. J. Brenner, A. G. Steigerwalt, and the Brazilian Purpuric Fever Study Group, Microbiology of Brazilian purpuric fever and diagnostic tests, *J. Clin. Microbiol. 27*:605 (1989).
88. R. S. Weyant, W. F. Bibb, D. S. Stephens, B. P. Holloway, W. F. Moo-Penn, K. A. Birkness, L. O. Helsel, and L. W. Mayer, Purification and characterization of a pilin specific for Brazilian purpuric fever-associated *Haemophilus influenzae* biogroup aegyptius (*H. aegyptius*) strains, *J. Clin. Microbiol. 28*:756 (1990).
89. K. Irino, F. Grimont, I. Casin, P. A. D. Grimont, and the Brazilian Purpuric Fever study group, rRNA gene restriction patterns of *Haemophilus influenzae* biogroup aegyptius strains associated with Brazilian purpuric fever, *J. Clin. Microbiol. 26*:1535 (1988).
90. S. R. M. Dobson, J. S. Kroll, and E. R. Moxon, Insertion sequence IS*1016* and absence of *Haemophilus* capsulation genes in the Brazilian purpuric fever clone of *Haemophilus influenzae* biogroup aegyptius, *Infect. Immun. 60*:618 (1992).
91. A. M. Whitney and M. M. Farley, Cloning and sequence analysis of the structural pilin gene of Brazilian Purpuric Fever-associated *Haemophilus influenzae* biogroup aegyptius, *Infect. Immun. 61*:1559 (1993).
92. R. K. Selander, R. M. McKinney, T. S. Whittam, W. F. Bibb, D. J. Brenner, F. S. Nolte, and P. E. Pattison, Genetic structure of populations of *Legionelle pneumophila*, *J. Bacteriol. 163*:1021 (1985).
93. A. Rosenau, P. Y. Sizaret, J. M. Musser, A. Goudeau, and R. Quentin, Adherence to human cells of a cryptic *Haemophilus* genospecies responsible for genital and neonatal infections, *Infect. Immun. 61*:4112 (1993).

94. J. M. Musser, A. R. Hauser, M. H. Kim, P. M. Schlievert, K. Nelson, and R. K. Selander, *Streptococcus pyogenes* causing toxic-shock-like syndrome and other invasive diseases: clonal diversity and pyrogenic exotoxin expression, *Proc. Natl. Acad. Sci. USA*. *88*:2668 (1991).
95. K. Nelson, P. M. Schlievert, R. K. Selander, and J. M. Musser, Characterization and clonal distribution of four alleles of the *speA* gene encoding pyrogenic exotoxin A (scarlet fever toxin) in *Streptococcus pyogenes*, *J. Exp. Med*. *174*:1271 (1991).
96. V. Kapur, K. Nelson, P. M. Schlievert, R. K. Selander, and J. M. Musser, Molecular population genetic evidence of horizontal spread of two alleles of the pyrogenic exotoxin C gene (*speC*) among pathogenic clones of *Streptococcus pyogenes*, *Infect. Immun*. *60*:3513 (1992).
97. J. M. Musser, V. Kapur, S. Kanjilal, U. Shah, D. M. Musher, N. L. Barg, K. H. Johnston, P. M. Schlievert, J. Henrichsen, D. Gerlach, R. M. Rakita, A. Tanna, B. D. Cookson, and J. C. Huang, Geographic and temporal distribution and molecular characterization of two highly pathogenic clones of *Streptococcus pyogenes* expressing allelic variants of pyrogenic exotoxin A (scarlet fever toxin), *J. Infect. Dis*. *167*:337 (1993).
98. J. M. Musser, K. Nelson, R. K. Selander, D. Gerlach, J. C. Huang, V. Kapur, and S. Kanjilal, Temporal variation in bacterial disease frequency: molecular population genetic analysis of scarlet fever epidemics in Ottawa, Canada, and eastern Germany, *J. Infect. Dis*. *167*:759 (1993).
99. V. Kapur, M. W. Majesky, L.-L. Li, R. A. Black, and J. M. Musser, Cleavage of interleukin 1β (IL-1β) precursor to produce active IL-1β by a conserved extracellular cysteine protease from *Streptococcus pyogenes, Proc. Natl. Acad. Sci. USA 90*:7676 (1993).
100. J. A. Mollick, G. G. Miller, J. M. Musser, R. G. Cook, D. Grossman, and R. R. Rich, A novel superantigen isolated from pathogenic strains of *Streptococcus pyogenes* with aminoterminal homology to staphylococcal enterotoxins B and C, *J. Clin. Invest. 92*:710 (1993).
101. V. Kapur, S. Topouzis, M. W. Majesky, L.-L. Li, M. R. Hamrick, R. J. Hamill, J. M. Patti, and J. M. Musser, A conserved *Streptococcus pyogenes* extracellular cysteine protease cleaves human fibronectin and degrades vitronectin, *Microb. Pathog*. 1993, (In press).
102. K. B. Reda, V. Kapur, J. A. Mollick, J. G. Lamphear, J. M. Musser, and R. R. Rich, Molecular characterization and phylogenetic distribution of the streptococcal superantigen gene (*ssa*) from *Streptococcus pyogenes, Infect. Immun*. 1994 (In press).
103. D. G. Higgins, and P. M. Sharp, Fast and sensitive multiple sequence alignments on a microcomputer, *Comp. Applic. Biol. Sci*. *5*:151 (1989).
104. D. L. Swofford, Phylogenetic analysis using parsimony version 3.0q, Illinois Natural History Survey, Champaign, Illinois, 1991.
105. J. Felsenstein, Confidence limits on phylogenies: an approach using the bootstrap, *Evolution 39*:783 (1985).

10

Molecular Basis of Antibody Diversity

William L. Carroll and Elisabeth E. Adderson

University of Utah, Salt Lake City, Utah

Alexander H. Lucas

Children's Hospital Oakland Research Institute, Oakland, California

Gregg J. Silverman

University of California—San Diego, La Jolla, California

Richard A. Insel

University of Rochester School of Medicine and Dentistry, Rochester, New York

Mitchell G. Scott, Moon H. Nahm, and Penelope G. Shackelford

Washington University School of Medicine, St. Louis, Missouri

I. INTRODUCTION

Recently our laboratories have examined the immune response to the capsular polysaccharide of *Haemophilus influenzae* type b (Hib) to study the molecular basis of antibody diversity in humans. Protective immunity to this major childhood pathogen is provided by antibodies against the organism's capsular polysaccharide, polyribosylribitol phosphate (PRP). The immune response to polysaccharide antigens provides a useful model to study the ontogeny and regulation of the antibody gene repertoire in the outbred human population. Although polysaccharide antigens may display multiple epitopes, they are antigenically much less complex than protein antigens (1). Furthermore, earlier studies in animals and in humans suggested a clonally restricted antibody response to polysaccharides as defined by light (L) chain preference and analysis of serum antibodies by isoelectric focusing (IEF) gels (2–4). Like many other polysaccharide antigens, immunity to Hib PRP develops relatively late in ontogeny, usually during the third year of life. Since studies in both animal and human fetuses show preferential use of certain variable (V) region genes, we questioned whether the restricted use of certain antibody genes early in development may explain the poor response of infants to many polysaccharide antigens. A further advantage of the Hib PRP system is the availability of different vaccine formulations permitting the analysis of the immunoglobulin (Ig) gene repertoire to both classic T-independent (plain PRP) and T-dependent (PRP protein conjugate) antigen formulations. In contrast to the plain PRP vaccine, the use of Hib PRP conjugated to protein carriers can induce protective antibody responses both in young infants and in patients with Ig subclass deficiency, and has been shown to prime for subsequent immunization with plain PRP (5–7). Presumably the recruitment of T-cell help to responding B cells plays a major role in these differential properties. In order to determine the molecular basis of immunity to Hib PRP, our laboratories have relied on a variety of experimental approaches to analyze the antibody genes used in this physiologically important immune response.

II. MOLECULAR MECHANISMS OF ANTIBODY DIVERSITY

It has been estimated that the antibody repertoire may be capable of generating up to 10^{14} B-cell clones, each secreting an antibody with a unique antigen specificity. This remarkable diversity is achieved by molecular diversifiers unique to antigen receptor genes expressed in T and B lymphocytes. Amino-terminal portions of the L and heavy (H) chains of the Ig molecule together comprise the antigen-binding domain (V region), whereas the carboxy-terminus of these molecules [constant (C) region] is responsible for effector functions. The V regions of Ig molecules contain three areas of extreme amino acid variability, called complementarity-determining regions (CDRs), which form the actual antigen contact domains.

The V regions of Ig molecules are encoded by individual members of two or three groups of discontinuous gene segments (Fig. 1). For the H chain one of up to 300 V-gene segments recombines with one out of approximately 30 diversity (D) segments and one of six joining (J) genes to form the gene segment encoding the variable portion of the IgH protein (8,9). This process occurs in a predictable temporal order with DJ joining occurring first, followed by V to DJ fusion (10,11). A similar process occurs at the L chain loci, although D segments are absent. Additional diversity is created at junction boundaries by nucleotide deletion (exonuclease action) and single base addition ("N addition"), presumably by the enzyme terminal deoxynucleotidyl transferase, TdT (12). The addition of mono- or dinucleotides is also accomplished by "P addition" resulting

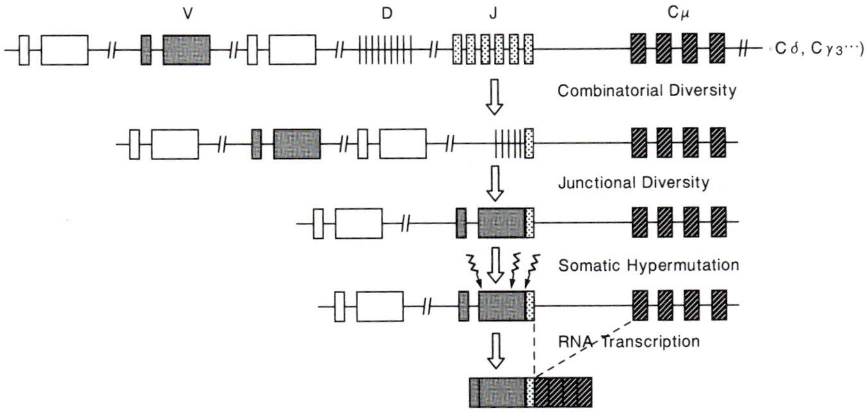

Figure 1 Antibody gene assembly. Individual members of three groups of germline elements recombine to form the gene segment encoding the antigen-binding domain of the Ig heavy chain. DJ recombination precedes V-to-DJ rearrangement. Imprecise joining of segments leads to diversity at segment boundaries, and rearranged genes are substrates for somatic hypermutation. Similar rearrangements occur at the light chain loci although D segments are absent. (From Ref. 69).

from the nicking of the terminal 5′ coding sequence followed by its inversion and joining to the 3′ end of the complementary strand (13). Finally, rearranged genes are substrates for further diversification, which is primarily the result of a striking degree of somatic hypermutation (14).

Most of what is known about Ig gene rearrangement and repertoire development comes from the study of B-cell development in experimental animals. Despite great similarity in overall Ig gene structure in chickens, rabbits, and mice, each of these organisms had relied on alternative molecular strategies to generate diversity (15–19). Although the human system may be most similar to the mouse, important differences are apparent making simple extrapolation of data problematic. For example, the murine IgH locus may contain up to 1000 V_H segments, which are for the most part clustered in discrete families with members sharing greater than 80% nucleic acid sequence homology. In contrast, individual members of the six or seven human V_H families are highly interspersed throughout the locus (15). Moreover, the immune response of highly inbred laboratory animals to simple haptens may not be comparable to the response in the outbred human population to physiologically more complex pathogens. For these reasons direct examination of the human antibody gene repertoire to defined pathogens is imperative.

III. LIGHT CHAIN TYPE AND CLONOTYPE ANALYSIS OF SERUM ANTI-PRP ANTIBODIES

Early analysis of serum anti-PRP antibodies by immunochemical techniques suggested a relatively restricted immune profile. The normal serum IgL chain distribution is 60% kappa and 40% lambda. Antibody to PRP is dominated by the disproportionate expression of kappa L chains. Seventy-five percent of postimmunization sera predominately express antibodies utilizing kappa chains, and 30% almost exclusively express kappa L chains (2,20). Kappa/lambda ratios of anti-PRP Ab in different studies have varied from 2.8 to 5.8. This preference for kappa L chains in the anti-PRP immune response persists for many years after infection or immunization (20).

Analytical IEF gels can be used to resolve serum antibodies derived from individual B cell clones. This technique separates proteins on the basis of charge. Post immunization serum can be applied to these gels and after appropriate separation of serum proteins, radiolabeled antigen will bind to anti-PRP antibodies. Initial analysis of post immunization sera from healthy volunteers yielded surprising results. Most individuals display a very restricted antibody repertoire to PRP with the detection of antibodies from only 1 to 4 clones (spectrotypes or clonotypes). In addition, certain clonotypes appear to be shared by unrelated individuals (3). Since the charge differences detected by this technique may be present in both V and C regions, and since adults usually generate both IgG_1 and IgG_2 antibodies, these results indicate a striking degree of antibody restriction. The immune response after immunization with conjugate vaccines appears to be as restricted as that seen for the response to plain PRP (4). In most cases the predominant clonotype detected shortly after primary immunization persists after secondary immunization and for many years later. The fixed nature of this immune response contrasts with the generation of increasing antibody diversity over time seen in the murine response to a variety of haptens.

IV. ANTI-IDIOTYPIC ANALYSIS OF THE SERUM ANTI-PRP REPERTOIRE

Anti-idiotypic antibodies (anti-Id Abs) are antibodies directed against the V region (idiotype, Id) of another antibody. As such, they are potentially serological markers for particular IgV regions of antibodies secreted from a single B-cell clone. Polyclonal and monoclonal anti-Id Abs have been generated against serum anti-Hib antibodies. Initially murine and goat anti-Id anti-sera were prepared by immunization with affinity purified $F(ab)'_2$ anti-

PRP antibodies isolated from the sera of unrelated immunized individuals. An inhibition assay was used to measure Id expression on anti-PRP antibodies in pre- and postimmunization sera of adults and children (21). The anti-Id antisera detected the expression of a cross-reactive idiotype (CRI) in the majority of subjects (76%) studied after vaccination (21,22). CRI expression was detected in prevaccination serum in most individuals and appeared to be associated with the majority of expressed anti-Hib antibodies (>50% inhibition). After vaccination, anti-Id inhibition increased to 85% and 71% in individuals positive and negative, respectively, for the CRI prior to immunization. Similar results were seen in postvaccination sera of children immunized between 2 months and 6 years of age (22). In this study infants had been immunized with a conjugate vaccine, whereas older individuals had received the PRP vaccine. These results indicate that the V region(s) identified by the anti-Id reagent forms a portion of most anti-PRP antibodies confirming the restricted Ig repertoire in this immune response. Furthermore, the repertoire directed to the conjugate vaccine appeared to be qualitatively similar to that generated in response to the plain polysaccharide (see below).

Since the accuracy of anti-Id analysis may be limited by the use of polyclonal antisera, monoclonal anti-Id (mAb) antibodies specific for anti-PRP antibodies were developed. Again, antibodies purified from post-PRP vaccination sera of two unrelated subjects served as an immunogen to prime mice. A single hybridoma clone was isolated secreting mAb which inhibited the binding of serum antibodies to ^{125}I-PRP (23). This clone was designated LuC9 and inhibition of anti-PRP Ab binding suggested that LuC9 mAb recognized an idiotype near the antigen combining site. LuC9 recognizes a CRI that is present in postimmunization sera of a majority of older children and adults (71–90%) after vaccination with the plain polysaccharide or conjugate vaccine (PRP coupled to diptheria toxoid, PRP-D). This CRI is present on a majority of anti-Hib antibodies since LuC9 inhibits an average of 60% of serum binding to PRP. This CRI has been designated HibId-1, and analysis of clonally purified anti-PRP antibodies indicates that HibId-1 is a marker for the expression of a particular V kappa germline gene, $V\kappa$II-A2 (24). HibId-1 is also expressed by patients recovering from invasive Hib disease and vaccine failures (25). The selective use of a single $V\kappa$II gene segment in the outbred human population is another striking example of restriction in the human immune response to PRP.

A major question relevant to the induction of protective immunity is whether age or vaccine formulation affects repertoire development. The development of a second mAb reagent, LuC1O, which is targeted to a CRI encoded by a subset of $V\lambda$ VII germline genes, made it possible to examine the expression of two major L-chain genes in response to conjugate vaccines among different age groups (26). The use of Vλ VII L chains correlates with anti-PRP antibody cross-reactivity with the structurally related polysaccharide of *Escherichia coli* K100 (27,28). Thus, colonization by this cross-reactive enteric organism may provide protective immunity for young infants prior to contact with pathogenic Hib. The lack of prior environmental contact with antigen makes infants an ideal target population in order to study de novo repertoire development after vaccination. Initial studies focused on measurement of idiotype expression in sera of infants immunized with one of three different conjugate vaccines: high molecular weight (mw) PRP coupled to meningococcal outer membrane protein complex (PRP-OMPC), high mw PRP coupled to tetanus toxoid (PRP-T), or PRP oligosaccharide coupled to a mutant diptheria toxin (Oligo-CRM). Vaccine formulation had a profound effect on expression of L chain–associated Id expression. HibId-1 (VκII-A2) was detected in 33% of the PRP-OMPC group compared to 68% and 64% of infants immunized with oligo-CRM or PRP-T. In contrast, HibId-2 (Vλ VII) was seen in 47% of PRP-OMPC immunized infants compared with 18% and 10%, respectively, in other two groups. Infrequently, subjects were positive for both idiotypes. The basis for differences in the expressed antibody repertoire to these different conjugate vaccine formulations is unknown. It is possible that the differences in V gene expression may be related to the variable contribution of the T-dependent and T-independent arms of the immune system. The PRP-OMPC may have a greater T-independent character (29,30).

More recently the V_L repertoire to PRP-OMPC was examined as a function of age of immunization (31). A single dose of this vaccine can induce protective immunity in young infants in contrast to other Hib PS conjugate vaccines (6). In addition to HibId-1 and HibId-2 expression, the use of VκIII L chains was detected by a murine VκIII-specific mAb, B12 (32). Postvaccination sera of 2-month-old infants, 18-month-old infants, and adults were analyzed (Fig. 2). HibId-1 was detected in all age groups, although the frequency of patients synthesizing HibId-1 (VκII-A2) antibodies was lower in 2-month-old infants (35%) compared to 18-month-old infants (80%) and adults (66%). In contrast, HibId-2 (Vλ VII) antibodies were significantly more prevalent among 2-month-old infants (43%) compared to 18-month-old subjects (6%) and adults (0%). None of the postvaccination samples of infants continued anti-PRP antibodies composed of VκIII L chains, whereas 26% and 69% of sera from 18-month old and adults, respectively, contained VκIII encoded anti-PRP antibodies.

The basis of these striking differences in the anti-PRP V_L repertoire at different ages is uncertain. The response of 2-month-old infants is probably

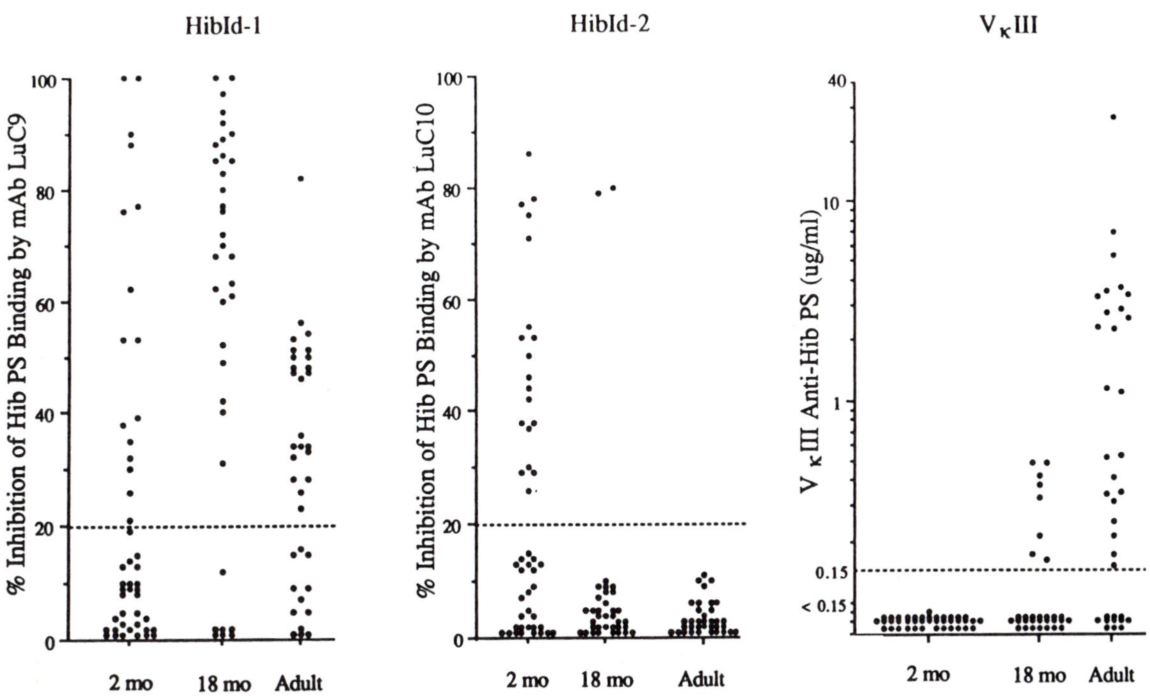

Figure 2 Expression of HibId-1, HibId-2, and VκIII light chains by anti-Hib PS antibodies in the postvaccination sera of 2-month-old infants ($n = 46$), 18-month old infants ($n = 35$), and adults ($n = 35$) after a single injection of the PRP-OMPC vaccine. Each circle represents a single subject, and values above the dotted line are considered positive. (From Ref. 31.)

representative of a primary immune repertoire, in contrast to older infants and adults, where a preexisting repertoire has been expanded by prior exposure to PRP or other cross-reactive antigens. Thus antigen-driven hypermutation of B-cell clones or the selection of rare clones with high affinity for antigen in older infants and adults may account for the expression of different idiotypes as a function of age (31,33,34).

V. AMINO ACID SEQUENCE ANALYSIS OF CLONALLY PURIFIED SERUM ANTI-PRP ANTIBODIES

Sequence analysis of individual anti-PRP antibodies provided more detailed information on V-region family assignment and determined the usage of D and J segments. Initial efforts focused on amino acid sequencing of affinity purified serum antibodies from adults imunized with the PRP vaccine (35). Monoclonal preparations of IgG_1 or IgG_2 anti-PRP antibodies were obtained by affinity chromatography and preparative IEF. Partial sequence revealed that all H chains utilized members of the V_H3 gene family (36). The V_H3 family is one of the larger families with at least 30 members (37). Although this large family size may contribute to its increased representation, its exclusive use in the anti-PRP response is remarkable. Since amino acid sequencing was limited to framework regions, it was not clear from this data whether certain members of the V_H3 family were used preferentially over others. In contrast to the restriction in V_H gene usage, 10 kappa L chains utilized $V\kappa$II segments, three $V\kappa$I, and one $V\kappa$III (36). Sequence analysis of lambda L chains was unsuccessful because a major portion of these L chains are known to be N-terminally blocked.

Classification of anti-PRP antibodies according to fine antigenic specificity correlated with V_L family usage. Cross-reactivity of anti-PRP antibodies with the structurally similiar capsular polysaccharide of *E. coli* K100 PS can be used as a marker of V gene heterogeneity. Three groups of antibodies can be identified: (a) cross-reactive antibodies utilizing kappa L chains, (b) non–cross-reactive antibodies associated with kappa L chains, and (c) cross-reactive antibodies with lambda L chains (38). Kappa cross-reactive antibodies utilize $V\kappa$I or $V\kappa$III genes but not $V\kappa$II (39). Non–cross-reactive kappa antibodies belong almost exclusively to the $V\kappa$II family and, as described in the preceding section, a major cross-reactive idiotype (HibId-1) is associated with these $V\kappa$II L chains. Thus, while it appears that a major requirement for PRP binding is mediated through the use of V_H3 sequences, fine specificity and idiotype expression can be modulated by the associated L chain.

Further characterization of the predominant $V\kappa$II-encoded L chains was performed by analyzing more extensive variable regions of sequence, including the entire CDR2 and CDR3 (40). Surprisingly, five such clonally purified anti-PRP VκII L chains were completely identical in CDR1 and CDR2. There was only a single amino acid difference in CDR3 in one of the antibodies. The almost complete identity of VκII-associated L chains in different individuals suggests that a single VκII gene with little or no somatic mutation dominates the anti-Hib immune response. A single germline gene A2 appears to encode the great majority of anti-PRP VκII L chains (24). This gene, which was previously localized to the Aa region of the human Vκ locus, matches all anti-PRP VκII L chains sequenced at the protein level to date with the only exception being a Thr94 substitution in a single L chain (40). In contrast to the restriction stated above, both Jκ1 and Jκ2 segments were found to contribute to CDR3. However, arginine is always present at the VJ junction, a result indicating some importance in antigen recognition. Alternative joining between codon 95 (CCT) of the A2 gene and the 5′ codon 96 (TGG) of Jκ1 could account for this arginine (CGG). Single nucleotide addition after exonuclease cleavage is necessary to explain the arginine in Jκ2-encoded CDR3 regions.

Non-A2–encoded anti-PRP L chains appear to be derived from a diverse group of gene families. Among 15 such antibodies from 12 vaccinated adults, four were Vλ, five VκI, one non-A2 VκII, four VκIII, and one VκIV (39). Formal assignment of these expressed sequences to parental germline genes is complicated because although the kappa locus has been extensively mapped and sequenced, unknown germline genes may be present. Moreover, polymorphism among human Vκ genes makes sequence comparison between L chains from different individuals complex. It does appear, however, that at least a portion of non-A2–encoded L chains represent mutated versions of previously characterized germline genes (39).

Serological analysis of anti-PRP antibodies using antisera specific for certain V genes confirmed amino acid sequencing data. A panel of serological reagents specific for the primary amino acid sequences of V genes was used to analyze circulating anti-PRP antibodies (41). All individuals studied displayed a major population of antibodies derived from the V_H3 gene family (42). Most of these antibodies appeared to be derived from genes structurally related to two previously cloned germline genes, V_H26 and 9.1 (43,44). Some subjects also showed a minor portion of their anti-PRP repertoire to be derived from the V_H1 and V_H4 family. L-chain reagents again demonstrated that most individuals secreted kappa antibodies with a major population dominated by the use of VκII genes, specifically A2-derived L chains. Some individuals also utilized VκIII L chains and a minor portion of the repertoire appeared to be derived from VκI genes.

VI. NUCLEOTIDE SEQUENCE ANALYSIS OF THE ANTI-PRP REPERTOIRE

Determination of the nucleic acid sequence of human anti-PRP antibody V regions provides additional information about the nature of this immune response. It allows more precise comparison of the relatedness of individual members of the anti-PRP V-region repertoire, permits the assignment of genes to well-defined germline elements (subfamilies), allows analysis of D and J segment usage, and more definitively evaluates the influence of somatic hypermutation in the clonal evolution of this response. To obtain such information a panel of human hybridomas secreting anti-PRP monoclonal antibodies was developed (45). Immune lymphocytes were harvested from the peripheral blood of patients immunized with the plain PRP vaccine or different Hib conjugate vaccines. Lymphocytes were fused to the nonsecreting mouse myeloma SP2/O-Ag14, and hybridoma supernatants were screened for anti-PRP antibody production by an ELISA method (46). Antibody genes were cloned by a modified polymerase chain reaction (45,47). Table 1 provides a description of a portion of this panel of hybridomas. The isotype of secreted antibodies mirrors that of the peripheral blood immune response 7 days following immunization (48). All patients had preexisting serum antibody prior to immunization, suggesting the isolated gene products are representative of a secondary or memory immune response (Table 1).

All anti-PRP H-chain genes cloned from this panel are members of the V_H3 family and are 71.0–100% homologous to one another. The nucleotide sequence of the first 5 V_H genes cloned is illustrated in Figure 3. Nine of 15 Ig V_H genes analyzed to date are members of the V_H3b subfamily, which is distinguished by an additional two codons in CDR2. The V_H3b subfamily accounts for approximately 20% of V_H3 genes (43). These V_H3b anti-PRP H chains are highly homologous to two germline genes LSG6.1 and LSG12.1 isolated from the subject LS from whom hybridoma LSF2 was generated (49). The LSG6.1 sequence was also isolated as a cDNA (M85) from a fetal cDNA library (50). A closely related germline gene 9.1/20P1 is also highly homologous to this subset of V_H3b anti-PRP antibodies (43). The anti-PRP V_H3a genes are most closely related to the well-characterized $V_H26/30P1$ germline gene (44).

Amino acid translation of the nucleic acid sequences of the anti-PRP V_H genes shows that about 60% of differences in nucleic acid sequence from the putative germline genes result in amino acid replacements. An increased ratio of amino acid replacement to silent mutations (R/S ratio) is characteristic of somatically mutated antibodies participating in a T-dependent secondary immune response. When compared to candidate

Table 1 Characteristics of anti-Hib PS Hybridoma Cell Lines[a]

Hybridoma	Isotype	Age	Vaccine form	Total anti-PRP Ab (μg/ml) pre	Total anti-PRP Ab (μg/ml) post	V_H	V_L	Hibid-1 expression	Hibid-2 expression	K100 PS binding
SB5/D6	IgA_1/λ	adult	PRP-D	3.0	688	VH3 LSG6.1	VλVII 4A	−	+	+
RAY4	IgA_2/λ	adult	PRP-D	1.9	28	VH3 LSG6.1	VλVII 4A	−	+	+
CB20	IgA_2/λ	adult	HbOC	21.0	75	VH3 LSG6.1	VλIII III.1	−	−	+
JB32	IgA_1/λ	adult	PRP	4.1	200	VH3 LSG6.1	VλVII 4A	−	−	+
JB21	IgG_2/λ	adult	PRP	4.1	200	VH3 LSG6.1	VλII 2.1	−	−	−
RC3	IgA/κ	adult	PRP-D	1.1	300	VH3 LSG6.1	VκII A2	ND	ND	−
LSF2	IgA_1/λ	adult	PRP	ND[b]	138	VH3 LSG6.1	VλVII 4A	−	+	+
SB1/D8	IgG_1/κ	adult	PRP-D	3.0	688	VH3 LSG12.1	NK[c]	+/−	−	−
ED6.1	IgG_2/κ	4 yr	PRP-D	0.8	22	VH3 LSG12.1	VκI clone KC-1	−	−	−
CB6	IgA/κ	adult	HbOC	21.0	75	VH3 VH26	NK	ND	ND	+
ED8.4	IgM/κ	4 yr	PRP-D	0.8	22	VH3 VH26	NK	+	−	−
SD15	IgA_2/κ	11 yr	PRP-D	0.4	550	VH3 VH26	NK	+	−	−
Ann2	IgA_1/κ	adult	HbOC	1.7	110	VH3 VH26	VκII A2	+	−	−
Ann6	IgA/κ	adult	HbOC	1.7	110	VH3 VH26	NK	ND	ND	−
16M3C8	IgG_2/λ	adult	PRP	ND	ND	VH3 VH26	VλII 2.1	ND	ND	
LD21	IgA_2/κ	adult	PRP	0.7	58	NK	VκIII Humhv328/L16	−	−	+

[a]Columns show name of hybridoma cell line, isotype of anti-PRP Ab secreted, age of subject at immunization, type of vaccine (PRP is plain, PRP-D is PRP conjugated to diphtheria toxoid, HbOC is PRP conjugated to CRM^{197} mutant diphtheria protein), concentration of total serum anti-PRP Ab immediately before and one month postimmunization, most closely homologous germline V_H and V_L genes, reactivity with the anti-idiotypic antibodies Hibid-1 and Hibid-2, and cross-reactivity with *E. coli* K100 capsular polysaccharide.

[b]Not done.

[c]Not known.

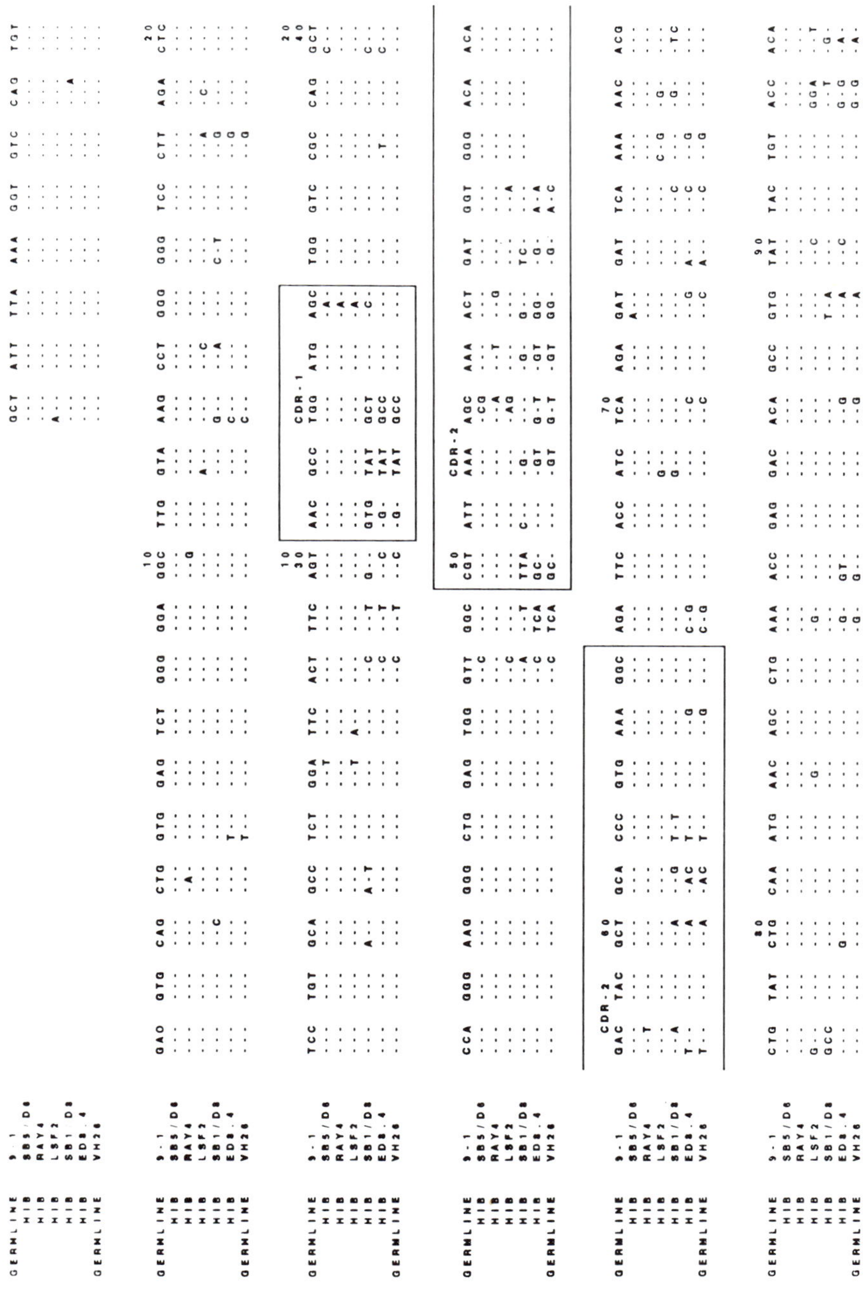

Figure 3 Nucleotide sequence of anti-PRP V_H genes. The nucleotide sequence of five anti-PRP V_H genes is compared to two homologous germline genes, 9.1 and V_H26. CDR1 and CDR2 are boxed. (From Ref. 45.)

genes LSG6.1, LSG 12.1, and V_H26, the R/S ratio of anti-PRP hybridoma genes are generally low but exceed 3:1 in the CDR regions of ED6.1, SB1/D8, and Ann2. Although formal assignment of parental germline genes to expressed cDNA sequences is problematic, these high R/S ratios suggest that some anti-PRP genes are mutated. Recently, antibodies to the capsular polysaccharide of other bacterial pathogens, *Streptococcus pneumoniae* and *Streptococcus pyogenes* (group A beta-hemolytic streptococcus), have been demonstrated to be encoded by V_H3 genes similar to the anti-PRP response (51–52). Although the V_H3 locus is quite polymorphic, certain germline elements such as 9.1/20P1 and V_H26/30P1 are highly conserved (53,54). This conservation may be related to their importance in the immune response to a variety of polysaccharide targets on the capsule of bacterial pathogens.

The anti-PRP V_H genes are homologous to V genes selectively expressed in the fetus. V_H3 genes are expressed in early fetal development disproportionately to their genomic representation. The 9.1/20P1, LSG6.1/M85, and V_H26/30P1 genes are among those identified in the fetal repertoire (50,55). It has been hypothesized that these well-conserved V_H genes provide a preassembled immune repertoire for defense prior to antigen contact or, alternatively, these antibodies form part of a regulatory network (via idiotypic interaction) to shape the developing immune repertoire (56,57). The use of these V_H segments early in development indicates that lack of expression of certain V_H genes is not responsible for anergy to PRP seen in infants.

Anti-PRP V_H genes are also homologous to V-gene segments encoding autoantibodies. An anti-Sm Ab has a nucleic acid sequence identical to the 9.1 germline sequence (43). The V_H26 gene has been shown to encode autoantibodies with rheumatoid factor activity as well as antibodies reactive with DNA, thyroglobulin, and myelin (58,59). This gene also encodes the lupus-associated idiotypic marker 16/6 (60). Preliminary work suggests that a small portion of anti-PRP hybridomas secrete antibodies capable of binding self antigens such as ssDNA and dsDNA (61). However, the affinity for these substrates is markedly lower than their affinity for PRP. Previous work also has linked the immune response to bacterial polysaccharides with the generation of anti-DNA antibodies. The immune response to S. *pneumoniae* and *Klebsiella* is associated with the expression of anti-DNA associated idiotypes (62,63). The basis for cross-reactive immune recognition of bacterial polysaccharides and DNA may be the structurally similar repetitive phosphodiester linkage common to both macromolecules (64). The autoimmune disease of NZB/W mice is diminished in a germ-free environment and animals homozygous for the xid mutation demonstrate a significant reduction in both antipolysaccharide and autoantibodies (65,66). It is possible that under conditions of immune dysregulation, autoantibody-producing B cells may be stimulated or perpetuated by exposure to microorganisms.

Examination of CDR3 in H-chain sequences demonstrates that a variety of combinations are sufficient for antigen binding (Fig. 4). Considerable diversity exists among segments and their length varies from 1 to 34 bp. Because of the short length of many of these regions, comparison with known germline or rearranged genes is problematic. Short CDR3 regions are characteristic of fetally derived heavy chains, and it is possible that some anti-PRP B cell clones may have been generated early in development (67). Five different J regions are used by anti-PRP H-chain genes. Despite this heterogeneity, certain D and J_H combinations appear to be preferentially utilized. Five pairs of hybridomas were obtained from unrelated subjects. In three cases, each hybridoma utilizes a distinct V_H segment and a unique VDJ joint indicating distinct clonal origins. In one case, the hybridomas have identical VDJ joints and highly homologous V_H segments, suggesting that they may have arisen from the same B-cell clone. Somatic hypermuation may account for the small number of base differences. In the final case, analysis of Ig genes shows identical V_H genes but differences in H-chain isotype and L-chain usage. Two explanations could account for these findings. A single pre-B cell may have generated two progeny each with different L chain rearrangements. Alternatively, V_H usage and VDJ association may be so restricted that expression of identical V_H genes in different anti-PRP B cell clones may be much more common than expected.

In contrast to the restricted nature of V_H gene usage, a variety of L-chain V genes participate in the anti-PRP immune response (Table 1). However, as summarized previously, a single kappa germline gene, A2, encoding the HibId-1 idiotype, appears to dominate the response. This gene has been cloned from two hybridomas, and these sequences are compared to the germline gene in F.5 (68). RC3 bears a $V\kappa$ gene identical to the A2 germline gene, whereas Ann2 differs at 5 positions. Although four of these five changes occur in CDR regions, only one results in an amino acid substitution. Therefore, this pattern is not typical of the antigen-driven pattern of somatic mutation. However, neither polymorphism of the A2 gene nor the existence of another germline gene more homologous to Ann2 than A2 has been reported. These results suggest that the observed changes in the Ann2 sequence may be the result of somatic mutation. Seven mAbs to PRP bind the structurally similar polysaccharide of *E. coli* K100, and this property appears to be mediated by L-chain expression. Three L-chain families conferring this property have been sequenced: $V\lambda$VII, $V\lambda$III, and $V\kappa$III (Table 1). Some $V\lambda$VII genes encode proteins bearing the HibId-2 idiotype as described above (26,68).

	VH	D	JH	
Germline LSG6.1	--			
Hib SB5/D	-G	G GGA GGG GTC	GGC TA primer	J4
Hib RAY4	-G	G GGT GCG GCC	GGC TA primer	J4
Hib JB32	-G	G GGG CAA CTG CCC C	TC GAC CC primer	J5a
Hib JB21	-G	G GGG CAA CTG CCC C	TC GAC CC primer	J5a
Hib RC3		AGG	GAC TA primer	J4
Hib LSF2		AGG	GAC TA primer	J4
Hib SB1/D8	--	T AAG ACG GGT TGT GCA TCT AGT GCC TAC GCT TGT	GCT TTT GGA AT primer	J3
Hib ED8.4	-G	T	TAC GGT ATG GAC GT primer	J6
Hib SD15	-G	T	TAC GGT ATG GAC GT primer	J6
Hib CB6	-G	T	TAC GGT ATG GAC GT primer	J6
Hib Ann2	-G	G	TAT GGT TTT GAC TC primer	J4
Hib Ann6	-G	G	TAT GGT TTT GAC TC primer	J4
Hib ED6.1	C-	C GGT ACT AGA CAC AGC CC	T GAC TA primer	J4
Hib CB20	C-	C TGT GTT AGT ACC AGG TGT AAT CGT CCA	CA primer	J1
Hib 16M3C8	--	T CCG AGC GGT GGG AGG ACG ACA GGC GGG CGC GCA	TTT GAG TTC TGG GGC CAG GGA primer	J4b
Germline VH26	--			

Figure 4 CDR3 of anti-PRP H chains. VDJ joining regions of 15 anti-PRP H chains. Segment boundaries are boxed.

```
                                                    10                                                      20
Germline A2   GAT ATT GTG ATG ACC CAG ACT CCA CTC TCT CTG TCC GTC ACC CCT GGA CAG CCG GCC TCC ATC TCC TGC AAG
RC3           --- --- --- --- --- --- --- --- --- --- --- --- --- --- --- --- --- --- --- --- --- --- --- ---
Ann2          --- --- --- --- --- --- --- --- --- --- --- --- --- --- --- --- --- --- --- --- --- --- --- ---

                     CDR-1                                  30                                            40
Germline A2   TCT AGT CAG AGC CTC CTG CAT AGT GAT GGA AAG ACC TAT TTG TAT TGG TAC CTG CAG AAG CCA GGC CAG CCT
RC3           --- --- --- --- --- --- --- --- --- --- --- --- --- --- --- --- --- --- --- --- --- --- --- ---
Ann2          --- --- --- --- --- --- --- --- --- --- --- --G --- --- --- --- --- --- --- --- --- --- --- T--

                                        50      CDR-2                                 60
Germline A2   CCA CAG CTC CTG ATC TAT GAA GTT TCC AAC CGG TTC TCT GGA GTG CCA GAT AGG TTC AGT GGC AGC GGG TCA
RC3           --- --- --- --- --- --- --- --- --- --- --- --- --- --- --- --- --- --- --- --- --- --- --- ---
Ann2          --- --- --- --- --- --- --- --- -TT --- --- --- --- --- --c --- --- --- --- --- --- --- --- ---

                        70                                       80                                         90
Germline A2   GGG ACA GAT TTC ACA CTG AAA ATC AGC CGG GTG GAG GCT GAG GAT GTT GGG GTT TAT TAC TGC ATG CAA AGT
RC3           --- --- --- --- --- --- --- --- --- --- --- --- --- --- --- --- --- --- --- --- --- --- --- ---
Ann2          --- --- --- --- --- --- --- --- --- --- --- --- --- --- --- --- --- --- --- --- --- --- --- --C

                   CDR-3
Germline A2   ATA CAG CTT CCT CC
RC3           --- --- --- --- -GA  TGG ACT TTC GGC CCT GGG ACC AAA GTG GAT ATC AAA CGA   Jκ3
Ann2          --- --- --- --- AGG  --- --G --- --- -AA --- --- --G --- --A --- --- ---   Jκ1
```

Figure 5 Nucleotide sequence of VKII anti-PRP L chains. Nucleotide sequences of anti-Hib PS hybridomas RC3 and Ann2 are compared to the germline A2 gene. CDR regions are outlined.

	V_κ	V_κ or 'N'	J_κ	
germline A2	L P			
HIB RC3	- -	R	W T F G P G T K V D I K R	
			F - - - - - - - - - - - -	germline $J_\kappa 3$
HIB ED6.1	T L	P	L - - - G - - - - - - - -	
			L - - - G - - - - - - - -	germline $J_\kappa 4$

	$V\lambda$	$V\lambda$ or 'N'	$J\lambda$	
HIB RAY4	G A	R	V F G G G T K L T V L	
HIB SB5/D6	- -	-	- - - - - - - - - - -	
HIB LSF2	- -	-	- - - - - - - - - - -	
HIB JB32	A D	-	- - - - - - - - - - -	
HIB JB21	T V	-	- - - - - - - - - - -	
HIB 16M3C8	T T	-	- - - - - - - - - - -	
			- - - - - - - - - - -	germline $J_\lambda 2/3$

Figure 6 Anti-PRP light-chain VJ junctions. Amino acid sequence at VJ junction of two kappa and six lambda anti-PRP antibodies. (From Ref. 28.)

Examination of CDR3 of L chains is notable for the presence of an arginine at the VJ joint in the majority of cases (Fig. 6). In some cases comparison with germline sequences indicates that this amino acid could only have arisen by N-segment addition or somatic mutation (28). The frequent finding of an arginine residue at this location, and particularly its presence in both kappa and lambda anti-PRP Abs, implies this residue is of considerable importance in antigen binding.

VII. SUMMARY

The antibody repertoire to PRP is encoded by a relatively small group of V genes with particular restriction in V_H gene usage. Similarly, selection at both the V_H DJ_H and V_LJ_L joints suggests that the CDR3 region of the H and L chains plays a particular role in antigen binding. Light-chain usage is associated with binding to the related polysaccharide of *E. coli* K100, and the preliminary finding that the same group of V_H genes encode antibodies to the capsular polysaccharide of other bacteria also indicates that CDR3 regions or L-chain usage may modulate fine antigen specificity. The V_H gene repertoire to PRP does not appear to be influenced by vaccine formulation, although L-chain usage may be affected. Similarly age-related differences in idiotype expression indicate expression by anti-PRP antibodies of VλVII L chains in early infancy followed by later expression of VκIII V regions and dominance of the VκII-A2 L chains in older infants and adults. Somatic mutation characterizes a portion of these genes, while other anti-PRP genes are expressed in their germline form. The presence of mutation does not appear to correlate with vaccine formulation (61). Ongoing research will focus on elucidating a possible relationship between the immune response to capsular polysaccharides and autoimmunity. The identification of B-cell subsets responsible for secreting antibody and the mechanism of anergy need to be explored further. The availability of cloned antibody segments will allow the development of chimeric antibodies to analyze structure-function relationships of both variable and constant regions. Finally, purified mAbs can be used to determine the nature of the oligosaccharide-binding pocket.

ACKNOWLEDGMENTS

The authors gratefully acknowledge Dr. Dan Granoff for support and advice throughout all phases of this work and for critical reading of this manuscript. We are also grateful to Ms. Laura Whitehead for manuscript preparation.

REFERENCES

1. E. A. Padlan and E. A. Kabat, Model-building study of the combining site of two antibodies to α (1,6) dextran, *Proc. Natl. Acad. Sci. USA 85*:6885 (1988).
2. D. M. Ambrosino, V. A. Barrus, G. G. Delange, and G. R. Siber, Correlation of Km(1) immunoglobulin allotype with anti-polysaccharide antibodies in caucasion adults, *J. Clin. Invest. 78*:361 (1986).
3. R. A. Insel, A. Kittelberger, and P. Anderson, Isoelectric focusing of human antibody to the *Haemophilus influenzae* b capsular polysaccharide: Restricted and identical spectrotypes in adults, *J. Immunol. 4*:2810 (1985).
4. R. A. Insel and P. W. Anderson, Oligosaccharide-protein conjugate vaccines induce and prime for oligoclonal IgG antibody responses to the *Haemophilus influenzae* b capsular polysaccharide in human infants, *J. Exp. Med. 163*:262 (1986).
5. P. Anderson, M. Pichichero, K. Edwards, C. R. Porch, and R. Insel, Priming and induction of *Haemophilus influenzae* type b capsular antibodies in early infancy by Dpo 20, an oligosaccharide protein conjugate vaccine, *J. Pediatr. 111*:644 (1987).
6. D. M. Granoff, E. L. Anderson, M. T. Osterholm, S. J. Holmes, J. E. McHugh, R. B. Belshe, F. Medley, and T. V. Murphy, Differences in the immunogenicity of three *Haemophilus influenzae* type b conjugate vaccines in infants, *J. Pediatr. 121*:187 (1992).

7. R. A. Insel and P. Anderson, Response to oligosaccharide-protein conjugate vaccines against *Haemophilus influenzae* b in two patients with IgG2 deficiency unresponsive to capsular polysaccharide vaccine, *N. Engl. J. Med. 315*:499 (1986).
8. S. Tonegawa, Somatic generation of antibody diversity, *Nature 302*:575 (1983).
9. F. W. Alt, T. K. Blackwell, and G. D. Yancopoulos, Development of the primary antibody repertoire, *Science 238*:1079 (1987).
10. H. Sakano, R. Maki, Y. Kurosawa, W. Roeder, and S. Tonegawa, Two types of somatic recombination are necessary for the generation of complete immunoglobulin heavy chain genes, *Nature 286*:676 (1980).
11. F. W. Alt, G. D. Yancopoulos, T. K. Blackwell, L. Wood, E. Thomas, M. Boss, R. Coffman, N. Rosenberg, S. Tonegawa, and D. Baltimore, Ordered rearrangement of immunoglobulin heavy chain variable region segments, *EMBO J. 3*:1209 (1984).
12. S. V. Desiderio, G. D. Yancopoulos, M. Paskind, E. Thomas, M. A. Boss, N. Landau, and F. W. Alt, Insertion of N regions into heavy-chain genes is correlated with expression of terminal deoxytransferase in B cells, *Nature 311*:752 (1984).
13. J. J. Lafaille, A. DeCloux, M. Bonneville, Y. Takagaki, and S. Tonegawa, Functional sequences of T cell receptor $\gamma\delta$ genes: Implications for $\gamma\delta$ T cell lineages and for a novel intermediate of V-(D)-J joining, *Cell 59*:859 (1989).
14. D. L. French, R. Laskov, and M. D. Scharff, The role of somatic hypermutation in the generation of antibody diversity, *Science 244*:1152 (1989).
15. J. E. Berman, S. J. Mellis, R. Pollack, C. L. Smith, H. Suh, B. Heinke, C. Kowal, U. Surti, L. Chess, C. R. Cantor, and F. W. Alt, Content and organization of the human Ig VH locus families and linkage to the Ig CH locus, *EMBO J. 7*:727 (1988).
16. M. A. Walter, H. M. Dosch, and D. W. Cox: A deletion map of the human immunoglobulin heavy chain variable region, *J. Exp. Med. 174*:335 (1991).
17. D. J. Kemp, B. Tyler, O. Bernard, N. Gough, S. Cerondakis, J. M. Adams, and S. Cory: Organization of genes and spacers within the mouse immunoglobulin VH locus, *J. Mol. Appl. Genet. 1*:245 (1981).
18. J. C. Weill and C. A. Reynaud, The chicken B cell compartment, *Science 238*:1094 (1987).
19. K. L. Knight and R. S. Becker, Molecular basis of the allelic inheritance of rabbit immunoglobulin VH allotypes: implications for the generation of antibody diversity, *Cell 60*:963 (1990).
20. R. A. Insel, P. Anderson, M. E. Pichichero, M. S. Amstey, G. Ekbury, and D. H. Smith, Anticapsular antibody to *Haemophilus influenzae,* (S. H. Sell and P. F. Wright, eds.), Elsevier Publishing Co. Inc., 1982, p. 155.
21. A. H. Lucas, Expression of crossreactive idiotypes by human antibodies specific for the capsular polysaccharide of *Haemophilus influenzae* b, *J. Clin. Invest. 81*:480 (1988).
22. A. H. Lucas and D. M. Granoff, A major crossreactive idiotype associated with human antibodies to the *Haemophilus influenzae* b polysaccharide: Ex-

pression in relation to age and immunoglobulin G subclass, *J. Clin. Invest* *85*:1158 (1990).
23. A. H. Lucas, R. J. Langley, D. M. Granoff, M. H. Nahm, M. Y. Kitamura, and M. G. Scott, An idiotype marker associated with a germline encoded k light chain variable region that predominates the vaccine-induced human antibody response to the *Haemophilus influenzae* b polysaccharide, *J. Clin. Invest.* *88*:1811 (1991).
24. B. Straubringer, E. Huber, W. Lorenz, E. Osterholzer, W. Pargen, M. Pech, H. D. Pohlenz, F. J. Zimmer, and H. G. Zachau, The human Vk locus: Characterization of a duplicated region encoding 28 different immunoglobulin genes, *J. Mol. Biol.* *199*:23 (1988).
25. Holmes S. J., Lucas A. H., Osterholm M. T., Froeschle J. E., and Granoff D. M., Immunoglobulin deficiency and idiotype expression in children developing *Haemophilus influenzae* type b disease after vaccination with conjugate vaccine, *JAMA* *66*:1960 (1991).
26. D. M. Granoff, P. G. Shackelford, S. J. Holmes, The Collaborative Vaccine Study Group, and AH Lucas, Variable region expression in the antibody responses of infants vaccinated with *Haemophilus influenzae* type b polysaccharide-protein conjugates: Description of a new λ light chain-associated idiotype and the relation between idiotype expression, avidity and vaccine formulation, *J Clin. Invest.* *91*:788 (1993).
27. R. A. Insel and P. W. Anderson, Cross reactivity with *Escherichia coli* K100 in the human serum anticapsular antibody response to *Haemophilus influenzae* type b, *J. Immunol.* *128*:1267 (1982).
28. E. E. Adderson, P. G. Shackelford, R. A. Insel, A. Quinn, P. M. Wilson, and W. L. Carroll, Immunoglobulin light chain variable region gene sequences for human antibodies to *Haemophilus influenzae* type b capsular polysaccharide are dominated by a limited number of Vκ and Vλ segments and VJ combinations, *J. Clin. Invest.* *89*:729 (1992).
29. J. J. Donnelly, R. R. Deck, and M. A. Liu, Immunogenicity of *Haemophilus influenzae* b polysaccharide-Neisseria meningitidis outer membrane protein complex conjugate vaccine, *J. Immunol.* *145*:3071 (1990).
30. K. Stein, Thymus-independent and thymus-dependent responses to polysaccharide antigens, *J. Infect. Dis* *165*:S49 (1992).
31. A. H. Lucas, F. H. Azmi, C. M. Mink, and D. M. Granoff, Age-dependent V region expression in the human antibody response to the *Haemophilus influenzae* type b polysaccharide, *J. Immunol.* *150*:2056 (1993).
32. A. Mageed, M. R. Walker, and R. Jeffries, Restricted light chain subgroup expression on human rheumatoid factor paraproteins determined by monoclonal antibodies, *Immunology* *59*:473 (1986).
33. M. Kaurtinen, G. M. Griffiths, A. F. Markham, and C. Milstein, mRNA sequences define an unusually restricted IgG response to 2-phenyloxazolone and its early diversification, *Nature* *304*:320 (1983).
34. C. Berek, G. M. Griffiths, and C. Milstein, Molecular events during maturation of the immune response to oxazolone, *Nature* *316*:412 (1985).

35. M. G. Scott, D. L. Crimmins, D. W. McCourt, J. J. Tarrand, M. C. Eyerman, and M. H. Nahm, A simple *in situ* cyanogen bromide cleavage method to obtain internal amino acid sequence of proteins electroblotted to polyvinyldifluoride membranes, *Biochem. Biophys. Res. Commun. 155*:1353 (1988).
36. M. G. Scott, J. J. Tarrand, D. L. Crimmins, D. W. McCourt, N. R. Siegel, C. E. Smith, and M. H. Nahm, Clonal characterization of the human IgG antibody repertoire to *Haemophilus influenzae* type b polysaccharide. II IgG antibodies contain VH genes from a single VH family and VL genes from at least four VL families, *J. Immunol. 143*:293 (1989).
37. M. A. Walter, U. Surti, M. H. Hofker, and D. W. Cox, The physical organization of the human immunoglobulin heavy chain gene complex, *EMBO J. 9*:3303 (1991).
38. J. J. Tarrant, M. G. Scott, P. A. Takes, and M. H. Nahm, Clonal characterization of the human IgG antibody repertoire to *Haemophilus influenzae* type b polysaccharide. Demonstration of three types of V regions and their association with H and L chain isotypes, *J. Immunol. 142*:2519 (1989).
39. M. G. Scott, D. L. Crimmins, D. W. McCourt, G. Chung, K. F. Schäble, R. Thiebe, E. M. Quenzel, H. G. Zachau, and M. H. Nahm, Clonal characterization of the human IgG antibody repertoire to *Haemophilus influenzae* type b polysaccharide IV. The less frequently expressed VL are heterogenous, *J. Immunol. 147*:4007 (1991).
40. M. G. Scott, D. L. Crimmins, D. W. McCourt, R. Thiebe, H. G. Zachau, and M. H. Nahm. Clonal characterization of the human IgG antibody repertoire to *Haemophilus influenzae* type b polysaccharide III. A single VκII gene and one of several Jκ genes are joined by an invariant arginine to form the most common L chain V region, *J. Immunol. 143*:4110 (1989).
41. G. J. Silverman, R. D. Goldfien, P. Chen, R. A. Mageed, R. Jefferis, F. Goni, B. Frangione, S. Fong, and D. A. Carson, Idiotypic and subgroup analysis of human monoclonal rheumatoid factors: implications for structural and genetic basis of autoantibodies in humans, *J. Clin. Invest. 82*:469 (1988).
42. G. J. Silverman and A. H. Lucas, Variable region diversity in human circulating antibodies specific for the capsular polysaccharide of *Haemophilus influenzae* type b. Preferential usage of two types of VH3 heavy chains, *J. Clin. Invest. 88*:911 (1991).
43. J. Sanz, H. Dang, M. Takei, N. Talal, and J. D. Capra, VH sequence of a human anti-Sm antibody, *J. Immunol. 142*:883 (1989).
44. H. Dersimonian, R. S. Schwartz, K. J. Barrett, and B. J. Stollar, Relationship of human variable region heavy chain germline genes to genes encoding anti-DNA antibodies, *J. Immunol. 139*:2496 (1987).
45. E. E. Adderson, P. G. Shackelford, A. Quinn, and W. L. Carroll: Restricted IgH chain V gene usage in the human antibody response to *Haemophilus influenzae* type b capsular polysaccharide, *J. Immunol. 147*:1667 (1991).
46. P. G. Shackelford, D. M. Granoff, S. J. Nelson, M. G. Scott, D. S. Smith, and M. H. Nahm, Subclass distribution of human antibodies to *Haemophilus influenzae* type b capsular polysaccharide, *J. Immunol. 138*:587 (1987).

47. R. K. Saiki, D. H. Gelfand, S. Stoffel, S. J. Scharf, R. Higuchi, G. T. Horn, K. B. Mullis, and H. A. Erlich, Primer directed enzymatic amplification of DNA with a thermostable DNA polymerase, *Science 239*:487 (1988).
48. A. Tarkowski, C. Lue, Z. Molodoreanu, H. Kiyano, J. R. McGhee, and J. Mestecky, Immunization of humans with polysaccharide vaccines induced systemic, predominantly polymeric IgA_2 subclass antibody response, *J. Immunol. 144*:3770 (1990).
49. E. E. Adderson, F. H. Azmi, P. M. Wilson, P. G. Shackelford, and W. L. Carroll, The human VH3b gene subfamily is highly polymorphic, *J. Immunol 151*:800 (1993).
50. H. W. Schroeder and J. Y. Wang, Preferential utilization of conserved immunoglobulin heavy chain variable region gene segments during human fetal life, *Proc. Natl. Acad. Sci. USA 87*:6146 (1990).
51. D. J. Barrett, M. M. Goodenow, T. O. Harville, J. W. Steason, and G. B. White: IgH chain usage in human antibody to pneumococcal polysaccharide. *Pediatr. Res. 31*:147A (1992).
52. G. J. Silverman and E. Rapaport, Variable region restriction in circulating human antibodies specific for pneumococcal capsular polysaccharides, *FASEB J. 6*:1137 (1992).
53. K. W. van Dijk, H. W. Schroeder, R. M. Perlmutter, and E. C. B. Milner, Heterogeneity in the human immunoglobulin VH locus, *J. Immunol. 142*:2547 (1989).
54. E. H. Sasso, K. Willems van Dijk, and E. C. B. Milner, Prevalence and polymorphism of human VH3 genes, *J. Immunol. 145*:2751 (1990).
55. H. W. Schroeder, J. L. Hillson, and R. M. Perlmutter, Early restriction of the human antibody repertoire, *Science 238*:791 (1987).
56. D. Holmberg, High connectivity natural antibodies prefertially use 7183 and Q52 VH families, *Eur. J. Immunol. 17*:399 (1987).
57. P. Casali and A. L. Notkins, $CD5^+$ B lymphocytes, polyreactive antibodies and the human B-cell repertoire, *Immunol. Today 10*:364 (1989).
58. P. P. Chen, M. Liu, S. Sinka, and D. A. Carson, A 16/6 idiotype anti-DNA antibody is encoded by a conserved VH gene with no somatic mutation, *Arthritis Rheum. 31*:1429 (1988).
59. I. Sanz, P. Casali, J. W. Thomas, A. L. Notkins, and J. D. Capra, Nucleotide sequences of eight human autoantibody VH regions reveals apparent restricted use of VH families, *J. Immunol. 142*:4054 (1989).
60. F. Young, L. Tucker, D. Rubinstein, T. Guillaume, J. Andre Schwartz, K. J. Barrett, R. S. Schwartz, and T. Loghtenberg, Molecular analysis of a germ line encoded idiotypic marker of pathogenic human lupus autoantibodies, *J. Immunol. 145*:2454 (1990).
61. E. E. Adderson, P. G. Shackelford, A. Quinn, P. M. Wilson, M. W. Cunningham, R. A. Insel, and W. L. Carroll, Restricted immunoglobulin VH usage and VDJ combinations in the human response to *Haemophilus influenzae* type b capsular polysaccharide-nucleotide sequences of monospecific anti-*Haemophilus* antibodies and polyspecific antibodies cross-reactive with self antigens, *J. Clin. Invest. 91*:2734 (1993).

62. A. El-Roiey, O. Sela, D. A. Isenberg, R. Feldman, B. C. Colaco, R. C. Kennedy, and Y. Schoenfield, The sera of patients with *Klebsiella* infection contain a common anti-DNA idiotype (16/6 Id) and anti-polynucleotide activity, *Clin. Exp. Immunol. 67*:507 (1987).
63. A. Grayzel, A. Solomon, C. Ardnow, and B. Diamond, Antibodies elicited by pneumococcal antigens bear an anti-DNA associated idiotype, *J. Clin. Invest. 87*:842 (1991).
64. E. A. Kabat, K. G. Nickerson, J. Liao, L. Grosshard, E. F. Osserman, E. Glickman, L. Chess, J. B. Robbings, R. Schnerson, and Y. Yang, A human monoclonal macroglobulin with specificity for α (2→8) linked poly-N-acetyl neuraminic acid, the capsular polysaccharide of group B meningococci and *Escherichia coli* K1 which cross reacts with polynucleotides and with denatured DNA, *J. Exp. Med. 164*:642 (1986).
65. K. K. Lenni, K. E. Holley, F. L. McDuffie, and J. L. Titus, Comparative study of NZB mice under germ free and conventional conditions, *J. Rheumatol. 2*:36 (1975).
66. B. J. Steinberg, P. A. Smathers, K. Fredericksen, and A. D. Steinberg, Ability of the xid gene to prevent autoimmunity in (NZB x NZB) F1 mice during the course of their natural history, after polyclonal stimulation or following immunization with DNA, *J. Clin. Invest. 70*:587 (1982).
67. F. M. Raaphorst, E. Timmers, M. J. H. Kenter, M. J. D. Van Tol, J. M. Vossen, and R. K. B. Schuurman, Restricted utilization of germ-line V_H3 genes and short third complementarity-determining regions (CDR3) in human fetal B lymphocyte immunoglobulin heavy chain rearrangements, *Eur. J. Immunol. 22*:247 (1992).
68. E. E. Adderson, P. G. Shackelford, A. Qinn, P. M. Wilson, and W. L. Carroll, Diversity of immunoglobulin light chain usage in the human immune response to *Haemophilus influenzae* type b capsular polysaccharide, *Pediatr. Res. 33*:307 (1993).
69. E. E. Adderson, J. M. Johnston, P. G. Shackelford, and W. L. Carroll, Development of the human antibody repertoire, *Pediatr. Res. 32*:257 (1992).

11

Epidemiology in Developed Countries

Constance M. Vadheim and Joel I. Ward

Harbor-UCLA Medical Center UCLA School of Medicine, Torrance, California

I. INTRODUCTION

Invasive *Haemophilus influenzae* type b (Hib) disease was a leading infectious disease health problem for young children prior to the widespread use of Hib conjugate vaccines in infancy. In developed countries in the prevaccine era, invasive Hib disease occurred endemically, and more than 95% of all invasive *H. influenzae* clinical isolates were serotype b (1–4). The most common serious manifestation, meningitis, accounts for more than half of all recognized cases of invasive Hib infection (1,2,4,5). Other manifestations include bacteremia/sepsis, pneumonia, epiglottitis, septic arthritis, osteomyelitis, cellulitis, pericarditis, empyema, and endophthalmitis (1–5).

Despite early diagnosis and the availability of effective antimicrobial therapies for invasive Hib disease, about 5% of children with Hib meningitis die (6). Neurological sequelae of varying severity are relatively common in Hib meningitis, occurring in 15–30% of the children who survive (7–14).

II. DISEASE DISTRIBUTION

A. Incidence

The incidence of *H. influenzae* disease in various developed countries is summarized in Table 1. Inevitably, these rates underestimate the true inci-

Table 1 Comparison of Rates of *Haemophilus influenzae* Meningitis and Other Invasive Disease Among Children Younger Than 5 Years of Age

Geographic area	Study period	Annual incidence of *H. influenzae*[a] Meningitis	Annual incidence of *H. influenzae*[a] All invasive disease	Ref.
	Prior to infant immunization			
Fresno Co., CA	1976–1978	60	90	20
Alaska (non-Natives)	1980–1982	69	129	15
Colorado (6 mo)	1981–1982	68	112	16
Jefferson Co., AL	1981–1983	62	NA	26
Monroe Co., NY	1982–1983	55	86	17
Dallas Co., TX	1982–1984	67	109	18
Minnesota	1982–1984	45	67	18
Atlanta, GA	1983–1984	57	82	19
Los Angeles Co., CA	1983–1988	NA	33–43	102
Sweden	1971–1983	27–31	NA	29,31
Finland	1976–1981	27	41	32,33
Geneva, Switzerland	1976–1989	NA	60	27
France	1980–1989	15	21	28
Israel	1988–1990	18	34	23
Manitoba, Canada	1981–1984	32	NA	22
The Netherlands	1977–1982	22	NA	34
Wales	1988–1990	22	35	25
	After infant immunization			
Los Angeles Co., CA	1991	NA	12.9	103
N CA Kaiser, CA	1991	NA	5.7	104
Connecticut	1991	3	4	24
Greater Pittsburgh, PA	1991	2	3	24
Minnesota	1991	NA	11 (7–15)	105
Dallas, TX	1991	NA	9 (5–14)	105
United States[b]	1991	NA	11	106
Helsinki, Finland	1990–1991	2.9[c]	NA	107

[a]Rate per 100,000 children per year
[b]National Bacterial Meningitis Survey
[c]Age 0–4 yr
NA, Not Available.

dence of Hib disease because case documentation depends on isolation of the organism from a normally sterile site such as blood or CSF, and such cultures are frequently not obtained prior to antimicrobial treatment. The most recent U.S. studies prior to vaccine availability (Table 1) demonstrate an annual attack rate of all Hib disease of 33–129 cases per 100,000 and for meningitis ranging from 45 to 69 cases per 100,000 children less than 5 years of age per year, with little change over time (15–20). In studies from the 1960s and early 1970s, reported rates of meningitis were less than 40/100,000 in some U.S. populations (21). It is not known whether higher rates of disease reported in the United States since the mid 1970s represent a true increase in disease incidence due to changes in risk factors, such as increased use of day-care facilities, or are due to improvements in diagnosis and surveillance.

Most studies from other developed countries in the prevaccine era suggest incidence rates substantially lower (one third to two thirds) than in the United States (see Table 1) (15,20,22–28). In Sweden (29–31), Finland (32,33), and the Netherlands (34) *H. influenzae* was, until recently, the most common cause of bacterial meningitis. Hib also ranked as the leading cause of bacterial meningitis in Canada, with an incidence similar to that in the United States (35). In other parts of Europe, including the United Kingdom prior to 1980 (36,37) and Norway, meningococcal disease was reported to be more common than Hib meningitis. Limited data from the United States and Scandinavian countries suggest that Hib incidence may have increased in the prevaccine era (30).

High rates of invasive Hib disease (200–1100 cases per 100,000 children <5 years of age per year) have been reported for selective populations in developed countries, including aboriginal children in central Australia (38–40), Navajo Indians, Native Alaskans (Indians and Eskimos), and Apache, Yakima, Athabascan, and Canadian Indians (15,41–47). While these populations reside in developed countries, it should be noted than the living conditions under which these populations reside may more closely approximate those found in developing regions of the world.

With the licensure and widespread use of Hib conjugate vaccines in infancy, dramatic decreases in Hib disease incidence occurred. Table 1 summarizes these data for the United States as a whole (National Bacterial Meningitis Reporting System), for seven specific U.S. populations, and for Helsinki, Finland. In each of these populations, Hib incidence decreased by 60–80% between the late 1980s and 1991. The greatest decrease in disease incidence was in children less than 2 years of age.

In unvaccinated populations, the most important epidemiological feature of invasive Hib disease is its age-related incidence, a feature which has been appreciated for more than half a century (48). Risk is highest between the ages of 6 and 12 months (see Table 2) (15,18,19). Approximately 85% of all invasive *H. influenzae* disease occurs in children under 5 years of age and in this age group is almost exclusively type b disease. Invasive disease is relatively uncommon in infants less than 6 months of age (<15% of cases),

Table 2 Age-Specific Incidence of Invasive *H. influenzae* Disease, U.S. Population-Based Studies, 1976–1984

Age (months)	Incidence[a]				Cumulative[b] percent of disease
	Meningitis only		All invasive disease		
	Median	Range	Median	Range	
0–5	101	59–141	148	98–197	10–15
6–11	179	143–279	275	218–452	37–43
12–17	146	88–184	223	123–248	60–61
18–23	62	20–64	92	57–107	64–68
24–35	31	18–39	50	37–70	75–78
36–47	17	5–26	31	7–39	80–83
48–59	4	2–16	11	7–41	84–86
≥ 60[b]	0.2	0.1–0.2	1.3	1.2–2.4	100

[a]Cases per 100,000 population/year. Range of point estimates from 5 studies, including Alaska 1980–1982 (excluding Eskimos, Indians), Atlanta 1983–1984, Fresno County 1976–1978, Dallas 1982–1984, Minnesota 1982–1984.
[b]Cumulative percent and incidence data for ages ≥ 60 months are based on studies from Alaska, Atlanta, and Fresno County, where active surveillance for all age groups was conducted.

presumably because of less exposure, transplacental acquisition of maternal antibodies, and protection conferred by breast-feeding.

B. Seasonal Distribution

In several studies a characteristic bimodal seasonal pattern has been observed, with one peak between September and December, and a second between March and May (15,49–51). In contrast, the peak incidence of both pneumococcal and meningococcal meningitis is between January and March (49). The reason for the seasonal effect is unknown and cannot be entirely explained by seasonal factors in birth cohorts. There may be factors related to crowding or exposure to school-age children involved.

III. RISK FACTORS

A. Factors Related to Increased Exposure

1. Socioeconomic Factors/Household Exposure

The interplay of multiple factors affecting exposure to the Hib organism and host susceptibility appears to determine the risk of developing invasive Hib disease (see Chapter 19). Socioeconomic factors that increase the likelihood of exposure to Hib among children include large household size (52–55), the presence of young siblings in the home, household crowding (56), and greater population density (57). Other socioeconomic factors, possibly surrogates for increased exposure, include low family income (58–62) and low parental education level (54,58,62).

Three recent studies assess the independent effects of multiple exposure-related risk factors using multivariate analyses. In a case-control study in Atlanta (19), household crowding (i.e., ≥1 person per room) was significantly associated with Hib and a trend toward increased risk was associated with low family income and low maternal education level, although these were not independent risk factors. In a primarily white population in Colorado (16), the risk of Hib disease was increased in households with at least one member of elementary school age, suggesting that such children may be the primary sources of introduction of Hib organisms into a household for acquisition by their susceptible younger siblings. In Los Angeles (55), the risk of Hib disease was increased by household size of more than six persons and by the presence of more than two smokers in the house.

2. The Day-Care Setting

Population-based studies (16,17,19) of day-care attendance and Hib disease have found that children attending day-care are at significantly higher risk for invasive Hib disease than children not in day-care. One study estimated that up to 50% of all invasive Hib disease may be attributable to day-care attendance (19). This topic is covered more extensively in Chapter 19.

B. Factors Increasing Susceptibility to Invasive Disease

1. Age

Each type of invasive disease has a characteristic age occurrence, but as a group the clinical syndromes, other than meningitis and cellulitis, tend to occur at older ages (2,15). In most U.S. populations studied, the peak incidence of meningitis occurs in children 6–9 months of age and declines markedly after 2 years of age (58,59,63,64). Hib cellulitis tends to occur during the first year of life, and epiglottitis generally occurs in children over 2 years of age. Interestingly, meningitis accounts for a relatively small proportion of episodes of invasive disease in adults, while pneumonia is more common.

In populations with an especially high disease incidence, such as Native Americans, the age-specific incidence is shifted towards younger children (15,41–43,47). Among Native Americans in southwestern Alaska, the incidence of Hib disease peaks in children 4–7 months of age, with similar peak attack rates of meningitis observed in Navajo Indian (4–5 months) and

Apache Indian (4–6 months) children (41,43). In populations with low incidence of Hib disease, the age-specific incidence may be shifted towards older preschool children (29–34). In Finland, the peak incidence of Hib meningitis is reported in children at about 12 months of age (4), and approximately 60% of childhood invasive Hib disease occurs in children older than 18 months of age (33). Such a shift to an older age of peak occurrence suggests less intense exposure to Hib than in high-risk populations, although other factors cannot be ruled out.

In unvaccinated populations in developed countries, approximately 15% of invasive *H. influenzae* disease occurs in persons 5 or more years of age. About half of the invasive disease in older individuals is due to *H. influenzae* type b, with the remainder caused by other serotypes or nontypeable strains (65–67). The incidence rates in older children and adults are low compared to those in children <6 years of age (1–6/100,000 population per year) (65,67,68). Most adults who develop invasive *H. influenzae* disease have an underlying condition such as chronic obstructive pulmonary disease, HIV infection, alcoholism, pregnancy, or malignancy (65,68,69). In the elderly, case-fatality rates can be as high as 10–30% of cases (65,68).

2. Gender

Although many studies show approximately equal rates of disease in boys and girls, several population-based studies (15,19,61) and national surveillance data from passively reported cases of meningitis (49) found attack rates in boys to be 1.2- to 1.5-fold higher than in girls.

3. Underlying Disease

Several hematological and immunological disorders are associated with increased risk for Hib disease, including sickle cell anemia (70–72), asplenia or splenectomy (73), antibody deficiency syndromes (74,75), complement deficiencies (76,77), and malignancies, especially Hodgkin's disease during chemotherapy (78–80). The precise mechanisms placing such immunocompromised patients at risk have yet to be determined. Reduced reticuloendothelial clearance of bacteria in blood by macrophages in the spleen and liver may be involved. Clearly, complement and antibody are needed to clear bacteremia and to maintain bactericidal activity in blood.

4. Breast-Feeding

Breast-feeding appears to be protective against invasive Hib disease in infants <6 months of age (16,19,81–83). Although the mechanism for protection is not known, it may be due to immune or nutritional factors in human milk. These findings are biologically plausible, based on studies demonstrating that human milk contains low levels of secretory antibody to the Hib polysaccharide capsule (PRP), which persist for 1–6 months after the onset of lactation (84). In women immunized at 34–36 weeks gestation with PRP vaccine, both the colostrum and milk, measured at either 3 or 6 months after delivery, had an anti-PRP antibody titer more than 20 times higher than that observed in nonimmunized women (85).

5. Antecedent Viral Respiratory Infection

Viruses have been implicated in the pathogenesis of bacterial infections for many years, and in experimental animal models, respiratory viruses increase susceptibility to Hib meningitis (86,87). Antecedent or concurrent viral respiratory infection may alter mucosal immunity or the bacterial flora, thereby increasing host susceptibility to invasive Hib disease. While at least one study suggests increased rates of viral infection prior to invasive Hib disease (88), the problems of conducting prospective studies with appropriate controls have made it difficult to determine conclusively whether antecedent viral respiratory illness predisposes to invasive Hib diseases (see Chapter 19).

C. Other Risk Factors

1. Race and Ethnicity

Population-based active surveillance studies have identified blacks as having increased risk for invasive Hib disease. The incidence of Hib meningitis has consistently been shown to be two or four times higher for black as compared to white children less than 5 years of age (58–62,89,90). Also, the incidence of all invasive Hib disease was 1.6- to 4-fold higher in blacks compared with whites (19,20). High incidences of invasive Hib disease have also been observed in Hispanics (20,90) and Native Americans (15,41–43,45–47,91). Studies in Dallas and Los Angeles, however, found no difference in the incidence of Hib disease between white and Hispanic children (18,55).

The hypothesis that racial and ethnic differences in incidence of Hib disease may be due to genetically determined differences in host susceptibility (92) is unproven because of confounding socioeconomic variables that are associated both with race/ethnicity and with disease. Factors that may increase exposure to Hib, such as household crowding, number of siblings, and day-care, are exceedingly difficult to separate from host susceptibility factors, such as an increased predisposition to Hib disease. Socioeconomic factors affect family size and structure, and therefore could influence the likelihood of exposure to Hib. Studies are needed that analyze both host susceptibility factors and exposure risk factors, including socioeconomic factors, using multivariate analysis to assess the independent effects of potential risk factors that may be highly correlated with each other, such as black race and household crowding. In a study in Atlanta (19), there was no increased risk in blacks compared with whites once the independent effects of household crowding, day-care, and family income on risk were accounted for by multivariate analysis, though in Los Angeles (55), black maternal race was an independent risk factor.

2. Genetic Factors

Selected genetic markers have been associated with invasive Hib disease risk (20,53,93–101), but the results are difficult to interpret. Earlier studies did not control for multiple cross-comparisons, and, hence, studies of multiple genetic markers may have shown significant results due to chance. It has been nearly impossible to separate the effects of genetic and exposure differences in the high-risk groups in whom genetic studies have been conducted. And even in high-risk Alaskan Eskimos, in whom some genetic factors have been associated with disease risk, the majority of patients with Hib disease still do not possess the genetic marker in question (98,101). Therefore, it remains to be determined whether known genetic factors play a significant role in the risk of population groups.

3. Lack of Vaccination/Under Vaccination

Lack of vaccination is clearly the most important risk factor for Hib disease in highly vaccinated populations. Chapters 18, 19, 22, and 23 of this volume discuss the effects of immunization with Hib conjugate vaccines on disease incidence and carriage rates in greater detail.

IV. SUMMARY

Prior to the widespread use of Hib conjugate vaccine in infancy, invasive Hib disease was an important health problem in developed countries. Incidence rates in children less than 5 years of age have decreased dramatically (fivefold) in several populations since 1990, presumably due to increased vaccination rates.

The development of invasive Hib disease in a given individual is a consequence of the complex interaction of a variety of factors, including events leading to exposure, as well as characteristics of the organism, the environment, and the host, all acting together in a multifactorial interrelationship (64) (see Table 1 in Chapter 19). The factors can be divided into those affecting likelihood of exposure to the Hib organism ("extrinsic exposure factors"; see Chapter 19) and those affecting the host's susceptibility to Hib disease, whether inherently through regulation of the host immune response or by contributing to a change in the host's ability to defend against the disease ("intrinsic host-susceptibility factors"). Some exposure factors, such as household crowding and day-care attendance, are fairly direct measures of increased exposure to Hib bacteria, while others, such as low family income and low parental education levels, are only indirect measures for increased exposure. Other risk factors cannot be so easily categorized, such as the association of black, Alaskan Eskimo, or Native American race with increased risk for Hib disease. Although abundant evidence suggests that more intense and early exposure to Hib may be the primary factors affecting risk in these populations, other lines of evidence suggest that genetic factors may also affect other susceptibility factors or the antibody response to Hib.

As the incidence of invasive Hib disease declines witth use of conjugate vaccines in developed countries, it will be interesting to note the effects on disease distribution.

REFERENCES

1. J. K. Todd and F. W. Bruhn, Severe *H. influenzae* infections: spectrum of disease, *Am. J. Dis. Child. 129*:607 (1975).
2. A. S. Dajani, B. I. Asmar, and M. C. Thirumoorthi, Systemic *H. influenzae* disease: an overview, *J. Pediatr. 94*:355 (1979).
3. E. O. Mason, S. L. Kaplan, L. B. Lambeth, Serotype and ampicillin susceptibility of *H. influenzae* causing systemic infections in children: three years of experience, *J. Clin. Microbiol. 15*:543 (1982).
4. H. Peltola, M. Virtanen, Systemic *H. influenzae* infection in Finland, *Clin. Pediatr. 5*:275 (1984).
5. D. M. Granoff, M. Basden, *H. influenzae* infections in Fresno County, California: a prospective study of the effects of age, race and contact with a case on incidence of disease, *J. Infect. Dis. 140*:40 (1980).
6. S. L. Cochi, C. V. Broome, A. W. Hightower, Immunization of U.S. children with *H. influenzae* type b polysaccharide vaccine: a cost-effectiveness model of strategy assessment, *JAMA 253*:521 (1985).
7. H. G. Taylor, R. H. Michaels, P. M. Mazur, C. B. Liden, Intellectual, neuropsychological and achievement outcomes in children six to eight years after recovery from *H. influenzae* meningitis, *Pediatrics 74*:198 (1984).
8. R. D. Feigin, B. W. Stechenberg, M. J. Chang, Prospective evaluation of treatment of *H. influenzae* meningitis, *J. Pediatr. 88*:542 (1976).
9. S. H. W. Sell, R. E. Merrill, E. O. Doyne, E. P. Zinsky, Long-term sequelae of *H. influenzae* meningitis, *Pediatrics 42*:206 (1972).
10. E. T. Sproles, III, J. Azerrad, C. Williamson, R. E. Merrill, Meningitis due to *H. influenzae*: long-term sequelae, *J. Pediatr. 75*:782 (1969).
11. P. R. Dodge, M. N. Swartz, Bacterial meningitis—a review of selected aspects. II. Special neurologic problems, post-meningitis complications and clinicopathological correlations, *N. Engl. J. Med. 272*:1003 (1965).

12. P. C. Ferry, J. L. Culbetson, J. A. Cooper, Sequelae of *H. influenzae* meningitis, Haemophilus influenzae (S. H. Sell and P. F. Wright, eds.), Elsevier Science, New York, 1982.
13. S. L. Pomeroy, S. J. Holmes, P. R. Dodge, R. D. Feigin, Seizures and other neurologic sequelae of bacterial meningitis in children, *N. Engl. J. Med. 323*:1651 (1990).
14. H. G. Taylor, E. L. Mills, A. Ciampi, et al., The sequelae of *Haemophilus influenzae* meningitis in school-age children, *N. Engl. J. Med. 323*:1657 (1990).
15. J. I. Ward, M. K. Lum, D. B. Hall, Invasive *H. influenzae* type b disease in Alaska: background epidemiology for a vaccine efficacy trial, *J. Infect. Dis. 153*:17 (1986).
16. G. R. Istre, J. S. Conner, C. V. Broome, Risk factors for primary invasive *H. influenzae* disease: increased risk from day care attendance and school age household members, *J. Pediatr. 106*:190 (1985).
17. S. R. Redmond, M. E. Pichichero, *H. influenzae* type b disease: an epidemiologic study with special reference to day care centers, *JAMA 252*:2581 (1984).
18. T. V. Murphy, M. T. Osterholm, L. M. Pierson, et al. Prospective surveillance of *H. influenzae* type b disease in Dallas County, Texas, and in Minnesota, *Pediatrics 79*:173 (1987).
19. S. L. Cochi, D. W. Fleming, A. W. Hightower, Primary invasive *H. influenzae* type b disease: a population-based assessment of risk factors, *J. Pediatr. 108*:887 (1986).
20. D. M. Granoff, E. Boies, J. Squires, et al., Interactive effect of genes associated with immunoglobulin allotypes and HLA specificities on susceptibility to *Haemophilus influenzae* disease, *J. Immunogenet. 11*:181 (1984).
21. G. W. Hammond, B. E. Rutherford, R. Malazdrewicz, et al., *Haemophilus influenzae* meningitis in Manitoba and the Keewatin District, NWT: potential for mass vaccination, *Can. Med. Assoc. J. 139*:743 (1988).
22. R. Dagan, The Israeli Pediatric Bacteremia Meningitis Group, A two-year prospective, nationwide study to determine the epidemiology and impact of invasive childhood *Haemophilus influenzae* type b infection in Israel, *Clin. Infect. Dis. 15*:720 (1992).
23. E. D. Shapiro, E. R. Wald, A. G. Margolis, M. E. Ortenzo, The decreasing incidence of *Haemophilus influenzae* type b disease in both Connecticut and greater Pittsburgh, Pa, *Pediatr. Res. 31*:100A (Abstract 587) (1992).
24. A. J. Howard, K. T. Dunkin, J. M. Musser, S. R. Palmer, Epidemiology of *Haemophilus influenzae* type b invasive disease in Wales, *Br. Med. J. 303*:441 (1991).
25. W. J. Alexander, J. F. Shaw, Results of a prospective population-based study of the incidence of invasive *Haemophilus influenzae* disease in children. Symposium on *Infectious Diseases in Day Care: Management and Prevention 1984*, Minneapolis, Abstract 7, June 1984.
26. A. Gervaix, S. Suter, Need for prevention of invasive *Haemophilus influenzae* type b infections in Geneva, Switzerland, *Vaccine 11* (Suppl. 1):S34 (1993).

27. P. Reinert, A. Liwartowski, H. Dabernat, C. Guyot, J. Boucher, C. Carrere, Epidemiology of *Haemophilus influenzae* type b disease in France, *Vaccine 11* (Suppl. 1):S38 (1993).
28. B. Claesson, B. Trollfors, U. Jodal, Incidence and prognosis of *Haemophilus influenzae* meningitis in children in a Swedish region, *Pediatr. Infect. Dis. J. 3*:35 (1984).
29. K. M. Salwen, T. Vikerfors, P. Olcen, Increased incidence of childhood bacterial meningitis: a 25-year study in a defined population in Sweden, *Scand. J. Infect. Dis. 19*:1 (1987).
30. B. Trollfors, B. A. Claesson, K. Strangert, J. Taranger, *Haemophilus influenzae* meningitis in Sweden, 1981–1983, *Arch. Dis. child. 62*:1220 (1987).
31. P. Valmari, M. Kataja, H. Peltola, Invasive *Haemophilus influenzae* and meningococcal infections in Finland. A climatic, epidemiologic and clinical approach, *Scand. J. Infect. Dis. 19*:19 (1987).
32. H. Peltola, H. Kayhty, M. Virtanen, P. H. Makela, Prevention of *H. influenzae* type b bacteremic infection with the capsular polysaccharide vaccine, *N. Engl. J. Med. 310*:1566 (1984).
33. L. Spanjaard, P. Bol, W. Ekker, H. C. Zanen, The incidence of bacterial meningitis in The Netherlands—a comparison of three registration systems, 1977–1982, *J. Infect. 11*:259 (1985).
34. P. Varaghese, *Haemophilus influenzae* infection, in Canada, 1969–1985, *Can. Dis. Wkly. Rep. 12*:37 (1986).
35. S. J. Broughton, R. E. Warren, A review of *Haemophilus influenzae* infections in Cambridge, 1975–1981, *J. Infect. Dis. 9*:30 (1984).
36. P. G. Davey, J. K. Cruikshank, I. C. McManus, B. MaHood, M. H. Snow, A. M. Geddes, Bacterial meningitis—ten years experience, *J. Hyg. 88*:383 (1982).
37. J. N. Hanna, B. E. Wild, Bacterial meningitis in children under five years of age in Western Australia, *Med. J. Aust. 155*:160 (1991).
38. J. N. Hanna, The epidemiology of invasive *Haemophilus influenzae* infections in children under five years of age in the Northern Territory: a three-year study, *Med. J. Aust. 152*:234, 238, 24 (1990).
39. D. Hansman, J. Hanna, F. Morey, High prevalence of invasive *Haemophilus influenzae* disease in central Australia, 1986, *Lancet 2*:927 (1986).
40. G. A. Losonsky, M. Santosham, V. M. Sehgal, et al., *H. influenzae* in the White Mountain Apaches: molecular epidemiology of a high risk population, *Pediatr. Infect. Dis. J. 3*:539 (1984).
41. J. L. Coulehan, R. H. Michaels, K. E. Williams, et al., Bacterial meningitis in Navajo Indians, *Public Health Rep. 91*:464 (1976).
42. J. L. Coulehan, R. H. Michaels, C. Hallowell, et al., Epidemiology of *H. influenzae* type b disease among Navajo Indians, *Public Health Rep. 99*:404 (1984).
43. P. R. Ostroy, Bacterial meningitis in Washington State, *West J. Med. 131*:339 (1979).
44. K. A. Wotton, H. G. Stiver, J. A. Hildes, Meningitis in the central Arctic: a 4-year experience, *Can. Med. Assoc. J. 124*:887 (1981).

45. J. R. Gilsdorf, Bacterial meningitis in southwestern Alaska, *Am. J. Epidemiol. 106*:388 (1977).
46. J. I. Ward, M. K. Lum, H. S. Margolis, et al., *H. influenzae* disease in Alaskan Eskimos: characteristics of a population with an unusual incidence of invasive disease, *Lancet 1*:1281 (1982).
47. L. D. Fothergill, J. Wright, Influenzal meningitis: the relation of age incidence to the bactericidal power of blood against the causal organism, *J. Immunol. 24*:273 (1933).
48. W. F. Schlech, J. I. Ward, J. D. Band, Bacterial meningitis in the United States 1978–1981: the national bacterial meningitis surveillance study, *JAMA 253*:1749 (1985).
49. G. R. Istre, J. S. Conner, M. P. Glode, R. S. Hopkins, Increasing ampicillin-resistance rates in H. influenzae meningitis, *Am. J. Dis. Child. 138*:366 (1984).
50. C. V. Broome, W. F. Schlech, III, Recent developments in the epidemiology of bacterial meningitis, *Bacterial Meningitis* (M. A. Sande, A. Smith, and R. D. Root, eds.), Churchill Livingstone, Edinburgh 1985, pp. 1–10.
51. C. Ounsted, *H. influenzae* meningitis: a possible ecological factor, *Lancet 1*:161 (1950).
52. D. M. Granoff, E. G. Boies, J. E. Squires, et al., Histocompatibility leukocyte antigen and erythrocyte MNS specificities in patients with meningitis or epiglottitis due to *H. influenzae* type b, *J. Infect. Dis. 149*:373 (1984).
53. R. H. Michaels, W. F. Schultz, The frequency of *H. influenzae* infections: analysis of racial and environmental factors, Haemophilus influenzae (S. W. Sell and D. T. Karzon, eds.), Vanderbuilt University Press, Nashville, 1973.
54. C. M. Vadheim, D. P. Greenberg, N. Bordenave, et al., Risk factors for invasive *Haemophilus influenzae* type b in Los Angeles county children 18-60 months of age, *Am. J. Epidemiol. 136*(2):221 (1992).
55. R. H. Michaels, F. E. Stonebraker, J. B. Robbins, Use of antiserum agar for detection of *H. influenzae* type b in the pharynx, *Pediatr. Res. 9*:513 (1975).
56. D. M. Ambrosino, W. Greif, C. Thompson, G. R. Siber, Kappa and lambda light chain composition of antibody to the capsular polysaccharide of *Haemophilus influenzae* type b, *J. Infect. Dis. 161*:922 (1990).
57. D. W. Fraser, C. E. Hencke, R. A. Feldman, Changing patterns of bacterial meningitis in Olmsted County, Minnesota, *J. Infect. Dis. 238*:300 (1973).
58. D. W. Fraser, C. C. Geil, R. A. Feldman, Bacterial meningitis in Bernalillo County, New Mexico: a comparison with three other American populations, *Am. J. Epidemiol. 100*:29 (1974).
59. P. I. Tarr, G. Peter, Demographic factors in the epidemiology of *H. influenzae* meningitis in young children, *J. Pediatr. 92*:884 (1978).
60. M. Santosham, C. H. Kallman, J. M. Neff, E. R. Moxon, Absence of increasing incidence of meningitis caused by *H. influenzae* type b, *J. Infect. Dis. 140*:1009 (1979).
61. R. F. Floyd, C. F. Federspiel, W. Schaffner, Bacterial meningitis in urban and rural Tennessee, *Am. J. Epidemiol. 99*:395 (1974).

62. D. W. Fraser, J. E. Mitchell, L. P. Silverman, R. A. Feldman, Undiagnosed bacterial meningitis in Vermont children, *Am. J. Epidemiol. 102*:394 (1975).
63. D. W. Fraser, *Haemophilus influenzae* in the community and in the home, Haemophilus influenzae (S. H. Sell and P. F. Wright, eds.), Elsevier, Amsterdam, 1982, pp. 11–22.
64. M. M. Farley, D. S. Stephens, P. S. Brachman, et al., Invasive *Haemophilus influenzae* disease in adults. A prospective, population-based surveillance, *Ann. Intern. Med. 116*:806 (1992).
65. H. M. Crowe, R. E. Levitz, Invasive *Haemophilus influenzae* disease in adults, *Arch. Intern. Med. 147*:241 (1987).
66. B. Trollfors, B. Claesson, T. Lagergard, T. Sandberg, Incidence, predisposing factors and manifestations of invasive H. influenzae infections in adults, *Eur. J. Clin. Microbiol. 3*:180 (1984).
67. H. B. Simon, F. S. Southwick, R. C. Moellering, Jr., E. Sherman, *H. influenzae* in hospitalized adults: current perspective, *Am. J. Med. 69*:219 (1980).
68. A. K. Takala, J. Eskola, L. van Alphen, Spectrum of invasive Haemophilus influenzae type b disease in adults, *Arch. Intern. Med. 150*:2573 (1990).
69. J. I. Ward, A. L. Smith, *H. influenzae* bacteremia in children with sickle cell disease. *J. Pediatr. 88*:261 (1976).
70. D. Powars, G. Overturf, E. Turner, Is there an increased risk of *H. influenzae* septicemia in children with sickle cell anemia? *Pediatrics 71*:927 (1983).
71. H. S. Zarkowsky, D. Gallagher, F. M. Gill, et al., Bacteremia in sickle hemoglobinopathies, *J. Pediatr. 109*:579 (1986).
72. R. Chilcote, R. Baehner, D. Hammond, Septicemia and meningitis in children splenectomized for Hodgkin's disease, *N. Engl. J. Med. 295*:798 (1976).
73. F. S. Rosen, C. A. Janeway, The gamma globulins: III. The antibody deficiency syndromes, *N. Engl. J. Med. 275*:709 (1966).
74. R. J. Farrand, Recurrent *Haemophilus* septicemia and immunoglobulin deficiency. *Arch. Dis. Child. 45*:582 (1970).
75. J. E. Figueroa, P. Densen, Infectious diseases associated with complement deficiencies, *Clin. Microbiol. Rev. 4*:359 (1991).
76. S. C. Ross, P. Densen, Complement deficiency states and infection: epidemiology, pathogenesis, and consequences of neisserial and other infections in an immune deficiency, *Medicine 63*:243 (1984).
77. G. R. Siber. Bacteremias due to *H. influenzae* and *Streptococcus pneumoniae*: their occurence and course in children with cancer, *Am. J. Dis. Child. 134*:668 (1980).
78. A. V. Bartlett, J. Zusman, R. S. Daum, Unusual presentations of *H. influenzae* infections in immunocompromised patients, *J. Pediatr. 102*:55 (1983).
79. S. Weitzman, A. C. Aisenberg, Fulminant sepsis after the successful treatment of Hodgkin's disease, *Am. J. Med. 62*:47 (1977).
80. M. K. Lum, J. I. Ward, T. R. Bender, Protective influence of breast feeding on the risk of developing invasive *H. influenzae* type b disease (Abstract), *Pediatr. Res. 16*(Part 2):436 (1982).
81. A. K. Takala, J. Eskola, J. Palmgren, Risk factors of invasive *Haemophilus*

influenzae type b disease among children in Finland, *J. Pediatr. 115*:694 (1989).

82. G. M. Petersen, D. R. Silimperi, C. Y. Chiu, J. I. Ward, Effects of age, breast feeding, and household structure on *Haemophilus influenzae* type b disease risk and antibody acquisition in Alaskan Eskimos, *Am. J. Epidemiol. 134*:1212 (1991).
83. M. E. Pichichero, A. E. Sommerfelt, M. C. Steinhoff, R. A. Insel, Breast milk antibody to the capsular polysaccharide of *Haemophilus influenzae* type b, *J. Infect. Dis. 142*:694 (1980).
84. R. A. Insel, M. Amstey, M. E. Pichichero, Postimmunization antibody to the *Haemophilus influenzae* type b capsule in breast milk, *J. Infect. Dis. 152*:407 (1985).
85. R. L. Myerowitz, C. W. Norden, Immunology of the infant rat experimental model of *H. influenzae* type b meningitis, *Infect. Immun. 16*:218 (1977).
86. R. H. Michaels, R. L. Myerowitz, R. Klaw, Potentiation of experimental meningitis due to *Haemophilus influenzae* by influenza virus, *J. Infect. Dis. 135*:641 (1977).
87. K. Krasinski, J. D. Nelson, S. Butler, J. P. Luby, H. Kusmiesz, Possible association of mycoplasma and viral respiratory infections with bacterial meningitis, *Am. J. Epidemiol. 125*:499 (1987).
88. J. C. Parke, Jr., R. Schneerson, J. B. Robbins, The attack rate, age incidence, racial distribution, and cae fatality rate of *H. influenzae* type b meningitis in Mecklenburg County, North Carolina, *J. Pediatr. 81*:765 (1972).
89. L. J. Baraff, P. F. Wehrle, Epidemiology of pediatric meningitis: Los Angeles County, 1975 (abstracted), *Pediatr. Res. 11*:434 (1977).
90. G. C. Yost, A. M. Kaplan, R. Bustamante, C. Ellison, A. F. Hargrave, D. L. Randall, Bacterial meningitis in Arizona American Indian children, *Am. J. Dis. Child. 140*:943 (1986).
91. D. M. Granoff, P. G. Shackelford, J. P. Pandey, E. G. Boies, Antibody responses to H. influenzae type b polysaccharide vaccine in relation to Km(1) and G2m(23) immunoglobulin allotypes, *J. Clin. Invest. 257*:264 (1986).
92. D. M. Granoff, B. K. Suarez, J. P. Pandey, P. G. Shackelford, Genes associated with the G2M(23) immunoglobulin allotype regulate the IgG subclass responses to *Haemophilus influenzae* type b polysaccharide vaccine, *J. Infect. Dis. 157*:1142 (1988).
93. A. A. Lenoir, J. P. Pandey, D. M. Granoff, Antibody responses of black children to *Haemophilus influenzae* type b polysaccharide-Neisseria meningitidis outer-membrane protein conjugate vaccine in relation to the Km(1) allotype, *J. Infect. Dis. 157*:1242 (1988).
94. J. K. Whisnant, D. L. Mann, G. N. Rogentine, J. B. Robbins, Human cell-surface structures related to *H. influenzae* type b disease, *Lancet 2*:895 (1971).
95. J. K. Whisnant, G. N. Rogentine, M. A. Gralnick, et al., Host factors and antibody response in *H. influenzae* type b meningitis and epiglottitis, *J. Infect. Dis. 133*:448 (1976).

96. A. Tejani, R. Mahadevan, B. Dobias, et al., Occurrence of HLA types in *H. influenzae* type b disease, *Tissue Antigens 17*:205 (1981).
97. G. M. Petersen, D. R. Silimperi, J. I. Rotter, et al., Genetic factors in *H. influenzae* type b disease susceptibility and antibody acquisition, *J. Pediatr. 110*:229 (1987).
98. D. M. Granoff, J. P. Pandley, E. G. Boies, et al., Response to immunization with *H. influenzae* type by polysaccharide-pertussis vaccine and risk of *Haemophilus* meningitis in children with the Km(1) immunoglobulin allotype, *J. Clin. Invest. 74*:1708 (1984).
99. D. M. Ambrosino, G. Schiffman, E. C. Gotschlich, et al., Correlation between G2m(n) immunoglobulin allotype and human antibody response and susceptibility to polysaccharide encapsulated bacteria, *J. Clin. Invest. 75*:1935 (1985).
100. G. M. Petersen, D. R. Silimperi, E. M. Scott, et al., Uridine monophosphate kinase 3: a genetic marker for susceptibility to *H. influenzae* type b disease, *Lancet 2*:417 (1985).
101. D. P. Greenberg, C. M. Vadheim, N. Bordenave, Protective efficacy of *Haemophilus influenzae* type b polysaccharide and conjugate vaccines in children 18 months of age and older, *JAMA 265*:987 (1991).
102. C. M. Vadheim, D. P. Greenberg, E. Eriksen, et al., Reduction of Hib disease in southern California, 1983–1991. Program and Abstracts of the 32nd ICAAC, 1992, Abs 1726, Anaheim (abstract).
103. S. B. Black, H. R. Shinefield, Immunization with oligosaccharide conjugate *Haemophilus influenzae* type b (HbOC) vaccine on a large health maintenance organization population: extended follow-up and impact on *Haemophilus influenzae* disease epidemiology, *Pediatr. Infect. Dis. J. 11*:610 (1992).
104. T. V. Murphy, K. E. White, P. Pastor, et al., Declining incidence of *Haemophilus influenzae* type b disease since introduction of vaccination, *JAMA 269*:246 (1993).
105. W. G. Adams, K. A. Deaver, S. L. Cochi, et al., Decline of childhood *Haemophilus influenzae* type b (Hib) disease in the Hib vaccine era, *JAMA 269*:221 (1993).
106. H. Peltola, T. Kilpi, M. Anttila, Rapid disappearance of *Haemophilus influenzae* type b meningitis after routine childhood immunisation with conjugate vaccines, *Lancet 340*:592 (1992).

12

Epidemiology of *Haemophilus influenzae* Invasive Disease in Developing Countries and Intervention Strategies

Henk A. Bijlmer

Bronovo Hospital, The Hague, The Netherlands

I. INTRODUCTION

Haemophilus influenzae type b (Hib) invasive disease is an ubiquitous illness occurring mainly in children. Subsequently it can be assumed that developing countries, which have a population structure with a large proportion of children, have their share of this often debilitating disease. Whereas the Western world has reached the stage of completion of epidemiological studies on *H. influenzae* invasive disease and the implementation of universal vaccination against Hib has been initiated, a shortage of data from third world countries hampers progress towards the same goal. Lack of resources and a shortage of facilities are prohibitive in many developing countries for doing research on a wider scale than in a single laboratory or hospital.

Fortunately, many laboratory or hospital-based studies on *H. influenzae* invasive disease have been carried out over the years. These data can be very helpful in combination with the few prospective field studies that have been done in developing countries. Altogether an impression can be formed of the epidemiology of *H. influenzae* invasive disease in developing countries, and the patchy data can be compared with the vast amount of scientific data from the Western world on this subject. In this chapter several parameters in the epidemiology of *H. influenzae* invasive disease that have been investigated in developing countries are described, in particular those parameters that differ from those in the Western world.

Obviously a description of the epidemiology of *H. influenzae* invasive disease in developing countries is subject to severe constraints. The "developing world" is such a vast area of different populations living under diverse conditions that one hardly dare to make generalizations. What may be valid for areas in West Africa may be entirely different in East Africa. This may be even more the case in comparing data from Africa with those from developing countries in Asia or Latin America. Extrapolation of results to countries that are so different and have only a low economic standard and a low grade of industrialization in common has to be done with extreme caution. Alternatively, one must realize that many developing countries do not have the means or the infrastructure to do the sort of scientific research the Western world is able to do and that they will not have them in the near future.

In spite of these shortcomings and restrictions, several important questions have to be answered: In view of the potential of vaccination against Hib disease, what are the differences in epidemiology of *H. influenzae* invasive disease between Western countries and developing countries that can have an impact on the efficacy rate of vaccination against Hib disease? And second, with regard to the stringent economic situation in the developing world, can a more favorable cost-benefit balance for Hib immunization be achieved for the developing world by using alternative vaccination schemes?

This chapter will discuss some of the discrepancies between the epidemiology of Hib disease in developing countries compared with that of the Western world and also the impact of the observations in the developing world on the available intervention strategies.

II. CLINICAL SYNDROMES

The plethora of clinical syndromes that can be caused by *H. influenzae* is well known and has been described elsewhere. The most common clinical syndromes—meningitis, septicemia, upper and lower respiratory tract infections, cellulitis, and arthritis—occur in developing countries as they do in developed countries (1). The more rare presentations of *H. influenzae* invasive disease, e.g., infective pericarditis or osteomyelitis at a single location, probably do occur, but have not been reported due to less available detection facilities in these countries.

Epiglottitis due to Hib may be a notable exception in that it has *not* been reported from developing countries. Epiglottitis was represented abundantly in the series from Finland (29% of Hib invasive disease before the introduction of Hib vaccination), the United States (2,3) and the Australian Capital Territory (4) (32% of *H. influenzae* invasive disease). The incidence of epiglottitis is age related: mainly children older than 2 years were affected. In populations with a high incidence of Hib-invasive disease and a low mean age at which Hib-invasive disease occurs, epiglottitis is not seen (5,6). Apart from genetic differences, the absence of reports on epiglottitis from developing countries probably reflects a similar high incidence and low age at which Hib invasive disease occurs. Indeed, in one survey in The Gambia, West Africa, epiglottitis was specifically looked for and was reported as being absent from the array of clinical syndromes (1). In the same survey a high incidence of *H. influenzae* meningitis was recorded (7). It is possible that the clinical picture of epiglottitis will emerge in developing countries when the incidence of Hib-invasive disease has declined due to intervention measures and the mean age of patients with *H. influenzae* invasive disease has increased.

A new clinical syndrome of *H. influenzae* invasive disease that has recently emerged is confined to a restricted area outside the Western world. Brazillian purpuric fever (BPF) was recognized for the first time during 1984 in Sao Paulo (8), and it was found more recently in the state of Mato Grosso outside Sao Paulo (9). The disease presents as a triad of hemorrhagic conjunctivitis, fever, and septicemia in previously healthy children. BPF is caused by an unencapsulated *H. influenzae* strain, biogroup *aegyptius,* and has an extremely high mortality (60%).

III. INCIDENCE, CASE FATALITY RATE (CFR), AND SEQUELAE RATE

Incidence, sequelae rate, and CFR are prime parameters in the measurement of a disease as a health problem. The results of some of the best documented surveys on *H. influenzae* meningitis are summarized in Table 1. Only two sets of incidence rates come from "developing countries": one from The Gambia and one from Senegal, two neighboring countries in West Africa. Both show a high incidence rate, in particular in the age group under 1 year of age. High incidence rates of *H. influenzae* meningitis are also found in "developing societies" living within the boundaries of "Western" countries. These societies all have a culture distinct from the Western culture, and they have another family structure. Genetically these communities are very different from Caucasians, but they are genetically also dissimilar to each other. They all live in less affluent areas, and their societies are "nonindustrialized." A division is made in Table 1 between the "Western" and the "non-Western" societies. The high incidence rates are found in the "non-Western" societies. In the survey from Western Australia, the incidence of *H. influenzae* meningitis was distinctly higher among Aboriginal children than among non-Aboriginal children living in the same

Table 1 Age-Specific Annual Incidence of *Haemophilus influenzae* Meningitis in Developed and Developing Populations of the World

Population location	Annual incidence per 100,000 population at age		Ref.
	<5 years	<1 year	
Developed populations			
Australia			
Capital Territory	30[a]		4
Western, non-Aboriginal	27		10
United States			
Dallas County	67[b]	190	3
Minnesota	45[b]	118	3
Fresno County	60[b]	113	11
Mecklenburg County	63		12
Bernalillo County	39		13
Charleston County	38		14
Baltimore	19	51	15
Europe			
Finland	26[b]		2
UK, Oxford	24[b]		16
The Netherlands	22		17
Sweden	31		18
Middle East			
Israel	34[b]		19[c]
Developing populations			
Australia			
Western, Aboriginals	150		10
United States			
Alaska Eskimos	282[b]	871	5
White Mountain Apaches	254		20
Navajo Indians	152		6
Africa			
The Gambia	60[b]	297	7
Senegal, Dakar	132		21

[a]Calculated from reported incidence of invasive disease.
[b]Prospective population-based studies.
[c]Hib invasive disease.

territory (4). The same was found in Alaska among Eskimo children versus non-Eskimo children (5).

Thus, an embarrassing lack of data on incidence from developing countries exists—the larger part of the Third World is blank as far as this parameter is concerned. However, the compilation of data from all "developing societies" (Table 1) seems to indicate that the incidence of *H. influenzae* meningitis is high in those "developing" populations compared to Western societies. Further collection of data in other parts of the developing world is needed in order to obtain a much better picture, but there is no need to await the results of those surveys before taking further steps in prevention of *H. influenzae* invasive disease.

The latter statement may be supported by the data on case fatality rate (CFR) and sequelae rate. In contrast to data on incidence, much more is known about CFR of *H. influenzae* meningitis in developing countries. Although hospital-based studies may give a biased view on the actual CFR, a fairly accurate picture can be made from these sources. The CFR is uniformly and depressingly high in the developing world compared to the Western world, even compared with those parts of the Western world that have an extremely high incidence rate (Table 2).

The high CFR figures do not include the rate of permanent sequelae following *H. influenzae* meningitis. In the field study from The Gambia a sequelae rate of 17% was recorded, using only a coarse method of testing neurological and auditory functions. This sequelae rate might well be an

Table 2 Case Fatality Rates (CFR) for *Haemophilus influenzae* Meningitis in Western Countries Versus Developing Countries

Location	CFR (%)	Ref.
Western		
The Netherlands	1.95	22
United States, Alaska	3	5
Finland	3.3	2
United States, Navajo Indians	4	6
United States (overall)	5	14
Israel	3.3	23
Developing		
Ivory Coast	22	24
Nigeria, Ibadan	26	25
Ghana, Kumasi	30	26
Senegal, Dakar	33	27
The Gambia	37	7
Egypt, Cairo	40	28

underestimate since Letson recorded in Alaskan Eskimos a sequelae rate of 29% for motor abnormalities and 7% hydrocephalus (29).

IV. AGE DISTRIBUTION

H. influenzae invasive disease is a disease of young children, but this seems to be even more so in developing countries. In the field study in The Gambia, 84% of all recorded cases of *H. influenzae* meningitis occurred before the age of 1 year and 44% of patients was younger than 6 months old (7). The age at which the highest incidence is recorded appears to be inversely correlated with the overall incidence rate; the higher the incidence, the lower the age at which the highest age specific incidence is found. The "division" between the populations with a high proportion of patients at a very young age and those with a low proportion is marked by the level of "development" (Table 3). Those with a high overall incidence and the peak of age-specific incidence at a low age are all situated in developing areas. An interesting observation was made by Dagan (19), who recorded a relatively high proportion of children under 6 months of age and a high proportion of children under 12 months of age with Hib invasive disease in Israel (Table 3), which is not a developing country.

Table 3 Proportion of Children with *Haemophilus influenzae* Meningitis or Hib Invasive Disease Occurring Before the Age of 6 Months or before the Age of 1 year in Developed and Developing Areas of the World

Location	Incidence (%) at age		Ref.
	<6 months	<1 year	
Developed countries			
Finland	5		2
Australia, Sydney	9		30
The Netherlands	12	37	22
United States, Fresno		38	11
United Kingdom, Oxford		42	16
Israel	22	69	19
Developing areas			
United States, Alaskan Eskimos	34	67	5
Senegal	32	69	27
United States, Navajo Indians		81	6
Nigeria		83	25
The Gambia	44	84	7

Again, only three of these observations regarding age (Table 3) have been made in Africa, and none of them come from Asia. All three point in the same direction: a high proportion of children suffering from Hib meningitis are younger than 6 months old. There are no reports that indicate the opposite. As the age distribution is strongly correlated with the efficacy rate of Hib conjugate vaccines, it is of paramount importance that more data be published on the age distribution of children with Hib invasive disease in developing countries. The age distribution may influence the choice between the available Hib conjugate vaccines and the decision whether or not to consider an alternative vaccination scheme.

V. CARRIAGE

Carriage of *H. influenzae* and in particular that of the more virulent serotype b is a prerequisite for becoming afflicted by disease. Nonetheless, the carriage rate is low (<5%) in Western countries, even in populations with a very high incidence rate of disease such as Alaskan Eskimos and Navajo Indians (5,6). In contrast, several surveys in developing countries showed a considerably higher Hib carriage rate in healthy children than in Western countries: in one survey from The Gambia the overall carriage rate of Hib was 10% in healthy non–household-contact children ($n = 1240$), and it was shown that transmission from Hib carrier to non–Hib carrier and vice versa occurred rapidly (30). In Papua New Guinea a similar figure was found by Gratten et al. (31) and more recently by Montgomery et al. (32). In a prospective study from Santiago, Chile, however, only 3% carriage was found in community controls (33). There are no data from other field studies on Hib carriage in the general population from developing countries.

These observations may be of importance in preparing a strategy for vaccination against Hib-invasive disease in developing countries for several reasons. First, a significant reduction in carriage of Hib in the oropharynx was recorded in Finland after immunization with Hib conjugate vaccine (34). If a high carriage rate in healthy children is correlated with a high incidence of Hib invasive disease at a young age, as it is in populations in The Gambia and in Papua New Guinea, immunization may reduce the transmission of Hib organisms substantially and may therefore enhance the efficacy of vaccination considerably in those countries. Second, a reduction of the number of Hib cases was seen in the United States in an age group younger than 18 months old after vaccination with conjugated Hib vaccine had been started in children older than 18 months (35). This effect has been attributed to the reduction of Hib carriage in the vaccinated older children and a subsequent reduction of transmission to the younger, susceptible children. If such an effect can be measured in populations with a low carriage rate, a substantial effect could be expected in populations with a high carriage rate. A one-dose immunization of older children, although far from optimal, might be taken into consideration as an alternative Hib-vaccination scheme rendering some effect if the optimal vaccination regimens are not feasible for economic reasons. However, the correlation between carriage of Hib and high incidence of Hib invasive disease needs further confirmation from surveys to be carried out in other developing countries. Apart from those studies, the effect of vaccination on Hib carriage will be assessed in the Hib vaccine trial initiated recently in The Gambia (Mulholland, personal communication).

VI. SERO-SUBTYPE DISTRIBUTION OF *H. INFLUENZAE* IN DEVELOPING COUNTRIES

A. Serotype Distribution

The six known serotypes of *H. influenzae,* as characterized by polysaccharide capsule, are not equally pathogenic in humans. Serotype b is by far the most prevalent serotype of *H. influenzae* invasive disease throughout the world. In the United States, in The Netherlands, in Denmark and Norway, in Sweden, and in Finland approximately 99% of *H. influenzae* invasive disease is caused by serotype b (18,22,36–38). Some significant contradictory observations have been made in developing countries. Serotype a was found in a high proportion of lung aspirates in infants in The Gambia (39) and in 7 and 10% of blood isolates in two studies from Papua New Guinea (40,41). In these studies a high proportion of nonserotypable (NT) *H. influenzae* was recorded. Also, over a period of 10 years, 82% of *H. influenzae* meningitis cases in Papua New Guinea were due to type b (42). In another study from The Gambia, 5.8% of isolates from *H. influenzae* invasive disease was serotype a (1). A similar figure was found in Senegal (27). In a small series of blood isolates from Pakistan only 64% was serotype b (43).

The conclusion from these data seems to be that in developing countries, too, type b is the predominant serotype, but to a much lesser extent that it is in Western countries. In estimating the expected efficacy rate of a vaccine against serotype b in developing countries, the lower prevalence of type b has to be taken into account. Also, in view of the wide variation of serotype distribution in the published series from developing countries, it seems wise to collect more data from different areas in the third world.

B. OMP Subtyping

On the subcapsular level, the distribution of outer membrane (OMP) subtypes in developing countries is different from that in the Western world. In

The Gambia only one of the less prevalent OMP subtypes was identical to a subtype found in Europe and in the United States. Four other subtypes were unique (1). A similar observation was made in Pakistan (43). No other reports in OMP subtyping in developing countries are known. Therefore, unlike the situation in Europe, Australia, and New Zealand where a single OMP subtype is responsible for more than 80% of *H. influenzae* invasive disease (44–46) and the United States where three OMP subtypes are responsible for most of Hib invasive disease (47), the outer-membrane composition of *H. influenzae* in developing countries could be less homogeneous. This observation has to be confirmed by analysis of more *H. influenzae* invasive strains from other developing countries. If so, the heterogeneity could have consequences for any vaccine based on the outer-membrane structure of *H. influenzae*. On the other hand, heterogeneity of OMP subtypes does not necessarily mean that these strains do not have a conserved P-epitope in common.

VII. INTERVENTIONS

The high incidence of *H. influenzae* type b meningitis in several developing countries and in particular the high case fatality rate (CFR) and sequelae rate warrant intervention. However, developing countries have a rather different list of health care priorities than do Western countries. Burdened by many diseases with devastating effects, such as malaria, filariasis, schistosomiasis, tuberculosis, and AIDS, the Ministry of Health of a developing country does not put the eradication or control of Hib invasive disease at the top of its list. With limited resources in most of the developing countries, the very first step in any discussion about intervention in Hib invasive disease is to decide whether or not to pursue any intervention other than for the individual patient who will be treated at a health center or hospital with any treatment available.

No cost-benefit analysis for prevention of Hib disease in developing countries has been done so far as was done in the United States and in The Netherlands before the introduction of Hib vaccine in those countries (48,49). It would be wise to do such a study at least once using parameters that are valid for the situation in developing countries.

Intervention can be done on many levels, some of which may seem obvious and a simple means to improve the poor outcome of Hib invasive disease in developing countries. It seems appropriate to discuss some of these alternatives in order to give an estimate of their impact on the outcome of Hib invasive disease in developing countries.

Expanding the health care facilities and making the system more accessible can be expected to reduce the CFR. At the same time, the improvement of transport and communication would have a beneficial impact on the high CFR. Of course these improvements have to be pursued, but reality dictates that it be a long-term goal for many developing countries. The efforts to improve transport, communication, and health care facilities in developing countries are not expected to have much impact in the short term.

A similar comment could be made on Hib-invasive disease–associated risk factors. The factors that have been investigated, such as malnutrition, sickle cell disease, concurrent pneumonia, anemia, and racial factors, are likely to have an impact on the severity of *H. influenzae* invasive disease in comparison to Western countries. The influence of racial factors and sickle cell disease obviously need to be accepted as unchangeable risk factors. It seems unrealistic that the other associated factors can be expected to change in the short term in developing countries.

Will improvement of antibiotic treatment be a more attainable goal then? Countries with limited resources cannot afford the full range of antibiotics that developed countries can. Oral treatment with chloramphenicol or intravenous treatment with ampicillin are the first-line treatments in many developing countries, as they were in Western countries until resistance became a major problem. The high CFR in developing countries, however, cannot be explained by inadequate antibiotic therapy, as resistance of *H. influenzae* to these antibiotics is not yet a major problem in some of the countries with a high CFR. In a series from The Gambia, none of 164 Hib strains produced beta-lactamase, and only 1.8% was resistant to chloramphenicol due to chloramphenicol acetyl transferase production (H. A. Bijlmer, unpublished), while the CFR in that survey was 37% (7). Also, in Papua New Guinea, ampicillin resistance was still rare and chloramphenicol resistance to Hib was nonexistent [42]. Cases of disease cause by strains with chloramphenicol resistance have been reported though (50).

Thus, affordable treatment of Hib meningitis is still possible in some developing countries, and the introduction of third-generation cephalosporins as first-line treatment may affect the health care budget, but will not diminish the death toll of Hib invasive disease. In fact, the high CFR can increase still more if resistance to ampicillin and chloramphenicol emerge on a large scale in developing countries, while third-generation cephalosporins are not available. In one area in India a resistance of 43% to ampicillin and chloramphenicol was reported. However, the exception of one case, all children that had not been treated with a third-generation cephalosporin died (51).

Monitoring of resistance patterns to the drugs available in the third world is important and should be done in many locations. The consequences of the results thereof are less promising.

VIII. VACCINATION

The best and most feasible approach to changing the epidemiological pattern of Hib disease in the developing world is to alter the susceptibility of the host. Hib conjugate vaccines in the Finnish trial (52) and the Californian trial (53) were protective from the age of 7 months onwards. These two trials were done in developed societies with a low to medium-high incidence of *H. influenzae* invasive disease.

It may be apparent that those age limits are not good enough for developing countries. Indeed, one of the earliest trials with the first Hib conjugate vaccine failed in a population with a high incidence—the Alaskan Eskimos (54). Conversely, the results of a vaccine trial with a newer and different Hib conjugate vaccine (PRP-OMPC) in the Navajo population showed an efficacy rate of ~95% in children vaccinated at 2 and 4 months of age (55). Therefore, the prospects for immunization of populations in which a high proportion of the patients with *H. influenzae* invasive disease is younger than 6 months of age are promising. It is nonetheless debatable whether extrapolation of these results to other populations, living in different environments and of different genetic origin (Africa, Papua New Guinea, Aborigines in Australia), is valid. It has been documented that genetic differences, such as the presence or absence of the Km(1) allotype in a black population, have a significant impact on the antibody response to an unconjugated Hib vaccine (56). It seems warranted to carry out at least one vaccination trial in Africa prior to the initiation of a large vaccination campaign in such a vast area.

In conjunction with a vaccination trial using a vaccination scheme that preferably does not interfere with the existing extended program of immunization (EPI) in developing countries, it can be strongly recommended to test alternative immunization schemes. The cost-benefit balance in developing countries will be different than it is in developed countries. Many developing countries will not be able to meet the costs involved in a full immunization scheme if proven efficacious, and a lack of funds may put severe restrictions to the optimal immunization scheme. If only the optimal vaccination scheme is going to be tested in the third world, the final result may well be that no children in the developing world are going to be vaccinated against Hib-invasive disease for many years to come, simply because that scheme is not affordable to a developing country. The WHO-initiated EPI is successful in many developing countries. The program achieved a vaccine coverage of approximately 67% in developing countries (57). Part of its success is related to the fact that it manages to purchase the full set of vaccination doses against measles, tuberculosis, diphtheria, tetanus, pertussis, and poliomyelitis for about $.50 per child. All these vaccines are long-used vaccines in contrast to the Hib conjugate vaccines, which will cost many times more than all of the vaccines involved in the EPI program. Until the time has arrived in developing countries that the optimal immunization scheme with one of the conjugated vaccines against Hib-invasive disease can be implemented, the third world may be better served by using an alternative and obviously cheaper vaccination scheme than no vaccination at all. It may be obvious that if no alternative regimen has been tested, there is no point in settling for it.

Which alternative immunization schemes could be tested in developing countries? First is maternal immunization. In developing countries like The Gambia and Senegal, 44% (7) and 32% (27), respectively, of all Hib meningitis cases were in infants less than 6 months old. Under these circumstances, an induction of anti-PRP antibodies in pregnant women by immunization could result in a substantial reduction of Hib-invasive disease. This approach has been successful in control of other infectious diseases such as tetanus neonatorum in which the passively transferred maternal antibodies cover the relatively short period of exposure long enough to prevent disease (58). For Hib meningitis in developing countries the period to be covered would be the first 12 months after birth. Almost all children have then acquired protective anti-PRP antibody levels, and the anti-PRP IgG serum level curve in healthy children is almost exactly inversely related to the disease incidence curve (59).

The IgG levels of full-term neonates are a reflection of those of their mothers and are approximately at the same level at birth (60). The IgG1 concentrations in the newborn are higher than those in the mother, due to active transport of antibody across the placenta (61). The rate of decline of maternally acquired IgG levels varies widely from one infant to another but reaches a nadir around the age of 6 months (62), the half-life of maternally derived IgG being approximately 25 days. Amstey et al. have shown that vaccination of women 34–36 weeks pregnant with the unconjugated PRP vaccine resulted in a 100-fold higher anti-PRP serum titer which persisted for 12 months in their newborns when compared to control newborns (63). In a study by Glezen, mothers were vaccinated in the third trimester of pregnancy with a single dose of PRP. Children born to these mothers had a significantly higher serum level of anti-PRP antibodies. It was estimated that these children would be protected for approximately 4 months compared to 2 months for children of mothers who received a placebo (64). Hib conjugate vaccines such as PRP-D in a single dose elicited a much higher antibody response in adults than plain PRP did (65). The response of adults to vaccination with PRP or Hib conjugate vaccine is predominantly IgG1 (66). A strategy whereby pregnant mothers would be given a single injection of conjugate vaccine should elicit very high antibody concentrations, predominantly IgG1. A one-dose vaccination of the pregnant mother with one of the older Hib conjugate vaccines would result in a higher IgG anti-PRP antibody level curve of the first 7 months of life in an upwards direction, with a subsequent reduction of the susceptibility of the young infants. This vaccination scheme would definitely not be optimal, but in developing countries it may achieve a substantial reduction of cases of Hib-invasive disease with a single dose of the oldest and therefore probably cheapest Hib conjugate vaccine.

The second alternative vaccination regimen to be investigated is the effect of a single dose with Hib conjugate vaccine at the age of 12 months old. As has been pointed out under the heading carriage, a significant reduction of Hib meningitis in one region in the United States was observed in the age group younger than 18 months old whereas the age group older than 18 months old had been vaccinated (35). A significant reduction in carriage of Hib in healthy children in developing countries could result in a substantial decrease of incidence of disease in areas with a high carriage rate. A single dose with one of the newer Hib conjugate vaccines could theoretically induce that reduction and deserves further investigation in the third world.

IX. SUMMARY

Haemophilus influenzae invasive disease in developing countries is very similar in presentation as that found in the Western world. The epidemiology shows nonetheless some distinct differences, although the published information from the third world is scanty and insufficient for such a vast area. More surveillance data are needed, but the general picture shows a high incidence of *H. influenzae* invasive disease with a depressingly high case fatality rate (CFR). Although the great majority of *H. influenzae* isolates are of serotype b, a substantial proportion of serotype a is found in developing countries. Also the subtype distribution seems less homogeneous than in the industrialized countries. The very young age at which most of the cases occur challenges the efficacy rate of the Hib conjugate vaccines. Action seems warranted, and a vaccination trial with a Hib conjugated vaccine in very young children such as one initiated in The Gambia is of paramount importance for the developing world. The financial situation of many developing countries calls for alternative solutions too. Suboptimal vaccination schemes should be tested, which may turn out to give a better cost-benefit balance for developing countries. These strategies include immunization of pregnant mothers and the reduction of carriage by vaccinating older children.

REFERENCES

1. H. A. Bijlmer, L. Van Alphen, L. Geelen-ven den Broek, B. M. Greenwood, H. A. Valkenburg, and J. Dankert, Molecular epidemiology of *Haemophilus influenzae* type b in The Gambia, *J. Clin. Microbiol. 30*:386 (1992).
2. A. K. Takala, J. Eskola, H. Peltola, and P. H. Mäkelä, Epidemiology of invasive *Haemophilus influenzae* type b disease among children in Finland before vaccination with *Haemophilus influenzae* type b conjugate vaccine, *Pediatr. Infect. Dis. J. 8*:297 (1989).
3. T. V. Murphy, M. T. Osterholm, L. M. Pierson, K. E. White, J. A. Breedlove, G. B. Seibert, J. N. Kuritsky, and D. M. Granoff, Prospective surveillance of *Haemophilus influenzae* type b disease in Dallas County, Texas, and in Minnesota, *Pediatrics 79*:173 (1987).
4. A. R. McGregor, J. M. Bell, I. M. Abdool, and P. J. Collignon, Invasive *Haemophilus influenzae* infection in the Australian Capital Territory region, *Med. J. Aust. 156*:569 (1992).
5. J. I. Ward, M. K. W. Lum, D. B. Hall, D. R. Silimperi, T. R. Bender, Invasive *Haemophilus influenzae* type b disease in Alaska: background epidemiology for a vaccine efficacy trial, *J. Infect. Dis. 153*:17 (1986).
6. J. L. Coulehan, R. H. Michaels, C. Hallowel, R. Schults, T. K. Welty, and J. S. C. Kuo, Epidemiology of *Haemophilus influenzae* type b disease among Navajo Indians, *Public Health Rep. 99*:404 (1984).
7. H. A. Bijlmer, L. Van Alphen, B. M. Greenwood, J. Brown, G. Schneider, A. Hughes, A. Menon, H. C. Zanen, and H. A. Valkenburg, The epidemiology of *Haemophilus influenzae* infections in children under five years of age in The Gambia, West Africa, *J. Infect. Dis. 161*:1210 (1990).
8. D. J. Brenner, L. W. Mayer, G. M. Carlone, L. H. Harrison, W. F. Bibb, M. C. Brandileone, F. O. Sottnek, K. Irino, M. W. Reeves, J. M. Swenson, et al., Biochemical, genetic, and epidemiologic characterization of *Haemophilus influenzae* biogroup aegyptius (Haemophilus aegyptius) strains associated with Brazilian purpuric fever, *J. Clin. Microbiol. 26*:1524 (1988).
9. The Brazilian Purpuric Fever Study Group, Brazilian purpuric fever identified in a new region of Brazil, *J. Infect. Dis. 165*:16 (1992).
10. J. Hanna, and B. E. Wild, Bacterial meningitis in children under five years of age in Western Australia, *Med. J. Aust. 155*:160 (1992).
11. D. M. Granoff, and M. Basden, *Haemophilus influenzae* infections in Fresno County, California: a prospective study of the effects of age, race, and contact with a case on incidence of disease, *J. Infect. Dis. 141*:40 (1980).
12. J. C. Parke Jr, R. Schneerson, and J. B. Robbins, The attack rate, age incidence, racial distribution, and case fatality rate of *Haemophilus influenzae* type b meningitis in Mecklenburg County, North Carolina, *J. Pediatr. 81*:765 (1972).
13. D. W. Fraser, C. C. Geil, and R. A. Feldman, Bacterial meningitis in Bernalillo County, New Mexico: a comparison with three other American populations, *Am. J. Epidemiol. 100*:29 (1974).

14. D. W. Fraser, Ch. P. Darby, R. E. Koehler, C. F. Jacobs, and R. A. Feldman, Risk factors in bacterial meningitis: Charleston County, South Carolina, *J. Infect. Dis. 127*:271 (1973).
15. M. Santosham, C. H. Kallman, J. M. Neff, and E. R. Moxon, Absence of increasing incidence of meningitis caused by *Haemophilus influenzae* type b, *J. Infect. Dis. 140*:1009 (1979).
16. G. Tudor-Williams, J. Frankland, D. Isaacs, R. T. Mayon-White, J. A. MacFarlane, M. P. E. Slack, E. Anderson, D. G. Rees, and E. R Moxon, *Haemophilus influenzae* type b disease in the Oxford region, *Arch. Dis. Child. 64*:517 (1989).
17. L. Spanjaard, P. Bol, W. Ekker, and H. C. Zanen, The incidence of bacterial meningitis in the Netherlands—a comparison of three registration systems, *J. Infect. 11*:259 (1985).
18. B. Trollfors, B. A. Claesson, K. Strangert, and J. Taranger. *Haemophilus influenzae* meningitis in Sweden 1981–1983, *Arch. Dis. Child. 62*:1220 (1987).
19. R. Dagan, A two-year prospective, nationwide study to determine the epidemiology and impact of invasive childhood *Haemophilus influenzae* type b infection in Israel. The Israeli Pediatric Bacteremia and Meningitis Group, *Clin. Infect. Dis. 15*:720 (1992).
20. G. A. Losonsky, M. Santosham, V. M. Sehgal, A. Zwahlen, and E. R. Moxon. *Haemophilus influenzae* disease in the White Mountain Apaches: molecular epidemiology of a high risk population, *Pediatr. Infect. Dis. 3*:539 (1984).
21. M. Cadoz, F. Denis, and I. Diop Mar, Etude épidémiologique des cas de méningites purulentes hospitalisés à Dakar pendant le décennie 1970–1979, *Bull. WHO 59*:575 (1981).
22. P. Bol, Epidemiology of bacterial meningitis in the Netherlands, Ph.D. thesis, University of Amsterdam, 1987.
23. P. E. Slater, M. Roitman, and C. Costin, Epidemiology of *Haemophilus influenzae* type b meningitis in Israel, 1981–90, *Publ. Health Rev. 18*:307 (1990–91).
24. J. B. De Bary, B. Soro, V. Synaeve, L. Schuermann, and J. L. Rey, Purulent meningitis at a semi-rural hospital in the forest area of the Ivory coast, *Bull. Soc. Pathol. Exot. Filiales 83*:460 (1990).
25. V. A. Nottidge, *Haemophilus influenzae* meningitis:a 5 year study in Ibadan, Nigeria, *J. Infect. 11*:109 (1985).
26. E. J. Mackie, P. Shears, E. Frimpong, and S. N. Mustafa-Kutana, A study of bacterial meningitis in kumasi, Ghana, *Ann. Trop. Paediatr. 12*:143 (1992).
27. E. Autret, I. Diop Mar, F. Denis, J. P. Chiron, M. Cadoz, and A. Sow, Méningite purulente à *Haemophilus influenzae* b. Analyse de 248 observations dakaroises, *Med. Afr. Noire. 26*:861 (1979).
28. N. I. Girgis, J. E. Sippel, M. E. Kilpatrick, W. R. Sanborn, I A. Mikhil, E. Cross, M. W. Erian, Y. Sultan, and Z. Farid, Meningitis and encephalitis at the Abbassia Hospital, Cairo, Egypt, from 1966 to 1989, *Am. J Trop. Med. Hyg. 48*:97 (1993).
29. G. W. Letson, B. G. Gellin, L. R. Bulkow, D. J. Parks, and J. I. Ward,

Severity and frequency of sequelae of bacterial meningitis in Alaska Native infants. Correlation with a scoring system for severity of sequelae, *Am. J. Dis. Child. 146*:560 (1992).

30. H. A. Bijlmer, N. Lloyd Evans, H. Campbell, L. Van Alphen, H. A. Valkenburg, and H. C. Zanen, Carriage of *Haemophilus influenzae* in healthy Gambian children, *Trans. R. Soc. Trop. Med. Hyg. 83*:831 (1989).
30. P. B. McIntyre, S. R. Leeder, and L. M. Irwig, Invasive *Haemophilus influenzae* type b disease in Sydney children 1985–1987: a population-based study, *Med. J. Aust. 154*:832 (1991).
31. M. Gratten, T. Lupiwa, J. Montgomery, and G. Gerega, Distribution and relationship to serotype of *Haemophilus influenzae* biotypes isolated from upper respiratory tracts of children and adults in Papua New Guinea, *J. Clin. Microbiol. 19*:526 (1984).
32. J. M. Montgomery, D. Lehmann, T. Smith, A. Michael, B. Joseph, T. Lupiwa, C. Coakley, V. Spooner, B. Best, I. D. Riley, and M. P. Alpers, Bacterial colonization of the upper respiratory tract and its association with lower respiratory tract infections in Highland children of Papua New Guinea, *Rev. Infect. Dis. 12*:S1006 (1990).
33. R. Lagos, A. Avendano, I. Horwitz, J. M. Musser, S. K. Hoiseth, D. R. Maneval Jr, M. J. Jones, M. M. Levine, J. P. Dattas, and I. Prenzel, Molecular epidemiology of *Haemophilus influenzae* within families in Santiago, Chile, *J. Infect. Dis. 164*:1149
34. A. K. Takala, J. Eskola, M. Leinonen, H. Kayhty, A. Nissinen, E. Pekkanen, and P. H. Mäkelä. Reduction of oropharyngeal carriage of *Haemophilus influenzae* type b (Hib) in children immunized with an Hib conjugated vaccine, *J. Infect. Dis. 164*:982 (1991).
35. T. V. Murphy, K. E. White, P. Pastor, L. Gabriel, F. Medley, D. M. Granoff, and M. T. Osterholm, Declining incidence of *Haemophilus influenzae* type b disease since introduction of vaccination, *JAMA 269*:246 (1993).
36. D. M. Granoff, S. J. Barenkamp, and R. S. Munson, Outer membrane protein subtypes for epidemiologic investigation of *Haemophilus influenzae* type b disease. In: H. influenzae: *Epidemiology, Immunology and Prevention of Disease*, S. H. Sell and P. F. Wright, Eds., Elsevier, Amsterdam, 1982, pp. 43–45.
37. M. Kilian, I. Sorensen, and W. Frederiksen, Biochemical characteristics of 130 recent isolates from *Haemophilus influenzae* meningitis, *J. Clin. Microbiol. 9*:409 (1979).
38. H. Peltola, and M. Virtanen, Systemic *Haemophilus influenzae* infection in Finland, *Clin. Pediatr. 23*:275 (1984).
39. R. A. Wall, D. C. W. Mabey, and P. T. Corrah, *Haemophilus influenzae* non type b, *Lancet 2*:845 (1985).
40. J. Barker, M. Gratten, I. Riley, D. Lehmann, J. Montgomery, M. Kajoi, H. Gratter, D. Smith, T. F. deC. Marshal, and M. P. Alpers, Pneumonia in children in eastern highlands of Papua New Guinea: a bacteriologic study of patients selected by standard clinical criteria, *J. Infect. Dis. 159*:348 (1989).
41. F. Shann, M. Gratten, S. Germer, V. Linneman, D. Hazlett, and R. Payne,

Aetiology of pneumonia in children in Goroka Hospital, Papua New Guinea, *Lancet* 1984;2:537–541.

42. M. Gratten and J. Montgomery, The bacteriology of acute pneumonia and meningitis in children in Papua New Guinea: assumptions, facts and technical strategies, *Papua New Guinea Med. J. 34*:185 (1991).
43. G. A. Weinberg, A. Ghafoor, Z. Ishaq, N. K. Nomani, M. Kabeer, F. Anwar, M. I. Burney, A. W. Qureshi, J. M. Musser, R. K. Selander, and D. M. Granoff, Clonal analysis of *Haemophilus influenzae* isolated from children from Pakistan with lower respiratory tract infections. *J. Infect. Dis. 160*:634 (1989).
44. L. Van Alphen, L. Geelen, K. Johsdottir, A. K. Takala, H. Käyhty, and H. C. Zanen, Distinct geographical distribution of subtypes of *Haemophilus influenzae* b in Western Europe, *J. Infect. Dis. 126*:216 (1987).
45. D. A. Clements, S. J. MacInnes, and G. L. Gilbert, Outer membrane protein subtypes of *Haemophilus influenzae* type b isolates causing invasive disease in Victoria, Australia, from 1988 to 1990, *J. Clin. Microbiol. 30*:1879 (1992).
46. G. A. Saravani, D. R. Martin, and M. T. Arriesgado, *Haemophilus influenzae* in New Zealand: subtyping of isolates from invasive disease using outer membrane protein profiling, *N. Z. Med. J. 105*:218 (1992).
47. S. J. Barenkamp, R. S. Munson, and D. M. Granoff, Comparison of outer-membrane protein subtypes and biotypes of isolates of *Haemophilus influenzae* type b, *J. Infect. Dis. 144*:480 (1981).
48. J. W. Hay and R. S. Daum, Cost-benefit analysis of two strategies for prevention of *Haemophilus influenzae* type b infection, *Pediatrics 80*:319 (1987).
49. L. L. Martens, G. H. M. Ten Velden, and P. Bol, De kosten en baten van vaccinatie tegen *Haemophilus influenzae* type b, *Ned. Tijdschr. Geneesk. 135*:16 (1991).
50. A. W. Johnson, O. A. Mokuolo, and B. A. Onile, Chloamphenicol-resistant *Haemophilus influenzae* meningitis in young urban Nigerian children, *Acta Pediatr. 81*:941 (1992).
51. R. Singh, S. Thomas, C. Kirubakaran, M. K. Lalitha, and P. Raghupathy, Occurrence of multiple antimicrobial resistance among *Haemophilus influenzae* type b causing meningitis, *Indian J. Med. Res. 95*:230 (1992).
52. J. Eskola, H. Kayhty, A. K. Takala, et al., A randomized, prospective field trial of a conjugate vaccine in the protection of infants and young children against invasive *Haemophilus influenzae* type b disease, *N. Engl. J. Med. 323*:1381 (1990).
53. S. B. Black, H. R. Shinefield, B. Fireman, et al., Efficacy in infancy of oligosaccharide conjugate *Haemophilus influenzae* type b (HbOC) vaccine in a United States population of 61,080 children, *Pediatr. Infect. Dis. J. 10*:97 (1991).
54. J. Ward, G. Brenneman, G. W. Letson, and W. L. Heyward. Limited efficacy of a *Haemophilus influenzae* type b conjugate vaccine in Alaska Native infants. The Alaska *Haemophilus influenzae* Vaccine Study Group, *N. Engl. J. Med. 323*:1393 (1990).

55. M. Santosham, M. Wolff, R. Reid, et al., The efficacy in Navajo infants of a conjugate vaccine consisting of *Haemophilus influenzae* type b polysaccharide and *Neisseria meningitidis* outer-membrane protein complex, *N. Engl. J. Med. 324*:1767 (1991).
56. D. M. Granoff, I. P. Pandey, E. Boies, J. Squires, R. S. Munson, Jr, and Suarez B, Response to immunization with *Haemophilus influenzae* type b polysaccharide-pertussis vaccine and risk of Haemophilus meningitis in children with the Km(1) immunoglobulin allotype, *J. Clin. Invest. 74*:1708 (1984).
57. S. E. Robertsen, C. Chan, R. Kim-Farley, and N. Ward, World-wide status of poliomyelitis in 1986, 1987 and 1988, and plans for its global eradication by the year 2000, *World Health Stat. Q. 43*:80 (1990).
58. K. W. Newell, A. Duenas Lehman, D. R. LeBlanc, and N. Garces Osioro, The use of toxoid for the prevention of tetanus neonatorum. Final report of a double-blind controlled field trial, *Bull. WHO 35*:863 (1966).
59. H. A. Bijlmer, *Haemophilus influenzae* meningitis in The Gambia, West Africa, a prospective field study, Ph.D. thesis, Amsterdam, 1992.
60. C. Y. Yeung and J. R. Hobbs, Serum-gamma G-globulin levels in normal, premature, post-mature and "small-for-dates" newborn babies, *Lancet 1*:1167 (1968).
61. M. S. Einhorn, D. M. Granoff, M. H. Nahm, A. Quinn, and P. G. Schackelford. Concentrations of antibodies in paired maternal and infant sera: relationship to IgG subclass, *J. Pediatr. 111*:783 (1987).
62. E. R. Stiehm and H. H. Fudenberg, Serum levels of immune globulins in health and disease—a survey, *Pediatrics 37*:715 (1966).
63. M. S. Amstey, R. Insel, J. Munoz, and M. Pichichero, Fetal-neonatal passive immunization against *Haemophilus influenzae* type b, *Am. J. Obstet. Gynecol. 153*:607 (1985).
64. W. P. Glezen, J. A. Englund, G. R. Siber, H. R. Six, C. Turner, D. Shriver, C. M. Hinkley, and O. Falcao, Maternal immunization with the capsular polysaccharide cvaccine for *Haemophilus influenzae* type b, *J. Infect. Dis. 165*:S134 (1992).
65. D. M. Granoff, E. G. Boies, R. S. Munson, Jr., Immunogenicity of *Haemophilus influenzae* type b polysaccharide-diphtheria toxoid in adults, *J. Pediatr. 105*:22 (1984).
66. P. G. Shackelford, D. M. Granoff, S. J. Nelson, M. G. Scott, D. S. Smith, and M. H. Nahm, Subclass distribution of human antibodies to *Haemophilus influenzae* type b capsular polysaccharide, *J. Immunol. 138*:587 (1987).

13

Principles for Designing Vaccine Clinical Studies

Vincent I. Ahonkhai

Robert Wood Johnson Pharmaceutical Research Institute, Raritan, New Jersey

I. INTRODUCTION

A *Haemophilus influenzae* type b (Hib) vaccine composed of the Hib capsular polysaccharide, polyribosyl ribitol phosphate (PRP) was first licensed in the United States in 1985 for use between the ages of 18 and 71 months. Because the preponderance of cases of invasive Hib disease occurs in infants under 18 months of age, only a limited impact on this disease was anticipated. In contrast, Hib conjugate vaccines represent a veritable success story from several points of view. As the first conjugate vaccines ever to be developed, this class of vaccines lent technological practicality to a long-appreciated immunological principle of immunopotentiation that results from the coupling of a polysaccharide antigen to a carrier protein (1). Response from the pharmaceutical sector was rapid, with formulation of three vaccines in the United States (PRP-D, HbOC, PRP-OMPC) and one in France (PRP-T).

Next, prompt incorporation of these vaccines into routine pediatric immunization schedules signaled tremendous prospects for significant public health benefits. Indeed, evidence is emerging that invasive Hib disease is on the decline (2). This success profile is the driving force behind current research and development efforts on conjugate vaccines against other diseases such as pneumococcal infections.

Although proof of safety and efficacy is the ultimate requirement for regulatory approval of any vaccine, including Hib conjugate vaccines, the time frame to garner the supporting data and the resources needed are subjects

Table 1

General Principles	
	Disease epidemiology
	Vaccine characteristics
	Serological testing
	CBER and other regulatory agencies
Preclinical	
	Animal model
	Relevant in vitro activity of antibody
	Surrogate markers
	Vaccine characteristics
Clinical	
	Clinical development plan
	IRB/Investigator
	Parent/Guardian, subject
	Site selection
	Handling test samples
	Publication activities

that must be handled by vaccine developers. Accordingly, each firm bears responsibility for designing a research and development program that desirably should be expeditious, while minimizing resource expenditure. This author's leading role in the development of a Haemophilus b conjugate vaccine by Merck is the experience base upon which this chapter is built.

Numerous factors are relevant when considering the design and implementation of clinical studies as in those conducted during the development of Hib conjugate vaccines. Beginning with early preclinical studies through the filing of a registration data package with regulatory agencies, the principles involved may vary with the stage of the development. Moreover, while certain principles may be limited to a specific phase of the clinical program, other principles may be relevant to all phases. Above all, it is important to recognize that the success of clinical studies, as ultimately the entire vaccine development program, depends on preclinical, clinical as well as nonclinical factors. A list of key principles that should be considered in the clinical studies on Hib vaccines is shown in Table 1.

II. GENERAL PRINCIPLES

A. Disease Epidemiology

If there was a *sine qua non* in the clinical development of Hib conjugate vaccines, a well-characterized epidemiological profile of the disease fits that distinction. The growth and expansion of epidemiology data on Hib disease served as a major driving force that heightened the awareness of researchers and pediatricians of the need for vaccine control of the disease. As a result, in an environment that was awaiting scientific breakthrough on this subject, acceptance of a new investigational vaccine was enhanced by the generation of relevant epidemiological data. Without a well-defined epidemiological profile the pace of clinical development might have been slower. Furthermore, specific aspects of disease epidemiology, such as the characteristics of age, race, and socioeconomic background, clearly identified the key targets or subpopulations wherein candidate vaccines should be evaluated so that the potential benefits from vaccination would be maximized in the general population.

B. Vaccine Characteristics

While the most desirable attribute of a candidate vaccine is that it be highly immunogenic, other characteristics influence its acceptance. A good safety and tolerability profile, ease of administration with a minimum of vaccine reconstitution procedures, storage requirements that can be met at any potential investigative study site, and adequate stability to assure that expiration dates are long enough to obviate frequent replacement of unused supplies such as when subject enrollment is slow, are important points to keep in mind. Placing studies in less accessible sites including sites outside the United States or those in developing countries requires a vaccine with stable composition to withstand the rigors of shipment.

The availability of facilities to manufacture large lots of vaccine is critical to ascertaining that adequate sample sizes are available for statistical evaluation of consistency in vaccine immunogenicity by lot. For a similar reason, the need to achieve lot-to-lot consistency in vaccine composition is especially important during Phase III pivotal studies.

C. Serological Tests

The Farr assay (3) and modifications of it have been the mainstay for quantifying the immunogenicity of Hib conjugate vaccines. More recently, an ELISA technique has been used, albeit less commonly (4). Because it is often difficult to obtain adequate volumes of serum from infants, a microassay procedure that can operate on fractional serum volumes will guarantee that virtually every subject's sample is usable. Reproducibility of any assay is important in order to permit comparisons of immunogenicity among different subject groups for a given vaccine and among different vaccine formulations. Optimum standardization of the serological assay additionally is important to minimize intra- and interlaboratory variability in results (5).

D. Center for Biologics Evaluation and Research (CBER)

The U.S. Food and Drug Administration (FDA) regulates the development of vaccines through CBER. As such, vaccine developers are fully aware of the regulatory role of the agency. Significant opportunities exist for partnership with CBER in design and implementation of clinical trials. This partnership ranges from protocol development to interpretations of controversial results. These issues are critical during Phase III efficacy field trials. Comprehensive interactions with the agency are necessary to reach a common understanding on key aspects of pivotal trials including selection of an independent data-monitoring committee, efficacy and safety endpoints, study stopping rules, and overall data analysis plan. Prospectively establishing these parameters reduces confusion and disagreements during FDA advisory committee review of product data for FDA approval.

Outside the United States, regulatory bodies may be structured and may function differently, but the importance of proactive interaction remains vital prior to filing a product license application. Local experts and opinion leaders serve as a useful bridge between the vaccine developer and the regulatory body.

III. PRECLINICAL PRINCIPLES

Availability of relevant information from preclinical studies enhances success in initiating studies in humans. Such information should be derived from:

1. Animal model of disease
2. Relevant biological activity of vaccine-induced antibody
3. Establishing surrogate markers (where possible) for vaccine efficacy and safety

A. Animal Model

Demonstration of T-cell dependence as reported in athymic nude mice and infant rhesus monkeys (6,7) provided supporting evidence that conjugate vaccines would be immunogenic in human infants. Furthermore, the rabbit model for pyrogenicity was useful in evaluating the safety and tolerability of PRP-OMPC prior to initiation of clinical trials. Detail of animal models for preclinical studies can be found elsewhere in this book.

B. Biological Activity of Vaccine-Induced Antibody

While stimulation of anti-PRP antibody is an important endpoint for the activity of a new Hib vaccine, evidence that the antibody mediates biological activity is also important. In vitro, the antibody should be bactericidal and show opsonic activity (8,9). In vivo, protection of experimentally induced Hib bacteremia with or without meningitis in an infant rat model is often regarded as standard for biological activity of vaccine-induced antibody (10).

C. Establishing Surrogate Markers

Considerable controversy existed on the subject of surrogate markers for efficacy of Hib conjugate vaccines early on in their clinical development. Although levels of anti-PRP antibody require to protect against Hib disease had been estimated from passive protection studies (11) and plain PRP vaccine studies (12), the issue became less clear when the first conjugate vaccine (PRP-D) was studied in a field trial (13). It has taken full evaluation of additional conjugate vaccines in field trials to show that evidence of a significant primary antibody response coupled with a memory (anamnestic) response may be appropriate surrogate markers for efficacy. In addition, demonstration of the in vitro and in vivo activities mentioned above should be considered ancillary surrogate markers. In today's environment where effective Hib conjugate vaccines are available, it would be ethically inappropriate and fiscally inadvisable to conduct a controlled efficacy field trial with a new Hib conjugate vaccine. However, it would be reasonable to evaluate such a vaccine using these surrogate markers.

To date an acceptable surrogate marker for safety is lacking.

D. Vaccine Characteristics

To enhance worldwide acceptance and public health benefit, a candidate vaccine should be compatible with as many components as possible of the World Health Organization (WHO) expanded program on immunization (EPI). This means that the conjugate vaccine should maintain satisfactory immunogenicity and safety when administered concurrently in the same syringe or at different sites. In developing countries the convenience, cost savings, and compliance engendered in concurrent administration of different vaccines are of paramount interest as documented in different geographic regions such as The Gambia, West Africa.

IV. CLINICAL PRINCIPLES

A. Clinical Development Plan

Formulating a clinical development plan is a necessary first step for successful clinical studies, including those for Hib conjugate vaccines. A comprehensive plan serves as a blueprint that defines key target milestones in the program from Phase 1 through Phase 4. The salient features to emphasize in each phase include:

Phase 1. Evaluation of vaccine safety, tolerability, and pilot immunogenicity, in small groups of children, typically one to two dozen subjects.

Phase 2. For determination of the most immunogenic tolerable vaccine dose through dose-ranging studies in larger groups of children. Inclusion of different age groups and subjects of different racial and ethnic backgrounds was instrumental to defining the differences in their antibody response to Hib conjugate vaccine. Phase 2 studies additionally provide valuable information on short-term longevity of vaccine-induced antibody and safety. One to two hundred subjects may be adequate to garner these data.

Phase 3. To establish the protective efficacy of a given vaccine, several points must be considered. The most desirable study population is one with a high incidence of disease. Appropriate statistical parameters such as sample size, clear endpoints, stopping rules, etc. must be specified in the study protocols. Several thousand subjects may be required to complete Phase 3 trials.

Phase 4. For further definition of safety and efficacy in an open population setting. Although several more thousands of subjects may be needed for this postmarketing surveillance phase, the strict criteria employed in Phase 3 studies are considerably relaxed here.

The clinical development plan additionally lays out resource needs in considerable details and sets a timeline for filing a product license application.

B. Study Approval: Role of Investigator and Review Committees

It is one thing for the vaccine developer to have a sound rationale for developing a new vaccine, but it is quite another issue for the investigator to be sufficiently convinced about the rationale and be willing to participate in a clinical trial, especially early in the program (Phase 1). It is thus necessary to include key potential investigators at the planning stages of a protocol and clinical strategy. An experienced investigator can provide invaluable insight into the general and special requirements of the Institutional Review Board (IRB) in regard to a study protocol and informed consent statement. Specific questions for the investigator should include dates and frequency of IRB meetings for protocol approval, what other local approvals are required, whether grants and budgets need special and separate approvals and how to obtain them, and the procedure for obtaining approval for protocol amendments. An elaborate procedure may be required in certain circumstances; underappreciation of this fact could result in unexpected delays in established timelines. For instance, field trials in Native American or Alaskan populations require multiple levels of approval that include the investigator's university IRB, community boards, and state and federal agencies (14). Adequate time must be set aside to meet such special needs.

A formal review committee may not exist in some places where the vaccine is designated for investigation. In such circumstances, sponsoring pharmaceutical companies must insist on at least two objectives:

1. To uphold the scientific standards being applied to protect the safety of the subject in the United States (or the company's country of origin)
2. To fully include local authorities, such as the national government, or its appropriate agency in decisions on the proposed clinical trial

The WHO, Medical Research Council (United Kingdom), Centers for Disease Control (CDC), and agencies of the U.S. government can provide information on how to conduct local trials in nonindustrialized countries. To sum up issues on study protocol approval, it is important to build in flexibility into the protocol and always maintain the highest standards of ethics.

C. Parent/Guardian and Subject Issues

Regulations protecting the safety of human participants in biomedical research are well defined on international and local levels. In addition to complying with such regulations, attention to a variety of nonregulatory issues can accelerate or delay clinical studies. The informed consent statement should be simple and comprehensive. Simplification includes use of the first language (not necessarily English) spoken by the parent or guardian of the minor subject, or working through an interpreter with medical background. Subjects from the inner cities or rural areas may need transportation assistance to the study site or incentives to return for follow-up. Other appropriate incentives may be welcome when subjects from indigent households are involved. Suitable group presentations of the research study should be considered as a means of reaching a large pool of study subjects. Establishing rapport with parents based on sincerity on the part of the investigator further enhances willingness to participate and compliance among parents. Not unexpectedly, initiating the first (Phase 1) clinical studies is more challenging since demonstration of encouraging clinical data progressively raises interest among potential study subjects.

D. Study Site Selection

The principal objective of a study site is the timely completion of subject enrollment, an end that can be accomplished at study sites of diverse composition. It should be recognized that study sites at academic institutions are not necessarily the most efficient in conducting vaccine clinical studies. On the other hand, pediatric practice groups and state/city public health clinics may not have the expertise or facilities for conducting clinical studies. Sites should be selected from suitable geographic locales that will assure a broad mix of socioeconomic and racial groups as well as inclusion of investigators with specialty on Hib disease. Outpatient clinics are most suitable, but provisions should be made for study coordinators to supervise the research. Adequate storage facilities for vaccine and other supplies, and personnel and equipment for management of medical emergencies must be available.

E. Handling Test Samples

The test sample, the ultimate source of laboratory proof of vaccine potency, demands special attention and protection with regard to quantity and quality. Spillage and loss of part or all of the sample should be avoided by using containers and lids of high quality. To maintain good-quality samples, packaging in dry ice to keep them frozen is necessary. The study site and the testing laboratory should discuss plans for sample shipment to permit prompt delivery, receipt, and inventory of samples.

As far as possible, a common procedure should be adopted for all study sites and test samples to eliminate any variability that could hinder interpretation of unexpected results. To this end it is desirable to test all samples in one laboratory. When practical, a single delivery service should be employed for shipment of test samples. Samples from foreign countries may pose an unique problem that requires even more elaborate planning. Specifics such as airline departure and arrival schedule, customs, and immigration regulations, if properly planned, will prevent sample packages from being left too long at the airport. When direct flights from study-site country to the testing-laboratory country are limited, it may be necessary to route samples to an intermediate country to preserve or reinforce the packaging.

F. Publication Activities

Dissemination of new information about an investigational vaccine is essential prior to and during clinical development as well as postlicensure. Publications in peer-reviewed journals and presentation at professional meetings are the most effective means of bringing new information to the awareness of individuals or groups that make the decisions governing the conduct of clinical trials. Thus, investigators, their support staff, and, indeed, IRB members are more likely to embrace and expedite approval of clinical studies if they have some degree of familiarity with the subject matter. As studies progress and evidence of promising efficacy accumulates, progressive acceptance is engendered such that, not infrequently, solicitation for study subject is replaced by parental requests for participation. Occasionally, requests come from locales beyond those with ongoing clinical studies. This is the genesis of compassionate use studies, which can be a source for valuable information about safety and efficacy. Thus, it is important to encourage meritorious publications as a means of facilitating the conduction of clinical studies.

V. SUMMARY

Four Hib conjugate vaccines have become commercially available in a relatively short period of time since 1987. This represents an unprecedented record in the history of vaccine development. That these vaccines are products of technological breakthrough lends more spectacle to their development. One or more of the vaccines witnessed considerable rapidity in development due to implementation of clinical research strategies driven by some of the principles outlined. The principles are broad based, being nonclinical, preclinical, or clinical. They are applicable to different stages of clinical development and may be suitable for nonconjugate vaccines as well as nonvaccine pharmacological products. Attention to these principles is likely to enhance success in developing future conjugate vaccines or related products.

REFERENCES

1. R. Schneerson, O. Barrera, A. Sutton, et al., Preparation, characterization and immunogenicity of Haemophilus influenzae type b polysaccharide-protein conjugates, *J. Exp. Med. 152*:361 (1980).
2. E. D. Shapiro, E. R. Wald, A. G. Margolis, et al., The decreasing incidence of Haemophilus influenzae type b (Hib) disease in both Connecticut and Greater Pittsburgh, PA., *Pediatr. Res. 31*:100A (1992).
3. R. S. Farr, A quantitative immunochemical measure of the primary interaction between I*BSA and antibody, *J. Infect. Dis. 103*:239 (1958).
4. A. Sutton, W. F. Vann, A. B. Karpas, et al., An avidin-biotin-based ELISA for quantitation of antibody to bacterial polysaccharides, *J. Immunol. Meth. 82*:215 (1985).
5. J. I. Ward, D. P. Greenberg, P. W. Anderson, et al., Variable quantitation of *Haemophilus influenzae* type b anticapsular antibody by radioantigen-binding assay, *J. Clin. Microbiol. 26*:72 (1988).
6. R. Schneerson, J. B. Robbins, C. Y. Chu, et al., Serum antibody responses of juvenile and infant rhesus monkeys injected with *Haemophilus influenzae* type b and pneumococcus type 6A capsular polysaccharide-protein conjugates, *Infect. Immun. 45*:582 (1984).

7. P. P. Vella, J. M. Staub, and R. W. Ellis, Biological activity of Hib conjugates, *Vaccine 9*(Suppl.):S26 (1991).
8. R. Scheerson, L. P. Rodriguez, J. C. Parke, Jr., et al., Immunity to disease caused by *Haemophilus influenzae* type b II. Specificity and some biologic characteristics of "natural," infection-acquired and immunization-induced antibodies to the capsular polysaccharide of *Haemophilus influenzae* type b, *J. Immunol. 107*:1081 (1971).
9. K. L. Cates, H. K. Marsh, and D. M. Granoff, Serum opsonic activity after immunization of adults with *Haemophilus influenzae* type b PRP-D conjugate vaccine, *Infect. Immun. 48*:183 (1985).
10. N. A. Halsey, T. L. Johansen, L. C. Bowman, et al., Evaluation of the protective efficacy of *Haemophilus influenzae* type b vaccines in an animal model, *Infect Immun 39*:1196 (1982).
11. M. Santosham, R. Reid, J. M. Ambrosino, et al., Prevention of *Haemophilus influenzae* type b infections in high-risk infants treated with bacterial polysaccharide immune globulin, *N. Engl. J. Med. 317*:923 (1987).
12. H. Peltola, H. Kayhty, M. Virtanem, et al., Prevention of *Haemophilus influenzae* type b bacteremic infections with the capsular polysaccharide vaccine, *N. Engl. J. Med. 310*:1561 (1984).
13. J. Eskola, H. Peltola, A. K. Takala, et al., Efficacy of *Haemophilus influenzae* type b polysaccharide-diphtheria-toxoid conjugate vaccine in infancy, *N. Engl. J. Med. 317*:717 (1987).
14. M. Santosham, M. Wolff, R. Reid, et al., The efficacy in Navajo infants of a conjugate vaccine consisting of *Haemophilus influenzae* type b polysaccharide and *Neisseria meningitidis* outer membrane protein complex, *N. Engl. J. Med. 324*:1767 (1991).

14

Antibody Assays

Philip P. Vella*

Merck Research Laboratories, West Point, Pennsylvania

Antibody assays for *Haemophilus influenzae* type b (Hib) conjugate vaccines can generally be divided into those measuring antibody to an essential functional activity (i.e., serum bactericidal, opsonin, and a passive protection test in infant rats) and those not specifically measuring functional activity such as radioimmunoassay (RIA) and enzyme-linked immunosorbant assay (ELISA). Those assays not specific for functional activity measure total antibody (RIA, ELISA) or isotype and subclass (ELISA). The capsular polysaccharide of Hib, polyribosyl ribitol phosphate or PRP, is associated with virulence, and antibody against PRP (anti-PRP) is protective against Hib disease (1,2) (see Chapter 1). The ideal serological assay is quantitative, reproducible, specific, sensitive, and capable of high throughput of test samples. Passive hemagglutination, immunofluorescence, or immunodiffusion do not meet all of these requirements.

I. ANTI-PRP IN VITRO ASSAY METHODS

A. RIA

The RIA, which measures total antibody to the target antigen (PRP), has gained wide acceptance among research laboratories and is the serological

*Retired.

assay upon which data were required for the licensure of PRP and Hib conjugate vaccines. Assay results among different research laboratories have been quite variable, and collaborative studies have been performed to provide a more uniform assay (3,4).

For performing the assay, blood samples are collected directly into serum separator tubes (e.g., Vacutainer or Microtainer tubes from Becton Dickinson) and, after gentle inversion several times, are allowed to clot for 30 minutes, centrifuged at 1000–3000 × *g* for 10 minutes and stored at 2–8°C for short-term for use in serological assays (1–2) or ≤−20°C for long-term storage in the serum separator tubes. The RIA procedure can use PRP labeled with ^{125}I or ^{3}H, either intrinsically labeled, i.e., the radiolabel is incorporated or chemically attached to a growth medium component of the organism from which the test antigen is to be isolated subsequently, or extrinsically labeled, i.e., chemically attached to the antigen after it has been isolated from the organism or culture medium. The type of radiolabeling does not appear to be a critical parameter of variability among assays, but PRP purity and size appear to be more crucial (3). Briefly, the standarized procedure utilizes ^{125}I-labeled PRP (chloramine-T method, described in Appendix 1) in which a fixed level of counts per minute (cpm) of antigen is incubated overnight with serial dilutions of test serum at 2–8°C. After the addition of a saturated ammonium sulfate solution (500 grams into 555.5 ml of distilled water) to salt out the antigen-antibody complexes and incubation for 1 hour at 2–8°C, the reaction mixture is centrifuged, the supernatant is decanted, and the bound antigen cpm are read from a standard curve (Fig. 1) prepared with a quantitatively defined FDA (Food and Drug Administration) standard for anti-PRP concentration. Table 1 outlines the RIA procedures used by various laboratories. Subsequently the FDA (4) developed a uniform procedure, utilizing a 0.1 M dibasic sodium phosphate-buffered saline diluent for diluting the radiolabeled antigen, which was employed by all laboratories seeking licensure for Hib conjugate vaccines. The test procedure works well when assaying human vaccinnee sera, but when assaying the sera of mice injected with the PRP-OMPC, the phosphate buffer appears to inhibit anti-PRP titers (P. P. Vella, unpublished; P. Anderson, personal communication).

A number of human serum controls are used in the assay in addition to the standard curve: five dilutions of a human control serum pool (obtained from adults vaccinated with PRP vaccine) are included at the beginning, middle, and end of the unknown test samples being run in the assay (c.a. 15 dilutions total), and two other adult PRP vaccinee pools (one dilution each) and an infant Hib conjugate vaccinee pool are included at the beginning of each assay, making a total of 18 controls run (in duplicate). In addition, 9 dilutions (in duplicate) of the FDA control serum are included in each assay to construct the standard curve.

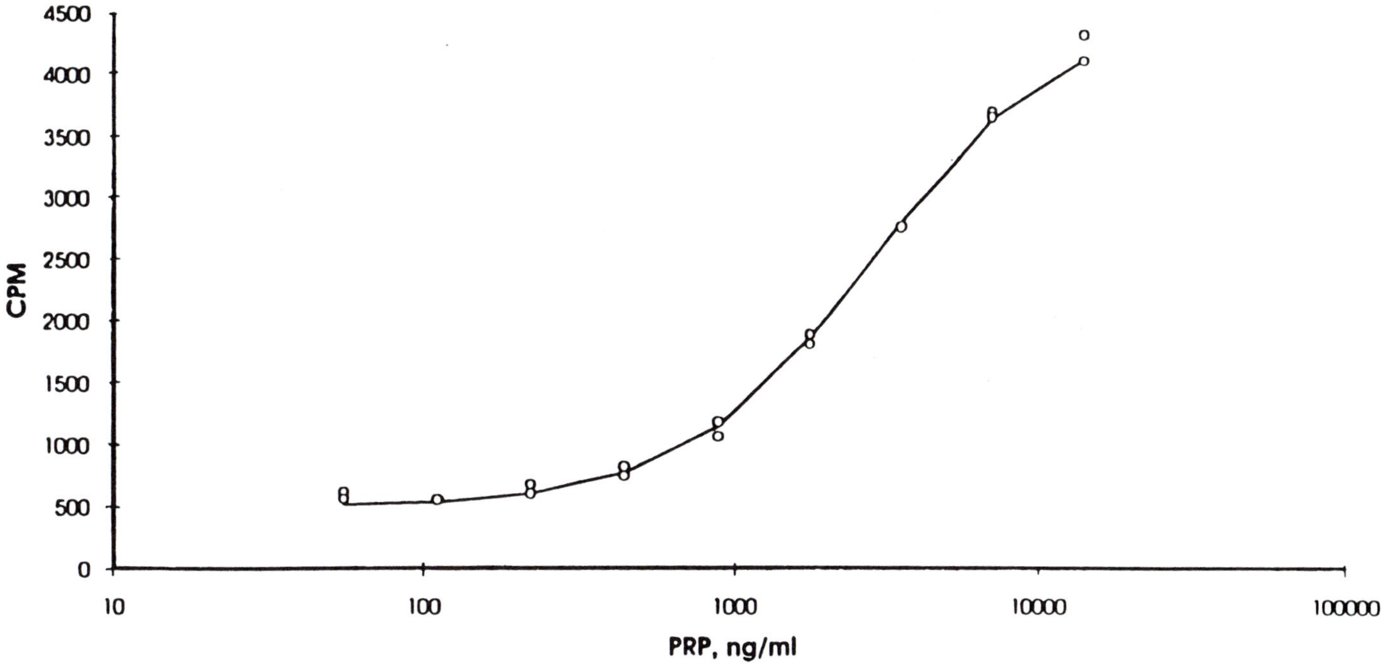

Figure 1 RIA standard curve (Hib). Each point represents a known standard serum dilution with each dilution run in duplicate. Single points reflect the identical value for both duplicates.

Table 1 Summary of Radioimmunoassay Methods for Detection of *H. Influenzae* Type b Capsular Antibody

Assay	Antigen label	Size of antigen[a]	Assay vol. (μl)	Antigen concn[b] (ng/ml)	Vol of serum (μl)	Incubation (temp [°C]/ duration [min])	Separation of bound and free antigen[c]	Radioactivity counting	Volume correction	Standard serum
Finland (ext)	^{125}I	UNK	75	20	25	4/ON[d]	SAS	Pellet	No	OBRR
UCLA (ext)	^{125}I	0.4–0.5	75	6.7	25	37/30; 4/ON	SAS	Pellet	No	OBRR
U-Roch. (ext)	^{125}I	0.4–0.5	75	6.7	25	37/30; 4/ON	SAS	Pellet	No	OBRR
MSD (ext)	^{125}I	0.65	60	50	50	2–8/ON	SAS	Supernatant	No	OBRR
UCLA (int)	^{3}H	0.6–0.7	50	20	25	4/ON	SAS	Pellet	Yes(^{36}Cl)	OBRR
Lederle (int)	^{3}H	0.45	500	2.5–3.0	25–50	37/60; 4/ON	PEG	Pellet	No	OBRR
U. Roch. (int)	^{3}H	0.25–0.40	75	3	25	4/ON	SAS	Pellet	Yes(^{36}Cl)	OBRR
Connaught (int)	^{3}H	0.6–0.7	50	20	25	4/ON	SAS	Pellet	Yes(^{36}Cl)	Pool 3

[a]K_d of the midpoint of the distribution of radiolabeled antigen on sepharose 2B. Molecular size of extrinsically labeled antigen refers to size after tyramination and iodination. UNK, Unknown.
[b]Concentration of labeled antigen in the assay mixture.
[c]SAS, saturated ammonium sulfate; PEG, polyethylene glycol.
[d]ON, Overnight.

Source: Ref. 3.

Because of the relatively lower molecular weight of the radiolabeled PRP [<200 kilodaltons (kD) on Sepharose 4B vs. nonlabeled PRP at ~ 550 kD] used in the RIA method, fetal calf serum must be used as a diluent for test serum dilutions in order to provide a sufficient mass of protein matrix to enable the precipitation of PRP-antibody complexes with saturated ammonium sulfate. Although the sensitivity of the assay is approximately 25–50 ng anti-PRP/ml serum, it has been more appropriate in the author's opinion to employ a cut-off of 125 ng anti-PRP/ml because of the considerable variation in that portion of the curve. This means that a negative serum is arbitrarily assigned a value of <125 ng anti-PRP/ml for the calculation of geometric mean titer (GMT) in a set of sera. Relatively small changes in cpm will cause moderate shifting of values on a percentage basis. Only those anti-PRP values that fall within the 20–80% binding range of the standard curve are employed unless undiluted sera bind <20%, in which case that value is used. Extrapolation of data is avoided because of the potential error from the plateauing of the low or high end of the antibody standard curve. The prozone phenomenon has been observed with some sera containing high levels of anti-PRP and assayed undiluted, i.e., when tested at increased dilution the anti-PRP value increases and subsequently plateaus. It is more appropriate with postvaccination sera to assay sera at dilutions in order to minimize serum use and to avoid any type of prozone phenomenon. A sufficient number of dilutions of each test serum should be made to assure that one or more dilutions will bind a sufficient amount of radiolabeled antigen to fall within the 20–80% antigen-binding range of the standard curve so that a value in the linear portion of the curve is obtained. On the example in Figure 1, this would correspond to the portion approximately between 700 and 7000 ng. The amount of radiolabeled PRP used in the assay can influence the measured level of the anti-PRP titer, since high-affinity antibody would bind preferentially to limiting quantities of the labeled PRP. Higher levels of radiolabeled PRP have been used with resultant increases in calculated anti-PRP titers (5), thus providing sufficient antigen for binding by both high- and low-affinity antibody. The human serum standard from the FDA has been assigned a value of 70 μg anti-PRP/ml; IgG and IgM standards also are available from the FDA, and these have been used to calibrate other assays in the users' laboratory. The disadvantages of the RIA method include the use of a radioactive reagent and ensuing environmental and disposal problems, short half-life of the ^{125}I isotope (necessitating new preparations every 4 weeks), and the inability to measure isotype or IgG subclass responses. Antibody avidity is the functional affinity of antibody to the antigen (7) and is a parameter that has been used to compare anti-PRP elicited by various Hib conjugate vaccines (5). The assay is based on the percentage of antigen measured in each of two RIA procedures, one using excess antibody and the other using excess radiolabeled antigen. Bound antigen is calculated in the antibody-excess method, and the functional antibody constant is given by the formula $K = P/[(1-P) \times (Ab)]$, where K is the avidity constant (5). P is the fraction of antigen-bound molecules, and Ab is the total antibody concentration. The total antibody concentration is obtained by using the radiolabeled antigen-excess RIA method, and the avidity value is expressed as nM^{-1}.

A GMT is calculated as being more representative of overall antibody response for a test group of individuals rather than an arithmetic mean titer (AMT). The GMT minimizes the skewing effect that occurs when a small percentage of the responders in a group have unusually high titers. A GMT is a simple average appropriate for log-normally distributed data. The larger the test group number, the less likely a skewing effect would be observed if a small percentage of the responders were unusually high. One would probably be correct in assuming that the distribution in a test group of, e.g., 6–10 cases would be very similar for a larger group if there was not an extreme bias in the smaller group. A more in-depth discussion of GMT has been reviewed (6).

B. ELISA

ELISA methods are being utilized more frequently because they are less expensive, do not require radioisotopes and the necessary counters, and have the ability to measure isotype and IgG subclass. Currently efforts are in progress among various research laboratories and the FDA to establish standardized ELISA procedures to replace RIA methodology. A variety of ELISA procedures have been in use to measure anti-PRP responses, with one of these methods described in detail as follows. Since PRP as a solid-phase antigen does not adhere well to the surface of microtiter plates, a conjugate of PRP to human serum albumin (PRP-HSA) was prepared as described previously (8). The PRP-HSA antigen in 0.05 M sodium bicarbonate buffer (pH 9.5) was used to coat microtiter wells in 0.1-ml volumes of 5.0 μg PRP/ml. Plates were placed on a rocker platform at 20–25°C overnight and washed three times with a phosphate-buffered saline (see Appendix 2) containing 0.05% Tween 20 (PBST). Sera, including standards, are diluted in PBST containing 1.0% (w/v) bovine serum albumin (BSA) and added to microtiter plate wells, incubated for 2 hours at 20–25°C, and washed three times (PBST). Subsequently 0.1 ml of an optimally determined dilution (the appropriate level of conjugate for use in the system has to have been determined in a separate set of experiments where several dilutions of the conjugate are tested to find the dilution(s) that gives the appropriate color reaction over the 30- to 40-minute reaction time normally used) of alkaline phosphatase-conjugated goat anti-human IgG (heavy- and light-chain specific) is added. Plates are washed in PBST, then incubated with 0.1 ml of 1.0 μg P-nitrophenyl phosphate in 1.0 M diethanolamine, pH 9.8. Color development is allowed to proceed until the highest concentration of the standard curve serum reaches an optical density (measured at 405 nm, i.e., A^{405} of 1.0–1.5), after which the reaction is stopped with 3.0 M sodium hydroxide. Anti-Ig conjugate sera can be from polyclonal or monoclonal (mAb) sources, with monoclonal being preferred because of greater specificity and reproducibility. As in any other assay system, a variety of test parameters must be optimized and the test system validated for sensitivity, specificity, parallelism, reproducibility, and linearity.

The subclass procedure employed in the author's laboratory is one utilizing ELISA procedures very similar to the one described for anti-PRP IgG responses (9). The subclass assays utilize mouse mAb antihuman IgG_1 and IgG_2 conjugate sera (vs. polyclonal for the Ig class assays). At this time the mAb antihuman IgG and IgM conjugate sera are available commercially, and it would be most appropriate to stay with the mAb antibody conjugates, in terms of sensitivity and uniformity.

C. Functional Antibody Assays

1. Bactericidal

Assays that measure antibody that binds to the surface of the bacterial cell resulting ultimately in cell lysis are key indicators of the effectiveness of the antibody response raised to the immunogen in question. In the case of gram-negative organisms, such as Hib, a complement (C′)-mediated serum bactericidal antibody (SBA) response is an indicator of protection against disease (10,11). It is important to assure that the antibody of Hib conjugate vaccinees can mediate functional activity (SBA, opsonin, or passive protection) against Hib organisms. Nevertheless, since it would be impossible to validate these assays and have high throughput, they are not routinely performed on all sera.

Complement components C′1–9 are required for complete lysis of the bacterial cell (12). A variety of C′ sources are satisfactory for use in the SBA assay but must be screened for nonspecific cell killing before use. Standard practice in the author's laboratory has been to screen several lots of C′ and order a sizable quantity of a lot that does not kill nonspecifically in order to minimize variable antibody responses that might be attributable to various C′ lots. The absorption of adult rabbit serum with whole killed organisms to eliminate nonspecific lytic activity is less satisfactory unless the bacterial cells are tanned (e.g., gluteraldehyde fixation) to eliminate the contamination of the rabbit serum C′ source with released bacterial components, thereby reducing the sensitivity of the test. The SBA employed in the author's laboratory has routinely used adult rabbit C′ (ARC′, Pel Freeze Labs) (12). ARC′ has been used successfully for measuring anti-Hib responses in rabbit sera, infant Rhesus monkey sera, and human infant and children sera. This test method is a modification of one described previously (13) where test serum (0.1 ml), organism in exponential-growth phase (0.1 ml), an excess of C′ (0.2 ml adult rabbit serum), and Gey's diluent (0.6 ml, see Appendix 3) are added in that order. The diluent must contain a sufficient level of magnesium ion, which if varied can cause variations in titers (13). Briefly, organisms are grown in Mueller-Hinton broth that has been inoculated with Hib organisms removed from an isolated growth area of an overnight culture at 37°C on chocolate agar plates. The initial A^{600} is 0.04–0.06, and organisms replicate until an $A^{600} = 0.10–0.12$ is reached ($\sim 10^{8.5}$ colony forming units [CFU]/ml). Hib organisms and other components described above are added to each tube. The reaction mixture (test sera are not preheated) is allowed to incubate for 30 minutes at 37°C, after which samples are placed on chocolate agar plates, incubated overnight at 37°C and 50% endpoint killing determined (all serum dilutions that kill at least 50% of the organisms when compared to a plating of organisms without serum, the organism control, are considered to be positive or have SBA activity). Appropriate controls including test sera without C′ as well as negative and positive sera should be included with every test. Positive sera are obtained by immunizing rabbits with whole, inactivated [3.0% formalin, final concentration, after the organisms were shown to be inactivated by plating samples on agar medium; the cultures were washed three times with phosphate-buffered saline to eliminate the formalin] Hib organisms intravenously every other day for 3 weeks with blood samples taken just prior to the first injection and 7–10 days after the last injection; the preimmunization blood sample serves as the negative control. The test organism is plated on chocolate agar at the beginning and end of the 30-minute reaction period in order to assure that the viable CFU count does not decrease during this time period for nonspecific reasons, e.g., a decrease in organism viability indicates organism instability or nonspecific killing that might otherwise be attributed to the test serum. Initial serum dilutions of hyperimmune rabbit anti-Hib sera < 1:100 do not mediate substantial kill of the organisms, but higher dilutions are extremely bactericidal at initial serum dilutions as high as 1:5000. This inhibitory effect (prozone effect) has been reported previously (14) and appears to be due to excessive antibody interference with C′ function. It has not been possible to quantitate antibody in the SBA assay, and titers are reported as reciprocal serum dilutions. Variation in titers among different laboratories can be attributable to different C′ lots, diluents, incubation conditions, and the challenge level of organisms used in the assay. A review of SBA activity mechanisms and assay requirements for gram-negative bacteria is available (15).

2. Opsonins

Another C′-dependent assay measuring functional anti-Hib activity is the opsonin assay (16,17), which detects antibodies that mediate opsonization (uptake of bacteria) by polymorphonuclear leukocytes (PMNs). Opsonin-mediating antibodies are distinct from serum bactericidal antibodies (18) in requiring only the first four components of C′ (19), compared to SBA, which requires the entire C′ cascade. Opsonins are considered to be the prime protective antibody in Hib disease (20). The major technical challenge in performing this assay is obtaining a suitable source of PMNs. A human opsonin procedure described previously (16)* uses Hib organisms harvested in exponential growth phase, washed, resuspended in a 15% glycerol buffer, and stored at −70°C for up to 4 weeks. The organisms (10 μl, 1000–2000 CFU) are mixed with the test or control serum (40 μl) for 30 minutes at 20–25°C in plastic microwell plates. Baby rabbit C′ (10 μl, confirmed to lack opsonic activity based on prior screening) and adult human PMN leukocytes (10^6 PMN/40 μl) are used in the assay. The procedure for preparing PMN involves collecting blood in a heparinized syringe followed by the addition of 3% dextran T500 in physiological saline and mixing. The syringe stands upright for 15–20 minutes, and the needle is replaced with a blunt end 17-gauge needle; the needle is bent to a 135° angle without disturbing the cells. A percoll density gradient (75 and 60%) is prepared in sterile, conical centrifuge tubes. After the red blood cells (RBCs) have settled, the plasma is gently layered over the percoll gradient by allowing it to run slowly down the wall of the conical centrifuge tube. Following centrifugation at 800 × *g* for 20 minutes, a sterile pipet is used to draw off the top two layers (lymphocyte and plasm-dextran), which are discarded. As much as possible of the 60% percoll layer is removed without disrupting the neutrophil layer. To eliminate most of the percoll and RBCs, nine volumes of cold potassium-Ringer's phosphate–dextrose-bovine serum albumin diluent (KRPDA, composition described in Appendix 4) are added to the neutrophils, mixed gently, and centrifuged at 400 × *g* for 5 minutes. One milliliter of KRPDA is added to each pellet of neutrophils and resuspended by vortexing. The neutrophil preparation is now ready for use.

The plates are vibrated constantly on a microplate mixer for 60 minutes. A 10-μl sample of the reaction mixture from each well is spread on Levinthal agar plates, incubated overnight at 37°C in 5% CO_2, and CFU counted to

*Reprinted in part with permission from *Pediatrics*, April 1990, pp. 694 and 695.

determine the percent kill when compared to a C′ control. Some test sera with poor opsonic activity were observed to have anti-PRP RIA titers up to 1–2 μg/ml, which may be attributable to the isotype or avidity of the antibody induced. IgM may be less efficient in opsonizing Hib organisms (21). The conditions of the opsonin assay promote growth and appear to eliminate any bacteriolytic effect not associated with phagocytosis.

II. ANTI-PRP IN VIVO ASSAY METHOD

A passive protection test in infant rats has been used as a measurement of protective anti-PRP activity (22). When infected with virulent Hib organisms, infant rats develop a histopathology similar to that observed in human infants (23). Five- to 7-day old rats are injected intraperitoneally (IP) with 0.1 ml of test serum 20–24 hours prior to an IP injection of virulent Hib organisms (10–30 CFU/0.1 ml). Although intranasal instillation of the organisms can be used, it normally involves multiple administration (e.g., twice daily for 2 days) of 10^6–10^7 CFU. Since the organism must ultimately gain entrance to the blood, the IP route is more direct and minimizes handling of the rat pups. Forty-eight hours postchallenge, blood cultures are obtained, placed on chocolate agar plates and incubated at 37°C overnight, and CPU are counted. The CFU observed in blood of rats treated with the test serum are quantitated relative to the CFU obtained in rats receiving a saline placebo in place of test serum. An ≥ 85% reduction in CFU between test and control groups has been set arbitrarily as a cutoff indicating protection. In many instances CFU reductions of greater than 95% were observed. If ≥ 50% of the animals in a test group have a ≥ 85% reduction in CFU, then that test serum dilution is considered protective. Human vaccinee sera with anti-PRP titers of ≥0.1 μg/ml have protected infant rats from bacteremia and subsequent meningitis (24).

III. ANTICARRIER IN VITRO ASSAY METHODS

The measurement of antibody directed against the carrier protein, while of no consequence with respect to activity against Hib, provides useful data to fully characterize the immune response to each vaccine. In addition, anticarrier antibodies may have biological activity against the bacterial source for each carrier.

A. OMPC

Anti-OMPC responses (IgG and IgM) are determined in an ELISA procedure very similar to the one described in Section I.B. for anti PRP, except that microtiter plate wells are coated with 4 μg OMPC/ml. A standard curve serum has been quantitated with respect to specific IgG anti-OMPC by relative potency comparisons to affinity-purified human anti-OMPC prepared from serum from an adult PRP-OMPC vaccinee. The assay results are expressed μg anti-OMPC/ml; the responses for human infants normally are ≥ 50 μg/ml after two doses of PRP-OMPC.

B. Serum Bactericidal Assay

SBA activity has correlated with immunity to meningococcal disease (25), and repeated meningococcal infections have been observed in individuals lacking some of the terminal C′ proteins (26,27).

Functional activity elicited by OMPC can be demonstrated in an SBA test that is very similar to the one described in Section I.C. for Hib, except that higher levels of baby rabbit C′ are utilized for NMB. Both infant Rhesus monkey and human vaccinee sera can be demonstrated to contain anti-NMB bactericidal activity (26,28). Since the OMPC is derived from an NMB serotype 2a strain, the bacterial antibody induced is cross-reactive only with those NMB strains sharing one or more of the P1.2, P2a, or P4 major outer membrane proteins in OMPC.

C. DT and TT Assays

Standarized ELISA procedures designed to measure antitoxin unit activity against the carrier proteins for the other conjugates utilizing diphtheria (PRP-D, HbOC) or tetanus toxoid (PRP-T) are employed. Because of the low concentration of the toxoid carrier proteins (relative to DTP vaccine) as well as their steric hindrance or possible antigenic alteration as a consequence of the conjugation process, their contribution to anti-D and anti-T levels relative to those elicited by the D and T toxoids in the standard DTP vaccination regimen is low. Diphtheria toxoid (DT, 62 kD) and tetanus toxoid (TT, 150 kD) are relatively poor immunogens per se as evidenced by the three-dose pediatric regimen during the first year of life plus two additional boosters, all employing aluminum adjuvants. The ELISA procedures (R. N. Hamburger, personal communication) used for antitoxin activity involve adsorption of the toxoids to the polyvinyl surface of microtiter plates. After reaction with human test sera, an alkaline phosphatase–conjugated antihuman IgG is added and after incubation the *p*-nitrophenyl phosphate substrate. The O.D. is read from a standard curve, and the antibody titer is reported in units (u)/ml. The antitoxin units (any level) generally correlate with biologically active, neutralizing antibody that is indicative of protection against *Clostridium tetani* and *Corynebacterium diphtheriae* disease.

APPENDIX 1: CHLORAMINE-T METHOD

The radiolabeling of the PRP proceeds as follows: PRP is dissolved in distilled water at 20–25°C and then placed at 2–8°C overnight with constant stirring. The dissolved PRP is placed in a wet ice bath, and the pH (6.5) is adjusted to 10.5 with 0.1 N NaOH followed by the addition of 10% (w/v) CNBr and mixed; the pH must be adjusted constantly using 0.1 N NaOH to keep it at 10.5–10.7. Tyramine hydrochloride in a 0.5 M bicarbonate buffer, pH 8.5–8.8, is added to the solution (this must be preheated in a boiling water bath to dissolve). The vial containing the reaction mixture is tumbled overnight (2–8°C storage). Following centrifugation, ethanol with 2 M calcium chloride is added to the pellet and mixed. Following centrifugation, phosphate-buffered saline (PBS) is added to the pellet and mixed. The preparation then is passed through a Sepharose 4 B column (1.6 cm by 38 cm), and 50 1-ml fractions are collected at the rate of approximately one cut every 5 minutes. Every third cut is assayed for ribose; those found positive are pooled and dialyzed against distilled water overnight at 20–25°C. The material in the dialysis bag is quick-frozen in a methanol–dry ice bath and lyophilized, completing the tyramination phase. To this product is added ^{125}I [100 millicuries (mCi)/ml] followed by 5.0 mg chloramine-T/ml in 0.4 M phosphate buffer for 1 minute, after which sodium metabisulfite is added and then sodium iodide, thus stopping the reaction. The reaction mixture is passed through a coarse G-50 column (13-ml size) that is eluted with 0.1 M phosphate buffer, and the peak fractions are identified.

After storage at 2–8°C, 4.8 ml of ethanol and 10 μl of saturated sodium acetate are added to each cut, mixed, centrifuged, and resuspended in PBS. The resulting product is desalted over a Sepharose CL-4B column (50 cm × 8 mm), and the selected cuts are stored in 5% bovine serum albumin and stored at −70°C.

APPENDIX 2: PHOSPHATE-BUFFERED SALINE SOLUTION*

Component	g/liter
NaCl	8.85
Na_2HPO_4 (anhydrous)	0.68
$NaH_2PO_4 \cdot H_2O$	0.20

*Adjust pH to 7.2

APPENDIX 3: GEY'S BALANCED SALT SOLUTION

Component	g/liter
$CaCl_2$ (anhydrous)	0.17
KCl	0.37
KH_2PO_4	0.03
$MgCl_2 \cdot 6H_2O$	0.21
$MgSO_4 \cdot 7H_2O$	0.07
NaCl	7.00
$NaHCO_3$	2.27
D-Glucose	1.00

APPENDIX 4: KRPDA SOLUTION

KRP stock:
- 7.02 g NaCl
- 0.36 g KCl
- 0.30 g $MgSO_4 \cdot 7H_2O$
- 0.47 g NaH_2PO_4 (monobasic)
- 2.22 g Na_2HPO_4 (dibasic)
- To a final volume of 1 liter distilled H_2O, adjust pH to 7.2–7.4; filter sterilize as needed

KRPDA (add components listed together):

6 ml Ca-BSA-Dex(add 0.5 bovine serum albumin, 0.5 g dextrose into 6 ml of 0.6% [w.v.] $CaCl_2$, filter sterilize)

250 ml KRP

REFERENCES

1. J. C. Hill, Summary of a workshop on *Haemophilus influenzae* type b vaccines, *J. Infect. Dis. 148*:167 (1983).
2. H. Peltola, H. Kayhty, A. Sivonen, and P. H. Mäkelä, *Haemophilus influenzae* type b capsular polysaccharide vaccine in children: a double-blind field study of 100,000 vaccinees 3 months to 5 years of age in Finland, *Pediatrics 60*(5):730 (1977).
3. J. I. Ward, D. P. Greenberg, P. W. Anderson, K. S. Burkart, P. D. Christenson, L. K. Gordon, H. Kayhty, J. S. C. Kuo, and P. Vella, Variable quantitation of *Haemophilus influenzae* type b anticapsular antibody by radioantigen binding assay, *J. Clin. Microbiol. 26*:72 (1988).

4. C. E. Frasch, Workshop on *H. influenzae* type b, U.S. FDA, Bethesda, MD, March 21, 1986.
5. Y. Schlesinger, D. M. Granoff, and the Vaccine Study Group, Avidity and bactericidal activity of antibody elicited by different *Haemophilus influenzae* type b conjugate vaccines, *J. Amer. Med. Assoc. 267*:1489 (1992).
6. G. Snedecor and W. Cochran, *Statistical methods*, 6th Ed. Iowa State University Press, Ames, IA, 1967, pp. 329–330.
7. W. R. Griswold, A. H. Lucas, J. F. Bastian, and G. Garcia, Functional affinity of antibody to the *Haemophilus influenzae* type b polysaccharide, *J. Infect. Dis. 159*:1083 (1989).
8. S. Marburg, D. Jorn, R. L. Tolman, B. Arison, J. McCauley, P. J. Kniskern, A. Hagopian, and P. P. Vella, Biomolecular chemistry of macromolecules: Synthesis of bacterial polysaccharide conjugates with *Neisseria meningitidis* membrane protein, *J. Am. Chem. Soc. 108*:5282 (1986).
9. K. T. Dolan, J. M. Staub, T. L. Schofield, V. I. Ahonkhai, R. W. Ellis, and P. P. Vella, An enzyme-linked immunosorbant assay for quantitation of *Haemophilus influenzae* type b polysaccharide-specific IgG_1 and IgG_2 in human and infant Rhesus monkey sera, *J. Immunoassay 12*:543 (1991).
10. L. D. Fothergill and J. Wright, Influenzal meningitis: the relation of age incidence to the bactericidal power of blood against the causal organism, *J. Immunol. 24*:273(1933).
11. R. D. Feigin, D. Richmond, M. W. Hosler, and P. G. Shackelford, Reassessment of the role of bactericidal antibody in *Haemophilus influenzae* infection, *Am. J. Med. Sci. 262*:338 (1971).
12. G. J. Noel, S. Katz, and P. J. Edelson, Complement-mediated early clearance of *Haemophilus influenzae* type b from blood is independent of serum lytic activity, *J. Infect. Dis. 157*:85 (1988).
13. L. H. Muschel and H. P. Treffers, Quantitative studies on the bactericidal actions of serum and complement, *J. Immunol. 76*:1 (1956).
14. L. H. Muschel, L. Gustafson, and L. J. Larsen, Re-examination of the Neisser-Wechsberg (antibody prozone) phenomenon, *Immunology 17*:525 (1969).
15. P. W. Taylor, Bactericidal and bacteriolytic activity of serum against Gram-negative bacteria, *Microbiol. Rev. 47*:1 (1983).
16. B. M. Gray, Opsonophagocidal activity in sera from infants and children immunized with *Haemophilus influenzae* type b conjugate vaccine (Meningococcal protein conjugate), *Pediatr.* (Suppl.): *85*:694 (1990).
17. G. W. Fischer, K. W. Hunter, and S. R. Wilson, Type III group B streptococcal strain differences in susceptibility to opsonization with human serum, *Pediatr. Res. 15*:1525 (1981).
18. S. L. Newman, B. Waldo, and R. B. Johnston, Jr., Separation of serum bactericidal and opsonizing activities for *Haemophilus influenzae* type b. *Infect. Immun. 8*:488 (1973).
19. R. B. Johnston, Jr., M. B. Klemperer, C. A. Alper, and F. S. Rosen, The enhancement of bacterial phagocytosis by serum: the role of complement components and two cofactors, *J. Exp. Med. 129*:1275 (1969).

20. J. Amir, M. G. Scott, M. H. Nahm, and D. M. Granoff, Bactericidal and opsonic activity of IgG_1, and IgG_2 anticapsular antibodies to *Haemophilus influenzae* type b, *J. Infect. Dis. 162*:163 (1990).
21. J. R. Schreiber, V. Barrus, K. L. Cates, and G. R. Siber, Functional characterization of human IgG, IgM, and IgA antibody directed to the capsule of *Haemophilus influenzae* type b, *J. Infect. Dis. 153*:8 (1986).
22. D. Ambrosino, J. R. Schreiber, R. S. Daum, and G. R. Siber, Efficacy of human hyperimmune globulin in prevention of *Haemophilus influenzae* type b disease in infant rats, *Infect. Immun. 39*:709 (1983).
23. A. L. Smith, D. H. Smith, D. R. Averill, Jr., J. Marino, and E. R. Moxon, Production of *Haemophilus influenzae* b meningitis in infant rats by intraperiotoneal inoculation, *Infect. Immun. 8*:278 (1973).
24. P. P. Vella, J. M. Staub, J. Armstrong, K. T. Dolan, C. M. Rusk, S. Szymanski, W. E. Greer, S. Marburg, P. J. Kniskern, T. L. Schofield, R. L. Tolman, F. Hartner, S. Pan, R. J. Gerety and R. W. Ellis, Immunogenicity of a new *Haemophilus influenzae* type b conjugate vaccine (meningococcal protein conjugate) (PedvaxHIB®), *Pediatrics 85*:668 (1990).
25. I. Goldschneider, E. C. Gotschlich, and M. S. Artenstein, Human immunity to the meningococcus. I. The role of humoral antibodies, *J. Exp. Med. 129*:1307 (1969).
26. D. Lim, A. Gewurz, T. F. Lint, M. Ghase, B. Sepheri, and H. Gewurz, Absense of the sixth component of complement in a patient with repeated episodes of meningococcal meningitis, *J. Pediatr. 89*:42 (1976).
27. G. Peter, M. B. Weigert, A. R. Bissel, R. Gold, D. Kreutzer, and R. H. McLean, Meningococcal meningitis in familial deficiency of the fifth component of complement, *Pediatrics 67*:882 (1981).
28. V. I. Ahonkhai, L. J. Lukacs, L. Jonas, H. Matthews, P. P. Vella, R. W. Ellis, J. M. Staub, K. T. Dolan, C. M. Rusk, G. B. Calandra, and R. J. Gerety, *Haemophilus influenzae* type b conjugate vaccine (meningococcal protein conjugate) (PedvaxHIB®): clinical evaluation, *Pediatrics 85*:676 (1990).

15

Lessons from the Evaluation of Immunogenicity

Robert S. Daum

University of Chicago, Chicago, Illinois

Dan M. Granoff*

Washington University School of Medicine, St. Louis, Missouri

More than 50 years ago, Landsteiner and van der Scheer (1) and Goebel and Avery (2–4) demonstrated that the immunogenicity of a hapten could be enhanced by covalently coupling it to an immunogenic protein. In 1980, Schneerson et al. (5) prepared investigational conjugates of polyribosyl ribitol phosphate (PRP) to protein and reported enhanced immunogenicity of these conjugates in mice when compared to that achieved by immunization with unconjugated PRP. Subsequently, investigators at Connaught Laboratories prepared PRP conjugated to diptheria toxoid (D) suitable for evaluation in humans (6).

Much new information has been learned since these early studies about *Haemophilus influenzae* type b (Hib) conjugate vaccines. This chapter will focus on the interpretation of antibody concentrations to capsular polysaccharide (anti-PRP) produced by immunization with these vaccines. Specifically addressed will be the assessment of immunogenicity as a means for understanding the immunological differences among the various conjugate vaccines, the relationship between conjugate vaccine priming, circulating anti-PRP concentrations and efficacy, and the assessment of immuno-

**Present affiliation:* Chiron Corporation, Emeryville, California, and Children's Hospital Oakland Research Institute, Oakland, California

genicity as a means for the investigation of geographic and genetic differences in antibody responses among populations.

I. THE PROTECTIVE CONCENTRATION OF ANTI-PRP ANTIBODY: AN HISTORICAL PERSPECTIVE

The notion that a specific concentration of anti-PRP antibody could be identified that would serve as a surrogate for protective efficacy has taken on new complexity in consideration of the immune response to conjugate vaccines (see Chapter 1). At first glance, the problem seems simple. The idea that serum antibody to the Hib capsular polysaccharide is protective was derived from observations in experimental animals (7) and patients when immune globulin containing anti-PRP at high concentration was administered passively (8). Further support came from Finland where, during an efficacy trial with unconjugated PRP, protection against invasive disease was related to the production of circulating anti-PRP antibody (9).

Given the importance of anti-PRP antibody in protection against Hib disease, many researchers have occupied themselves with attempts at estimating the protective threshold. Until 1983, a serum concentration of about 0.1 μg/ml or greater, based on a Farr-type radioimmunoassay (see Chapter 14), was assumed to confer protection against invasive Hib infection in unimmunized individuals (10). However, during a field trial with PRP vaccine in Finnish infants, it was deduced that an anti-PRP concentration ≥ 1.0 μg/ml measured 3 weeks after immunization correlated better with efficacy (11), although Anderson suggested that this higher value might simply predict a time span during which a subject retains a concentration ≥0.1 μg/ml (12). These two estimates have persisted in the literature, the lower estimate often cited as 0.15 μg/ml. Many investigators have dealt with the uncertainty by reporting the percentage of children with anti-PRP antibody concentrations ≥0.15 and ≥1.0 μg/ml.

The importance of these estimates may not be relevant to immunity induced by conjugate vaccines. In Finland, Eskola and colleagues (13) demonstrated that a three-dose regimen of PRP-D administered at 3, 4, and 6 months was highly protective (VE = 94%, 95% CI = 83–98) against invasive infection. However, the immunogenicity of PRP-D was surprisingly poor. The geometric mean anti-PRP concentration after the three doses was only 0.53 μg/ml, and only 40 and 70% of 7-month-old infants had an anti-PRP concentration ≥1.0 and ≥0.15 μg/ml, respectively.

The results of this trial challenged the dogma that 1.0 μg/ml was the protective concentration and necessitated new hypotheses to account for protection associated with conjugate vaccine administration. With unconjugated PRP vaccine, the immune response does not appear to require the cooperation of T lymphocytes. The poor immunogenicity of this carbohydrate antigen in infants and the lack of booster antibody response to revaccination (14) suggested that PRP behaves as a thymus-independent type 1 (TI-1) antigen (15). Since immunological memory is not thought to be elicited by immunization with this vaccine, protection is dependent on the concentration of circulating antibody. In contrast, as described below, conjugate vaccines appear to act as thymus-dependent (TD) antigens (see Chapters 4 and 6) and both elicit serum antibody and prime for memory antibody responses upon subsequent encounter with PRP (16,17). This ability to generate memory responses is probably important in the protection of infants against invasive disease and precludes the designation of a minimum "protective" concentration of circulating antibody.

II. ANTI-PRP ANTIBODY RESPONSES IN INFANTS AFTER ADMINISTRATION OF CONJUGATE VACCINES

Four conjugate vaccines are currently licensed in the United States. Three (HbOC, PRP-OMPC, and PRP-T) have labeling approved by the Food and Drug Administration for administration to children as young as 2 months of age. The fourth, PRP-D, has labeling approved for children 12 months of age and older. All four vaccines consist of the type b saccharide capsule covalently linked to a protein carrier. Because of differences in their chemical structure detailed elsewhere (see Chapter 3), it might be anticipated that there would be differences in the antibody responses to the different vaccines. These differences in response also have clinical and immunological implications.

A. PRP-D

PRP-D was the first conjugate vaccine to be licensed in the United States (December 1987) and, therefore, played an important historical role in the development of effective strategies for the prevention of Hib disease. At the time of licensure, concern was being voiced regarding the inconsistent efficacy of the PRP vaccines in the United States (18,19) and a possible increased relative risk of invasive Hib disease in the first week after immunization (20).

At the time of licensure of PRP-D, efficacy data from U.S. studies were not available. However, its superior immunogenicity compared to that of unconjugated PRP in children 15–24 months of age (21) was accepted as a surrogate. PRP-D was initially recommended for administration to children at 18 months of age (22,23). The recommended age was lowered in 1990 to 15 months (24) and in 1993 to 12 months (25). Postlicensure case-control studies revealed efficacy estimates ranging from 74 to 88% in children 18 months of age or older (reviewed in Ref. 26).

Despite the excellent performance of PRP-D in children immunized at 18 months of age or older and excellent efficacy in Finnish infants vaccinated at 3, 4, and 6 months of age (13), approval of labeling for immunization beginning in early infancy was not obtained in the United States. PRP-D is substantially less immunogenic than the other Hib conjugate vaccines subsequently licensed (Fig. 1). In one study (27) in subjects who received a three-dose regimen of PRP-D initiated at 2 months of age, the geometric mean anti-PRP concentration was 0.28 μg/ml after the third injection given at 6 months of age, and only 29% had a concentration exceeding 1.0 μg/ml. A second reason that PRP-D has not been licensed for use in infants younger than 12 months of age is the poor efficacy of this vaccine in a trial conducted among Alaskan Eskimos, Indians, and Aleuts vaccinated at 2, 4, and 6 months of age (VE = 35%, 95% CI −57–73%) (28).

The reasons for the disparity in the efficacy of PRP-D in Alaska and Finland are uncertain (see Chapter 18). In both trials, the immunogenicity of PRP-D was low (13,28). However, immunological memory was demonstrated in vaccinated Finnish infants (29) but was not assessed in the Alas-

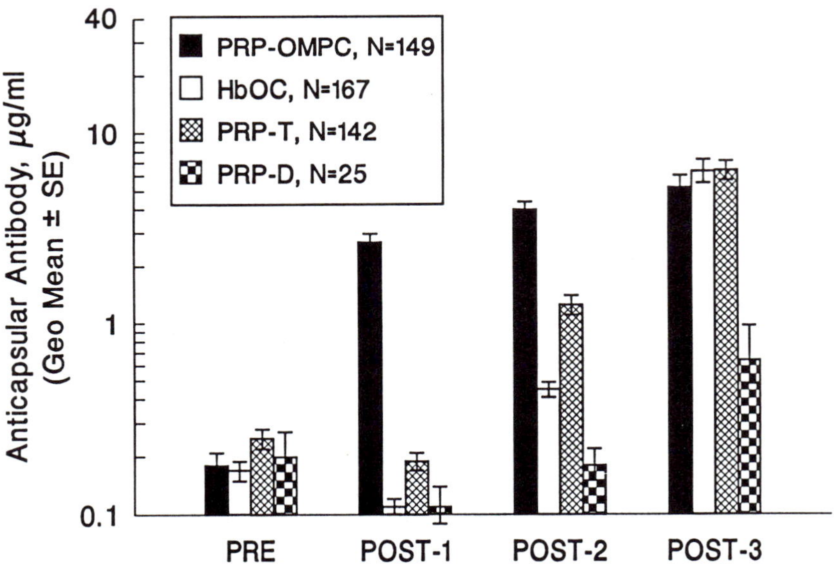

Figure 1 Immunogenicity of four Hib conjugate vaccines in infants vaccinated at 2, 4, and 6 months of age. Data are from a randomized, comparative immunogenicity trial performed in Minneapolis, St. Louis and Dallas. (Reprinted with permission of the American Academy of Pediatrics, Ref. 25.)

kan children. Given the likely importance of priming for memory antibody responses in the protection conferred by PRP-D, it is possible that poor memory responses accounted for the low protective efficacy observed in Alaska. It is also possible that differences in epidemiology with a higher incidence of disease at a younger age in Alaska than in Finland may hold the explanation for the differences in efficacy observed.

Taken together, the conflicting results of the two efficacy trials and the relatively poor immunogenicity of PRP-D in infants immunized at 2, 4, and 6 months of age have continued to raise concern about recommending its use in infants younger than 12 months of age in the United States. However, PRP-D has been effective in preventing disease when administered to infants younger than 12 months of age in Iceland (30) and Germany (31). In retrospect it seems likely that PRP-D also would have conferred protection to many U.S. infants of this age. However, given the uncertainty and greater diversity of the U.S. population, a more protective vaccine was needed.

B. PRP-OMPC

The mechanism by which this vaccine elicits an antibody response in infants appears to differ from that of the other licensed conjugate vaccines based on the following evidence:

1. PRP-OMPC elicits a significant increase in IgG1, IgM, and total antibody concentration after one dose administered to infants at 2 months of age (32–34), whereas the other conjugate vaccines require repeated injections (Fig. 1)
2. With PRP-OMPC, after second and third injections at 4 and 6 months of age, only modest, additional increases in antibody concentration occur (27,33,35).
3. After three injections, the antibody elicited by PRP-OMPC is of lower avidity and uses different light-chain V regions than those elicited by HbOC or PRP-T (36,37).
4. PRP-OMPC but not HbOC was a mitogen for murine B cells (15), a property usually attributed to TI-1 antigens (38).

In addition to its TI characteristics, PRP-OMPC also has properties attributable to TD antigens, such as the ability to induce immunological memory (39,40), even after one (33) or two doses (40) given at 2 and 4 months of age. Thus, the immune response to PRP-OMPC is complex and has immunological features common to both TI and TD antigens (see also Chapter 4).

One important advantage of PRP-OMPC is its demonstrated ability to protect 2-month-old infants after a single injection (8) for at least 2 months.

Another may lie in the unique carrier protein being immunologically unrelated to other currently licensed vaccines, and thus the immunogenicity of the conjugate is not dependent on the simultaneous administration of the carrier protein (41). However, one potential disadvantage is that the antibody produced by PRP-OMPC is of lower avidity and has lower bactericidal activity than the antibody elicited by HbOC or PRP-T (36).

C. HbOC

HbOC appears to act as a typical TD antigen. It is poorly immunogenic after one or two doses in infants vaccinated at 2 and 4 months of age but elicits substantial antibody responses after a third dose given at 6 months of age (Fig. 1) (27,35) The antibody elicited by this vaccine is predominantly IgG (IgG1 in infants) (34,40,42) and is active in assays of complement-mediated bactericidal activity (36). In infants, HbOC elicits antibody of higher avidity than that elicited by PRP-OMPC or, to a lesser extent, PRP-T (36). The higher avidity may result from selective stimulation of B cells expressing high-affinity anti-PRP antibody by the relatively low-molecular-weight saccharide oligomer in HbOC.

HbOC also primes for a memory antibody response to unconjugated PRP vaccination (17,40). Interestingly, priming occurs even among those with minimal antibody responses measured after two injections of HbOC given at 2 and 4 months of age (35) (Fig. 2). Thus, HbOC appears to be a highly immunogenic vaccine that elicits high-quality anti-PRP antibody and primes for memory antibody responses. Its major disadvantage is its low immunogenicity after one or two doses administered at 2 and 4 months of age (Fig. 1).

D. PRP-T

PRP-T appears to be somewhat more immunogenic after two doses given at 2 and 4 months of age than HbOC (27,35,43) (Fig. 1). However, compared with HbOC, a three-dose regimen of PRP-T administered at 2, 4, and 6 months yields otherwise similar kinetics of appearance of anti-PRP antibody (Fig. 1), isotype distribution (40,43) antibody avidity (36), V-region/idiotypic expression (37), and bactericidal activity (36). PRP-T vaccination also primes for memory antibody responses to subsequent PRP vaccination (29,40).

PRP-T is the most recent conjugate to receive licensure in the United States (1993) (25). Licensure was based primarily on immunogenicity data (see Chapter 24). Two efficacy trials in the United States were terminated prematurely because licensure of other Hib conjugate vaccines precluded

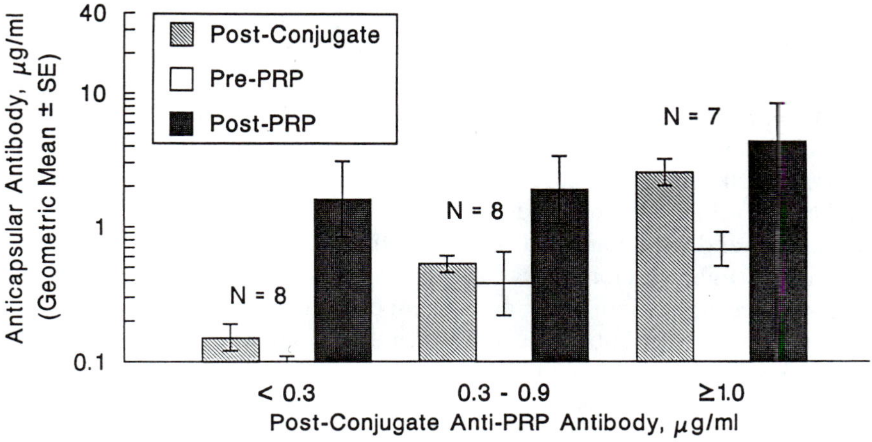

Figure 2 Memory response to PRP vaccination at 9 months of age in infants given two doses of HbOC at 2 and 4 months of age. The subjects were stratified based on the magnitude of the anti-PRP antibody response after the second dose of HbOC. Differences in the magnitude of the anti-PRP antibody response were not significant. (From Ref. 88.)

the continued use of placebo controls (44,45). In the two incomplete trials, no cases of invasive Hib disease occurred in about 6000 infants vaccinated with PRP-T (see Chapter 18). The results of another trial done in the United Kingdom demonstrated efficacy of PRP-T when administered at 2, 3, and 4 months of age (46).

III. DURATION OF ANTIBODY ELICITED BY IMMUNIZATION REGIMENS ADMINISTERED IN THE FIRST SEVERAL MONTHS OF LIFE

Following a priming series of any of the licensed conjugate vaccines at 2 and 4 or at 2, 4, and 6 months of age, antibody concentrations decline rapidly so that, at 12 months of age, they are three to six times less than their respective peak concentration (40). The meaning of the decline with respect to susceptibility to invasive Hib disease is uncertain. Despite low serum anti-PRP concentrations, subjects immunized with conjugate vaccines are likely primed for the ability to rapidly develop a serum antibody response to unconjugated PRP vaccination (40). It is likely, therefore, but unproven that an anamnestic response also could be mounted rapidly upon environmental encounter with *H. influenzae* type b. Thus, although there are few explicit data to prove that memory antibody responses alone are sufficient to confer protection, antibody decline after conjugate priming in early infancy may not be associated with substantial risk of invasive disease.

At least upon occasion, however, a decline in circulating antibody was associated with development of invasive disease, perhaps because priming did not occur. For example, invasive Hib disease occurred in a 15.5-month-old Navajo child who received two doses of PRP-OMPC at 2 and 4 months of age (8) and whose antibody concentration was known to have declined from 1.49 μg/ml 1 month after the second dose to 0.14 μg/ml 3 months prior to hospitalization. Thus, assessment of the duration of immunity after immunization with Hib conjugate vaccines is a complex problem. Additional insight may be gained from long-term follow-up of immunized individuals and the immunological study of patients who develop invasive disease despite immunization.

IV. INTERCHANGEABILITY OF Hib CONJUGATE VACCINES: THE SO-CALLED "MIX-AND-MATCH" TRIALS

Beginning with the initial recommendations for multidose Hib conjugate vaccine regimens, there has been interest in the immunogenicity and effectiveness of using different vaccines licensed for sequential doses. There are several reasons for this. The increasing mobility of society often results in the use of multiple health-care facilities for completion of a vaccine regimen. Since only a single Hib conjugate vaccine may be available at a given facility, knowledge about the interactions between the different Hib conjugate vaccines is necessary to plan a continuing immunization regimen.

Decker et al. (47) randomized infants at 2 months of age to receive one of the four licensed Hib conjugate vaccines in a three-dose priming series. At 15 months of age, irrespective of which vaccine was received in the primary series, the children were again randomized to receive the priming vaccine or PRP-D. Boosting with PRP-D produced concentrations that equaled or exceeded the antibody concentrations produced by boosting with the primary series vaccine. Indeed, when PRP-D was employed to boost children "primed" with PRP-OMPC, the response to PRP-D boosting significantly exceeded that produced by PRP-OMPC boosting. The investigators concluded that PRP-D is an appropriate choice for a booster vaccine no matter what the priming regimen and that PRP-OMPC may be less well suited as a boosting Hib conjugate vaccine in children primed with PRP-OMPC.

Differences in the kinetics of anti-PRP appearance and the quality of the antibody elicited in the primary series by different conjugate vaccines suggested other reasons to investigate "mix-and-match" protocols. If, for example, PRP-OMPC administered at 2 months of age primed for an anamnestic response to HbOC or PRP-T administration at 4 months or at 4 and 6 months of age, the overall effect might be an increased "area under the curve" when age is plotted against anti-PRP concentration, i.e., appearance of a substantial antibody response after the first dose followed by a further substantial increase after subsequent conjugate vaccine administration. Further, in infants given one dose of PRP-OMPC, boosting with HbOC or PRP-T might result in increased antibody avidity compared to that elicited by PRP-OMPC injection.

Preliminary reports of several studies indicate that "mixed-sequence" regimens, e.g., employing PRP-OMPC for the first dose and HbOC or PRP-T for the second and third dose administered at 4 and 6 months of age, may result in the earlier appearance of a substantial antibody response when compared to three-dose regimens in which the same vaccine was used for all three doses (48–50), and, possibly, higher antibody concentrations after the three-dose regimen. Completion and analysis of the several trials in progress will be required to be certain of the validity of these tentative conclusions and to speculate regarding their clinical implications.

V. RESPONSES TO Hib CONJUGATE VACCINES IN INDIVIDUALS AT INCREASED RISK FOR INVASIVE DISEASE

Children with certain chronic illnesses or genetic phenotypes associated with increased risk of invasive Hib disease, such as human immunodeficiency virus (HIV) infection, immunoglobulin deficiency, or sickle cell anemia, have been evaluated for their antibody responses to Hib conjugate vaccines. The available information is summarized below.

In children infected with HIV, existing data that define the response to Hib conjugate vaccines are limited. Five infants vaccinated at 2, 4, and 6 months of age with HbOC had a geometric mean of 3.78 μg/ml after the third dose (51); four had a concentration ≥ 1 μg/ml. In adults, the response to HbOC immunization correlated with the concentration of CD4 lymphocytes in blood and, therefore, with the severity of HIV-associated disease and ranged from high antibody concentrations occuring in HIV-infected, asymptomatic individuals to relatively low concentrations occurring in those with AIDS (52).

Children with IgG2 subclass deficiency have impaired responses to unconjugated PRP vaccine (53,54). Responses to Hib conjugate vaccines can, however, be elicited in these children, although several doses may be required, even in children 18 months of age or older. The explanation for the ability of infants with IgG2 subclass deficiency to respond to conjugated but not to unconjugated PRP vaccines is unknown.

Children with sickle cell anemia immunized with HbOC (55), PRP-T (56), PRP-OMPC (57), or PRP-D (58–60) generally respond to Hib conjugate vaccine administration with production of substantial levels of anti-PRP antibody. For PRP-D, in one study, the mean anti-PRP concentration among 15 patients with sickle cell disease immunized at a mean age of 35 months was 2.9 μg/ml, significantly lower than that found in age- and race-matched controls (60); three of the 15 children with sickle cell disease had an antibody concentration <0.37 μg/ml. This suggests that older children with sickle cell disease immunized with this vaccine may have relatively impaired antibody responses.

Children, and possibly adults, undergoing transplantation procedures may be at increased risk for Hib infection, and, therefore, their responses to conjugate vaccination are of interest. Allogeneic bone marrow transplantation recipients, adult and pediatric (aged 10–54 years), were immunized with PRP-T, 4–83 months after transplantation when all had engrafted. The geometric mean anti-PRP concentration increased more than 10-fold one month later; 70% had a concentration ≥1.0 μg/ml (61). These findings should be interpreted with some caution since the anti-PRP response may increase with time elapsed after transplantation (62), and the response to a single dose given shortly after transplantation may be minimal. Administration of a two-dose regimen may overcome this problem. When HbOC was given to allogeneic or autologous transplant recipients, 2–45 years of age, at various times after transplantation, a two-dose regimen, administered 12 and 24 months after the transplantation procedure, produced the highest concentrations of anti-PRP. Such two-dose regimens are currently being evaluated to determine whether they may be initiated earlier after transplantation.

Certain populations of children including Alaskan Eskimos, Indians, and Aleuts (63), Canadian Inuit (64), Navajo (65), and Apache (66) are at greater risk of invasive Hib infections, and perhaps other infections, than white children. The reason for their increased susceptibility is not known. At least some of these populations also have impaired responses to immunization with Hib vaccines. For example, when 18- to 25-month-old Apache children were immunized with unconjugated PRP vaccine (67), the concentrations of anti-PRP antibody were about 10-fold lower than those obtained in white children of similar age. Antibody responses to diphtheria toxoid were also significantly lower in the Navajo infants, although the magnitude of the difference was less. Others have made similar observations (68,69). The suggestion that the increase in risk for Hib infections in several populations may be associated with decreased immunological responsiveness to PRP, whether presented as an unconjugated polysaccharide vaccine or conjugated to a carrier protein, is of potential interest; the immunological mechanisms underlying these differences will require further clarification. In this light, the success of PRP-OMPC in protecting Navajo infants (8) from Hib disease is particularly gratifying and demonstrates that a conjugate vaccine can be effective even in a high-risk population that has impaired responses to at least some Hib vaccines.

VI. CLINICAL CONSIDERATIONS RELATED TO CARRIER IMMUNITY

With some conjugate vaccines, there may be an absolute requirement for vaccination with unconjugated carrier protein to elicit an anti-PRP response to the hapten component of the conjugate vaccine molecule (41). For example, when HbOC was administered at 2 and 4 months to children who did not receive diphtheria and tetanus toxoids, normally administered in DPT vaccine at those ages, there was no increase in serum anti-PRP at 5 months of age. In contrast, infants given PRP-OMPC in the absence of DTP responded normally to the conjugate. It may be possible, therefore, to generalize that in infants not being vaccinated with DTP, there may be an impairment of the antibody response to conjugate vaccines employing carrier proteins related to diphtheria or tetanus toxoids such as PRP-T, PRP-D, or HbOC.

Enhanced antibody responses in mice to immunization with protein conjugate vaccines after priming with the unconjugated protein carrier were first described for a Hib conjugate vaccine by Schneerson et al. (5). This phenomenon, termed carrier priming, i.e., the effect on production of anti-PRP antibody in response to conjugate vaccine administration after prior immunization with the carrier protein, has been the focus of recent interest to evaluate whether it might suggest a strategy for improved protection against Hib disease. Several observations are of interest. In children who received diphtheria and tetanus toxoids (DT vaccine) at one month of age followed by HbOC or PRP-T (and DTP) at 2 and 4 months of age, the anti-PRP antibody responses after two doses of conjugate were higher in the primed subjects than in the controls who received only the two doses of the Hib conjugates (70). In the DT-primed HbOC recipients, this enhanced immunogenicity was absent after the third dose at 6 months of age, but in the PRP-T recipients it persisted at least one month beyond the booster dose of PRP vaccine administered at 12 months of age (D. M. Granoff, unpublished data).

In contrast, Lieberman et al. administered DT vaccine at birth and a standard three-dose regimen of HbOC or PRP-T with DTP beginning at 2 months of age. In this instance, enhancement of the anti-PRP response was not observed (71) but, rather, suppression, at least of the antibody response to HbOC. Taken together, these studies suggest that the age at which the carrier is administered may play an important role in the subsequent response to PRP-conjugate administration, but by what mechanism? One hypothesis invokes inhibition of the response to a hapten-carrier conjugate by passive transfer of antibody to the carrier protein (72). If correct, it would be expected that the likelihood of an enhanced anti-PRP response in infants primed with carrier might increase with postnatal age. Another hypothesis concerns the non–epitope-specific suppression of the response to antigens presented as part of conjugate vaccines in adults primed with the carrier protein. When tetanus or diphtheria toxoid was administered followed by PRP-T or PRP-D (73), suppression of the antibody response to both the polysaccharide and protein components of the conjugate vaccines was observed. The mechanism is uncertain but may relate to the expanded number of B cells specific for the priming carrier (74) and the relatively few B cells committed to responding to the polysaccharide moiety. The implication of this observation for pediatric populations is uncertain but suggests that strategies for improving the competition between carrier-specific and hapten-specific B cells for the conjugate may be necessary if carrier priming can be exploited as a tool for enhancing the immune responses to Hib and other conjugate vaccines.

VII. IMMUNOGENICITY OF Hib CONJUGATE VACCINES IN THE POSTLICENSURE ERA

Despite careful monitoring of individual lots of Hib conjugate vaccines and assurance by vaccine manufacturers and the Food and Drug Administration of strict adherence to defined chemical specifications, several unanticipated changes occurred in the immunogenicity of conjugate vaccines after licensure.

Attention was called to a problem regarding the immunogenicity of PRP-OMPC when several investigators alerted the manufacturer regarding the poor antibody responses they observed with lot 0498T. The geometric mean anti-PRP concentration after three doses of that lot was only 0.15 μg/ml (75) compared to an expected value, based on prelicensure studies, of about 2–6 μg/ml. Subsequent studies by the manufacturer suggested that the decreased immunogenicity was related to inadvertent excessive conjugation of PRP to the outer membrane protein complex (OMPC) carrier (J. Hennessey, personal communication). Since a novel amino acid, S-(carboxymethyl) homocysteine (S-CMHC), is formed by the conjugation of PRP to the OMPC carrier, this amino acid can be monitored to assess the kinetics of the conjugation reaction and the degree of conjugation (see Chapter 3). High S-CMHC/PRP monomer ratios appeared to characterize the lots with decreased immunogenicity and allow a strategy to prevent recurrence of this problem. Twenty-three percent of the doses of PRP-OMPC distributed between August 1990 and May 1992 had high ratios; 16 lots were ultimately known to have been involved. In Los Angeles where about 55% of the doses of PRP-OMPC distributed from February 1991 to July 1992 were from "high-ratio lots" (D. Greenberg, personal communication), postmarketing surveillance of 85,000 children indicated that only two vaccine failures occurred (75), although both occurred in children who received vaccine from lots subsequently identified as hypoimmunogenic. The authors cautiously concluded that the hypoimmunogenicity of these lots was probably not associated with an increased occurrence of invasive Hib disease. If correct, protection in these infants may have reflected priming to PRP that occurred even after immunization with hypoimmunogenic conjugate vaccines.

An unexplained change has also occurred in the immunogenicity of HbOC. Prior to licensure, Madore et al. (42) vaccinated infants with a three-dose regimen administered at 2-month intervals, beginning at 1–2 months of age. The geometric mean anticapsular antibody concentrations were 0.2 μg/ml prior to immunization and 0.3, 5.1, and 16.8 μg/ml after one, two, and three doses, respectively. Subsequently, the results of several studies employing multiple postlicensure lots of HbOC have demonstrated up to 10-fold lower antibody concentrations occurring after the second dose (0.45 vs. expected 5.1 μg/ml) (27,35) and three- to fourfold lower concentrations after the third dose (e.g., 3.1 vs. 16.8 μg/ml). However, the clinical importance of the lower antibody response to HbOC vaccination is uncertain since after the third dose most subjects had an anti-PRP concentration that exceeded 1.0 μg/ml (27,35) and even those who do not are probably primed for a memory response to native PRP should an environmental encounter with Hib occur. Moreover, because Hib conjugate vaccination appears to decrease asymptomatic pharyngeal colonization, such encounters likely have become less frequent (76,77).

VIII. COMBINED VACCINES

Combined vaccines have the advantage of decreasing the number of injections a child must endure and the potential to lower the cost of a vaccine program. Accordingly, considerable effort has been undertaken in their development. In 1993, Lederle-Praxis Biologicals and Connaught Laboratories-Institut Mérieux obtained approval from the U.S. Food and Drug Administration for the use of a combined vaccine with a Hib conjugate-vaccine component.

The Lederle-Praxis vaccine (Tetramune™) consists of HbOC and DTP (Lederle). In prelicensure evaluations, administration of the combined HbOC/DTP elicited antibody concentrations to PRP, diphtheria and tetanus toxoids, and four pertussis antigens that were as high or higher than those obtained after separate, simultaneous injections of HbOC and DTP (78).

The Connaught-Mérieux vaccine consists of PRP-T and DTP (U.S. Connaught). Prelicensure evaluation of this combination included a study in Chile (79) in which PRP-T and DTP (Pasteur-Mérieux) were administered to healthy infants in the same syringe or separately. The combination recipients had lower antibody responses to PRP (79) and three pertussis antigens (80) than did recipients of the separate injections. However, all children in both groups had an anti-PRP concentration that exceeded 1.0 μg/ml. In a second study, also performed among Chilean infants but with U.S. Connaught DTP (81), similar respective trends were observed but the differences were not statistically significant. Whether interference in the second study was small and statistically undetected or nonexistent is uncertain, as is the suggestion that the different DTP formulations used might account for the different conclusions of the two studies. The results of two studies in the United States (82, R. Daum et al., unpublished data) suggested that combining PRP-T and DTP (U.S. Connaught) produced no statistically significant differences in relevant antibody concentrations compared to those achieved by simultaneous, separate injections.

Simultaneous administration of PRP-OMPC with DTP also has received recent study. In Gambian infants (83), administration of PRP-OMPC with DTP (Connaught), either in the same or in separate syringes, produced respective concentrations of antibody directed against PRP, tetanus or diphtheria toxoids, or pertussis agglutinogens that did not differ significantly in the two groups.

The future challenge will be in the interpretation of studies such as these when antigens are combined and studied in different populations or administered in differing schedules. These issues were discussed at a recent workshop organized by the U.S. Food and Drug Administration (84). Further discussion will be necessary to formulate guidelines defining acceptable limits for the differences in safety and immunogenicity that will inevitably occur, particularly with respect to ascertaining the biological importance of altered immunogenicity in protecting against disease.

IX. CONCLUSION

The immunization programs with Hib conjugate vaccines have been highly successful in controlling Hib disease in the United States (85–87). Study of the immunogenicity of these vaccines has revealed important differences in the quantity of antibody and the pattern of antibody elicited by one, two, or three injections in infancy. The clinical importance, if any, of other differences such as the quality of the elicited antibody or its relative activity in complement-mediated bactericidal assays has yet to be determined. However, taken together, the experience gained from the study of these vaccines has provided important paradigms for rational evaluation of other conjugate vaccines, on the horizon or beyond. It is clear that our success in the control of Hib disease has resulted not only from the investigations summarized above and also from good fortune, since our understanding of how these vaccines elicit immune responses and protect against disease is still incomplete.

ACKNOWLEDGMENTS

This chapter is supported by a grant from the Blowitz-Ridgeway Foundation and grant R01 A117962 from the National Institute of Allergy, Immunology, and Infectious Diseases, National Institutes of Health.

REFERENCES

1. K. Landsteiner and J. van der Scheer, Serological differentiation of steric isomers (antigens containing tartaric acids), *J. Exp. Med.* 50:407 (1929).
2. W. F. Goebel and O. T. Avery, Chemo-immunological studies on conjugated carbohydrate proteins: I. The synthesis of *p*-aminophenol β-glucoside, *p*-aminophenol β-galactoside and their coupling with serum globulin, *J. Exp. Med.* 50:521 (1929).
3. O. T. Avery and W. F. Goebel, Chemo-immunological studies on conjugated carbohydrate proteins: II. Immunological specificity of synthetic sugar-protein antigens, *J. Exp. Med.* 50:533 (1929).
4. W. S. Tillet, O. T. Avery, and W. F. Goebel, Chemo-immunological studies on conjugated carbohydrate proteins: III. Active and passive anaphylaxis with synthetic sugar-proteins, *J. Exp. Med.* 50:551 (1929).
5. R. Schneerson, O. Barrera, A. Sutton, and J. B. Robbins, Preparation, characterization, and immunogenicity of *Haemophilus influenzae* type b polysaccharide-protein conjugates, *J. Exp. Med.* 152:361 (1980).
6. L. K. Gordon, Characterization of a hapten-carrier conjugate vaccine: *Haemophilus influenzae*-diphtheria conjugate vaccine, *Modern Approaches to Vaccines* (R. M. Chanock and R. A. Lerner, eds.), Cold Spring Harbor Laboratory, Cold Spring Harbor, NY, 1984.
7. D. Ambrosino, J. R. Schreiber, R. S. Daum, G. R. Siber, Efficacy of human hyperimmune globulin in prevention of *Haemophilus influenzae* type b disease in infant rats, *Infect. Immun.* 39:709 (1983).
8. M. Santosham, R. Reid, D. M. Ambrosino, M. C. Wolff, J. Almeido-Hill, C. Priehs, K. M. Aspery, S. Garrett, L. Croll, S. Foster, G. Burge, P. Page, B. Zacher, R. Moxon, G. R. Siber, Prevention of *Haemophilus influenzae* type b

infections in high-risk infants treated with bacterial polysaccharide immune globulin, *N. Engl. J. Med.* 317:923 (1987).

9. H. Peltola, H. Kayhty, M. Virtanen, P. H. Makela, Prevention of *Haemophilus influenzae* type b bacteremic infections with the capsular polysaccharide vaccine, *N. Engl. J. Med.* 310:1561 (1984).
10. J. B. Robbins, J. C. Parke Jr, R. Schneerson, J. K. Whisnant, Quantitative measurements of "natural" and immunization induced *Haemophilus influenzae* type b capsular polysaccharide antibodies, *Pediatr. Res.* 7:103 (1973).
11. H. Kayhty, H. Peltola, V. Karanko, P. H. Makela, The protective level of serum antibodies to the capsular polysaccharide of *Haemophilus influenzae* type b, *J. Infect. Dis. 147*:1100 (1983).
12. P. Anderson, The protective level of serum antibodies to the capsular polysaccharide of *H influenzae* type b, *J. Infect. Dis.* 149:1034 (1984).
13. J. Eskola, H. Peltola, A. K. Takala, et al, Efficacy of *Haemophilus influenzae* type b polysaccharide-diphtheria toxoid conjugate vaccine in infancy, *N. Engl. J. Med.* 317:717 (1987).
14. H. Kayhty, V. Karanko, H. Peltola, P. H. Makela, Serum antibodies after vaccination with *Haemophilus influenzae* type b capsular polysaccharide and responses to reimmunization: No evidence for immunologic tolerance or memory, *Pediatrics* 74:857 (1984).
15. K. E. Stein, Thymus-independent and thymus-dependent responses to polysaccharide antigens, *J. Infect. Dis.* 165:S49 (1992).
16. G. A. Weinberg, M. S. Einhorn, A. A. Lenoir, P. D. Granoff, D. M. Granoff, Immunologic priming to capsular polysaccharide in infants immunized with *Haemophilus influenzae* type b polysaccharide-*Neisseria meningitidis* outer membrane protein conjugate vaccine, *J. Pediatr.* 111:22 (1987).
17. P. Anderson, M. Pichichero, K. Edwards, C. R. Porch, R. Insel, Priming and induction of *Haemophilus influenzae* type b capsular antibodies by Dpo20, an oligosaccharide-protein conjugate vaccine, *J. Pediatr.* 111:644 (1987).
18. M. T. Osterholm, J. H. Rambeck, K. E. White, J. L. Jacobs, L. M. Pierson, J. D. Neaton, C. W. Hedberg, K. L. MacDonald, D. M. Granoff, Lack of efficacy of *Haemophilus* b polysaccharide vaccine in Minnesota, *JAMA* 260:1423 (1988).
19. E. D. Shapiro, T. C. Murphy, E. R. Wald, C. A. Brady, The protective efficacy of *Haemophilus* b polysaccharide vaccines, *JAMA* 260:1419 (1988).
20. S. K. Sood, R. S. Daum, *Haemophilus influenzae* type b disease in the period following homologous immunization, *Pediatrics* 85:698 (1990).
21. C. D. Berkowitz, J. I. Ward, K. Meier, J. O. Hendley, P. A. Brunell, R. A. Barkin, J. M. Zahradnik, J. Samuelson, L. Gordon, Safety and immunogenicity of *Haemophilus influenzae* type b polysaccharide and polysaccharide diphtheria toxoid conjugate vaccines in children 15 to 24 months of age, *J. Pediatr.* 110:509 (1987).
22. American Academy of Pediatrics, Committee on Infectious Diseases: *Haemophilus influenzae* type b conjugate vaccine, *Pediatrics* 81:908 (1988).

23. Immunization Practices Avisory Committee: Update: Prevention of *Haemophilus influenzae* type b disease, *MMWR* 37:13 (1988).
24. American Academy of Pediatrics, Committee on Infectious Diseases: *Haemophilus influenzae* type b conjugate vaccines. Immunization of children at 15 months of age, *Pediatrics* 86:794 (1990).
25. American Academy of Pediatrics, Committee on Infectious Diseases: *Haemophilus influenzae* type b conjugate vaccines: Recommendations for immunization with recently and previously licensed vaccines. *Pediatrics* 92:480 (1993).
26. A. M. Loughlin, C. D. Marchant, S. Lett, E. D. Shapiro, Efficacy of *Haemophilus influenzae* type b vaccines in Massachusetts children 18 to 59 months of age, *Pediatr. Infect. Dis. J.* 11:374 (1992).
27. M. D. Decker, K. M. Edwards, R. Bradley, P. Palmer, Comparative trial in infants of four conjugate *Haemophilus influenzae* type b vaccines, *J. Pediatr.* 20:184 (1992).
28. J. I. Ward, G. Brenneman, G. W. Letson, W. L. Heyward and the Alaska *H influenzae* Vaccine Study Group, Limited efficacy of a *Haemophilus influenzae* type b conjugate vaccine in Alaskan native infants. *N. Engl. J. Med. 323:*1393 (1990).
29. H. Kayhty, J. Eskola, H. Peltola, L. Saarinen, P. H. Makela, High antibody responses to booster doses of either *Haemophilus influenzae* capsular polysaccharide or conjugate vaccine after primary immunization with conjugate vaccines, *J. Infect. Dis.* 165:S165 (1992).
30. K. E. Jonsdottir, O. Steingrimsson, O. Olafsson, Immunisation of infants in Iceland against *Haemophilus influenzae* type b, *Lancet* 340:252 (1992).
31. S. Zeilen, Hib PRP-D vaccine post-marketing surveillance study in Germany. Proceedings of the International Congress for Infectious Diseases, Nairobi, Kenya, June 1992.
32. M. S. Einhorn, G. A. Weinberg, E. L. Anderson, P. D. Granoff, D. M. Granoff, Immunogenicity in infants of *Haemophilus influenzae* type b polysaccharide in a conjugate vaccine with *Neisseria meningitidis* outer-membrane protein, *Lancet* ii:299 (1986).
33. R. S. Daum, G. R. Siber, G. A. Ballanco, S. K. Sood, Serum antibody response in the first week after immunization with the *Haemophilus influenzae* type b-*Neisseria meningitidis* outer membrane protein complex conjugate vaccine, *J. Infect. Dis.* 64:1154 (1991).
34. D. M. Ambrosino, S. K. Sood, M. C. Lee, D. Chen, H. R. Collard, D. L. Bolon, C. Johnson, R. S. Daum, IgG1, IgG2 and IgM responses to two *Haemophilus influenzae* type b conjugate vaccines in young infants, *Pediatr. Infect. Dis. J.* 11:855 (1992).
35. D. M. Granoff, E. L. Anderson, M. T. Osterholm, S. J. Holmes, J. E. McHugh, R. B. Belshe, F. Medley, T. V. Murphy, Differences in the immunogenicity of three *Haemophilus influenzae* type b conjugate vaccines in infants, *J. Pediatr.* 121:187 (1992).
36. Y. Schlesinger, D. M. Granoff and the Vaccine Study Group. Avidity and

bactericidal activity of antibody elicited by different *Haemophilus influenzae* type b conjugate vaccines, *JAMA* 67:1489 (1992).
37. D. M. Granoff, P. G. Shackelford, S. J. Holmes, the Collaborative Vaccine Study Group, A. H. Lucas, Variable region expression in the antibody response of infants vaccinated with *Haemophilus influenzae* type b polysaccharide-protein conjugates: description of a new λ light chain-associated idiotype and the relationship between idiotype expression, avidity and vaccine formulation, *J. Clin. Invest.* 91:788 (1993).
38. D. E. Mosier, B. Subbarao, Thymus-independent antigens: complexity of B-lymphocyte activation revealed, *Immunol. Today* 3:217 (1982).
39. S. K. Sood, G. A. Ballanco, R. S. Daum, Duration of seum anticapsular antibody after a two-dose regimen of a *Haemophilus influenzae* type b-*Neisseria meningitidis* outer membrane protein conjugate vaccine and anamnestic response after a third dose, *J. Pediatr.* 119:652 (1991).
40. D. M. Granoff, S. J. Holmes, M. T. Osterholm, J. E. McHugh, A. H. Lucas, E. L. Anderson, R. B. Belshe, J. L. Jacobs, F. Medley, T. V. Murphy. Induction of immunologic memory in infants primed with *Haemophilus influenzae* type b conjugate vaccines, *J. Infect. Dis.* 168:663 (1993).
41. P. P. Vella, R. W. Ellis, Immunization with *Haemophilus influenzae* type b conjugate vaccines in infant rhesus monkeys, *Pediatr. Res.* 29:10 (1990).
42. D. V. Madore, C. L. Johnson, D. C. Phipps, Pennridge Pediatric Associates, L. A. Popejoy, R. Eby, D. H. Smith, Safety and immunogenic response to *Haemophilus influenzae* type b oligosaccharide-CRM197 conjugate vaccine in 1- to 6-month-old infants, *Pediatrics* 85:331 (1990).
43. S. J. Holmes, B. Fritzell, K. P. Guito, J. Esbenshade, M. M. Blatter, K. S. Reisinger, H. Keyserling, E. P. Rothstein, K. S. Bernstein, S. Feldman, D. M. Granoff, The immunogenicity of *Haemophilus influenzae* type b polysaccharide-tetanus toxoid conjugate vaccine in infants. *Am. J. Dis. Child.* (in press).
44. C. M. Vadheim, D. P. Greenberg, S. Partridge, J. Jing, J. I. Ward and Kaiser-UCLA vaccine study group, Effectiveness and safety of an *Haemophilus influenzae* type b conjugate vaccine (PRP-T) in young infants, *Pediatrics* 92:272 (1993).
45. B. Fritzell, S. Plotkin, Efficacy and safety of a *Haemophilus influenzae* type b capsular polysaccharide-tetanus protein conjugate vaccine, *J. Pediatr.* 121:355 (1992).
46. R. Booy, E. R. Moxon, J. A. MacFarlane, R. T. Mayon-White, M. P. E. Slack, Efficacy of *Haemophilus influenzae* type b conjugate vaccine in Oxford region, *Lancet* 340:847 (1992).
47. M. D. Decker, K. M. Edwards, R. Bradley, P. Palmer, Responses of children to booster immunization with their primary conjugate *Haemophilus influenzae* type b vaccine or with polyribosylribitol phosphate conjugated with diphtheria toxoid, *J. Pediatr.* 122:410 (1993).
48. D. P. Greenberg, J. M. Lieberman, S. M. Marcy, V. K. Wong, S. Partridge, S. J. Chang, C. Y. Chiu, J. I. Ward, Safety and immunogenicity of mixed

sequences of *Haemophilus influenzae* type b (HIB) conjugate vaccines in infants, *Pediatr. Res.* 33:169A (1993).

49. E. L. Anderson, M. D. Decker, K. M. Edwards, J. A. Englund, R. B. Belshe, Interchangeability of conjugated *Haemophilus influenzae* type b conjugate vaccines in infants, *Pediatr. Res.* 33:85A (1993).
50. R. S. Daum, W. M. Milewski, G. A. Ballanco, Interchangability of *H influenzae* type b vaccines for the primary series ("mix and match")—a preliminary analysis, *Pediatr. Res.* 33:166A (1993).
51. F. J. Indacochea, R. A. Insel, B. L. Hamilton, Immunogenicity of *Haemophilus influenzae* type b (Hib) CRM_{197} conjugate vaccine (HbOC) in young HIV infected (HIV+) infants, *Pediatr. Res.* 31:165A (abstract 974) (1992).
52. M. C. Steinhoff, B. S. Auerbach, K. E. Nelson, D. Vlahov, R. L. Becker, N. M. H. Graham, D. H. Schwartz, A. H. Lucas, R. E. Chaisson, Antibody responses to *Haemophilus influenzae* type b vaccines in men with human immunodeficiency virus infection, *N. Engl. J. Med.* 325:1837 (1991).
53. D. T. Umetsu, D. M. Ambrosino, I. Quinti, G. R. Siber, R. S. Geha, Recurrent sinopulmonary infection and impaired antibody response to bacterial capsular polysaccharide antigen in children with selective IgG-subclass deficiency, *N. Engl. J. Med.* 313:1247 (1985).
54. P. G. Shackleford, D. M. Granoff, S. H. Polmar, M. G. Scott, M. C. Goskowicz, J. V. Madassery, M. H. Nahm, Subnormal serum concentrations of IgG2 in children with frequent infections associated with varied patterns of immunologic dysfunction, *J. Pediatr.* 116:529 (1990).
55. F. Gigliotti, S. Feldman, W. C. Wang, S. W. Day, G. Brunson, Immunization of young infants with sickle cell disease with a *Haemophilus influenzae* type b saccharide-diphtheria CRM_{197} protein conjugate vaccine, *J. Pediatr.* 114:1006 (1989).
56. S. L. Kaplan, T. Duckett, D. H. Mahoney, L. L. Kennedy, C. M. Dukes, D. M. Schaffer, E. O. Mason, Immunogenicity of *Haemophilus influenzae* type b polysaccharide-tetanus protein conjugate vaccine in children with sickle hemoglobinopathy or malignanicies, and after systemic *Haemophilus influenzae* type b infection, *J. Pediatr.* 120:367 (1992).
57. W. Newcomer, M. Santosham, S. Bengston, S. Panny, G. Dover, Immunogenicity of *Haemophilus influenzae* type b polysaccharide-*Neisseria meningitidis* outer-membrane protein complex conjugate vaccine in infants and children with sickle cell anemia, *Pediatr. Infect. Dis. J.* (in press, 1994).
58. A. L. Frank, R. J. Labotka, S. Rao, L. R. Frisone, P. H. McVerry, J. S. Samuelson, H. Maurer, R. Yogev, *Haemophilus influenzae* type b immunization of children with sickle cell diseases, *Pediatrics* 82:571 (1988).
59. J. F. Marcinak, A. L. Frank, R. L. Labotka, S. Rao, L. Drawhorn, C. Dampier, L. R. Frisone, R. Yogev, P. McVerry, Immunogenicity of *Haemophilus influenzae* type b polysaccharide-diphtheria toxoid conjugate vaccine in 3- to 17-month-old infants with sickle cell diseases, *J. Pediatr.* 118:69 (1991).
60. P. G. Shackelford, M. H. Rathore, E. Vichinsky, A. H. Lucas, Antibody response and expression of cross-reactive idiotype (CRI) in children with

sickle cell anemia immunized with Hib polysaccharide (PS) or Hib-PS-diphtheria conjugate vaccines, *Abstracts of the 1990 Interscience Conference on Antimicrobial Agents and Chemotherapy,* Atlanta, Georgia, Abstract 65, p. 97 (1990).
61. A. Barra, C. Cordonnier, M. P. Preziosi, L. Intrator, L. Hessel, B. Fritzell, J. L. Prud'homme, Immunogenicity of *Haemophilus influenzae* conjugate vaccine in allogeneic bone marrow recipients, *J. Infect. Dis.* 166:1021 (1992).
62. E. C. Guinan, D. C. Molrine, J. H. Antin, H. J. Weinstein, S. E. Sallan, S. K. Parsons, C. Wheeler, W. Gross, C. McGarigle, P. Blanding, G. Schiffman, R. W. Finberg, G. R. Siber, M. C. Lee, D. Bolon, M. Wang, S. Carriati, D. M. Ambrosino, Polysaccharide conjugate vaccine responses in bone marrow transplant patients. *Transplantation* (in press, 1994).
63. J. I. Ward, H. S. Margolis, M. K. Lum, D. W. Fraser, T. R. Bender, P. Anderson, *Haemophilus influenzae* disease in Alaskan Eskimos: characteristics of a population with an unusual incidence of invasive disease, *Lancet* 1:1281 (1981).
64. K. A. Wotton, H. G. Stiver, J. A. Hildes, Meningitis in the central Arctic: a 4-year experience, *Can. Med. Assoc. J.* 124:887 (1981).
65. J. L. Coulehan, R. H. Michaesl, C. Hallowell, R. Schults, T. K. Welty, J. S. Kuo, Epidemiology of *Haemophilus influenzae* type b among Navajo Indians, *Public Health Rep.* 99:404 (1984).
66. G. A. Losonsky, M. Santosham, V. M. Sehgal, A. Zwahlen, E. R. Moxon, *Haemophilus influenzae* disease in the White Mountain Apache: molecular epidemiology in a high risk population, *Pediatr. Inf. Dis.* 539 (1984).
67. G. R. Siber, M. Santosham, R. Reid, C. Thompson, J. Almeido-Hill, A. Morell, G. deLange, J. K. Ketcham, E. H. Callahan, Impaired antibody response to *Haemophilus influenzae* type b polysaccharide and low IgG2 and IgG4 concentrations in Apache children, *N. Engl. J. Med.* 323:1387 (1990).
68. J. I. Ward, G. Brenneman, M. Lepow, M. Lum, K. Burkhart, C. Y. Chiu, *Haemophilus influenzae* type b anticapsular antibody responses to PRP-pertussis and PRP-D vaccines in Alaskan native infants, *J. Infect. Dis.* 158:719 (1988).
69. M. Santosham, B. Rivin, M. Wolff, R. Reid, W. Newcomer, G. W. Letson, J. Almeido-Hill, C. Thompson, G. R. Siber, Prevention of *Haemophilus influenzae* type b infections in Apache and Navajo children, *J. Infect. Dis.* 165:S144 (1992).
70. D. M. Granoff, S. J. Holmes, R. B. Belshe, E. L. Anderson, The effect of carrier priming on the anticapsular antibody response to *Haemophilus influenzae* type b (HIB) conjugate vaccines, *Pediatr. Res.* 33:169A (1993).
71. J. B. Lieberman, D. P. Greenberg, V. K. Wong, S. M. Marcy, S. Partridge, S. J. Chang, C. Y. Chiu, J. I. Ward, Does newborn immunization with diphtheria-tetanus toxoid (DT) prime for enhanced antibody responses to *Haemophilus influenzae* type b conjugate vaccines? *Pediatr. Res.* 33:174A (1993).
72. D. H. Katz, W. E. Paul, E. A. Goidl, B. Benacerraf, Carrier function in anti-

hapten immune responses. I. Enhancement of primary and secondary anti-hapten antibody responses by carrier preimmunization, *J. Exp. Med.* 132:261 (1970).

73. T. Barington, M. Skettrup, L. Juul, C. Heilmann, Non-epitope-specific suppression of the antibody response to *Haemophilus influenzae* type b conjugate vaccines by preimmunization with vaccine components, *Infect. Immun.* 61:432 (1993).
74. T. Barington, K. Kristensen, J. Henrichsen, Influence of pre-vaccination immunity on the human B-lymphocyte response to a *Haemophilus influenzae* type b (HIB) conjugate vaccine, *Infect. Immun.* 59:1057 (1991).
75. D. P. Greenberg, C. M. Vadheim, S. Partridge, S. J. Chang, C. Y. Chiu, J. I. Ward, Post-licensure evaluation of PRP-OMP vaccine lots with less than expected immunogenicity, *Pediatr. Res.* 33:169A (1993).
76. A. K. Takala, J. Eskola, M. Leinonen, H. Kayhty, A. Nissinen, E. Pekkanen, P. H. Makela, Reduction of oropharyngeal carriage of *Haemophilus influenzae* type b (Hib) in children immunized with an *Haemophilus influenzae* type b conjugate vaccine, *J. Infect. Dis.* 164:982 (1991).
77. T. V. Murphy, P. Pastor, F. Medley, M. T. Osterholm, D. M. Granoff, Decreased *Haemophilus* colonization in children vaccinated with *Haemophilus influenzae* type b conjugate vaccine, *J. Pediatr.* 22:517 (1993).
78. P. R. Paradiso, D. A. Hogerman, D. V. Madore, H. Keyserling, J. King, K. S. Reisinger, M. M. Blatter, E. Rothstein, H. H. Bernstein, Pennridge Pediatric Associates, J. Hackell, Safety and immunogenicity of a combined diphtheria, tetanus, pertussis and *Haemophilus influenzae* type b vaccine in young infants, *Pediatrics 92:*827 (1993).
79. C. Ferreccio, J. Clemens, A. Avendano, I. Horwitz, C. Flores, L. Avila, M. Cayazzo, B. Fritzell, M. Cadoz, M. Levine, The clinical and immunologic response of Chilean infants to *Haemophilus influenzae* type b polysaccharide-tetanus protein conjugate vaccine coadministered in the same syringe with diphtheria-tetanus toxoids-pertussis vaccine at two, four and six months of age, *Pediatr. Infect. Dis. J.* 10:764 (1991).
80. J. D. Clemens, C. Ferreccio, M. M. Levine, I. Horwitz, M. R. Rao, K. M. Edwards, B. Fritzell, Impact of *Haemophilus influenzae* type b polysaccharide-tetanus protein conjugate vaccine on responses to concurrently administered diphtheria-tetanus-pertussis vaccine, *JAMA* 267:673 (1992).
81. A. Avendano, C. Ferreccio, R. Lagos, I. Horwitz, M. Cayazzo, B. Fritzell, C. Meschievitz, M. Levine, *Haemophilus influenzae* type b polysaccharide-tetanus protein conjugate vaccine does not depress serologic responses to diphtheria, tetanus or pertussis antigens when coadministered in the same syringe with diphtheria-tetanus-pertussis vaccine at two, four and six months of age, *Pediatr. Inf. Dis. J.* 12:638 (1993).
82. S. L. Kaplan, M. A. Ward, B. A. Lauer, B. L. Wiedermann, C. M. Dukes, Immunogenicity and safety of *H. influenzae* type B-tetanus protein conjugate vaccine (PRP-T) alone or mixed with DTP in infants, *Pediatr. Res. 31:*166A (1992).

83. E. K. Mulholland, V. I. Ahonkhai, A. M. Greenwood, L. C. Jonas, L. J. Lukacs, C. M. Mink, J. M. Staub, J. Todd, P. P. Vella, B. M. Greenwood, Safety and immunogenicity of *Haemophilus influenzae* type B- *Neisseria meningitidis* group B outer membrane protein complex conjugate vaccine mixed in the same syringe with diphtheria-tetanus-pertussis vaccine in young Gambian infants, *Pediatr. Infect. Dis. J.* 12:632 (1993).
84. Department of Health and Human Services, *International Workshop: Combined vaccines and Simultaneous Administration: Current Issues and Perspectives,* National Institutes of Health, Bethesda, MD, July 1993.
85. L. E. Broadhurst, R. L. Erickson, P. W. Kelley, Decreases in invasive *Haemophilus influenzae* diseases in US Army children, 1984 through 1991, *JAMA* 269:227 (1993).
86. T. V. Murphy, K. E. White, P. Pastor, L. Gabriel, F. Medley, D. M. Granoff, M. T. Osterholm, Declining incidence of *Haemophilus influenzae* type b disease since introduction of vaccination, *JAMA* 269:246 (1993).
87. W. G. Adams, K. A. Deaver, S. Cochi, B. Plikaytis, E. R. Zell, C. V. Broome, J. D. Wenger, Decline of childhood *Haemophilus influenzae* type b (Hib) disease in the Hib vaccine era, *JAMA* 269:221 (1993).
88. D. M. Granoff, A. H. Lucas, Laboratory correlates of protection against *Haemophilus influenzae* type b disease: importance of assessment of antibody avidity and immunologic memory, *Ann. NY Acad. Sci.* (in press, 1994).

16

Clinical Studies in Developing Countries

E. Kim Mulholland and Brian M. Greenwood

Medical Research Council Laboratories, Banjul, The Gambia

I. INTRODUCTION

Haemophilus influenzae type b (Hib) is an important cause of serious infections in young infants in all countries in the world that do not have active Hib vaccination programs. The epidemiology of the infection in developing countries differs markedly from that in industrialized countries, and for this reason different vaccination strategies may be required in each epidemiological situation. In this chapter the special conditions that warrant the separate consideration of developing countries from developed countries with respect to Hib vaccination will be outlined. Immunogenicity studies in developing countries that have been completed or are underway will be described as will an efficacy study soon to commence in The Gambia. Finally, some alternative strategies that may have a role in the control of Hib disease in developing countries will be discussed.

II. FACTORS THAT WARRANT SEPARATE STUDIES OF Hib VACCINES IN DEVELOPING COUNTRIES

Until recently little was known about the epidemiology of Hib disease in developing countries. Several large blood culture studies from developing countries failed to detect Hib (1,2). As the pneumococcus was also infrequently found in those studies, it is likely that these negative results were due to inadequate bacteriology rather than to the absence of the organism. During the past few years, several studies have documented a high prevalence of Hib meningitis among hospitalized children in several parts of tropical Africa (3–5). High rates of Hib disease have also been reported from Papua, New Guinea (6). These and other studies have shown that, in developing countries, the epidemiology of Hib disease differs in a number of important respects from the pattern seen in developed countries.

In developing countries the peak incidence of infection is much younger than in industrialized societies, usually around the age of 6 months. This may be due to the exposure of children to high levels of the infective organism at a young age. Thus, by the end of the first year most infants are immune as a result of a period of nasopharyngeal carriage of Hib or from colonization by a cross-reacting organism. Alternatively, qualitative or quantitative aspects of maternally-derived immunity to Hib may differ in developing countries from industrialized countries rendering infants in those countries susceptible to infection by the organism at an earlier age. Regardless of the reason, most cases of Hib disease in developing countries occur during or very soon after a child's primary series of diphtheria, tetanus, and pertussis (DTP) vaccinations. Thus, in developing countries, the earlier protection can be achieved the better, and the time required to develop protective immunity after the first, second, or third dose of vaccine will be much more critical in determining the impact of a vaccine than in countries where the mean age of cases of Hib disease is higher.

In most developing countries, mortality for those cases of Hib disease that reach medical attention is high and survivors have a high rate of serious complications (7). This may be due to the younger age of those affected, larger infective doses, poorer immune responses, or external factors such as delays in reaching medical care and inadequacies in the quality of that care. Because of the greater cost of Hib disease in developing countries in terms of mortality and morbidity, the potential gains from a successful vaccination program are greater than in developed countries for a given incidence of disease.

The spectrum of Hib disease in developing countries is also different from that seen in developed countries, where meningitis and epiglottitis are the most frequent manifestations of Hib infection. In developing countries, pneumonia is a leading cause of early childhood death, and many studies have shown that Hib is the second most important cause of severe pneumonia (8). This means that for most developing countries, pneumonia is the most frequent manifestation of Hib disease. In contrast, acute epiglottitis due to Hib is extremely uncommon in developing countries. As the pathogenesis of pneumonia due to Hib is uncertain, it is by no means certain that a vaccine that protects against other manifestations of

Hib disease will protect against Hib pneumonia. Failure of a vaccine to protect against Hib pneumonia would adversely affect its potential value in developing countries. It would also have important implications for the pneumococcal conjugate vaccines currently undergoing development, as pneumonia is the most frequent manifestation of invasive pneumococcal disease.

Finally, there are genetic and environmental factors that could affect the performance of Hib vaccines in developing countries (Table 1). Studies of immunoglobulin allotypes have provided some evidence for genetic control over immune responsiveness to capsular polysaccharides (9), and HLA class 2 antigens are likely to have some influence on immune responsiveness also. The prevalence of individual HLA antigens, some of which may be associated with good or poor responses, varies substantially from community to community. In general, African populations show extensive HLA diversity (10), and some haplotypes that have a high prevalence in West Africa are found only rarely in Caucasians. However, it is likely that conjugate vaccines have several B- and T-cell epitopes so that genetic restriction is unlikely to be a major cause of variation in responsiveness between communities.

Immune responsiveness may be suppressed by malnutrition. Impaired cell-mediated immunity has been described in children with severe malnutrition, particularly kwashiorkor (11,12). However, most malnourished children appear to respond normally to standard EPI vaccines (13). In developing countries, Hib vaccines will be given before the age at which malnutrition is encountered frequently in breast-fed babies. However, in those urban areas of developing countries where bottle-feeding is common, malnutrition may be prevalent during the first few months of life.

Table 1 Reasons for Variations in Vaccine Efficacy Between Developing and Industrialized Countries

Variations in genetic control over responsiveness
HLA class 2–related
Other
Variations in the prevalence of environmental factors influencing responsivenss
Protein-calorie malnutrition
Micronutrient deficiencies
Suppressive effect of infections
Variations in the level of exposure
Route of exposure to infection
Infective dose

The protective effect of immunization may be influenced by the level of exposure to which immunized subjects are subsequently subjected and by the prevalence of other infections at the time of vaccination. The latter applies particularly to vaccines, such as polio vaccine, which are given orally. Several studies have shown that immune responsiveness to oral polio and to rotavirus vaccines is less in developing than in industrialized countries, presumably because of the higher prevalence of infection with other enteroviruses (14,15). Furthermore, immune responsiveness to capsular polysaccharide antigens can be depressed profoundly by malaria (16). This effect is likely to be less marked with conjugate than with pure polysaccharide vaccines, but the possibility remains that the immunogenicity of conjugate vaccines could be impaired in areas of high malaria endemicity. Fortunately, maternally-derived antibody provides some protection against malaria during the first few months of life, the time when conjugate vaccines are likely to be given. In some areas of Africa, perinatal transmission of HIV-1 is now widespread. Adult studies suggest that asymptomatic HIV infection does not affect the response to Hib conjugate vaccines (17), so it is unlikely that perinatally-acquired HIV infection will have an effect.

For all these reasons, new vaccines such as the protein-polysaccharide conjugate vaccines need to be evaluated in developing as well as industrialized countries before consideration can be given to their inclusion in Expanded Programme of Immunization (EPI) programs.

III. IMMUNOGENICITY STUDIES IN DEVELOPING COUNTRIES

There have been a number of studies of the immunogenicity of Hib conjugate vaccines in developing countries designed to determine whether children in developing countries respond differently from their counterparts in industrialized countries and to identify dosage schedules that can be incorporated into EPI schedules for developing countries, which differ from those for industrialized countries.

A. Effect of Age on Immune Response to Hib Conjugate Vaccines

Because of the young age of children affected by Hib disease in developing countries, it is important that a vaccination schedule provides protection at the youngest possible age. Two studies in The Gambia compared a 1- and 3-month dosage schedule with a 2- and 4- month schedule for both PRP-OMPC and PRP-T vaccines. In the first of these studies, 141 Gambian infants were vaccinated with PRP-OMPC (15 μg PRP/dose) at 1 and 3 months

(Group A) or at 2 and 4 months (Group B) (18). One month after the first dose, the geometric mean titer of anti-PRP antibody was 0.53 μg/ml (95% confidence interval 0.41, 0.70) in group A and 0.82 (0.57, 1.18) in group B (Fig. 1). After the second dose mean antibody titers had risen to 1.27 (0.89, 1.81) and 1.59 (1.01, 2.49) in groups A and B with 54 and 61%, respectively, achieving levels above 1.0 μg/ml, the level regarded as providing long-term protection. In both groups 84% had antibody levels greater than 0.15 μg/ml after the second dose, indicating some response to the vaccine. None of the differences between groups A and B were statistically significant.

The wide confidence intervals suggested that with this sample size only very large differences could be detected. However, the study did demonstrate that either of these regimens would induce a protective immune response in the majority of Gambian infants and some response in over 80%. Perhaps of greater importance is the fact that over 70% of children in both groups had antibody levels greater than 0.15 μg/ml after the first dose of vaccine. Infants in this study were followed up, and 124 vaccinated children and 33 controls were bled at 18 months of age (19). At the age of 18 months the geometric mean titer had fallen to 0.44 μg/ml in group A and

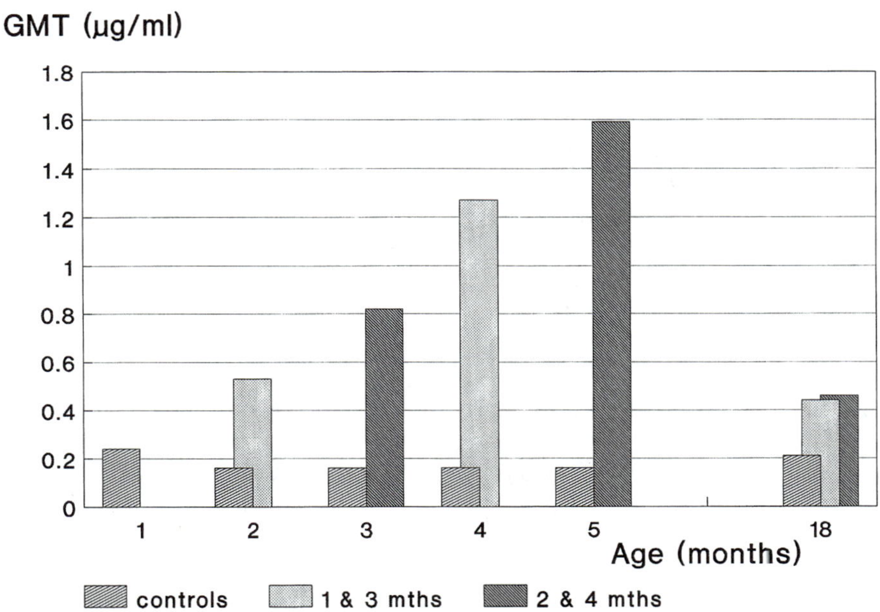

Figure 1 Antibody responses to PRP-OMPC given to Gambian infants at 1 and 3 months or 2 and 4 months.

0.46 in group B. About 60% of both groups still had levels greater than 0.15 μg/ml, and 25% had levels greater than 1.0 μg/ml. It is of interest that 23 of the vaccinated children who were bled at 18 months had antibody levels at least twice as high as those found at the one-month postvaccination bleed. These children are likely to have received environmental boosting either from a period of Hib carriage or from exposure to a cross-reacting organism.

Although declining antibody levels reflect declining production rather than clearance of a fixed amount of antibody, the concept of a half-life was used in this study to describe the persistence of antibody following vaccination. For most children the half-life was about 100 days. This appears to be lower than that found with PRP-T (20), suggesting that immunity derived from vaccination with PRP-OMPC is more short-lived. This is consistent with the qualitative differences in antibody induced by the two vaccines (21). On the other hand, the shorter half-life of antibody in the Gambian study may be a manifestation of enhanced turnover of IgG. This is a well-recognized feature of exposure to malaria, although the infants in this study were too young to have had significant exposure to that infection. Forthcoming data on the persistence of antibody following PRP-T vaccination in Gambian infants should clarify this point.

In the same Gambian community 88 infants were vaccinated with PRP-T (10 μg/dose, liquid form) at either 1 and 3 months or 2 and 4 months (E. K. Mulholland et al., manuscript in preparation). In both groups there was virtually no response to the first dose of vaccine, and after the second dose less than 20% of infants achieved antibody levels greater than 1.0 μg/ml. Subsequent studies with PRP-T have shown little or no response after the first dose, and it is now recognized that this vaccine is best given to infants in a 3-dose schedule. Despite the suboptimal dosage regimen this was a disappointing result, possibly due to instability of PRP-T in the liquid form. Subsequent studies of PRP-T have used lyophilized vaccine. A further study of Gambian infants evaluated that vaccine using the more optimal dosage regimen of 2, 3, and 4 months Again there was virtually no response after the first dose, but after three doses over 70% of children achieved antibody levels greater than 1.0 μg/ml.

A study of PRP-OMPC (7.5 μg/dose) in combination with DTP in Gambian infants using the 2-, 3-, and 4-month dosage schedule produced disappointing results, with just over 50% of infants achieving antibody levels of 1.0 μg/ml after three doses and almost half the infants actually having lower levels after the third dose than after the second (E. K. Mulholland et al., manuscript in preparation).

In all the Gambian studies, detailed side effect surveillance was carried out, and both vaccines were found to be free of serious side effects and to produce few minor side effects. These studies confirm that both PRP-T and PRP-OMPC are safe and immunogenic in young African infants. Only PRP-OMPC produces a response after the first dose, but PRP-T produces better antibody levels using a 2-, 3-, and 4-month regimen corresponding to the usual time of administration for DTP.

B. The Effect of Mixing Hib Vaccines with Other Vaccines

In recent years great progress has been made in developing countries towards the goals of universal vaccination of children. With the success of EPI programs in delivering the basic vaccines—diphtheria/tetanus/pertussis (DTP), polio, and measles—the pressure to include hepatitis B vaccine in the programs, and the development of new vaccines such as the protein-polysaccharide conjugate vaccines, there is an increasing need for combination vaccines in order to reduce the number of injections required to fully vaccinate a child.

In recognition of this, several studies have been undertaken to examine the effect of mixing an Hib conjugate vaccine with DTP vaccine, which is the most suitable candidate for combined administration with Hib vaccines. DTP was chosen because it is given at appropriate ages (three doses in the first 6 months of life) and it is given by injection. The other vaccine that would be suitable for mixing with the Hib vaccines is the hepatitis B vaccine, which is usually given at birth, 2 months, and 4 months. There are no published studies on the use of Hib conjugate vaccines at birth. A two-dose schedule of PRP-OMPC mixed with hepatits B vaccine at 2 and 4 months would be reasonable, but as yet no studies have been performed with this combination.

The mixture of two vaccines prior to their administration may affect the immunogenicity of any of the vaccine components, alter the reactogenicity of either vaccine, or result in some new side effect. The effect of mixing PRP-T with DTP (Pasteur-Mérieux) was first assessed by Ferreccio and Clemens (22,23). They randomized 278 Chilean infants to receive either DTP mixed with PRP-T, DTP administered separately but at the same time as PRP-T, or DTP alone. The vaccines were given at 2, 4, and 6 months of age. They found a higher rate of febrile responses in the group receiving the mixed vaccine compared to each of the other two groups. Otherwise, the incidence of adverse reactions in the three groups was similar.

The anti-PRP responses were excellent in both groups, with all children achieving antibody levels greater than 0.15 μg/ml after three doses and 89% of those receiving the mixed vaccine and 98% of those receiving the vaccines separately achieving levels greater than 1.0 μg/m. However, the geometric mean titer was significantly higher after both the second dose

(4.26 vs. 2.68 μg/ml) and the third dose (11.33 vs. 4.83 μg/ml) in the group who received the vaccines separately rather than mixed (Table 2). This suggests that while mixing PRP-T with DTP does not significantly affect the rate at which infants respond to PRP-T, it does negatively affect the magnitude of the response to that vaccine. No significant differences were found in responses to diphtheria and tetanus vaccines. However, responses to pertussis vaccine were depressed in both groups receiving DTP and PRP-T compared to those receiving DTP alone, more so in the group that received the vaccines mixed. This effect was seen in levels of antibody to pertussis agglutinins, pertussis toxin, and filamentous hemaglutinin. Unlike the anti-PRP effect, this effect produced a reduction in both the geometric mean titer and the proportion achieving the lower threshold titer of 320 IU/ml. The significance of this apparent reduction in the immunogenicity of pertussis vaccine is unclear. Prior to the study it was determined that the antipertussis potency of the DTP vaccine, as measured by the mouse intracerebral challenge test, was unaffected by incubation with PRP-T vaccine for 24 hours at 37°C. A similar study comparing the safety and immunogenicity of DTP and PRP-T given at the same time either separately or mixed in the syringe is nearing completion in The Gambia.

A study from Israel compared PRP-T and DTP (Pasteur-Mérieux) mixed in the syringe with DTP alone in 112 infants (24). The group receiving PRP-T had good anti-PRP responses with a geometric mean titer of 6.4 μg/ml and 94% achieving levels greater than 1.0 μg/ml after three doses. However, the group that received the mixed vaccine had lower antitetanus and antipertussis agglutinin responses than the controls, although these differences were not significant. The reactogenicity of DTP was not altered by the addition of PRP-T.

Table 2 Effect of Mixing PRP-T with DTP on the Immunogenicity of Each Component Vaccine as Measured by Geometric Mean Titers After Third Dose

	Group 1, PRP-T + DTP (*mixed*)	Group 2, PRP-T + DTP (*separate*)	Group 3, DTP only
Anti-PRP antibody	4.83 μg/ml*	11.33 μg/ml	0.06 μg/ml
Pertussis agglutinin antibody	929.6 IU/ml†	1962.0 IU/ml	3182.0 IU/ml
Diphtheria toxoid antibody	0.19 IU/ml	0.19 IU/ml	0.26 IU/ml
Tetanus toxoid antibody	4.79 IU/ml	5.62 IU/ml	5.75 IU/ml

* $p < 0.0001$ compared with Group 2.
† $p < 0.01$ compared with Group 3.
Source: Refs. 22, 23.

Preliminary results from a study of the PRP–diphtheria toxoid conjugate (PRP-D) mixed in the syringe with DTP (Connaught) suggest that the mixture of those two vaccines also diminishes responses to the pertussis and diphtheria components of DTP while the other components are unaffected (25).

The effect of mixing PRP-OMPC with DTP (Connaught) was studied in The Gambia (E. K. Mulholland et al., manuscript in preparation). In the study 126 infants were given PRP-OMPC and DTP (either by separate injection or mixed in the syringe at 2, 3, and 4 months of age. As the PRP-OMPC had to be drawn up in alum diluent prior to mixing with DTP, injection volume became a problem, and even with the dose of PRP-OMPC halved to 7.5 μg the volume per injection was 0.75 ml. In this study there were no differences between the groups with respect to antibodies to diphtheria, tetanus, pertussis, or PRP. However, the anti-PRP titers after the third dose in both groups were lower than in the previous Gambian study. This may be due in part to the narrow dose spacing, which has been shown in previous studies to produce lower titers (26). However, even after the first dose the geometric mean titer in the mixing study was significantly lower than that after the first dose at the same age in the earlier study, a result suggesting that the lower dose used may be a factor although earlier studies in North America showed that reducing the dose of PRP-OMPC from 15 to 7.5 μg did not diminish the response (27).

In the Gambian study side effect surveillance was carried out on days 1, 2, and 6 after vaccination. There were no significant differences between the groups with respect to symptoms reported. There was some increase in the local side effects seen in children receiving the combined vaccine, presumably due to the greater volume of injection. Otherwise the addition of PRP-OMPC did not appear to add to the known reactogenicity of DTP.

All the studies conducted so far affirm that the mixture of Hib conjugate vaccines with DTP is safe. However, for two of the three vaccines assessed in this way, mixture of vaccines led to a modest reduction in the immunogenicity of one or more of the components of combined vaccine. It is not known whether this is of any clinical significance.

C. The Effect of Nutrition on the Response to Hib Conjugate Vaccines

It has recently been suggested that immunization strategies in developing countries should be reviewed to take into account the high prevalence of malnutrition (28). A study by Steinhoff et al. (29) examined the antibody response to the HbOC Hib conjugate vaccine in 88 Kenyan children between 15 and 20 months of age, 42 of whom were clinically malnourished.

They found that those children who were wasted had normal antibody responses, but those who were stunted (low height for age, indicating chronic malnutrition) had poor antibody responses compared to those who were not stunted (GMT 0.34 vs. 0.65 μg/ml). As indicated above, the limited data available suggest that routine immunizations are not substantially affected by malnutrition; further data are required on the effect of malnutrition on the responses to conjugate vaccines. In most African countries malnutrition is usually associated with weaning, and thus it is most frequent during the second year of life. Thus if malnutrition were to have a negative effect on the response of children to Hib vaccination, it is unlikely that this would affect the primary course, which will generally be completed during the first 6 months of life.

IV. EFFICACY TRIALS IN DEVELOPING COUNTRIES

As yet no efficacy trials have been conducted in a developing country, although a double-blind trial of PRP-T is due to start in The Gambia early in 1993. Studies of the efficacy of Hib conjugate vaccines are costly and difficult. Studies from Finland and the United States have shown the efficacy of three of these vaccines, and these results have been backed up by dramatic reductions in the incidence of Hib disease in those countries. The trial of PRP-OMPC in the Navajo Indian population was conducted in a community in which living conditions and Hib epidemiology resemble those seen in developing countries (30). Why then are further studies being proposed in more difficult environments?

First, there are precedents for Hib vaccines working in some communities and not in others. PRP-D was highly efficacious in low-risk Finnish children (31) but offered no significant protection to high-risk Alaskan natives (32). It might be argued then that PRP-D is effective only in communities where carriage is infrequent and where infective doses are low. Such a description excludes the Alaskan natives and virtually all developing countries.

Second, in all efficacy trials conducted to date a late booster dose was given to all participants at 15–18 months, something that would be very difficult to achieve in many developing countries. Finally, none of the studies conducted so far have addressed the question of whether Hib conjugate vaccines offer protection against pneumonia due to Hib. Protection may be offered if Hib pneumonia is usually caused by bloodborne spread of the organism from a focus in the nasopharynx. Protection may also be offered if the vaccines prevent Hib disease by preventing nasopharyngeal carriage. However, if Hib pneumonia is often due to direct spread down the airways from the nasopharynx and Hib conjugate vaccines do not prevent carriage in the African environment, then the vaccines may be unable to prevent Hib pneumonia in children in developing countries.

V. THE GAMBIAN EFFICACY STUDY OF PRP-T

The Gambian efficacy study of PRP-T has been designed to address the above questions. In the study a major effort will be made to detect cases of Hib pneumonia, the effect on carriage will be examined, and no late booster dose will be used. The Gambia is a country with an excellent EPI program. Over 90% of Gambian children have received their third dose of DTP by the age of 12 months, and over 85% have received measles vaccination by that age. While the whole country is covered by a functioning primary health care program, only the western part of the country has curative health facilities of a standard such that most cases of Hib meningitis reaching the health facilities are likely to be confirmed. This is the area in which the proposed study will be conducted. For more than 2 years active surveillance has been undertaken in this area to determine the feasibility of the trial. The results of 1 year of surveillance are depicted in Figure 2.

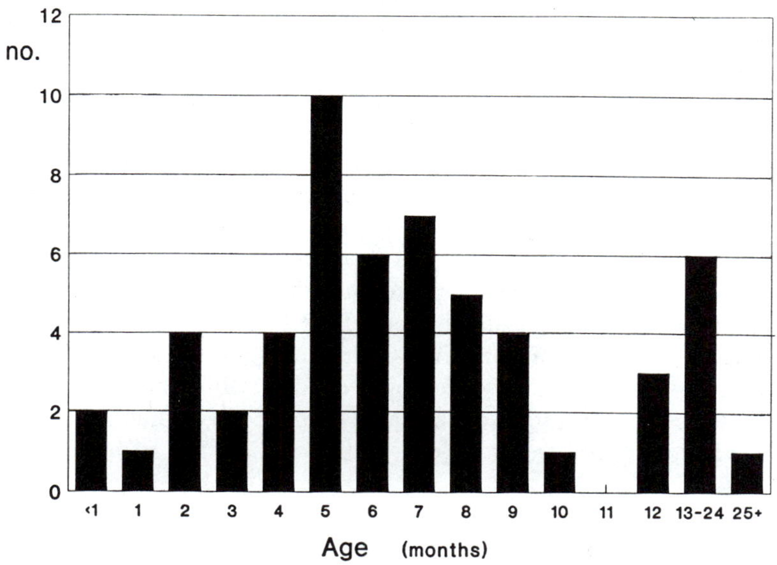

Figure 2 Invasive Hib cases detected over a 12-month period in children who had been vaccinated or were scheduled to be vaccinated within the study area of the proposed Gambian efficacy trial.

The trial will be a double-blind study with all participating children receiving either DTP mixed in the syringe with PRP-T or DTP mixed with a harmless powder. The vaccines will be given at 2, 3, and 4 months of age. This is the age at which Gambian infants are recommended to receive DTP, although experience suggests that the actual age of vaccination is more likely to be 11, 18, and 26 weeks. It is anticipated that 15,000 infants will be enrolled in each of 2 years. In addition to all cases of meningitis occurring in study infants, all cases of severe pneumonia and a sample of those with moderate pneumonia will be investigated bacteriologically including, when indicated, percutaneous lung aspirate. The power of this trial is such that it should give a more concise estimate of vaccine efficacy for the prevention of meningitis than previous trials. However, the difficulties inherent in the detection of Hib pneumonia mean that the power for this aspect of the trial is more problematic.

If the trial demonstrates efficacy against both pneumonia and meningitis, then pressure will mount on donor agencies for the inclusion of this vaccine in EPI programs in developing countries. Undoubtedly cost will then become a major consideration. At the current price few developing countries could consider these vaccines. However, these costs do not reflect the actual costs of production, and so there is considerable scope for cost reduction. Cost-benefit analyses of the effect of Hib vaccines have a role in developed countries where benefits can be measured in terms of the cost of managing a case of Hib meningitis. But how does one measure the cost of a case of Hib meningitis in countries where the likely outcome of the disease is death? In The Gambia, one third of patients with Hib meningitis who reach medical attention and survive do so with severe neurological sequelae. The costs of such children in developed countries are considerable, but in countries where there are no services for them and all care must be undertaken by the family, the costs are much more difficult to quantify.

These factors will need to be considered in any discussion of the cost of the introduction of Hib conjugate vaccines. Ignoring the financial aspects, the inescapable conclusion must be that the administration of an Hib conjugate vaccine to an infant in a developing country will produce greater benefits that the administration of the same vaccine to an infant in North America or Europe.

VI. ALTERNATIVE APPROACHES

The two factors most likely to obstruct the introduction of Hib conjugate vaccines into developing countries are the cost of the vaccine and the possibility of cases occurring in infants too young to be protected by vaccine-induced immunity. While vaccine costs are certain to fall, the Hib conjugate vaccines may still be too expensive to be incorporated into EPI programs in a three-dose schedule. A single dose of any of the Hib conjugate vaccines, except PRP-OMPC, does not produce protective antibody levels in young infants. However, as immunity derived from vaccination with Hib conjugate vaccines is believed to be T-cell mediated, it is possible that a single dose will prime an infant's immune system so that protective antibody levels may be generated on exposure to the organism. A single dose might, therefore, provide some protection. None of the studies carried out until now addresses this issue. Furthermore, there is evidence that immunity derived from Hib conjugate vaccines may be boosted with doses of the much cheaper plain PRP vaccine (33,34). Perhaps then an early dose of an Hib conjugate vaccine could be followed by a DTP vaccine that contains PRP. This concept could be taken one step further if meningococcal and pneumococcal conjugate vaccines, when available, were mixed with the Hib conjugate vaccine and given at 1 month. Then all the polysaccharides could be mixed with DTP and given at 2, 3, and 4 months of age.

Prevention of early cases may be achieved by earlier vaccination, although early studies of neonatal vaccination have not been encouraging. If carriage could be eliminated, as has happened in Finland, early cases would be prevented, but this seems an unlikely prospect in developing countries. An alternative approach to this, which may be applicable to other serious infections in young infants, is to augment maternally-derived immunity by vaccinating pregnant women or adolescant girls. This approach has been applied to the problem of neonatal tetanus with good effect, and in the future a composite maternal vaccine might contain vaccines against Hib, the pneumococcus, group B *Streptococcus*, and others in addition to tetanus toxoid. If this approach is to be effective, it is essential that infants of vaccinated mothers respond normally when they are vaccinated. Studies currently underway in Texas and The Gambia are examining this issue.

Invasive disease caused by encapsulated bacteria exact a terrible toll on children living in the poor countries of the world. If Hib disease can be effectively controlled, attention can be focused on the pneumococcus, and control of disease due to that organism may not be far away.

REFERENCES

1. D. Yardi, S. Galkwad, and L. Doedhar, Incidence, mortality and bacteriological profile of septicemia in pediatric patients, *Indian J. Pediatr. 51*:173 (1984).
2. N. Somu, M. V. Shetty, L. G. Moses, et al., A critical analysis of septicemia in infancy, *Indian Pediatr. 13*:443 (1976).

3. E. Autret, I. Diop Mar, F. Denis, et al., Meningites purulentes a *Haemophilus influenzae* b. Analyse de 248 observations Dakaroises, *Med. Afr. Noire 26*:861 (1979).
4. M. Ntihinyurwa, D. Shako, M. M. Muaka, et al., Meningites a *Haemophilus influenzae* (a propos de 116 cas), *Ann. Soc. Belge. Med. Trop. 59*:133 (1979).
5. H. A. Bijlmer, L. van Alphen, B. M. Greenwood, et al. The epidemiology of *Haemophilus influenzae* meningitis in children under 5 years of age in The Gambia, West Africa, *J. Infect. Dis. 161*:1210 (1990).
6. D. Lehmann, Epidemiology of acute respiratory tract infections, especially those due to *Haemophilus influenzae,* in Papua New Guinean children, *J. Infect. Dis. 165* (Suppl. 1):S20 (1992).
7. V. A. Nottidge, *Haemophilus influenzae* meningitis: a 5 year study in Ibadan, Nigeria, *J. Infect. 11*:109 (1985).
8. B. M. Greenwood, Epidemiology of acute lower respiratory tract infections, especially those due to *Haemophilus influenzae* type b, in The Gambia, West Africa, *J. Infect. Dis. 165* (Suppl 1):S26 (1992).
9. D. M. Granoff, P. G. Shackleford, J. P. Pandey, and E. G. Boies, Antibody responses to *Haemophilus influenzae* type b polysaccharide vaccine in relation to Km(1) and G2m(23) immunoglobulin allotypes, *J. Infect.. Dis. 154*:257 (1986).
10. A. V. S. Hill, C. E. M. Allsopp; D. Kwiatkowski, et al., common West African HLA antigens are associated with protection from severe malaria, *Nature 352*:595–600 (1991).
11. P. M. Smythe, M. Schonland, G. Brereton-Stiles, et al., Thymolymphatic deficiency and depression of cell-mediated immunity in protein-calorie malnutrition, *Lancet 2*:939 (1971).
12. J. Geefhuysen, E. U. Rosen, J. Katz, et al., Impaired cellular immunity in kwashiorkor with improvement after therapy, *Br. Med. J. 4*:527 (1971).
13. B. M. Greenwood, A. M. Bradley-Moore, A. K. Bradley, et al., The immune response to vaccination in undernourished and well nourished Nigerian children, *Ann. Trop. Med. Parisitol. 80*:537 (1986).
14. P. Hanlon, L. Hanlon, V. Marsh, et al., Trial of an attenuated bovine rotavirus vaccine (RIT 4237) in Gambian infants, *Lancet 1*:1342 (1987).
15. K. Chopra, S. Kundu, and D. S. Chowdhury, Antibody response of infants in tropics to five doses of oral polio vaccine, *J. Trop. Paediatr. 35*:19 (1989).
16. W. A. Williamson and B. M. Greenwood, Impairment of the immune response to vaccination after acute malaria, *Lancet 1*:1328 (1978).
17. M. C. Steinhoff, B. S. Auerbach, K. E. Nelson et al., Antibody responses to *Haemophilus influenzae* type b vaccines in men with human immunodeficiency virus infection, *N. Engl. Med. 325*:1837 (1991).
18. H. Campbell, P. Byass, V. I. Ahonkhai, et al., Serologic responses to an *Haemophilus influenzae* type b polysaccharide-Neisseria meningitidis outer membrane protein conjugate vaccine in very young Gambian infants, *Pediatrics 86*:102 (1990).
19. E. K. Mulholland, J. Todd, M. Rowe, et al., Persistence of antibody at 18

months following vaccination of young Gambian infants with PRP-OMPC *Haemophilus influenzae* type b conjugate vaccine, *Ann. Trop. Paediatr.* (in press).

20. B. A. Claesson, R. Schneerson, T. Lagergard, et al., Persistence of serum antibodies elicited by *Haemophilus influenzae* type b-tetanus toxoid conjugate vaccine in infants vaccinated at 3, 5 and 12 months of age, *Pediatr. Infect. Dis. J. 10*:560 (1991).
21. Y. Schlesinger, D. M. Granoff, and the Vaccine Study Group, Avidity and bactericidal activity of antibody elicited by different *Haemophilus influenzae* type b conjugate vaccines, *JAMA 267*:1489 (1992).
22. C. Ferreccio, J. Clemens, A. Avendano, et al., The clinical and immunologic response of Chilean infants to *Haemophilus influenzae* type b polysaccharide-tetanus protein conjugate vaccine coadministered in the same syringe with diphtheria-tetanus toxoids-pertussis vaccine at two, four and six months of age, *Pediatr. Infect. Dis. J. 10*:764 (1991).
23. J. D. Clemens, C. Ferreccio, M. M. Levine, et al., Impact of *Haemophilus influenzae* type b polysaccharide-tetanus protein conjugate vaccine on responses to concurrently administered diphtheria-tetanus-pertussis vaccine, *JAMA 267*:673 (1992).
24. N. Watemberg, R. Dagan, Y. Arbelli, et al., Safety and immunogenicity of *Haemophilus* type b-tetanus protein conjugate vaccine, mixed in the same syringe with diphtheria-tetanus-pertussis vaccine in young infants, *Pediatr. Infect. Dis. J. 10*:758 (1991).
25. E. P. Rothstein, H. H. Bernstein, R. P. Schiller, et al., Safety and immunogenicity of PRP-D and DTP administered concurrently at separate sites compared to PRP-D/DTP administered as a single injection, *Pediatr. Res. 29*:182A (Abstract) (1991).
26. A. A. Lenoir, P. D. Granoff, D. M. Granoff, et al., Immunogenicity of *Haemophilus influenzae* type b polysaccharide-*Neisseria meningitidis* outer membrane protein conjugate vaccine in 2 to 6 month old infants, *Pediatrics 80*:283 (1987).
27. V. K. Wong, R. Quagliata, R. Adler, and K. S. Kim, Dose-related immunogenicity of *Haemophilus influenzae* type b capsular polysaccharide-*Neisseria meningitidis* outer membrane protein conjugate vaccine, *Am. J. Dis. Child. 145*:742 (1991).
28. G. T. Keusch, Nutritional effects on response of children in developing countries to respiratory tract pathogens: implications for vaccine development, *Rev. Infect. Dis. 13* (Suppl 6):S486 (1991).
29. M. C. Steinhoff, F. Onyango, D. Mbori-Ngacha, and G. Siber, The effect of nutritional status on antibody response of Kenyan children to *Haemophilus influenzae* type b conjugate vaccine, Abstract 70. *Program and Abstracts of the Interscience Conference on Antimicrobial Agents and Chemotherapy*, 1991.
30. M. Santosham, M. Wolff, R. Reid, et al., The efficacy in Navajo infants of a conjugate vaccine consisting of *Haemophilus influenzae* type b polysaccharide

and *Neisseria meningitidis* outer membrane protein complex, *N. Engl. J. Med. 324*:1767 (1991).

31. J. Eskola, H. Kayhty, A. K. Takala, et al., A randomized prospective field trial of a conjugate vaccine in the protection of infants and young children against invasive *Haemophilus influenzae* type b disease, *N. Engl. J. Med. 323*:1381 (1990).
32. J. Ward, G. Brenneman, G. Letson, et al., Limited protective efficacy of a *Haemophilus influenzae* type b conjugate vaccine in Alaskan native infants, *N. Engl. J. Med. 323*:1393 (1990).
33. E. P. Rothstein, R. P. Schiller, J. A. Girone, et al., Response of 7 to 15 month old infants to sequential immunization with *Haemophilus influenzae* type b-CRM 197 conjugate and polysaccharide vaccines, *Am. J. Dis. Child. 145*:898 (1991).
34. D. M. Granoff, G. A. Weinberg, and P. G. Shackleford, IgG subclass response to immunization with *Haemophilus influenzae* type b polysaccharide-outer membrane protein conjugate vaccine, *Pediatr. Res. 24*:180 (1988).

17

Bacterial Polysaccharide Immune Globulin

Raymond Reid, Janné Croll, and Mathuram Santosham

The Johns Hopkins University, Baltimore, Maryland

George R. Siber and Claudette M. Thompson

Dana-Farber Cancer Institute, Boston, Massachusetts

I. INTRODUCTION

The most common causes of serious bacterial infections in children are due to three encapsulated bacteria: *Haemophilus influenzae* type b (Hib), pneumococci, and meningococci. In the past few years, Hib-polysaccharide-protein conjugate vaccines have been developed and are highly immunogenic and protective in infants.

Individuals who are particularly susceptible to infection by these encapsulated bacteria may not adequately respond to conjugate vaccines. These individuals include children receiving cancer chemotherapy (1) and children with AIDS (2). Pneumococci and Hib are the most common causes of bacteremia in patients with primary or secondary hypogammaglobulinemia caused by chronic lymphocytic leukemia (3), multiple myeloma, intensive treatment for Hodgkin's disease (4), or bone marrow transplantation (5). Apache and Navajo infants are known to be at high risk of infections due to Hib (6,7) and to have low antibody responses to Hib polysaccharide (8) and to Hib polysaccharide-protein conjugate vaccines (9). Preventing serious infections due to Hib, pneumococci, and meningococci in these high-risk groups by passive immunization with high-titered immune globulin offers an alternative to active immunization.

II. PREPARATION OF BACTERIAL POLYSACCHARIDE IMMUNE GLOBULIN

A human high-titered immune globulin, also called bacterial polysaccharide immune globulin (BPIG), is prepared from the plasma of donors immunized with Hib polysaccharide or conjugate vaccine, 14- or 23-valent pneumococcal vaccine, and 4-valent meningcoccal polysaccharide vaccine (10). High-titered BPIG, compared to conventional immune globulin, has 10–60 times higher antibody concentrations to Hib polysaccharide, and about 4 times higher antibody concentrations to pneumococcal and meningococcal polysaccharides. Hib antibody is functionally active in the complement-mediated bactericidal reaction and in opsonizing Hib for granulocyte-mediated killing (11). Hib antibody levels in BPIG, when maintained at $\geq$ 0.05–0.15 μg/ml, protect infant rats from intraperitoneal or intranasal Hib challenge (12).

III. PHARMACOLOGY OF Hib ANTIBODY AFTER BPIG ADMINISTRATION

For protection from serious Hib infection, most individuals require an estimated minimum level of passively acquired Hib antibody of 0.05–0.15 μg/ml (13). Whereas an intramuscular dose of 0.5 ml/kg of conventional immune globulin can result in levels of Hib antibody at >0.15 μg/ml for 1 month (14), the same dose of BPIG can result in this level of Hib antibodies for 3 months in infants (14,15) and for 4 months in older children (14,15).

Table 1 shows the kinetics of the rise in Hib antibodies in Apache infants who received BPIG intramuscularly at a dose of 0.5 ml/kg. Detectable increases of anti-Hib antibodies were noted in three of four infants 4 hours after BPIG and in five of six infants 6 hours after BPIG (16). These data demonstrate the potential for the use of BPIG in postexposure prophylaxis of susceptible individuals.

IV. EFFECT OF BPIG ON THE ACTIVE IMMUNE RESPONSE TO SIMULTANEOUSLY ADMINISTERED VACCINES

When BPIG is administered simultaneously (in a different site) with routine childhood diphtheria-tetanus-pertussis (DTP) vaccine at 2, 4, and 6 months of age, no interference with active antibody responses to these antigens is noted when measured at 10 months of age (Table 2) (16). It was found that BPIG recipients did not differ from placebo recipients in levels

Table 1 Increases in Antibody to *Haemophilus influenzae* Type b Polysaccharide After Administration of BPIG

	Antibody concentration (μg/ml) at time after BPIG administration				
Patient	Pre	4 hr	6 hr	24 hr	72 hr
1	0.28			0.86	3.00
2	0.54			1.76	
3	0.68		0.94	2.40	2.60
4	<0.10	0.51			
5	0.21		0.36	1.12	
6	0.28		0.94		
7	0.27	0.46		1.60	
8	0.56	0.48			
9	<0.10				
10	<0.10	0.37	1.18		
11	<0.10		0.68		
12	<0.10				4.20
13	<0.10				3.30
14	0.23				3.30
15	<0.10				3.55
16	0.32				4.10
17	<0.10				2.44
Mean Increase		0.22	0.57	1.15	3.10

Patients 1–7 received BPIG lot 5 and patients 8–17 received BPIG lot 7, 0.5 ml/kg, intramuscularly. Antibody concentrations were determined by radiolabeled antigen binding assay.

Source. Ref. 16.

Table 2 Concentrations of Antibodies in 10-Month-Old Apache Infants Immunized with Diphtheria and Tetanus Toxoids and Pertussis Vaccine and Either BPIG or Placebo

	Geometric mean antibody concentration				
	Tetanus toxoid		Diphtheria toxoid		Pertussis toxin
Treatment (*n*)	IgG	IgM	IgG	IgM	IgG
BPIG (44)	12.2	0.63	3.38	0.40	2.65
Placebo (41)	9.38	0.61	3.10	0.44	2.65

BPIG and placebo were given at 2 and 6 months simultaneously with vaccine but in separate sites. Antibody concentrations are ELISA units × 10^{-3}.

Source: Ref. 16

of IgG or IgM class antibodies to tetanus and diphtheria toxoids or in levels of IgG class antibodies to pertussis toxin. At 10 months of age, the concentrations of passively acquired IgG antibodies to all toxoids were calculated to be <0.5 ELISA units × 10^{-3}. Since BPIG is >95% IgG, the IgM antibodies represent only the active immune responses of the infants.

In a study among Navajo infants, simultaneous immunization at separate sites at 2 months of age with BPIG and Hib polysaccharide-diphtheria CRM conjugate vaccine (Praxis Biologics, Rochester, NY) followed by booster doses at 4 and 6 months of age of Hib conjugate vaccine showed active antibody responses to Hib polysaccharide that were similar to the response of infants who received only the active vaccine (9,17). However, only the group of infants who received the passive-active immunization regimen reliably had protective antibody levels between 2 and 4 months of age.

V. EFFECT OF BPIG ON MATURATION OF THE ANTIBODY RESPONSE TO Hib POLYSACCHARIDE

Among Apache children who received BPIG or placebo at 2, 6, and 10 months of age, no significant difference was noted in the natural acquisition

Table 3 Antibody Responses to *Haemophilus influenzae* Type b Polysaccharide (PRP) and PRP-Diphtheria Toxoid Conjugate Vaccine (PRP-D) in Apache Children

Vaccine, age at immunization, passive immunization (n)	Antibody concentration (μg/ml)			% with antibody	
	Pre	Post	Rise	>0.15 μg/ml	>1 μg/ml
PRP					
18 months					
BPIG (12)	0.045	0.128	2.78	42	8.3
Saline (17)	0.063	0.152	2.42	47	18
24 months					
BPIG (49)	0.117	0.339	2.33	65	14
Saline (43)	0.142	0.326	2.37	70	21
PRP-D, 18 months					
BPIG (18)	—	0.743*	—	94	33
Saline (28)	—	1.13*	—	96	54†

BPIG or saline was given at 2, 6, and 10 months of age and at 4 months in some. Antibody concentrations (determined by radiolabeled antigen binding assay) are geometric means.
*$p < 0.01$ compared with 18-month-old PRP recpients by t-test or Wilocoxon test for geometric means or by Fisher's exact test for proportions.
†$p < 0.05$ compared with 18-month-old PRP recipients by Fisher's exact test.
Source: Ref. 16.

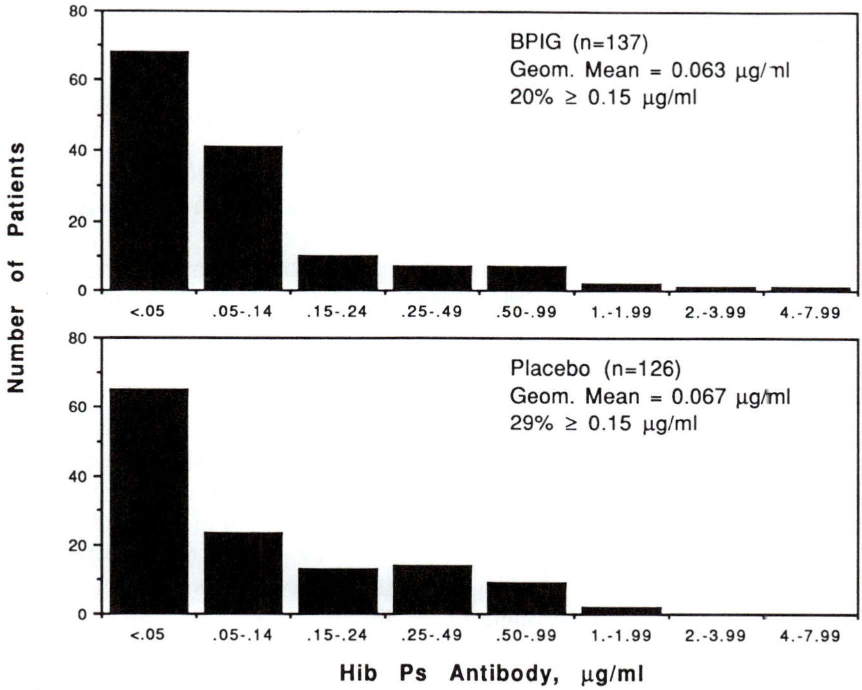

Figure 1. Distribution of naturally acquired antibody concentrations to *Haemophilus influenzae* b polysaccharide in 18-month-old Apache infants who have received BPIG or saline placebo at 2, 6, and 10 months of age.

of antibody to Hib at 18 months of age (Fig. 1). However, at 18 months of age, only a small proportion of Apache children (20% of BPIG recipients and 29% of placebo recipients) had acquired Hib antibody concentrations ≥ 0.15 μg/ml (16).

Apache infants who received BPIG or placebo showed similar antibody responses after active immunization at 18 or 24 months of age with Hib polysaccharide vaccine or with Hib conjugate vaccine (PRP-D) (Table 3). Significant differences were not noted between BPIG and placebo recipients in their geometric mean Hib antibody responses or in the proportion who achieved Hib antibody concentrations ≥ 0.15 or ≥ 1.0 μg/ml. However, PRP-D was significantly more immunogenic than PRP in 18-month-old Apache children (16).

The low responses of 18- to 24-month-old Apache children to PRP vaccine are of special note. These responses were found to be significantly lower than those of similarly aged Caucasian children (8,9). Also, the postimmunization Hib antibody levels after PRP-D appear lower than those reported for other U.S. children at 18 months (18), but no Caucasian controls were evaluated in those studies.

VI. EFFICACY OF BPIG IN PREVENTING INVASIVE Hib AND PNEUMOCOCCAL INFECTIONS

In a double-blind, randomized, placebo-controlled trial among two Apache tribal groups in which BPIG was compared to placebo [19], infants received BPIG at a dose of 0.5 ml/kg IM or placebo at 2, 6, and 10 months of age. As expected, BPIG recipients had a significantly lower frequency of bacteremic Hib infection. In addition, there was a trend for BPIG recipients to have a lower frequency of pneumococcal infections (Table 4). No episodes of Hib or pneumococcal bacteremia were noted within 3 months of receiving BPIG; on the other hand, placebo recipients had seven cases of subsequent Hib and four pneumococcal bacteremias within 3 months. In a subsequent study, BPIG was found to be 75% efficacious in preventing serious pneumococcal infections (20). During the fourth month after BPIG administration, however, several cases of Hib or pneumococcal infections were noted, but no compensatory increases in these infections were noted during further follow-up throughout childhood.

VII. EFFICACY OF BPIG IN PREVENTING OTHER INFECTIONS

While the studies among Apache infants were in progress, significant decreases were noted among BPIG recipients in the numbers of children with recurrent pneumonia (>3 episodes) and of children hospitalized with fever ≥ 39°C. However, there were no significant differences between BPIG or placebo-treated infants in the frequencies of all pneumonias (x-ray documented), otitis media (clinically diagnosed), or gastroenteritis (19).

Studies of experimental otitis media in chinchillas suggested that BPIG was effective in preventing pneumococcal otitis media (21). Treatment with BPIG also decreased the frequency of pneumococcal otitis media among infants in Cleveland at high risk for recurrent otitis media (22). Two doses of BPIG (0.5 ml/kg) or placebo were given one month apart to infants in Cleveland with an initial episode of otitis during the first 6 months of age or two or more episodes in the first 12 months of age. Infants were followed for a total of 4 months. Based on culture specimens obtained by tympanocentesis, a significant decrease in pneumococcal otitis media was noted in BPIG-treated infants (7 episodes in 37 BPIG recipients vs. 18 in 42 placebo recipients). However, the frequency of otitis associated with *H. influenzae* (nontypable), *Branhamella catarrhalis,* or negative cultures was

Table 4 Bacteremic *Haemophilus influenzae* Type b and Pneumococcal Infections in Apache Infants Treated with BPIG or Placebo

Infection, time after treatment	BPIG (n = 353)	Placebo (n = 353)	p^a
Invasive Hib			
1–90 days	0	7	.007
90–120 days	1	0	
After entire course	2	4	
Invasive pneumococcal			
1–90	0	4	.06
90–120 days	2	0	
After entire course	6	6	

BPIG was given at 2, 6, and 10 months of age (total doses, 858 in BPIG and 838 in placebo group).
[a]By two-sided Fisher's exact test.
Source: Refs. 16,19.

not decreased. Thus, BPIG did not significantly decrease the overall frequency of recurrent otitis media.

VIII. EVALUATION OF BPIG IN THE TREATMENT OF ESTABLISHED Hib MENINGITIS

The therapeutic effect of BPIG or conventional IVIG with or without ceftriaxone in the treatment of Hib meningitis and bacteremia was evaluated in an infant rat model (23). Immune globulin treatment was found to increase early mortality ($\leq$ 24 hours) compared to saline placebo. Significantly greater early mortality was noted in groups receiving IVIG and ceftriaxone than in groups receiving ceftriaxone alone. The effect on mortality was mediated by specific anticapsular antibodies rather than by high doses of nonspecific IgG. Higher concentrations of endotoxin in blood and CSF was found in antibody-treated animals than in controls that did not receive antibodies. Enhanced bacteriolysis and release of endotoxin may have mediated the increased early mortality found to be associated with specific antibody treatment in this model. BPIG and other immunoglobulins should not be used in the treatment of established Hib infections unless a benefit is established in well-controlled clinical trials.

IX. SUMMARY

In a study among Apache infants, passive immunization with BPIG at a dose of 0.5 ml/kg every 4 months decreased the frequency of bacteremic

Hib infections by about 85%. Protection was most reliable during the first 3 months after immunization as breakthrough infections occasionally occurred after 3 months. No detectable interference with the active antibody response to simultaneously administered DTP or Hib-diphtheria CRM conjugate vaccine was noted because of BPIG administration. Neither was BPIG noted to have delayed the acquisition of antibodies to Hib polysaccharide by natural exposure. Similarly, BPIG administration did not affect the maturation of the capacity to respond to purified Hib polysaccharide or PRP-D conjugate vaccine.

Although more expensive than active immunizations, BPIG immunoprophylaxis is likely to be more effective for the prevention of serious Hib infections in high-risk populations such as children with humoral immunodeficiencies, malignancies, and AIDS. Current preparations of BPIG are suitable only for intramuscular administration. An intravenous formulation of BPIG may be more desirable for these groups since such a preparations may allow use of higher doses of immunoglobulin/antibody and would facilitate repeated administration. For many high-risk infants, such as Native Americans, uninterrupted protection at modest cost may be provided by regimens combining passive and active immunization with more immunogenic conjugates.

ACKNOWLEDGMENTS

This study was supported by NIH grants AI18125, AI24996, and AI20738, and the Thrasher Research Fund Award #2792-6.

REFERENCES

1. G. R. Siber, Bacteremias due to *Haemophilus influenzae* and *Steptococcus pneumoniae*: Their occurrence and course in children with cancer, *Am. J. Dis. Child. 134*:668 (1980).
2. The National Institute of Child Health and Human Development Intravenous Immunoglobulin Study Group, Intravenous immune globulin for the prevention of bacterial infections in children with symptomatic human immunodeficiency virus infection, *N. Engl. J. Med. 325*:73 (1991).
3. Cooperative Group for the Study of Immunoglobulin in Chronic Lymphocytic Leukemia, Intravenous immunoglobulin for the prevention of infection in chronic lymphocytic leukemia, *N. Engl. J. Med. 319*:902 (1988).
4. G. R. Siber, C. Gorham, P. Martin, et al., Antibody response to pretreatment immunization and post-treatment boosting with bacterial polysaccharide vaccines in patients with Hodgkin's disease, *Ann. Int. Med. 104*:467 (1986).

5. D. J. Winston, G. Schiffman, D. C. Wang, et al., Pneumococcal infections after human bone-marrow transplantation, *Ann. Int. Med. 91*:835 (1979).
6. G. A. Losonsky, M. Santosham, V. M. Sehgal, A. Zwahlen, and E. R. Moxon, *Haemophilus influenzae* disease in the White Mountain Apaches: molecular epidemiology of a high risk population, *Pediatr. Infect. Dis. 84*:539
7. J. L. Coulehan, R. H. Michaels, C. Hallowell, et al., Epidemiology of *Haemophilus influenzae* type b among Navajo Indians, Public Health Rep. *99*:404 (1984).
G. R. Siber, M. Santosham, G. R. Reid, et al., Impaired anitbody response to *Haemophilus influenzae* type b polysaccharide and low IgG2 and IgG4 concentrations in Apache children, *N. Engl. J. Med. 323*:1387 (1990).
9. M. Santosham, B. Rivin, M. Wolff, et al., Prevention of *Haemophilus influenzae* type b infections in Apache and Navajo children, *J. Infect. Dis. 165*:S144 (1992).
10. G. R. Siber, D. M. Ambrosino, J. McIver, et al., Preparation of human hyperimmune globulin to *Haemophilus influenzae* b, *Streptococcus pneumoniae* , and *Neisseria meningitidis*, *Infect. Immun. 45*:248 (1984).
11. J. R. Schreiber, V. Barrus, K. L. Cates, and G. R. Siber, Functional characterization of human IgG, IgM and IgA antibody directed to the capsule of *Haemophilus influenzae* type b, *J. Infect. Dis. 153*:8 (1986).
12. D. Ambrosino, J. R. Schreiber, R. S. Daum, and G. R. Siber, Efficacy of human hyperimmune globulin in prevention of *Haemophilus influenzae* type b disease in infant rats, *Infect. Immun. 39*:709 (1983).
13. J. B. Robbins, J. C. Parke Jr. R. Schneerson, and J. K. Whisnant, Quantitative measurement of "natural" and immunization-induced *Haemophilus influenzae* type b capsular polysaccharide antibodies, *Pediatr. Res. 7*:103 (1973).
14. D. M. Ambrosino, S. H. Landesman, C. A. Gorham, and G. R. Siber, Passive immunization against disease due to *Haemophilus influenzae* type b: concentrations of antibody to capsular polysaccharide in high-risk children, *J. Infect. Dis. 153*:1 (1986).
15. J. I. Ward, D. Ambrosino, K. Burkhart, B. Sonne, J. Dengrove, and G. Siber, Passive protection for *Haemophilus influenzae* type b (Hib) disease: Antibody levels in infants given hyperimmune globulin, *Pediatr. Res. 18*:237A (Abstract #1151) (1984).
16. G. R. Siber, C. Thompson, R. Reid, et al., Evaluation of bacterial polysaccharide immune globulin for the treatment or prevention of *Haemophilus influenzae* type b and pneumococcal disease, *J. Infect. Dis. 165*:S129 (1992).
17. G. W. Letson, M. Santosham, R. Reid, et al., Comparison of active and combined active/passive immunization of Navajo children against *Haemophilus influenzae* type b, *Ped. Infect. Dis. J. 7*:747 (1988).
18. C. D. Berkowitz, J. I. Ward, K. Meier, et al., Safety and immunogenicity of *Haemophilus influenzae* type b polysaccharide and polysaccharide diphtheria toxoid conjugate vaccines in children 15 to 24 months of age, *J. Pediatr. 110*:509 (1987).

19. M. Santosham, R. Reid, D. M. Ambrosino, et al., Prevention of *Haemophilus influenzae* type b infections in high risk infants with bacterial polysaccharide immune globulin, *N. Engl. J. Med. 317*:923 (1987).
20. M. Santosham, R. Reid, J. Almeido-Hill, et al., Efficacy of bacterial polysaccharide immune globulin (BPIG) for prevention of bacteremic pneumococcal infections in Apache children, *Pediatr. Res.* 31:178A (Abstract #1055) (1992).
21. P. A. Shurin, G. S. Giebink, D. L. Wegman, et al., Prevention of pneumococcal otitis media in chinchillas with human bacterial polysaccharide immune globulin, *J. Clin. Microbiol. 26*:755 (1988).
22. J. Rehmus, C. Johnson, C. Marchant, et al., Bacterial polysaccharide immune globulin prophylaxis of otitis media in high-risk infants, 28th Interscience Conference on Antimicrobial Agents and Chemotherapy, Los Angeles, CA, October 1988 (Abstract #334).
23. J. Schreiber, C. Basker, C. Priehs, and G. Siber, Deleterious effect of immune globulin in the treatment of *H. influenzae* b infection in infant rats, *Pediatr. Res. 21*:334A (Abstract #961) (1987).

18

Protective Efficacy Trials

Eugene D. Shapiro

Yale University School of Medicine, New Haven, Connecticut

Although the immunogenicity of the different *Haemophilus influenzae* type b (Hib) conjugate vaccines has been studied extensively, there are many uncertainties about the correlation between concentrations of antibodies and clinical protection from Hib infection. Consequently, to assess the efficacy of a vaccine, it is necessary to do studies to determine how well the vaccine protects against clinical disease in patients.

I. ASSESSMENT OF A VACCINE'S PROTECTIVE EFFICACY

A vaccine's protective efficacy is defined as the proportionate reduction in the risk of infection among vaccinees (compared to controls) that is attributable to the vaccine (1–3). The "efficacy" of a vaccine, which refers to a vaccine's performance under optimal—e.g., experimental—conditions, should be distinguished from its "effectiveness," which refers to its ability to prevent infections in actual practice. For example, in clinical trials of an experimental vaccine, potential subjects might be excluded from the study if they are known to have an immunodeficiency or a different factor that is known to increase either their exposure to or their susceptibility to the infection. Thus, a vaccine with a protective efficacy of 96% under experimental conditions might have a much lower effectiveness in actual practice if the target population includes many individuals with factors that would have excluded them from the original experimental clinical trial of the vaccine's protective efficacy. Other factors that might limit the use of a vaccine in clinical practice, such as significant and frequent adverse side effects or extreme cost, could also result in limited effectiveness for a highly efficacious vaccine.

A vaccine's efficacy may be assessed either by experimental studies (such as randomized clinical trials, in which the subjects are assigned by chance to receive either the experimental vaccine or a control, usually a placebo, to which the experimental vaccine is being compared) or by observational studies (such as longitudinal cohort, case-control, or household-exposure studies). A longitudinal cohort study, which may be either prospective or retrospective, is similar to a clinical trial in that the subjects are followed forward from the time of enrollment. It differs in that the allocation of the subjects to receive or not to receive vaccine is determined not by the investigators but by many different practitioners in the course of normal medical care of the subjects. A household-exposure study is similar to a retrospective cohort study except that the subjects are selected because they are members of a household in which a member developed the infection of interest (and therefore are at increased risk of developing the infection). In a case-control study, in which subjects are *not* followed forward in time, subjects are selected based on their outcomes; the cases have had the infection of interest (e.g., invasive infections caused by Hib) and the controls have not had the infection. The vaccine's efficacy is calculated based on the proportion of each group that had received the vaccine.

However, since a vaccine generally must be used routinely in the population before an observational study of a vaccine's efficacy can be conducted, prelicensure testing of a vaccine's efficacy virtually always must be done through clinical trials. In a clinical trial of a vaccine's efficacy, subjects are assigned (ideally by randomization) to receive (vaccinees) or not to receive (controls) the vaccine that is being assessed. The subjects are then followed longitudinally and the frequency of target infections in both groups is determined. A vaccine's protective efficacy (PE) is defined as:

$$\text{PE} = \frac{\text{Risk of infection in controls} - \text{risk of infection in vaccinees}}{\text{Risk of infection in controls}}$$

This equation can be simplified to: 1 − (risk of infection in vaccinees/risk of infection in controls). Because the ratio in this equation is the relative risk of infection in vaccinees vs. controls, a vaccine's protective efficacy may also be expressed as 1 − the relative risk. The calculation of the protective efficacy of a vaccine against *H. influenzae* type b from a clinical trial is shown in Table 1.

Table 1 Calculation of the Protective Efficacy of a Vaccine Against *Haemophilus influenzae* Type b

	Haemophilus b infection	No *Haemophilus* b infection	Total
Vaccinated	a	b	N_1
Not vaccinated	c	d	N_2

$$\text{Protective Efficacy} = \frac{c/N_2 - a/N_1}{c/N_2} = 1 - \frac{a/N_1}{c/N_2}$$

Clinical trials that demonstrate a vaccine's efficacy are usually required before a vaccine is licensed because this kind of study, when properly conducted, provides the most reliable scientific evidence that a vaccine is efficacious. Randomized assignment of the subjects to either the vaccine or the control group assures that there is no bias in the selection of who receives the vaccine. If the size of the sample is sufficiently large, the distribution of important risk factors for infection should be approximately equal in the two groups. Furthermore, by conducting the trial in a double-blind fashion (i.e., neither the subjects nor the investigators are aware of the identity of the injection that subjects receive), bias in the assessment of the outcome can be minimized.

However, there are certain potential limitations of clinical trials. Because, for diseases that are relatively rare, the statistical power of clinical trials to assess the efficacy of vaccines is poor, it is necessary to enroll a very large number of subjects to have meaningful results. For this reason, and because the need for careful longitudinal follow-up of the subjects presents many additional logistical problems, such studies are quite expensive to conduct. Consequently, prelicensure clinical trials often are conducted in populations that are chosen because of certain logistical or financial advantages (such as an unusually high incidence of the infection, which permits the study to be conducted with a smaller sample), rather than because of the similarity of the sample to ultimate target populations for the vaccine. This can lead to problems with the generalizability of the results of the prelicensure clinical trial.

A good example of this phenomenon occurred with the polyvalent pneumococcal polysaccharide vaccine (3). Prelicensure clinical trials were conducted among ambulatory adults ≥45 years of age at Kaiser-Permanente in San Francisco and among young goldminers in South Africa (4–6). Although the adults in San Francisco were similar to the target population for the vaccine in the United States, the incidence of pneumococcal bacteremia in this group was so low that, even though a sizable number of subjects were enrolled in the study, the statistical power of the study was much too poor for the assessment of the vaccine's efficacy to be meaningful (4). By contrast, the incidence of pneumococcal bacteremia among the young African goldminers was very high. Well-conducted randomized clinical trials showed that the efficacy of the vaccine was excellent in this population (5,6). Pneumococcal polysaccharide vaccine was licensed in the United States based on those clinical trials. However, the target population in the United States was not young goldminers but rather persons who were at increased risk of pneumococcal bacteremia because they either were elderly or had certain chronic illnesses such as chronic obstructive pulmonary disease, congestive heart failure, or sickle cell disease. Subsequent reports of vaccine failures among persons in the United States for whom the vaccine was recommended, coupled with the lack of a definitive study that demonstrated that pneumococcal polysaccharide vaccine was efficacious in the target population, led to many years of controversy about both this vaccine's efficacy and the appropriateness of official recommendations for its use.

There was similar controversy about the protective efficacy of plain PRP vaccine in the United States (7–9). This vaccine was licensed based on clinical trials conducted in Finland (where the epidemiology of Hib disease differs from that in the United States), which indicated that its protective efficacy was 90% for children 18 months of age and older. However, the 95% confidence interval for the estimate of the vaccine's efficacy (the interval which, based on the data from the study, includes the true efficacy of the vaccine with 95% statistical probability) was wide and, for children 24–35 months of age (the ages at which universal immunization was recommended), the lower limit of the 95% confidence interval was only 5%. After it was licensed in the United States, the results of case-control studies of this vaccine's efficacy were conflicting (and ranged from −55 to 88%) and reflected differences in methodology and the different populations that were studied (7–9).

II. PRELICENSURE TRIALS OF CONJUGATE VACCINES AGAINST Hib

Many of these factors had to be considered when prelicensure trials of the conjugate vaccines against Hib were planned. Hib was both the most common cause of bacterial meningitis and a common cause of other serious invasive bacterial infections in children beyond the neonatal period in the United States and in many other developed countries. Nevertheless, in industrialized areas the absolute frequency of such infections still was relatively low, which made clinical trials of the efficacy of conjugate vaccines in most populations in the United States or in other developed countries both expensive and logistically difficult. The one circumstance that would make such a clinical trial feasible in a developed country would be to conduct the study in a large health-care system with a highly centralized administration. This would provide the opportunity to enroll a large number of subjects under the auspices of a single administrative entity and would also provide assurance of relatively complete longitudinal follow-up without a great deal of added expense.

Indeed, two of the prelicensure clinical trials were conducted under just such circumstances. In one trial of the PRP-D vaccine that was conducted in Finland, virtually the entire country participated because of its centralized, socialized health-care system (10). Praxis Biologics (later purchased by Lederle Laboratories) sponsored a prelicensure trial of their HbOC vaccine among the enrollees of Kaiser-Permanente of Northern California, a large prepaid health management organization in the San Francisco area, which made it possible to conduct the study through a single organization (11).

An alternative course, which was pursued both by Merck Research Laboratories and by investigators who conducted a clinical trial of the protective efficacy of PRP-D that was sponsored by the National Institutes of Health (NIH), was to choose a select population in which the risk of Hib disease was extremely high, thus making it possible to conduct the study with a smaller sample. Merck sponsored a study of the efficacy of PRP-OMPC vaccine among Native American (Navajo) infants in the southwestern United States (12), while the NIH sponsored a study of the efficacy of PRP-D among Native Alaskans (13). Each of these studies, as well as some others, will be reviewed in detail.

III. CLINICAL TRIALS

Although conjugate vaccines were first licensed in the United States for use in children $\geq$ 18 months of age (14) (and later for children $\geq$ 15 months of age), there were no clinical trials of the protective efficacy of the different conjugate vaccines for children of these ages before they were licensed. Licensure of the vaccines for children in this age group was based on their proved safety and their superior immunogenicity compared to the plain PRP vaccine (15). The controversy about the protective efficacy of the plain PRP vaccine after its licensure no doubt hastened the licensure of the conjugate vaccines for children 15 months of age and older (7–9). However, despite the well-documented immunogenicity of at least some of the conjugate vaccines, clinical trials of their protective efficacy in infants were required before the Food and Drug Administration would license them for infants.

A. PRP–Diphtheria Toxoid Conjugate Vaccine (PRP-D)

Clinical trials of the protective efficacy of PRP-D were conducted in Finland and in Native Alaskans. The epidemiology of Hib infections was very different in these two populations. The age-specific incidence of Hib infections in Finnish children peaked at 15 months of age (16,17), whereas the peak incidence among Native Alaskans occurred in much younger infants (18). In addition, the overall incidence of invasive Hib infections was dramatically higher among Native Alaskan infants $<$ 1 year of age (1702/100,000/year) than among Finnish infants $<$ 1 year of age (57/100,000/year). In part, this difference may be due to differences in the prevalence of risk factors for Hib infections in these populations (see Chapter 19). In Finland, the socioeconomic conditions are much better than among Native Alaskans. In addition, in Finland the average number of children in families is lower, there is less crowding, and the prevalence of breast-feeding is greater. Unlike in the United States, the use of group day care before one year of age is uncommon in Finland.

1. Clinical Trial in Finland

From October 1, 1985, through August 31, 1987, all children who were born in Finland were eligible to participate in the study (10). After obtaining oral informed consent, children who were born on odd days of the month received PRP-D (25 μg of PRP/dose) at 3, 4, 6, and 14–18 months of age. Children who were born on even days of the month served as controls. The controls were to receive PRP-D when they were 24 months of age. Since no placebo was administered, neither the investigators nor the parents were blinded to the allocation of the vaccine. Infants in both the experimental and the control groups received their other routine childhood immunizations at the normally scheduled times (diphtheria-tetanus-pertussis vaccine at 3, 4, 5, and 24 months of age, inactivated polio vaccine at 6, 12, and 24 months of age and measles-mumps-rubella vaccine at 14–18 months of age). Surveillance for invasive Hib infections in all of the microbiology laboratories in Finland was intensified.

The number and the allocation of enrollees were estimated by prospective and retrospective surveillance of certain "sentinel" health centers. Approximately 98% of the more than 116,000 children born in Finland during the period of the study were enrolled (approximately 58,000 were in the experimental group that received PRP-D and approximately 56,000 were in the control group, at least in part because there are 4% more odd-numbered than even-numbered days in the year). The median ages at which the children in the experimental group received the first, second, third, and fourth doses of PRP-D were 3.1, 4.2, 6.4, and 17.3 months, respectively.

The investigators chose to assess the protective efficacy of PRP-D by counting invasive Hib infections that occurred among vaccinees after they had received the first three doses of PRP-D and among the controls after the first dose of inactivated polio vaccine (administered at 6 months of age). For both groups the endpoint for follow-up was receipt of the fourth dose of diphtheria-tetanus-pertussis vaccine (administered at 24 months of age). Thus, the period of follow-up for invasive Hib infections was approximately from 6 through 23 months of age.

As of December 31, 1989, Hib organisms were isolated from cultures of normally sterile sites from 91 children born during the period of the study. Of these, 23 occurred either before (20) or after (3) the designated period of follow-up. Thus, the assessment of the vaccine's efficacy was based on the remaining 68 invasive infections that occurred in the enrollees. Of these, four occurred among vaccinees (all before the child had received the fourth dose of the vaccine) and 64 occurred among the controls (37 before and 27 after the administration of the measles-mumps-rubella vaccine, which had been scheduled to be administered between 14 and 18 months of age—the same ages at which the fourth dose of PRP-D had been scheduled for the children in the experimental group). By contrast, there was virtually no difference between the groups in the incidence of bacteremic infections caused by bacteria other than Hib during the same time period (170/100,000/year in the experimental group and 169/100,000/year in the control group).

Based on these data, the protective efficacy of PRP-D after three doses but before the fourth (booster) dose was 90% (95% C.I.: 70–96%; $p < 0.001$). (The p-value indicates the probability that the observed result would occur by chance alone.) After the booster dose, the vaccine's protective efficacy was 100%. Overall, between 7 and 24 months of age the protective efficacy of PRP-D was 94% (95% C.I.: 83–98%; $p < 0.001$).

Twelve cases of invasive Hib infections occurred in children who had received only a part of their initial series of immunizations. Four of these Hib infections occurred among children in the experimental group (three of whom had received one dose of PRP-D and one of whom had received two doses of PRP-D). Eight of these Hib infections occurred among controls. The protective efficacy of PRP-D for "partially vaccinated" children was 50% ($p = 0.25$).

Although the protective efficacy of PRP-D was excellent in this clinical trial, the concentration of anti-PRP induced in the vaccinees were modest at best. The geometric mean concentration of anti-PRP that were induced in a subsample of 120 healthy vaccinees was less than 0.1 than 0.1 μg/ml after the first and second doses of PRP-D and was only 0.53 μg/ml after the third dose. Furthermore, one month after the third dose of PRP-D only 40% of these infants had a concentration of anti-PRP that was 1.0 μg/ml or more and only 70% had a concentration of 0.15 μg/ml or more. However, after the fourth (booster) dose of the vaccine, all of the children had concentrations of anti-PRP that were >1.0 μg/ml (the geometric mean concentration was 45.22 μg/ml).

2. Clinical Trial in Native Alaskans

Another clinical trial of PRP-D was conducted among Native Alaskan infants (Eskimos, Aleuts, or Indians) who have an extremely high risk of invasive Hib infections (13). For this clinical trial, potential subjects who resided in six of the eight most populous Native Health Board service units were recruited from October 1984 through January 1988. Infants were eligible for the trial if they were ≤4 months of age and had not received their first dose of diphtheria-tetanus-pertussis vaccine. Enrollees were scheduled to receive either PRP-D (20 μg/dose) or a saline placebo at 2, 4, and 6 months of age, although the first dose could be administered at up to 4 months of age and there were no upper limits on the ages at which subsequent doses were administered. Other childhood vaccines were administered at the same visits at which PRP-D or placebo was administered. Follow-up surveillance for invasive Hib infections occurred through June 1988.

During the study period, 2102 (35%) of the 5982 Native Alaskan infants who were born in the six health districts were enrolled in the study. Of these, 1054 were randomly allocated to receive PRP-D and 1048 were randomly allocated to receive the placebo. The median ages at which the subjects received their immunizations were 1.7, 4.2, and 6.7 months for the first, second, and third doses, respectively. However, for each dose there was a considerable range of ages within which the subjects were immunized. For example, although 72% of the subjects received their third dose between 5 and 8 months of age, the range of ages at which the third dose was administered was 4.5–15 months.

There were 20 episodes of invasive Hib infections in subjects who had received three doses of PRP-D or placebo—8 occurred among the vaccinees (including one child who also had had an invasive Hib infection 48 days after the first dose of the vaccine) and 12 occurred among the controls. Based on these data, the vaccine's protective efficacy after three doses was either 43% (95% C.I.: −43 to 78%; $p = 0.16$) if the child with two episodes of invasive Hib infections is excluded after the first episode or 35% (95% C.I.: −57 to 73%) if the child's second episode is not censored from the analysis. There was little difference in the frequency of invasive Hib infections after one dose (three vs. four cases) or two doses (two vs. three cases) between the vaccinees or the placebo recipients, respectively. Thus, no statistically significant efficacy for PRP-D could be demonstrated in this population after any of the first three doses.

Because only 35% of the eligible subjects enrolled in the study, it was possible that the study sample was not representative of the entire study population. However, extensive analyses revealed only one significant difference between those who enrolled and those who refused to enroll in the study—the proportion of enrollees who were city residents was significantly lower ($p < 0.0001$). The overall incidence of Hib infections was higher among the placebo recipients (9.6 cases/1000 patient-years) than among those who did not participate in the study (6.0 cases/1000 person-years), but this difference was not statistically significant ($p = 0.08$).

The immunogenicity of PRP-D was assessed in a sample of enrollees. There was no significant difference in the geometric mean concentrations of anti-PRP between the vaccinees and the placebo recipients either before immunization or after the first injection. Although the concentrations of antibodies were statistically significantly higher ($p < 0.01$) among the vaccinees than among the controls after the second (0.10 μg/ml vs. 0.07 μg/ml) and the third (0.18 μg/ml vs. 0.07 μg/ml) doses, the magnitude of these differences was small. In addition, even after the third dose of PRP-D, only 15% and 48% of the vaccinees tested had concentrations of anti-PRP-D antibodies that were >1.0 μg/ml and >0.1 μg/ml, respectively.

PRP-D was highly efficacious in Finnish infants but was not found to have statistically significant efficacy in Native Alaskan infants. The reasons for the striking difference in the results of the two clinical trials of PRP-D are not clear. Certainly, the populations that were studied were dramatically different in both their socioeconomic and their racial backgrounds. Different lots of PRP-D were used in the studies. However, the immunogenicity of PRP-D was similar in both populations after adjusting for differences in the ages at which samples of serum were obtained for testing and in the statistical methods used to summarize the concentrations of antibodies. In addition, stratification by the degree of Caucasian, Eskimo, or Indian ancestry of the subjects in the Alaskan trial indicated that ethnic factors were not important in determining either the immunogenicity or the protective efficacy of the vaccine. The size of the Alaskan trial was substantially smaller than that of the trial that was conducted in Finland and, despite the higher incidence of Hib infections in Alaska, the statistical power of the Alaskan trial was only fair. Some investigators speculated that the exposure to Hib of Native Alaskan infants is either more frequent, more intense, or both, and that the immunogenicity of PRP-D was insufficient to provide adequate protection for these infants.

PRP-D was licensed by the U.S. Food and Drug Administration in December 1987 for use as a single dose only in children 18 months of age or older (14). Subsequently, the lower limit of the age for which PRP-D was licensed was changed to 15 months (19,20) and later to 12 months. Because of the conflicting results of the clinical trials of the protective efficacy of PRP-D in infants, as well as the knowledge that trials of more immunogenic conjugate vaccines were underway, PRP-D was not (and is unlikely ever to be) licensed in the United States for use in infants. However, PRP-D has been licensed for use in infants in both Germany and Iceland, countries in which the epidemiology of Hib infections is similar to that in Finland.

B. Haemophilus b–Oligosaccharide Conjugate Vaccine (HbOC)

1. Clinical Trial in Northern California

A clinical trial of the protective efficacy of HbOC was conducted at 16 different sites within the Northern California Kaiser-Permanente Medical Care Program from February 1988 to June 1990 (11). The study was neither randomized nor blinded. A dose of HbOC (containing 10 μg of the Hib capsular oligosaccharide) was administered to infants at (ideally) 2, 4, and 6 months of age, usually in conjunction with the administration of DTP and oral polio vaccines. In practice, infants were eligible to enroll for the first dose of the vaccine if they were between 6 weeks and 6 months of age. The series of three immunizations had to be completed by the time the child was a year old.

Beginning in April 1988, all children were offered HbOC except those who were born on one of the first 5 days of any month. In May 1989 children who were born on one of the first 6 days of any month were not offered HbOC. In June 1990, the interval was further expanded so that children born on one of the first 7 days of any month were not offered HbOC. Thus, there were three groups of subjects: children who received the vaccine (vaccinees), children who did not receive the vaccine since it was not offered to them because they were born on one of the designated days of the month (controls), and children who did not receive the vaccine because the parents refused when it was offered (refusers).

The vaccine's efficacy was assessed by comparing the incidence rate of invasive Hib infections among vaccinees (beginning 1 week after the third dose of the vaccine) to the incidence rate among the controls and the refusers (beginning 1 week after the average age at which the fully vaccinated children received the third dose of the vaccine—255 days of age). The subjects were followed until 2 years of age, the occurrence of an invasive Hib infection, departure from the Kaiser Health Plan as the source of medical care, the receipt of a different Hib vaccine, or June 30, 1990, whichever occurred first.

In the primary analysis of the vaccine's efficacy, follow-up was only until 18 months of age to assure that none of the children had received a dose of one of the Hib vaccines that was already licensed for use in children 18 months of age or older. In this analysis, the mean duration of follow-up was 7.5 months for the 20,800 fully vaccinated children, who had a mean age of 11.9 months at the end of the study and were followed for a total of 12,949 person-years), and 7.2 months for the unvaccinated children (controls and refusers), whose mean age was 12.1 months at the end of the study and who had been followed for a total of 11,335 person-years. There were no invasive Hib infections among the vaccinees during this follow-up period, while therre were 12 Hib infections among the unvaccinated controls and refusers (incidence: 105.9 cases/100,000 person-years). Based on these data, the protective efficacy of HbOC for children who had received three doses was 100% (95% C.I.: 68–100%; $p = 0.0002$).

An analysis of the efficacy of HbOC after one and two doses was also conducted. There were no episodes of Hib infection among children who had received at least two doses of HbOC, and there were three episodes among children who had received a single dose of HbOC. There were nine episodes of Hib infection among the comparison group during the comparable period, although the authors do not explain precisely how they defined the comparison group to estimate the vaccine's efficacy after one or two doses. Nevertheless, the investigators report that the vaccine's efficacy after two doses was 100% (95% C.I.: 47–100%) and after one dose was 26% (95% C.I.: −166 to 80%).

Because this study was neither randomized nor blinded and parents often were able to choose whether their child would receive the vaccine, it was more susceptible to bias than are most clinical trials of experimental vaccines. To try to assure that the results were not substantially affected by bias, numerous additional analyses were conducted. The data were analyzed after adjusting for age and seasonality. A matched case-control study with adjustments for race, attendance of group day-care, breast-feeding, and a variety of socioeconomic factors also was conducted. There was little difference between the results of these analyses and those of the primary analysis. In addition, an "intent-to-treat" analysis (a very conservative approach to assessing the vaccine's efficacy) was done in which the refusers (the children who were offered the vaccine but did not receive it—51.6% of all children who were offered the vaccine) were treated as though they had received the vaccine. All episodes of Hib infection (including those among partially immunized children) were included in this analysis. In the intent-to-treat analysis, the vaccine's protective efficacy was 84% (95% C.I.: 59–94%; $p = 0.0001$).

A major concern in any nonrandomized clinical trial is that the results are biased by confounders—that is, by factors (such as socioeconomic status) that may differ between the groups and that may be independently related both to the risk of developing Hib infection and the probability of being vaccinated. To address this issue, the investigators demonstrated that the rates at which blood cultures were obtained as well as the rates of pneumococcal bacteremia (an infection that should not be affected by HbOC vaccine but that could be a marker for confounding) were not substantially different among the vaccinated and the unvaccinated subjects.

The immunogenicity of HbOC in this trial paralleled its protective efficacy (21). In a sample of 144 vaccinees, 2–6 weeks after the third dose of HbOC the geometric mean concentration of anti-PRP antibodies was 18.9 μg/ml, and 97% of the vaccinees had an antibody concentration of 1.0 μg/ml or greater. The proportion of vaccinees with a concentration of anti-PRP that was 1.0 μg/ml or greater after receiving all three doses was 83% 1.5–6 months later, 84% 6–12 months later, 71% > 12 months later, and was 97% 1 month after the 18-month booster dose.

2. Clinical Study in Finland

In another study that was conducted in Finland beginning in 1988, all children received either HbOC vaccine or PRP-D vaccine (22). The immunization schedule for the vaccines (both were administered to children at 2, 4, and 14–18 months of age) differs from the current recommendations for children in the United States (19,20). Nevertheless, during the subsequent 3 years Hib infections among Finnish children were virtually eliminated. Among the approximately 55,000 children who received HbOC, one developed an Hib infection after one dose of the vaccine and two developed an Hib infection after two doses. There were no Hib infections among children who had received three doses of the vaccine. There were a total of 11 cases of invasive Hib infections among children who had received PRP-D: six cases among children who had received one dose, five cases among children who had received two doses, and none among children who had received three doses of the vaccine. Because there was no unvaccinated control group, the protective efficacy of the vaccines in this study could not be estimated. However, the incidence of infection among both groups of vaccinees was dramatically lower than the incidence had been among unvaccinated children in previous years (23).

In October 1990 HbOC became the first vaccine licensed in the United States for use in infants. It was recommended that it be administered at 2, 4, 6, and 15 months of age.

C. PRP–*Neisseria meningitidis* Outer Membrane Protein Complex Vaccine (PRP-OMPC)

This vaccine's protective efficacy was assessed in a classical double-blind placebo-controlled randomized clinical trial among Native American infants (Navajos and Hopi infants who lived on the Navajo reservation) conducted from July 1, 1988, through August 2, 1990 (12). The incidence of invasive Hib infections among children in this population is 5–10 times higher than that in the general population of American infants, and the infections tend to occur at younger ages (24). Infants were randomized to receive either PRP-OMPC vaccine (each dose of which contained 15 μg PRP) or placebo. Ideally the vaccines were to be administered to children at 2 and 4 months of age. In practice, the first dose of either the vaccine or the placebo was administered to infants between the ages of 42 and 90 days and was given with other routine immunizations of childhood. The second dose was given at least 28 days after the first and was administered to children between 70 and 146 days of age. A booster dose of PRP-D vaccine was administered when the child reached 18 months of age (after HbOC was licensed in April 1990, the booster was given at 15 months and was either PRP-D, PRP-OMPC, or HbOC vaccine). Follow-up was conducted until the child developed an invasive Hib infection, reached 18 months of age, died, or the study was stopped (August 2, 1990), whichever occurred first.

Approximately 64% of the potentially eligible infants were enrolled in the study. Of these, 2588 were randomized to receive PRP-OMPC and 2602 were randomized to receive the placebo. The mean age at which the subjects received the injections was 54.6 days for the first dose for both groups and, for the second dose, 124.7 days for the vaccinees and 125.7 days for the placebo recipients. Of the enrollees, 80% (2056 vaccinees and 2105 placebo recipients) had received a second dose before the study was terminated.

Among the children who had received two doses of either the vaccine (1913) or the placebo (1929), one vaccinee and 12 placebo recipients developed an invasive Hib infection. The vaccine's protective efficacy after two doses was 93% (95% C.I.: 53–98%; $p < 0.001$). After the first dose and before the second dose, an invasive Hib infection occurred in none of 2451 vaccinees and in six of 2430 placebo recipients. The estimate of the protective efficacy of a single dose of the vaccine was 100% (95% C.I.: 15–100%; $p = 0.014$).

The immunogenicity of PRP-OMPC was assessed in a large sample of the subjects who enrolled in the study. The geometric mean concentrations of anti-PRP as well as the proportion of each group with concentrations

>0.15 μg/ml and >1.0 μg/ml are shown in Table 2. The vaccine's immunogenicity paralleled its protective efficacy. Notably, the geometric mean concentration of anti-PRP 2 months after the *first* dose of PRP-OMPC was 0.97 μg/ml, and 90% of the vaccinees had a concentration of anti-PRP that was >0.15 μg/ml (the putative minimal concentration for short-term protection from Hib infections) (25,26). This relatively substantial immune response after a single dose of PRP-OMPC is consistent with its apparent clinical efficacy after a single dose and is quite different from the poor immunogenicity of a single dose of the other Hib conjugate vaccines when administered to young infants.

On the other hand, the concentrations of anti-PRP after the second dose of PRP-OMPC fell rather rapidly; 8 months after the second dose the geometric mean concentration of anti-PRP was 0.40 μg/ml and only 76% of the vaccinees had a concentration>0.15 μg/ml. In the clinical trial, the one vaccinee who had an invasive Hib infection developed osteomyelitis at 15½ months of age. The anti-PRP concentration of this child was 2.86 μg/ml after he received the second dose of PRP-OMPC, but the antibody concentration fell to 0.14 μg/ml when he was 1 year of age.

In December 1990, PRP-OMPC became the second Hib vaccine licensed in the United States for use in infants. It was recommended that PRP-OMPC be administered at 2, 4, and 12 months of age. The recommendation that a booster dose be administered at 12 months (rather than at 15 months, as for HbOC) was made because of the clinical data about the relatively rapid decline in the concentrations of anti-PRP after two doses of this vaccine. However, based on subsequent data on the persistence of

Table 2 Anti-PRP Antibody Responses of Children Immunized with PRP-OMPC

Time	Number of infants	Mean age (months)	Geometric mean concentration	Proportion with concentrations >0.15 μg/ml	Proportion with concentrations >1.0 μg/ml
Before Immunization	982	1.8	0.16 μg/ml	45%	10%
2 months after first dose	879	4.2	0.97 μg/ml	90%	51%
2 months after second dose	735	6.3	1.35 μg/ml	91%	59%
8 months after second dose	331	11.7	0.40 μg/ml	76%	24%

Source: Ref. 12.

antibodies after the two doses, the recommended age for a booster dose was changed to 12–15 months.

D. PRP–Tetanus Toxoid Vaccine (PRP-T)

A double-blind randomized clinical trial of PRP-T was begun in infants enrolled in 13 selected clinics in the Southern California Kaiser-Permanente Health Plan on August 28, 1989 (27). Infants were randomized to receive, at 2, 4, and 6 months of age (concurrent with DTP and oral polio vaccine), either PRP-T (10 μg of PRP/dose) or hepatitis B vaccine (the controls). Unfortunately, because of the licensure of HbOC, enrollment in this study was prematurely halted in October 1990, and the controls were recalled to be immunized with an Hib conjugate vaccine that was licensed for infants. Because the study was stopped early, only a few more than 5000 infants were enrolled in each group. Consequently, the statistical power of the study to assess the protective efficacy of PRP-T was extremely poor. Nevertheless, as in other studies of its immunogenicity (28,29), PRP-T induced substantial concentrations of anti-PRP in infants after three doses. The limited data on the vaccine's protective efficacy (there were three cases of invasive Hib infections among the controls and none among the vaccinees) was consistent with the vaccine's immunogenicity.

A similar randomized clinical trial of PRP-T was begun in North Carolina, but it too was aborted early because of the licensure of HbOC for infants (27). In that study, two cases of invasive Hib infections occurred among the controls and none occurred among the vaccinees (27–29).

Finally, since January 1990, the policy in Finland has been to immunize all infants with PRP-T at 4 and 6 months of age (23). This policy has been highly effective: in the Helsinki area (with a population of 5 million persons) there were only three cases of Hib meningitis in 1990 and none in 1991 (23).

It will be impossible to conduct a prelicensure clinical trial of the protective efficacy of PRP-T in the United States, since other Hib conjugate vaccines are licensed for infants and routine immunization is officially recommended. Consequently, PRP-T was evaluated by FDA based on its immunogenicity (see Chapter 24) and was licensed for use in infants and older children in 1993.

IV. SUMMARY

The estimates from the prelicensure trials of the protective efficacy of the Hib conjugate vaccines in fully vaccinated infants are shown in Table 3.

Table 3 Protective Efficacy of Conjugate Hib Vaccines in Fully Vaccinated Infants[a]

Vaccine	Approximate age interval of follow-up (months)	Number of Hib infections/ Number of subjects		Protective efficacy	95% C.I.	Ref.
		Vaccinees	Controls			
PRP-D	6.4–17.3	4/58,000	39/56,000	90%	70% to 96%	10
PRP-D	6.7–20+	7/915	12/883	43%	−43% to 78%	13
HbOC	8.5–18	0/12,949[b]	12/11,335[b]	100%	68% to 100%	11
PRP-OMPC	4–18	1/1913	14/1929	93%	53% to 98%	12

[a]In Finland, two other studies of the effectiveness of conjugate vaccines have been conducted. From 1988 to 1989, infants received either PRP-D or HbOC at 2, 4, and 14–18 months of age. Since January 1990, all infants have received PRP-T at 4 and 6 months of age. There has been a dramatic decrease in the incidence of Hib infections in Finnish infants. However, because there are no unimmunized controls, the protective efficacy of the vaccines cannot be determined from these studies (22,23).
[b]Person-years of follow-up.

PRP-D very likely will not be licensed for use in infants in the United States, although HbOC, PRP-OMPC, and PRP-T currently are licensed.

REFERENCES

1. W. A. Orenstein, R. H. Bernier, T. H. Dondero, et al., Field evaluation of vaccine efficacy, *Bull. WHO 63*:1055 (1985).
2. W. A. Orenstein, R. H. Bernier, and A. R. Hinman, Assessing vaccine efficacy in the field: Further observations, *Epidemiol. Rev. 10*:212 (1988).
3. J. D. Clemens and E. D. Shapiro, Resolving the pneumococcal vaccine controversy: Are there alternatives to randomized clinical trials? *Rev. Infect. Dis. 6*:589 (1984).
4. R. Austrian, Surveillance of pneumococcal infection for field trials of polyvalent pneumococcal vaccine, Report DAB-VDP-12-84, National Institutes of Health, Bethesda, MD, 1980, pp. 1–84.
5. P. Smit, D. Oberholzer, S. Hayden-Smith, et al., Protective efficacy of pneumococcal polysaccharide vaccines, *JAMA 238*:2613 (1977).
6. R. Austrian, R. M. Douglas, G. Schiffman, et al., Prevention of pneumococcal pneumonia by vaccination, *Trans. Assoc. Am. Phys. 89*:184 (1976).
7. E. D. Shapiro, A. T. Berg, Protective efficacy of *Haemophilus influenzae* type b polysaccharide vaccine, *Pediatrics 85*:S643 (1990).
8. R. S. Daum, E. K. Marcuse, G. S. Giebink, et al., *Haemophilus influenzae* type b vaccines: lessons from the past, *Pediatrics 81*:893 (1988).

9. J. I. Ward, C. V. Broome, L. H. Harrison, et al., *Haemophilus influenzae* type b vaccines: lessons for the future, *Pediatrics 81*:886 (1988).
10. J. Eskola, H. Kayhty, A. K. Takala, et al., A randomized, prospective field trial of a conjugate vaccine in the protection of infants and young children against invasive *Haemophilus influenzae* type b disease, *N. Engl. J. Med. 323*:1381 (1990).
11. S. B. Black, H. R. Shinefield, B. Fireman, et al., Efficacy in infancy of oligosaccharide conjugate *Haemophilus influenzae* type b (HbOC) vaccine in a United States population of 61,080 children, *Pediatr. Infect. Dis. J. 10*:97 (1991).
12. M. Santosham, M. Wolff, R. Reid, et al., The efficacy in Navajo infants of a conjugate vaccine consisting of *Haemophilus influenzae* type b polysaccharide and *Neisseria meningitidis* outer-membrane protein complex, *N. Engl. J. Med. 324*:1767 (1991).
13. J. Ward, G. Brenneman, G. W. Letson, et al., Limited efficacy of a *Haemophilus influenzae* type b conjugate vaccine in Alaska native infants, *N. Engl. J. Med. 323*:1393 (1990).
14. Update: Prevention of *Haemophilus influenzae* type b disease, *MMWR 37*:13 (1988).
15. G. A. Weinberg and D. M. Granoff, Polysaccharide-protein conjugate vaccines for the prevention of *Haemophilus influenzae* type b disease, *J. Pediatr. 113*:621 (1988).
16. H. Peltola, T. O. Rød, K. Jónsdóttir, et al., Life-threatening *Haemophilus influenzae* infections in Scandinavia: a five-country analysis of the incidence and the main clinical and bacteriologic characteristics, *Rev. Infect. Dis. 12*:708 (1990).
17. A. K. Takala, J. Eskola, H. Peltola, et al., Epidemiology of invasive *Haemophilus influenzae* type b disease among children in Finland before vaccination with *Haemophilus influenzae* type b conjugate vaccine, *Pediatr. Infect. Dis. J. 8*:297 (1989).
18. J. I. Ward, M. K. W. Lum, D. B. Hall, et al., Invasive *H. influenzae* type b disease in Alaska: Background epidemiology for a vaccine efficacy trial, *J. Infect. Dis. 108*:887 (1986).
19. Recommendations of the Immunization Practices Advisory Committee (ACIP). *Haemophilus* b conjugate vaccines for prevention of *Haemophilus influenzae* type b disease among infants and children two months of age and older, *MMWR 40*(RR1):1 (1991).
20. Committee on Infectious Diseases, American Academy of Pediatrics, *Haemophilus influenzae* type b conjugate vaccines: recommendations for immunization of infants and children 2 months of age and older: update, *Pediatrics 88*:169 (1991).
21. S. B. Black, H. R. Shinefield, D. Lampert, et al., Safety and immunogenicity of oligosaccharide conjugate *Haemophilus influenzae* type b (HbOC) vaccine in infancy, *Pediatr. Infect. Dis. J. 10*:92 (1991).
22. J. Eskola, H. Peltola, A. Takala, et al., Protective efficacy of the *Haemophilus influenzae* type b conjugate vaccine HbOC in Finnish infants, *Program and*

Abstracts of the 30th Interscience Conference on Antimicrobial Agents and Chemotherapy, Atlanta, GA, October 1990, American Society for Microbiology, Washington, DC, 1990 (Abstract No. 60).
23. H. Peltola, T. Kilpi, and M. Anttila, Rapid disappearance of *Haemophilus influenzae* type b meningitis after routine childhood immunisation with conjugate vaccines, *Lancet 340*:592 (1992).
24. J. L. Coulehan, R. H. Michaels, C. Hallowell, et al., Epidemiology of *Haemophilus influenzae* type b disease among Navajo Indians, Public Health Rep. *99*:404 (1984).
25. H. Kayhty, H. Peltola, V. Karanko, et al., The protective level of serum antibodies to the capsular polysaccharide of *Haemophilus influenzae* type b, *J. Infect. Dis. 147*:1100 (1983).
26. P. Anderson, The protective level of serum antibodies to the capsular polysaccharide of *Haemophilus influenzae* type b, *J. Infect. Dis. 149*:1034 (1984).
27. E. D. Shapiro, and J. I. Ward, The epidemiology and prevention of disease caused by *Haemophilus influenzae* type b, *Epidemiol. Rev. 13*:113 (1991).
28. B. Fritzell, and S. Plotkin, Efficacy and safety of a *Haemophilus influenzae* type b capsular polysaccharide-tetanus protein conjugate vaccine, *J. Pediatr. 121*:355 (1992).
29. J. C. Parke, R. Schneerson, C. Reimer, et al., Clinical and immunologic responses to *Haemophilus influenzae* type b-tetanus toxoid conjugate vaccine in infants injected at 3, 5, 7, and 18 months of age, *J. Pediatr. 118*:184 (1991).

19

Risk Factors in Transmission of *Haemophilus influenzae* Type b

Aino K. Takala

National Public Health Institute, Helsinki, Finland

I. INTRODUCTION

Haemophilus influenzae type b (Hib) is a major cause of serious invasive infections in childhood. Hib is a strictly human pathogen. Transmission of Hib occurs via droplet spread followed by oropharyngeal colonization with Hib (1). Asymptomatic colonization can last for months (2,3). In some cases colonization proceeds to invasive Hib infection via mechanisms that are still poorly understood.

The epidemiology of invasive Hib disease varies considerably among populations. Low incidence rates are found among Caucasian populations in Australia and Europe, whereas up to 10-fold greater rates are found among certain ethnic groups, such as Native American and Australian populations (4–9). In populations with high incidence rates of Hib disease, the age distribution is shifted towards younger age groups (7–9). In accordance with these differences, oropharyngeal carriage of Hib in Caucasian populations has been reported to be rare among young infants, increasing up to a point prevalence rate of 3–5% in preschool and school-aged children, and declining during later life (10–12). In contrast, among Apache and Navajo Indian infants, oropharyngeal carriage of Hib starts earlier in infancy, with carriage rates of 3% among infants as young as 3 months of age (13). Carriage rates among close contacts of patients with invasive Hib disease are considerably higher, up to 30–70% (2,11,14,15), and somewhat higher (10%) among day-care attendees (3).

As much as 99% of Hib disease in different populations is endemic (16), and factors associated with the risk of primary Hib disease and its spread are thus of major public health importance. Risk factors associated with secondary spread of invasive Hib disease are largely the same as those with primary Hib disease, and, thus, factors associated with transmission of primary and secondary Hib disease are here discussed jointly.

Of all risk factors for invasive Hib disease, young age is the most important (17). Most studies also show a predominance of males (4–6). Conditions that impair host defenses as well as several genetic and racial factors have been associated with increased risk of Hib disease (9,18–21). However,

Table 1 Risk Factors for *H. influenzae* Type b Colonization, Transmission, and Disease

Increased risk for colonization and transmission
Young age
Large, crowded households
Siblings of preschool age
Day-care attendance
Concurrent viral respiratory infections
Season
Smoking of parents and other respiratory irritants
Short duration of breast feeding
Increased risk for disease
Young age
Male sex
Frequent infections in general
Concurrent viral respiratory infections
Smoking of parents
Short duration of breast feeding
Genetic factors
Selected racial/ethnic groups
Eskimos
American Indians
Blacks
Hispanics
Antibody or complement deficiencies
Sickle cell anemia
Malignancies
Decreased risk for colonization and disease
Antimicrobial treatment
H. influenzae type b conjugate vaccines

evidence to date suggests that the contribution of these to the overall risk of Hib disease are minor and that socioeconomic risk factors that largely relate to factors associated with exposure to Hib are decisive (Table 1).

II. FACTORS ASSOCIATED WITH INCREASED EXPOSURE TO Hib

A. Factors Related to Increased Contact

Crowding and increased contact between young children have been related to increased risk of invasive Hib disease in several studies (22–30). In these circumstances the transmission of infectious agents including Hib bacteria is facilitated, and the infective dose is likely to be high.

1. Siblings and Crowded Households

Factors that have been associated with increased exposure to Hib in the family setting include the presence of siblings (23–25) and crowding (21,22,25). The presence of crowded large households and especially extended family groups has been reported to be a risk factor for Hib disease among Alaskan Eskimos (31) and is probably also an important risk factor among Navajo Indians, who traditionally live in extended family groups.

Presence of siblings of elementary school age (23) or preschool age (24,25) has been found to increase the risk for invasive Hib disease. This risk factor is most important among the youngest children, with a doubling of the risk with each additional sibling (24). Preschool-aged children have the highest oropharyngeal carriage rates of Hib (10). Thus, the more siblings of this age a susceptible infant has, the more likely he or she is to acquire Hib and subsequently contract invasive Hib disease. Furthermore, the closer in age the siblings are to the young child, the more intimate the contact and the more likely the transmission of Hib. Close contact also may increase the infectious dose. This scenario is supported by results from a study in which family contacts of patients were studied for oropharyngeal carriage of Hib (32). The highest carriage rates (86%) were found for siblings of the same age as the case, namely, healthy co-twins of twin patients, indicating an intimate contact and high rate of transmission between children of the same age. Lower rates were seen among other healthy siblings of the twin patients (29%) or among age-matched healthy siblings of nontwin patients (54%). The study also found an increased (threefold) risk of primary invasive Hib disease among twins, the risk being equally high for mono- and dizygotic twins (32).

2. Day-Care Attendance

Day-care attendance provides an increased exposure to many infectious agents, including Hib (33). Contact between infants and young children in day-care is close. Thus it is likely that infectious agents are shared, leading to increased pathogen transmission and probably to transmission of a high dose of the infectious agent. Thus, day-care attendance has been found to be an important risk factor for acquiring invasive Hib disease (22–25,34). The risk is highest for the youngest children and decreases with increasing age, so that there is little increased risk for children older than approximately 2 years of age (21,22,24,25,34,35). However, one study (23) has showed an increased risk with increasing age. That study did not address special day-care practices that might explain this difference: Wenger et al. found that the use of towels or handkerchiefs to wipe the children's noses was a specific day-care practice that increased risk of invasive Hib disease at day-care centers (36). In a study that evaluated the presence of Hib bacteria in different secretions of Hib carriers, nasal secretions were most consistently positive for Hib and contained the largest numbers of Hib bacteria (37). In addition Hib bacteria survived up to 48 hours on the surface of toys that had been mouthed by children colonized with Hib (37). Thus, sharing of uncleaned toys may also facilitate transmission of Hib.

An increased risk for invasive Hib disease with increasing size of the day-care groups and increasing time spent in day care has been demonstrated in several studies (22,23,25). However, such an effect was not detected in Finland, a result probably reflecting the small group size in day-care (maximum group size is 6 for infants and is 12 for 1–2 year olds in day-care centers, and 4 to 6 in family day-care) (24,38). Also, Finnish children start day-care later in childhood than children in the United States. In Finland, there was no difference between the risk from attendance at day-care centers and family day care. A conclusion from these studies is that several characteristics including both group size and other factors (36,37) influence the intensity of transmission, exposure, and risk of contracting Hib infection.

The start of day-care attendance is associated with intensive exposure to new infectious agents and thus, could be the time when a child is most vulnerable to developing Hib disease and probably also other infectious diseases. The risk for invasive Hib disease has been shown to be significantly higher during the first month of day-care attendance than the risk from day-care during later months (24). A practical conclusion is that preventive measures are most important just before and during the first month of a child's day-care attendance.

3. Other Crowded Conditions

Although cases of secondary spread of Hib disease have been reported in chronic care institutions for children (39) and in acute-care hospitals (40), overall, secondary Hib disease in these settings is rare. Thus the risk of transmission in such settings is negligible, a result suggesting that for the spread of Hib bacteria, the contact probably needs to be rather close and intense.

B. Factors Related to Enhanced Colonization and Spread

Changes in the respiratory mucosa may increase the potential of Hib bacteria to colonize the oropharynx and also may increase the development of respiratory secretions. With increased spread of secretions, transmission of Hib bacteria is facilitated. Conditions that can increase both the colonization rate and the likelihood of spread of secretions include viral respiratory infections and exposure to respiratory irritants, e.g., smoke.

1. Viral Respiratory Infections

Influenza A and other major respiratory viruses have been demonstrated to induce changes in the epithelium of pharyngeal cells (41). In human volunteers influenza A infection has been shown to enhance attachment of Hib to the pharyngeal epithemlium (42). During such an infection, the formation of respiratory secretions is enhanced, which facilitates the transmission of the virus as well as Hib bacteria. In addition, viral respiratory infections may damage the respiratory epithelium and, thereby, increase the likelihood of bacterial invasion by impairing host defense mechanisms. Thus, in a study conducted in Finland, it is not surprising that occurrence of frequent infections in general and a history of otitis media were found to be risk factors for invasive Hib disease (24,43).

Howard et al. (44) have reported an increased rate of oropharyngeal carriage of non–type b *Haemophilus influenzae* among children with viral respiratory infection. Michaels et al. (10) also found a higher Hib carriage rate among children with respiratory infection (5.7%) than among healthy children (3.6%), but the difference was not statistically significant (10). In a recent study among Apache and Navajo Indian infants and children, carriage of Hib was twofold greater among children with symptoms of respiratory infection compared to healthy children (OR 2.0; 95% CI 1.06–3.77) (13). This study also found that the rate of upper respiratory infection in this population was high: 30% of the children who came for a well-child visit had symptoms related to an upper respiratory infection (13). Similar high rates were found among children 3 months of age and older, but were lower among those less than 3 months of age (11%). The etiology of respiratory infections in this population was not determined, but it is likely that the majority of the symptoms was a result of infection from respiratory viruses. Unlike Caucasian infants (10,12,44), oropharyngeal carriage of Hib started to occur early, with carriage rates of 3% among infants as young as 3 months of age. Frequent viral respiratory infections that occur in early infancy may be one factor that increases transmission of Hib in this native population and increases the risk for development of invasive Hib disease at an earlier age than in lower-risk groups.

Concurrent viral respiratory infections may play a further role in the spread of secondary Hib disease: as a part of a case-control study of risk factors for invasive Hib disease, the occurrence of symptoms of upper respiratory infections among cases (N = 117) and their age-, sex-, and residence-matched controls (N = 225) as well as their family members, were evaluated (43). Occurrence of symptoms of upper respiratory symptoms (fever, cough, coryza, stomatitis, conjunctivitis, and headache) was significantly higher among cases during 4 weeks before the illness than among controls. Similarly, occurrence of respiratory illness was more common among family members of cases than among family members of controls. Viral (adenovirus, influenza A and B, RSV, parainfluenza types 1, 2, and 3) etiology of these infections was evaluated in paired sera of cases. Associated cases of Hib disease (i.e., either the primary or secondary case of a case pair) more often had serological evidence of recent viral infection (50%) than did sporadic cases (13%) (OR 7.0; 95% CI, 1.6–33; p = 0.006). These results suggest that some infectious agent(s) caused symptoms among the patients and circulated among the patients' closest contacts immediately before the development of invasive Hib disease. In addition, for the development of associated Hib disease among close contacts of an index case, viral respiratory infections may be important.

2. Parental Smoking

Parental smoking is more common among parents of patients with invasive Hib disease than parents of controls (22,24,25). In a study by Vadheim et al., presence of at least two persons in the household who smoked daily was significantly associated with an increased risk of Hib disease (OR 5.7; 95% CI, 1.4–23) (21). Parental, especially maternal, smoking increases the risk of both upper and lower respiratory infections (45,46) and impairs ventilatory function (47). In such circumstances, the transmission of Hib bacteria is likely to be enhanced. Exposure to tobacco smoke also may cause damage to the respiratory mucosa, which could enhance the attachment and invasion of Hib bacteria and lead to an increased risk of invasive Hib disease (48). This mechanism also may play a role among populations that traditionally use open fire for heating their homes, e.g., native American populations (49).

C. Factors Associated with Decreased Transmission of Hib

1. Breast Feeding

In studies conducted in the United States a protective effect of breast feeding was demonstrated among infants less than 6 months of age (22,23) and among Alaskan Eskimos less than 18 months of age (31). In Finland, breast feeding for at least 6 months was found to be protective (24). The effect of breast feeding among Finnish infants less than 6 months of age could not be analyzed because of the small number of patients in this age group (5,24) and the fact that the majority of infants are breast-fed up to at least 6 months of age (50).

The mechanism of the protective effect of breast feeding is not known; it may involve the presence of anti-PRP antibodies in human milk, an enhancement of the immune responses to Hib among breast-fed infants (51–53), or an effect related to the mother staying at home with a breast-fed child, which reduces the child's outside contacts and, thus, the likelihood of exposure to Hib bacteria. In addition, human breast milk has been shown to prevent oropharyngeal colonization with *Haemophilus influenzae* (54), independent of specific antibody content of the breast milk. This effect has been reported to be associated with the casein fraction of breast milk (55,56).

2. Antimicrobial Treatment

Intravenous antimicrobial treatment of patients with invasive Hib disease (see Chapter 20) has been reported to suppress oropharyngeal colonization with Hib after 24 hours of the start of therapy (57,58), a result indicating that 24 hours of respiratory isolation is sufficient for prevention of nosocomial spread of Hib disease (58,59). Orally administered rifampin treatment has been shown to eradicate oropharyngeal colonization with Hib (15,60–62) although reaquisition may occur after treatment (15). In the absence of rifampin prophylaxis, the risk of secondary Hib disease has been reported to be highest for household contacts of susceptible age, up to 6% among contacts less than 1 year of age (29,30,63–66). The use of rifampin prophylaxis has been shown to lower the risk of secondary spread among household members (16). Until recently, rifampin prophylaxis (orally once daily for 4 days in a 20 mg/kg dose, maximal dose 600 mg/day) was recommended for all household contacts in a family with at least one child less than 4 years old (59). Furthermore, the index case should receive rifampin treatment (67). However, the American Academy of Pediatrics now considers that an otherwise healthy child who is fully immunized with Hib conjugate vaccine is at minimal risk of acquiring disease, even if exposed to a child with *H. influenzae* type b disease. Therefore, rifampin prophylaxis is no longer indicated for management of households where all contacts younger than 4 years are fully immunized.

There has been considerable controversy about prophylactic rifampin use for day-care contacts of an index case with invasive Hib disease. Rifampin prophylaxis among day-care attendees was found to reduce significantly the risk of development of secondary cases of invasive Hib disease in several studies (16,68,69). However, in subsequent studies the risk of secondary Hib disease among day-care attendees was found to be similar to the base rate of primary disease in day care and, therefore, use of rifampin prophylaxis was questioned (27,28,66). The U.S. recommendations in 1990–91 still indicated that rifampin prophylaxis should be used for all day-care contacts of an index case if two or more cases occur in a center within 60 days and children less than 2 years of age have been exposed (59,67). However, since safe and effective Hib conjugate vaccines are available for use in infancy, the highest-risk group, the role of rifampin prophylaxis is becoming less important; primary prevention of endemic disease by routine vaccination offers the best control for secondary disease. If, however, high coverage of routine Hib vaccinations is not achieved, rifampin prophylaxis remains an effective means in the prevention of secondary cases among nonvaccinated contacts.

3. Hib Conjugate Vaccines

Hib conjugate vaccines have been shown to prevent or lower oropharyngeal colonization with Hib (12,13,70–72), an effect not seen with the plain PRP vaccine (17,70). (see Chapter 22).

The lower oropharyngeal carriage of Hib in the vaccinated population decreases the opportunity for transmission in the population at large. Immunization with Hib conjugate vaccines has led to a more rapid decrease of invasive Hib disease than expected based on the direct effect of Hib conjugate vaccines on those vaccinated (73–78). Also, a decline in the incidence has been documented among age groups that did not receive Hib conjuagte vaccine, i.e., young infants and older children (73,76–78).

REFERENCES

1. E. H. Beachey, Bacterial adherence: Adhesin-receptor interactions mediating the attachment of bacteria to mucosal surfaces, *J. Infect. Dis. 143*:325 (1981).
2. R. H. Michaels, and C. W. Norden, Pharyngeal colonization with *Haemophilus influenzae* type b: a longitudinal study of families with a child with meningitis due to *Haemophilus influenzae*, *J. Infect. Dis. 136*:222 (1977).
3. T. V. Murphy, D. M. Granoff, R. N. Chrane, K. D. Olsen, S. J. Barenkamp, S. F. Dowell, and G. H. McCracken, Pharyngeal colonization with *Haemo-*

philus influenzae type b in children in a day care center without invasive disease, *J. Pediatr. 106*:712 (1985).
4. G. L. Gilbert, D. A. Clements, and S. J. Broughton, *Haemophilus influenzae* type b infections in Victoria, Australia, 1985 to 1987, *Pediatr. Infect. Dis. J. 9*:252 (1990).
5. A. K. Takala, J. Eskola, H. Peltola, and P. H. Mäkelä, Epidemiology of invasive *Haemophilus influenzae* type b disease among children in Finland before vaccination with *Haemophilus influenzae* type b conjugate vaccine, *Pediatr. Infect. Dis. J. 8*:297 (1989).
6. S. L. Cochi, C. V. Broome, and A. W. Hightower, Immunization of U.S. children with *Haemophilus influenzae* type b polysaccharide vaccine. A cost-effectiveness model of strategy assessment, *JAMA 253*: 521 (1985).
7. J. I. Ward, M. K. Lum, D. B. Hall, D. R. Silimper, and T. R. Bender, Invasive *Haemophilus influenzae* type b disease in Alaska: background epidemiology for a vaccine efficacy trial, *J. Infect. Dis. 153*:17 (1986).
8. G. A. Losonsky, M. Santosham, V. M. Sehgal, V. M. Sehgal, A. Zwahlen, and E. R. Moxon, *Haemophilus influenzae* disease in the White Mountain Apaches: molecular epidemiology of a high risk population, *Pediatr. Inf. Dis. 3*:539 (1984).
9. P. H. Mäkelä, A. K. Takala, H. Peltola, and J. Eskola. Epidemiology of invasive *Haemophilus influenzae* disease, *J. Infect. Dis. 165*(Suppl.):S2 (1992).
10. R. H. Michaels, C. S. Poziviak, F. E. Stonebraker, and C. W. Norden, Factors affecting pharyngeal *Haemophilus influenzae* type b colonization rates in children, *J. Clin. Microbiol. 4*:413 (1976).
11. D. C. Turk, Naso-pharyngeal carriage of *Haemophilus influenzae* type b, *J. Hygiene 61*:247 (1963).
12. A. K. Takala, J. Eskola, M Leinonen, H. Käyhty, A. Nissinen, E. Pekkanen, and P. H. Mäkelä, Reduction of oropharyngeal carriage of *Haemophilus influenzae* type b (Hib) in children immunized with an Hib conjugate vaccine, *J. Infect. Dis. 164*:982 (1991).
13. A. K. Takala, M. Santosham, J. Almeido-Hill, M. Wolff, W. Newcomer, R. Reid, H. Käyhty, E. Esko, and P. H. Mäkelä, Vaccination with *Haemophilus influenzae* type b meningococcal protein conjugate vaccine reduces oropharyngeal carriage of Hib among American Indian children, *J. Pediatr. Infect. Dis. 12*:593 (1993).
14. R. Heikkilä, A. K. Takala, H. Käyhty, and M. Leinonen, Latex agglutination test for the screening of *Haemophilus infuenzae* type b carriers, *J. Clin. Microbiol. 25*:1131 (1987).
15. M. P. Glode, R. S. Daum, E. G. Boies, T. L. Ballard, M. Murray, and D. M. Granoff, Effect of rifampin chemoprophylaxis on carriage eradication and new acquisition of *Haemophilus influenzae* type b in contacts, *Pediatrics 76*:537 (1985).
16. J. Band, D. W. Fraser, and G. Ajello, Prevention of *Haemophilus influenzae* type b disease, *JAMA 251*:2381 (1984).
17. H. Peltola, H. Käyhty, A. Sivonen, and P. H. Mäkelä, *Haemophilus influ-*

enzae type b capsular polysaccharide vaccine in children. A double-blind field study of 100 000 vaccinees 3 months to 5 years of age in Finland, *Pediatrics 60*:730 (1977).

18. D. M. Granoff, J. P. Pandey, E. Boies, J. Squires, R. S. Munson, and B. Suarez, Response to immunization with *Haemophilus influenzae* type b polysaccharide-pertussis vaccine and risk of Haemophilus meningitis in children with the Km (1) immunoglobulin allotype, *J. Clin. Invest. 74*:1708 (1984).
19. G. M. Petersen, D. R. Silimperi, J. I. Rotter, et al., Genetic factors in *Haemophilus influenzae* type b disease susceptibility and antibody acquisition, *J. Pediatr. 110*:228 (1987).
20. P. I. Tarr, G. Peter, Demographic factors in the epidemiology of *Haemophilus influenzae* meningitis in young children, *J. Pediatr. 92*:884 (1978).
21. C. M. Vadheim, D. P. Greenberg, N. Bordenave, L. Ziontz, P. Christenson, S. H. Waterman, and J. I. Ward, Risk factors for invasive *Haemophilus influenzae* type b in Los Angeles County children 18–60 months of age, *Am. J. Epidemiol. 136*:221 (1992).
22. S. L. Cochi, D. W. Fleming, A. W. Hightower, K. Limpakarnjanarat, R. R. Facklam, J. D. Smith, R. K. Sikes, and C. V. Broome, Primary invasive *Haemophilus influenzae* type b disease: a population-based assessment of risk factors, *J. Pediatr. 108*:887 (1986).
23. G. R. Istre, J. S. Conner, C. V. Broome, A. Hightower, and R. S. Hopkins, Risk factors for primary invasive *Haemophilus influenzae* disease: increased risk from day-care attendance and school-aged household members, *J. Pediatr. 106*:190 (1985).
24. A. K. Takala, J. Eskola, J. Palmgren, P.-R. Rönnberg, E. Kela, P. Rekola, and P. H. Mäkelä, Risk factors of invasive *Haemophilus influenzae* type b disease among children in Finland, *J. Pediatr. 115*:694 (1989).
25. D. A. Clements, I. A. Guise, S. J. MacInnes, and G. L. Gilbert, *Haemophilus influenzae* type b infections in Victoria, Australia, 1985–1989, *J. Infect. Dis. 165*(Suppl. 1):S33 (1992).
26. A. K. Takala and D. A. Clements, Socio-economic risk factors for invasive *Haemophilus influenzae* type b disease, *J. Infect. Dis. 165*(Suppl. 1):S11 (1992).
27. T. V. Murphy, J. F. Clements, J. A. Breedlove, E. J. Hanson, and G. B. Seibert, Risk of subsequent disease among day-care contacts of patients with systemic *Haemophilus influenzae* type b disease, *N. Engl. J. Med. 316*:5 (1987).
28. M. T. Osterholm, L. M. Pierson, K. E. White, T. A. Libby, J. N. Kuritsky, and J. G. McGullough, The risk of subsequent transmission of *Haemophilus influenzae* type b disease among children in day care, *N. Engl. J. Med. 316*:1 (1987).
29. M. P. Glode R. S. Daum, D. A. Goldman, F. Leclair, and A. Smith, *H. influenzae* type b meningitis: A contagious disease of children, *Br. Med. J. 280*:899 (1980).
30. J. I. Ward, D. W. Fraser, L. J. Baraff, and B. D. Plikalytis. *Haemophilus influenzae* meningitis. A national study of secondary spread in household contacts, *N. Engl. J. Med. 301*:122 (1979).

31. G. M. Petersen, D. R. Silimperi, C. Y. Chiu, and J. I. Ward, Effects of age, breast feeding, and household structure on *Haemophilus influenzae* type b disease risk and antibody acquisition in Alaskan Eskimos, *Am. J. Epidemiol. 134*:1212 (1991).
32. A. K. Takala, P.-R. Rönnberg, E. Kela, and J. Eskola. Increased risk of primary invasive *Haemophilus influenzae* type b disease in twins, *Pediatr. Infect. Dis. J. 8*:799 (1989).
33. E. L. Wald, B. Dashefsky, C. Byers, N. Guerral, and F. Taylor, Frequency and severity of infections in day care, *J. Pediatr. 112*:540 (1988).
34. T. V. Murphy, K. White, D. M. Granoff, and M. T. Osterholm, Risk of *Haemophilus influenzae* type b disease (Hibdis) in children attending day care homes in Dallas Co, TX (Dal) and Minnesota (MN) (Abstract 1142), Presented at the 30th Interscience Conference on Antimicrobial Agents and Chemotherapy, Atlanta, GA, Oct. 1990.
35. S. R. Redmond and M. E. Pichichero. *Haemophilus influenzae* type b disease. An epidemiologic study with special reference to day-care centers, *JAMA 252*:2581 (1984).
36. J. D. Wenger, L. H. Harrison, M. S. Hightower, C. V. Broome, and the *Haemophilus influenzae* study group, Day care characteristics associated with *Haemophilus influenzae* disease, *Am. J. Public. Health 80*:1455 (1990).
37. T. V. Murphy, J. F. Clements, M. Petroni, S. Conry, and L. Stetler, *Haemophilus influenzae* type b in respiratory secretions, *Pediatr. Infect. Dis. J. 8*:148 (1989).
38. Lasten päivähoito 1983. Tilastotiedotus 1985:7. (Child-care arrangements 1983 statistical report 1985:7) Sosiaalihallitus suunnittelu-ja tilastotoimisto, Helsinki, Finland, 1985.
39. M. P. Glode, M. S. Schiffer, J. B. Robbins, et al., An outbreak of H. influenzae type b meningitis in an enclosed hospital population, *J. Pediatr. 88*:36 (1976).
40. L. L. Barton, D. M. Granoff, and S. J. Barenkamp, Nosocomial spread of *H. influenzae* type b infection documented by outer membrane subtype analysis, *J. Pediatr. 102*:820 (1983).
41. J. L. Carson, A. M. Collier, and S. S. Hu, Aquired ciliary defects in nasal epithelium of children with acute viral upper respiratory infections, *N. Engl. J. Med. 312*:463 (1985).
42. V. Fainstein, D. M. Musher, and T. R. Cate, Bacterial adherence to pharyngeal cells during viral infection, *J. Infect. Dis. 141*:172 (1980).
43. A. K. Takala, O. Meurman, M. Kleemola, E. Kela, P.-R. Rönnberg, J. Eskola, and P. H. Mäkelä, Preceding respiratory infection predisposing for primary and secondary invasive *Haemophilus influenzae* type b disease, *J. Pediatr. Infect. Dis. 12*:189 (1993).
44. A. J. Howard, K. T. Dunkin, and G. W. Millar, Nasopharyngeal carriage and antibiotic resistance of *Haemophilus influenzae* in healthy children, *Epidem. Inf. 100*:193 (1988).
45. D. W. Fleming, S. L. Cochi, A. W. Hightower, and C. V. Broome, Childhood upper respiratory tract infections: to what degree is incidence affected by day-care attendance? *Pediatrics 79*:55 (1987).
46. F. A. Pedreira, V. L. Guandolo, E. J. Feroli, G. W. Mella, and I. P. Weiss,

Involuntary smoking and incidence of respiratory illness during the first year of life, *Pediatrics 75*:594 (1985).
47. I. B. Tager, S. T. Weiss, A. Munoz, B. Rosner, and F. E. Speizer, Longitudinal study of the effects of maternal smoking on pulmonary function in children, *N. Engl. J. Med. 390*:699 (1983).
48. R. Wilson, Interaction of *Haemophilus influenzae* with mucus, cilia and respiratory epithelium, *J. Infect. Dis. 165*(Suppl.):S100 (1992).
49. K. Morris, M. Morganlander, J. L. Coulehan, S. Cahagen, and V. C. Arena, Wood-burning stoves and lower respiratory tract infections in American Indian children, *Am. J. Dis. Child. 144*:105 (1990).
50. P. Verronen, Imetys on muotia (Breast-feeding is popular), *Suom Lääkäril*; *39*:1078 (1984).
51. H. F. Pabst and D. W. Spady, Effect of breast-feeding on antibody response to conjugate vaccine, *Lancet 336*:269 (1990).
52. P. Brandzaeg, Humoral immune response patterns of human mucosae: induction and relation to bacterial respiratory tract infections, *J. Infect. Dis. 165*(Suppl.):S167 (1992).
53. D. Scheifele, G. Bjornson, R. Guasparini, B. Friesen, and W. Meekison, Breastfeeding and antibody responses to routine vaccination in infants, *Lancet 340*:1406 (1992).
54. B. Andersson, O. Porras, L. Å. Hanson, T. Lagergåard, and C. Svanborg-Eden, Inhibition of attachement of *Streptococcus pneumoniae* and *Haemophilus influenzae* by human milk and receptor oligosaccharides, *J. Infect. Dis. 153*:232 (1986).
55. G. Aniansson, B. Andersson, R. Lindstedt, and C. Svanborg, Anti-adhesive activity of human casein against *Streptococcus pneumoniae* and *Haemophilus influenzae*, *Microb. Pathogenesis 8*:315 (1990).
56. H. Sabharwal, B. Lönnerdal, and C. Svanborg, A new anti-bacterial glocoprotein in human milk, Abstract presented at European Research Conferences, Research Conference on Molecular Pathogenesis of Infectious Disease: Bacterial Meningitis, Eurovillage, Obernai, France, 17–21 October, 1992.
57. J. W. Ogle, G. P. Rabalais, and M. P. Glode, Duration of pharyngeal carriage of *Haemophilus influenzae* type b in children hospitalized with systemic infections, *Pediatr. Infect. Dis. 5*:509 (1986).
58. J. Gilsdorf, Dynamics of nasopharyngeal colonization with *Haemophilus influenzae* b during antibiotic therapy, *Pediatrics 77*:242 (1986).
59. Meningitis. IIB Haemophilus meningitis, *Control of Communicable Diseases in Man* (A. S. Beneson, ed.), An official report of the American Public Health Association, Washington, DC, 1990.
60. D. Granoff, J. Gilsdorf, C. Gessert, and M. Basden, *Haemophilus influenzae* type b disease in a day-care center: erradication of carrier state by rifampin, *Pediatrics 63:* 3971 (1979).
61. J. I. Ward, G. Goreman, C. Phillips, et al., *Haemophilus influenzae* type b disease in a day care center, *J. Pediatr. 92*:713 (1978).
62. E. Shapiro and E. Wald, Efficacy of rifampicin in eliminating pharyngeal carriage of *Haemophilus influenzae* type b, *Pediatrics 66:*5 (1980).

63. A. Tejani, B. Dobias, B. S. Nagia, et al., Intrafamily spread of *Haemophilus influenzae* type b infections, *Am. J. Dis. Child. 131*:778 (1977).
64. G. A. Filice, J. S. Andrews, Jr., M. P. Hudgins, et al., Spread of *Haemophilus influenzae*. Secondary illness in household contacts of patients with *H. influenzae* meningitis, *Am. J. Dis. Child. 132*:757 (1978).
65. L. R. Campbell, A. J. Zedd, and R. H. Michaels, Household spread of infection due to *Haemophilus influenzae* type b, *Pediatrics 66*:115 (1980).
66. A. K. Takala, Epidemiology and risk factors for invasive *Haemophilus influenzae* type b (Hib) disease among children in Finland, Publications of the National Public Health Institue, Helsinki, NPHI A2/1989.
67. *Haemophilus influenzae* infections, *Report of the Committee on Infectious Diseases*, American Academy of Pediatrics, Elk Grove, IL, 1991.
68. D. W. Fleming, M. H. Leibenhaut, D. Albanes, S. L. Cochi, A. W. Hightower, S. D. Helgerson, and C. V. Broome, Secondary *Haemophilus influenzae* type b in day-care facilities. Risk factors and prevention, *JAMA 254*:509 (1985).
69. S. Makintubee, G. R. Istre, and J. I. Ward, Transmission of invasive *Haemophilus influenzae* type b disease in day care settings, J. *Pediatr. 111*:180 (1987).
70. T. V. Murphy, P. N. Pastor, F. B. Medley, M. T. Osterholm, and D. M. Granoff, Decreased Haemophilus colonization in children vaccinated with *Haemophilus influenzae* type b conjugate vaccine, *J. Pediatr 122*:517 (1993).
71. M. L. Barbour, R. Booy, D. W. Crook, H. Griffiths, H. Chapel, E. R. Moxon, and R. T. Mayon-White, *Haemophilus influenzae* type b: carriage and immunity four years after conjugate vaccine, Abstract 978, 32nd Interscience Conference on Antimicrobial Agents and Chemotherapy, Anaheim, CA, 11–14 October, 1992.
72. J. Mohle-Boetani, G. Ajello, E. Breneman, K. Deaver, C. harvey, M. Farley, D. Stephens, and J. Wenger, Oropharyngeal carriage of *Haemophilus influenzae* type b in a heavily vaccinated population of 2–5-year-olds, Abstract 1729, 32nd Interscience Conference on Antimicrobial Agents and Chemotherapy, Anaheim, CA, 11–14 October, 1992.
73. J. Eskola, A. K. Takala, H. Käyhty, E. Koskenniemi, H. Peltola, and P. H. Mäkelä, Protection achieved by *Haemophilus influenzae* type b (Hib) conjugate vaccines is better than expected on the basis of efficacy trials, Abstract 979, 32nd Interscience Conference on Antimicrobial Agents and Chemotherapy, Anaheim, CA, 1992.
74. K. E. Jonsdottir, O. Steingrimsson, and O. Olafsson, Immunization of infants in Iceland against *Haemophilus influenzae* type b, Lancet 340:252 (1992).
75. S. B. Black, H. Shinefield, and the Kaiser Permanente Pediatric Vaccine Study Group, Immunization with oligosaccharide conjugate *Haemophilus influenzae* type b (HbOC) vaccine on a large health maintenance organization population: extended follow-up and impact on *Haemophilus influenzae* disease epidemiology, *Pediatr. Infect. Dis. J. 11*:610 (1992).
76. W. G. Adams, K. A. Deaver, S. L. Cochi, B. D. Plikalytis, E. R. Zell, C. V. Broome, and J. D. Wenger, Decline of childhood *Haemophilus influenzae* type b (Hib) disease in the Hib vaccine era, *JAMA 269*:221 (1993).

77. T. V. Murphy, K. E. White, P. Pastor, L. Gabriel, F. Medley, D. M. Granoff, and M. T. Osterholm, Declining incidence of *Haemophilus influenzae* type b disease since introduction of vaccination, *JAMA 269*:246 (1993).
78. L. E. Broadhurst, R. L. Erickson, and P. W. Kelley, Decreases in invasive *Haemophilus influenzae* diseases in US army children, 1984 through 1991, *JAMA 269*:227 (1993).

20

Pathogenesis and Treatment of Infants and Children

Sheldon L. Kaplan

Baylor College of Medicine and Texas Children's Hospital, Houston, Texas

I. PATHOGENESIS

As with other bacterial infections, the initial events leading to infection of the host by *Haemophilus influenzae* type b (Hib) involve colonization of the mucosal surface of the upper respiratory tract. Both pilin and nonpilin adhesins appear to contribute to the ability of Hib to adhere to respiratory epithelial tissue. Farley et al. have shown that after being added to a human nasopharyngeal organ culture, Hib initially are bound to or entangled by mucus above the epithelial surface (1). Hib also are seen attached to nonciliated cells. At this early stage piliated organisms have a growth advantage over nonpiliated isolates (2). In the infant rat model a preceding viral infection enhances the intensity of nasal colonization by Hib (3). A prior or concomitant viral upper respiratory infection is also very common in children with Hib meningitis (see Chapter 19) (4). In organ culture ciliary activity early on is diminished and ciliated cells are damaged and sloughed. These findings may be related to the lipopolysaccharide (LPS) of Hib, since no Hib are attached to the ciliated cells. Twelve hours into the organ culture infection, following invasion of the mucosal surface at the epithelial cell separation, Hib were noted intercellularly (Fig. 1). During invasion nonpiliated bacteria had a selective advantage over piliated Hib. Finally at 24 hours, bacteria were seen in the subepithelium adjacent to lymphoid follicles. Experiments in the infant rat model also suggest that

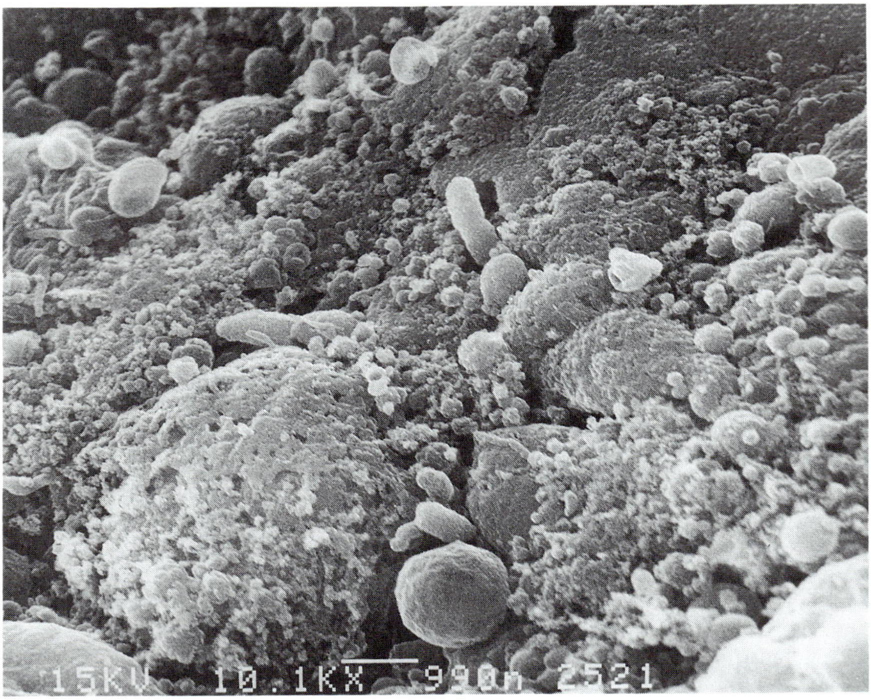

Figure 1 Scanning electron micrograph of nonpiliated *H. influenzae* type b (strain #1007) interaction with human nasopharyngeal organ culture. After 24 hours of incubation, intercellular invasion of the muscosal surface by Hib is observed. (Photograph courtesy of Monica M. Farley, M.D., Veterans Administration Medical Center and the Division of Infectious Diseases, Department of Medicine, Emory University School of Medicine, Atlanta, GA.)

Hib LOS contributes in some way to the ability of Hib to invade nasal epithelia (5,6). Phase variation for pilus production is probably an important means by which Hib optimally adhere, colonize, and ultimately invade respiratory epithelial barriers (7). Loss of piliation appears to be advantageous once Hib has entered into the bloodstream. What role the IgA_1 protease produced by Hib has in this sequence of events is unclear (see Chapter 8).

Once past the respiratory epithelium, Hib appears to penetrate pharyngeal vessels directly to lead to bacteremia (8). In the bloodstream Hib multiply intravascularly or are cleared depending upon the immune status of the host. Dissemination of Hib from the bloodstream to cause extravascular infection presumably occurs after a sufficient density of organisms in blood circulate for an adequate period of time (9). In the infant rat and primate models at least 10^3 organisms [colony-forming units (CFU)] per ml in blood for at least 6 hours are necessary before meningitis is observed (10,11). Similarly, in children LaScolea et al. noted that 50% of children with Hib meningitis had $>10^3$ CFU/ml of Hib on admission, whereas no child with uncomplicated epiglottitis had colony densities in this range (12).

II. MENINGITIS

H. influenzae type b organisms egress from the bloodstream to peripheral sites causing specific infections, although our understanding of this process is just beginning to develop. In several animal models Hib first enters the cerebrospinal fluid (CSF) of the central nervous system via the choroid plexus, where bacteria reach ventricular fluid through "leaky" inflamed capillaries (13). Patrick et al. have studied the effects of Hib on primary cultures of bovine brain microvascular endothelial cells (14). Both live Hib or Hib LOS caused marked cytotoxicity of the brain endothelial cells. This effect was blocked by a monoclonal antibody against CD14, a molecule involved with the interaction of LPS and monocytes, suggesting that CD14-dependent pathways are contributing to the effects of LPS to disrupt the blood-brain barrier. These findings may help one understand how Hib enters into ventricular fluid from choroid plexus capillaries, as well as the subsequent pathophysiological changes occurring during meningitis.

Once Hib organisms have entered the ventricular fluid, they are able to multiply in the relative absence of host defenses and spread throughout the CSF. Production of cytokines such as tumor necrosis factor (TNF) and interleukin-1*B* (IL-1) within the central nervous system is stimulated by Hib, especially the LOS component that is released to a greater degree following therapy with bactericidal antibiotics. These cytokines are instrumental in mediating the inflammatory response that leads to the characteristic CSF findings of Hib meningitis—increased white blood cell count, depressed glucose, and increased protein concentrations. Concentrations of TNF, IL-1, interferon, platelet-activating factor, and other mediators are elevated in the CSF of children with Hib meningitis and, in some studies, are correlated with the conventional parameters of meningeal inflammation (16–19). These molecular events are discussed in greater detail in Chapter 8 as well as review articles (20,21).

Alteration of the blood-brain barrier is primarily a result of the separation of tight junctions between endothelial cells. Protein and fluid enter past these intercellular junctions into brain parenchyma causing vasogenic edema. Cytotoxic edema (swelling of neural elements), presumably related to the effects of bacterial toxins or other factors, is also present. Impairment of CSF reabsorption via arachnoid villi leads to an increase in the volume of CSF within the intracranial vault. Transient ventricular dilation in children with bacterial meningitis can be detected by computed tomography and is evidence of these changes in CSF hydrodynamics (22).

The cerebral edema and increased CSF volume contribute to the development of the increased intracranial pressure (ICP) that is associated with bacterial meningitis. Since cerebral perfusion pressure is influenced by ICP, an increase in ICP may impair cerebral blood flow (23). In three infant primates with Hib meningitis blood flow to the cortex was decreased compared to two control animals (13). The only study of cerebral blood flow in children with bacterial meningitis measured total and regional cerebral blood flow (CBF) by stable xenon computed tomography (24). Measurements were obtained within 24–48 hours of hospitalization. Twenty children between 1 week and 8 years of age were included; eight children had Hib meningitis. Within the first 24 hours, signs and symptoms observed included seizures ($n = 15$), coma ($n = 12$), respiratory impairment ($n = 10$), cranial nerve dysfunction ($n = 8$), and herniation ($n = 4$). In 13 children CBF (62 ± 20 ml/min/100 g) was considered to be within the normal range for each age, although in many of the patients localized regions of decreased flow were noted (number not specified). In contrast, total and most regional blood flow were significantly decreased in 5 children. Thus, even in a group of children severely ill with bacterial meningitis, total CBF was within the normal range for the majority. Other findings in this study suggested that autoregulation of CBF was preserved. Hyperventilation in 6 of 7 children significantly decreased total CBF and the majority of regional flows. Questions regarding the optimal management of increased ICP during bacterial meningitis are raised by this study. Nevertheless, intubation and hyperventilation, along with mannitol administration, may be life saving for cerebral herniation. Major brain parenchymal injuries occur as a result of vasculitis and spasm of cerebral vessels, occlusion of the lumen, and subsequent infarction of supplied tissue (25). CT scan of the head may demonstrate such infarction associated with a hemiparesis.

Sensorineural hearing loss is an important sequela of Hib meningitis (26,27). The pathogenesis of this deafness includes the development of a bacterial labyrinthitis. In an infant rat model, Hib reach the cochlea via the cochlear aqueduct, a pathway connecting CSF and perilymphatic fluid (28). Bacteria also may invade around the eighth cranial nerve by way of the internal auditory canal with a subsequent inflammatory response in this region. Furthermore, bacterial toxins or alterations in blood flow may contribute to the destruction of the cochlear elements, such as the organ of Corti, or lead to calcification of the cochlear channels. This process appears to occur early in the course of Hib meningitis and is correlated with a low CSF glucose on admission and delayed sterilization of CSF following initiation of antimicrobial therapy (29). Since vestibular damage also may occur as a result of labyrinthitis, ataxia is very common in children with sensorineural hearing loss secondary to Hib meningitis (30).

III. SEPTIC ARTHRITIS

Prior to infant immunization with Hib conjugate vaccines, Hib was the most common etiology of septic arthritis in children under 2 years of age. Hib enters the joint space via a hematogenous route, but the details of this process are not known. The synovial membrane has a blood flow through vessels without a limiting basement membrane and, presumably, Hib egress from this area into the synovial fluid (31). Once in the joint space, events similar to those within the CNS appear to occur. Sáez-Llorens et al. injected various doses of purified Hib LOS into the knees of rabbits (32). A dose-dependent increase of the leukocyte count and protein concentration was observed. Intraarticular Hib LOS also was associated with detection of IL-1β and TNF activity in synovial lavage fluids. Concomitant injection of antibody to rabbit TNF and IL-1β blunted the inflammatory response within the joint space. Thus, in septic arthritis, Hib LOS also is an important stimulus for cytokine production and the resulting synovial inflammatory response. The same investigators detected both TNF and IL-1β in the synovial fluid from 5 of 5 children with Hib septic arthritis (33).

Reactive arthritis, in contrast to septic arthritis, also may develop during the course of Hib meningitis. In such patients, typically the onset of arthritis is several days into therapy, and cultures and Gram stain of synovial fluid are negative (34).

IV. CELLULITIS

The pathogenesis of Hib cellulitis is unclear. Cellulitis due to Hib is most commonly noted in the head and neck area, especially the buccal region. Some authors have proposed spread of infection via the lymphatics from the middle ear cavity to the ipsilateral buccal soft tissue. However, in one study only 23 of 72 children (32%) had buccal cellulitis with an ipsilateral otitis media. Another route of infection may be by direct invasion of the mucous membranes, although evidence of mucosal lesions is seen in only a minority of patients (35).

V. EPIGLOTTITIS

Epiglottitis is associated with marked swelling and edema of the epiglottis and surrounding structures (36). Although many organisms can cause epiglottitis, Hib was by far the leading cause in children. Again, the pathogenesis of the Hib epiglottitis is unclear but is thought to be due to direct invasion of the epiglottis. The facts that the mean age of children with epiglottitis is higher than that of children with other Hib infections and the density of Hib in blood is lower in children with Hib epiglottitis than observed in children with Hib meningitis suggest that some preceding immunity may play a role in the evolution of this infection. Similar inflammation and swelling of the uvula can occur, presumably following direct invasion of the uvula by Hib (37).

VI. PNEUMONIA

Acute Hib pneumonia is characterized by a variety of roentgenographic manifestations, including pleural effusions, which may be seen in up to 75% of patients (38,39). Upper respiratory infections such as otitis media are noted frequently in these children as well. It is thought that Hib colonizing the upper respiratory tract are aspirated or invade past local barriers (such as ciliated cells, secretory IgA, etc) to invade lung parenchyma. Bacteremia occurs secondary to the pulmonary infection. In normal adult C57BL/6 mice, a large inoculum of Hib placed directly into the trachea results in a progressive pneumonia (40). In the absence of antibiotic therapy in these animals, studies of pulmonary clearance of Hib revealed that the bacterial counts from lung tissue did not decrease over 54 hours, a result suggesting that normal defenses could contain, but not clear, this Hib infection. Bacteremia occurred following the development of sublethal or lethal pneumonia.

VII. OTHER INFECTIONS

Hib also has been associated with epididymitis, endophthalmitis, endocarditis, peritonitis, tracheitis, pericarditis, osteomyelitis, soft tissue abscesses, and CSF shunt infections (41). Most of these infections are related to spread of Hib from the bloodstream to the involved site. Besides direct tissue involvement by Hib, hematological alterations have been described due to Hib infections. Children with Hib meningitis have a lower hemoglobin at admission and develop lower hemoglobin concentrations during hospitalization than children with other forms of bacterial meningitis (42). The mechanisms by which anemia develop appear related to decreased deformability of erythrocytes and hemolysis and changes in iron metabolism by Hib infections (as with other infections) with subsequent decrease in erythrocyte production (43,44). Platelet function is also affected by Hib. Bleeding time and adenosine diphosphate–induced aggregation are altered in some children with Hib meningitis (45). Endotoxin from other bacteria are associated with similar platelet defects. Thrombocytosis is quite common at the end of therapy for Hib meningitis, but it has no implications with respect to an increased risk for thrombotic events.

VIII. ANTIMICROBIAL SUSCEPTIBILITY

Prior to 1972, isolates of Hib were always susceptible to ampicillin (46). However, in 1972 in Europe and in 1974 in the United States, the initial descriptions of ampicillin-resistant isolates of Hib were reported. Subsequently ampicillin resistance in Hib became widely recognized and appeared to become increasingly common (47). In some studies ampicillin-resistant isolates were recovered more commonly in patients who had received antibiotics prior to culture compared to children who had not received recent antimicrobial therapy (48). Ninety-five percent of ampicillin-resistant Hib isolates produce a plasmid-mediated β-lactamase enzyme (49). The remainder are resistant via alteration of penicillin-binding proteins; these organisms may be more difficult to detect in the routine microbiology laboratory.

Chloramphenicol resistance in Hib was first reported in 1977 and was subsequently shown to be due to an acetyl transferase enzyme (CAT) capable of inactivating chloramphenicol. Both β-lactamase and CAT enzymes are plasmid mediated and, thus, combined ampicillin-chloramphenicol resistance in Hib has become a problem, especially in Spain, which has the highest prevalence of β-lactamase-producing Hib in Europe.

Resistance to third-generation cephalosporins has not been a clinical concern (50). Isolates of Hib resistant to rifampin have been reported. In some instances resistance may have been related to failure of rifampin prophylaxis to prevent secondary cases of Hib infection.

The most recent U.S. collaborative study of antimicrobial resistance among clinical isolates of Hib was conducted in 1986 by 30 hospital-based microbiology laboratories and one national private, independent laboratory (51). Among 573 isolates recovered from children and 184 from adults, the overall rate of β-lactamase production was 32%. The rate of resistant strains that were β-lactamase-negative (MIC $\geq$ 2.0 μg/ml) was 1%. Two Hib isolates were resistant to both ampicillin and chloramphenicol, five were resistant to trimethoprim-sulfamethoxazole, and nine were considered resistant to rifampin.

The Centers for Disease Control conducted surveillance for invasive Hib infections in five states and Los Angeles County, California for 1986 (52). Hib was responsible for 964 cases of bacterial meningitis. Overall, 342 of 1019 (33.6%) Hib isolates from all systemic disease from children and adults were ampicillin-resistant. One combined ampicillin-chloramphenicol resistant isolate was reported. In a European collaborative study, 78 laboratories from 9 countries between 1988 and 1989 contributed 602 Hib isolates of which 10.5% were β-lactamase positive (53). The frequency of β-lactamase production varied between 0% in Italy to 31.2% in Spain. Only 54 and 60 Hib isolates were recovered from blood and CSF cultures, respectively.

IX. THERAPY

As in most cases, the antimicrobial therapy of infections due to Hib is based upon three major factors: (a) activity of the specific antibiotic against Hib isolates, (b) concentration of antibiotic achieved at the sites of interest, and (c) safety profile of the antibiotic (Table 1) (54–56). For many years ampicillin or chloramphenicol were the major agents employed for treating systemic Hib disease. Ampicillin and amoxicillin remain important agents in treatment of infections due to susceptible strains. Chloramphenicol is the drug of choice for children with a history of anaphylactic reactions to penicillins or cephalosporins. Chloramphenicol also can be administered orally for selected patients (58). However, because of the potential for adverse effects of chloramphenicol (bone marrow suppression, rare aplastic anemia, myocardial effects, interaction with many other drugs, etc.) and the need to monitor serum concentrations, other agents are currently considered first-line therapy for infections due to ampicillin-resistant Hib (59).

For the treatment of Hib meningitis, the efficacy of cefotaxime and ceftriaxone is equivalent to that of ampicillin or chloramphenicol (57). Cefotaxime and ceftriaxone are favored when ampicillin-resistant Hib are isolated. Cefotaxime is also effective when combined ampicillin-chloram-

Table 1 Minimal Inhibitory Concentrations Against *H. influenze* Type b and CSF Concentrations of Selected Antibiotics

	MIC (μg/ml)	CSF concentrations (μg/ml)
Ampicillin	0.5–1.0[a]	3.4 (0–50)
Cefotaxime	0.04	2.2–3.7
Ceftazidime	0.02	6.7 (0–32)
Ceftriaxone	<0.03	4.6 (1–9.1)
Chloramphenicol	2.0–8.0	6–13
Imipenem[b]	.02–0.8	1.9
Cefuroxime[b]	0.3–0.6	6.4 (11.1–18.8)

[a]Ampicillin-susceptible strains only.
[b]Do not use for meningitis.

phenicol–resistant Hib are encountered (60). In general, ceftriaxone is associated with gallbladder sludge and more frequent diarrhea than cefotaxime, but the former has the advantage of less frequent administration (one or two times daily). Cefuroxime should not be used for treatment of Hib meningitis since it is associated with delayed sterilization of CSF and more frequent hearing loss than these other agents (61). Imipenem/cilastatin is not recommended since this combination has an increased incidence of drug-related seizure activity (62). Although ceftazidime can be used successfully for treating Hib meningitis, experience with this agent is greatly limited compared to that for cefotaxime or ceftriaxone. The combination of ampicillin and sulbactam, a β-lactamase inhibitor, should also be avoided for treatment of meningitis and is not yet approved for use in children. In one unpublished study of ampicillin/sulbactam vs. standard therapy for bacterial meningitis in children, there appeared to more neurological sequelae in the ampicillin/sulbactam group, and the study was terminated.

For infections outside the central nervous system, several of the agents already discussed, including cefuroxime, can be administered parenterally. In many instances some combination of a third-generation cephalosporin, plus nafcillin or oxacillin, is provided to cover optimally the common pediatric pathogens until the culture results are known.

Surgical drainage is also key for several infections. Optimal management of Hib pericarditis includes surgically removing pericardium to promote adequate drainage, avoid tamponade, and prevent constrictive pericarditis (63). Surgical drainage of septic arthritis of the hip is recommended to protect the blood supply to the head of the femur, which can be compromised during this infection. Needle aspiration(s) is all that is generally required for management of Hib infections in other joints. Intubation is mandatory to manage children with Hib epiglottitis.

The optimal management of outpatients with fever and possible occult bacteremia remains uncertain. Retrospective reviews of occult Hib bacteremia are not in agreement as to the risk of continued bacteremia and subsequent development of focal infection, despite improvement in clinical appearance, loss of fever, and treatment with an appropriate oral antibiotic (64–66). The value of a single dose of an agent such as ceftriaxone followed by oral therapy in preventing invasive Hib disease in children with occult Hib bacteremia is not known. Certainly, close communication with the family and follow-up are necessary in an outpatient with a positive blood culture for Hib. Obviously, after the blood culture is reported to be growing possible Hib, the child should be seen as soon as feasible. If on follow-up the child is ill-appearing, febrile, or has developed focal infection(s), full evaluation, including performing a lumbar puncture and obtaining repeat blood cultures, hospitalization, and prompt initiation of treatment with intravenous antibiotics, is undertaken. Even if the child is afebrile and well appearing, close follow-up and repeated blood culture are recommended. Despite these reassuring clinical findings, bacteremia may persist and focal infection can develop.

X. DURATION OF ANTIMICROBIAL THERAPY

For many infections the duration of antibiotic therapy is based upon clinical experience and judgment, since studies to support such recommendations are limited. Nevertheless, for Hib infections these recommendations appear reasonable. Most uncomplicated infections are treated for 10 days. Septic arthritis is usually treated for 14 days. Some authorities recommend 7 days of treatment for Hib meningitis, although I prefer 10 days. Children with Hib meningitis may continue to be febrile for up to 8 or 9 days despite adequate treatment and still remain within a normal range for duration of fever. Usually, the magnitude of the fever begins to decrease. Also, as long as such a child is clinically improving and has no other manifestations of infection other than persistent fevers, I generally recommend continuing antibiotics for up to 14 days. Usually a CT scan does not help in determining the source of persistent fever in these instances. However, performing a complete physical examination may reveal another source of the fever, such as acquisition of a viral respiratory infection or an inflamed area around an intravenous site.

Antimicrobial therapy for Hib meningitis should be provided entirely by parenteral route (an exception is the use of oral chloramphenicol). For other infections, therapy can often be completed by continuing intravenous therapy on a home care program or by administering an acceptable oral antibiotic once the child has responded satisfactorily to parenteral therapy in the hospital. Guidelines for selecting patients and families who are suitable for outpatient management should be followed (67). Selection is less of a problem when an ampicillin-susceptible isolate is encountered, since oral therapy with amoxicillin is well tolerated and effective concentrations can be achieved to complete therapy for bacteremia or septic arthritis. With the exception of chloramphenicol, oral therapy for ampicillin-resistant Hib infection is not as certain. Trimethoprim-sulfamethoxazole, cefaclor, and amoxicillin-clavulanate have been used in these cases. Cefuroxime-axetil would seem ideal, but no pediatric suspension is available. The data regarding "step-down" therapy using cefixime, cefpodoxime, or other newer agents are too scanty to recommend their use for systemic Hib infections. Quinolone therapy should be avoided in growing children.

XI. ADJUNCTIVE THERAPY

Since the host's inflammatory response may, in part, be responsible for the pathogenesis of neurological sequelae related to Hib meningitis, attempts to modify this response have been undertaken. Two published studies have suggested that treatment with dexamethasone, when administered sometime after (up to 12–24 hours) or just before the first dose of parenteral antibiotics, may decrease overall neurological sequelae of Hib meningitis (68,69). In these studies, levels of some cytokines measured in CSF 18–30 hours after the initial doses were significantly decreased in children who received dexamethasone compared to the levels in the CSF from control children (16). Based on these studies, the Committee on Infectious Diseases of the American Academy of Pediatrics suggested that treatment with dexamethasone (dose 0.15 mg/kg/dose q 6h × 16 doses) may decrease the likelihood of developing deafness after *H. influenzae* type b meningitis and that "currently, individual consideration of dexamethasone is recommended for bacterial meningitis in infants and children 2 months and older after the physician has weighed the benefits and possible risks. The utility of dexamethasone in treating pneumococcal or meningococcal meningitis is not yet known" (70). If dexamethasone is administered, H_2-blockers such as ranitidine should be provided as well to decrease the likelihood of developing serious gastrointestinal bleeding. Furthermore, the physician should recognize that fever may recur once dexamethasone has been discontinued.

Three additional unpublished studies have been performed to determine the safety and efficacy of dexamethasone therapy in patients with bacterial meningitis. In the Swiss multicenter study, 115 children with bacterial meningitis received ceftriaxone with or without dexamethasone (0.4 mg/kg/dose) every 12 hours for 2 days (71). The first dose of placebo or dexamethasone was given 10 minutes prior to the ceftriaxone dose. *H. influenzae* type b, *N. meningitidis*, and *S. pneumoniae* were identified in 76, 27, and 11 children, respectively. At follow-up 5 of 55 placebo-treated and 3 of 60 dexamethasone-treated children had one or more neurological sequelae ($p = 0.07$). Three children in the placebo group and one child in the dexamethasone group were bilaterally deaf.

The placebo-controlled trial conducted in Canada enrolled 101 children with bacterial meningitis (72). The dexamethasone dose was the same as for the study by Lebel et al. (68) but was administered a mean of 11 hours after the first ceftriaxone dose. Approximately 60% of the children had *H. influenzae* type b meningitis, 20% had *S. pneumoniae* meningitis, and 12% had *N. meningitidis* meningitis. There were no differences in neurological abnormalities, including deafness, between the study groups. One child receiving dexamethasone developed a bowel perforation requiring surgery.

In the United States multicenter study, 74 children received placebo and 69 children received dexamethasone (dose as in the Lebel study) a mean of 2 hours (all within 4 hours) from the first ceftriaxone dose (73). Approximately 60% of the children had *H. influenzae* type b meningitis, 23% had *S. pneumoniae* meningitis, and 17% had *N. meningitidis* meningitis. Overall, there were no differences in neurological or audiological outcome, although for children with *H. influenzae* type b meningitis, no child receiving dexamethasone versus five in the placebo group were bilaterally deaf ($p = 0.02$). However, more children in the placebo than in the dexamethasone group had a hearing loss detected within 24 hours of admission by auditory brain stem response testing, which may have confounded this analysis.

My overall conclusion from these studies is that dexamethasone decreases hearing loss and possibly other neurological sequelae for children with *H. influenzae* type b meningitis. However, the numbers of children with other forms of bacterial meningitis in these studies were too small to come to any firm conclusion regarding the efficacy of dexamethasone. Use of other anti-inflammatory agents has been evaluated in animal models of Hib meningitis, but clinical trials of their efficacy in children with Hib meningitis probably can no longer be conducted in countries where Hib conjugate vaccines are routinely administered to infants, since the incidence of disease has fallen so dramatically (74,75).

Prior to introduction of vaccination, *H. influenzae* type b was a relatively common cause of septic shock in children. In one study Hib was the most common pathogen isolated from otherwise normal children in septic shock managed in a pediatric intensive care unit (76). Use of antibiotic treatment, appropriate fluid administration, and vasoactive drugs such as dopamine or dobutamine are critical for successful therapy of septic shock due to Hib. Adjunctive measures such as treatment with monoclonal antibodies to core lipopolysaccharide and lipid A have been studied in adults with life-threatening infections due to gram-negative enteric bacteria. One antibody, HA-1A, appeared to decrease mortality in adults with proven gram-negative bacteremia and septic shock (77). However, a second trial of HA-1A in adults did not confirm this finding. Whether this antibody or other agents may be beneficial in children with septic shock due to gram-negative organisms including *H. influenzae* type b is uncertain (78). In a multicenter study of the pharmacokinetics and safety of HA-1A conducted in children between December 1990 and November 1991, only one of 42 children with presumed gram-negative septic shock had disease due to *H. influenzae* type b (79). Perhaps HA-1A will prove to be efficacious for meningococcal sepsis, since it is very doubtful that any meaningful study can be completed for its use in Hib infection.

Much of what I have written in this chapter will be predominantly of historical interest to physicians caring for children in the post–Hib conjugate vaccine era. Indeed, it is likely that at some point our initial approach to empiric antimicrobial therapy will change such that including antibiotics to cover for Hib will not be automatic. This change will mark a truly remarkable event. Both pediatricians and the families for whom they care owe a debt of thanks to the individuals responsible for the development of the Hib conjugate vaccines. Much agonizing and suffering by both groups as a result of Hib infections can now be largely prevented.

REFERENCES

1. M. M. Farley, D. S. Stephens, M. H. Mulks, M. D. Cooper, J. V. Bricker, S. S. Mirra, and A. Wright, Pathogenesis of IgA1 protease-producing and nonproducing *Haemophilus influenzae* in human nasopharyngeal organ cultures, *J. Infect. Dis. 154*:752 (1986).
2. M. M. Farley, D. S. Stephens, S. L. Kaplan, and E. O. Mason, Jr., Pilus-and non-pilus-mediated interactions of *Haemophilus influenzae* type b with human erythrocytes and human nasopharyngeal mucosa, *J. Infect. Dis. 161*:274 (1990).
3. R. H. Michaels and R. L. Myerowitz, Viral enhancement of nasal colonization with *Haemophilus influenzae* type b in the infant rat, *Pediatr. Res. 17*:472 (1983).
4. S. L. Kaplan, L. H. Taber, A. L. Frank, and R. D. Feigin, Nasopharyngeal viral isolates in children with *Haemophilus influenzae* type b meningitis, *J. Pediatr. 99*:591 (1981).
5. A. P. Johnson and T. J. Inzana, Loss of ciliary activity in organ cultures of rat trachea treated with lipo-oligosaccharide from *Haemophilus influenzae*, *J. Med. Microbiol. 22*:265 (1986).
6. S. L. Kaplan, E. P. Hawkins, T. J. Inzana, C. C. Patrick, and E. O. Mason, Jr., Contribution of *Haemophilus influenzae* type b lipopolysaccharide to pathogenesis of infection, *Microb. Pathogenesis 5*:55 (1988).
7. S. L. Kaplan, E. O. Mason, Jr., and B. L. Wiedermann, Role of adherence in the pathogenesis of *Haemophilus influeanzae* type b infection in infant rats, *Infect. Immun. 42*:612 (1983).
8. L. G. Rubin and E. R. Moxon, Pathogenesis of bloodstream invasion with *Haemophilus influenzae* type b, *Infect. Immun. 41*:280 (1983).
9. L. G. Rubin, A. Zwahlen, and E. R. Moxon, Role of intravascular replication in the pathogenesis of experimental bacteremia due to *Haemophilus influenzae* type b, *J. Infect. Dis. 152*:307 (1985).
10. P. T. Ostrow, E. R. Moxon, N. Vernon, and R. Kapko, Pathogenesis of bacterial meningitis. Studies on the route of meningeal invasion following *Haemophilus influenzae* inoculation of infant rats, *Lab. Invest.* 40:678 (1979).

11. D. W. Scheifele, R. S. Daum, V. P. Syriopoulou, D. R. Averill, and A. L. Smith, *Haemophilus influenzae* bacteremia and meningitis in infant primates, *J. Lab. Clin. Med. 95*:450 (1980).
12. L. J. LaScolea, Jr., S. V. Rosales, R. C. Welliver, and R. L. Ogra, Mechanisms underlying the development of meningitis or epiglottitis in children after *Haemophilus influenzae* type b bacteremia, *J. Infect. Dis.* 151:1162 (1985).
13. A. L. Smith, J. E. Hass, M. C. Roberts, T. L. Stull, P. M. Mendelman, Mechanisms of *Haemophilus influenzae* type b meningitis, *Bacterial Meningitis* (M. A. Sande, A. L. Smith, and R. K. Root, eds.), Churchill Livingstone, New York, 1985, p. 11.
14. D. Patrick, J. Betts, E. A. Frey, R. Prameya, K. Dorovini-Zis, and B. B. Finlay, *Haemophilus influenzae* lipopolysaccharide disrupts confluent monolayers of bovine brain endothelial cells via a serum-dependent cytotoxic pathway, *J. Infect. Dis. 165*:865 (1992).
15. M. Arditi, L. Ables, and R. Yogev, Cerebrospinal fluid endotoxin levels in children with *H. influenzae* meningitis before and after administration of intravenous ceftriaxone, *J. Infect. Dis* 160:1005 (1989).
16. M. M. Mustafa, M. H. Lebel, O. Ramilo, K. D. Olsen, J. S. Reisch, B. Beutler, and G. H. McCracken, Jr., Correlation of interleukin-1β and cachectin concentrations in cerebrospinal fluid and outcome from bacterial meningitis, *J. Pediatr. 115*:208 (1989).
17. M. Arditi, K. R. Manogue, M. Caplan, and R. Yogev, Cerebrospinal fluid cachectin/tumor necrosis factor-α and platelet-activating factor concentrations and severity of bacterial meningitis in children, *J. Infect. Dis. 162*:139 (1990).
18. T. Chonmaitree and S. Baron, Bacteria and viruses induce production of interferon in the cerebrospinal fluid of children with acute meningitis: A study of 57 cases and review, *Rev. Infect. Dis. 13*:1061(1991).
19. M. K. Sharief, M. Ciardi, and E. J. Thompson, Blood-brain barrier damage in patients with bacterial meningitis: Association with tumor necrosis factor-α but not interleukin 1-β, *J. Infect. Dis. 166*:350 (1992).
20. X. Sáez-Llorens, O. Ramilo, M. M. Mustafa, J. Mertsola, and G. H. McCracken, Jr., Molecular pathophysiology of bacterial meningitis: Current concepts and therapeutic implications, *J. Pediatr. 116*:671 (1990).
21. V. Quagliarello and W. M. Scheld, Bacterial meningitis: Pathogenesis, pathophysiology, and progress, *N. Engl. J. Med. 327*:864 (1992).
22. J. Stovring and R. D. Snyder, Computed tomography in childhood bacterial meningitis, *J. Pediatr. 96*:820 (1980).
23. K. J. Goitein and I. Tamir, Cerebral perfusion pressure in central nervous system infections of infancy and childhood, *J. Pediatr. 103*:40 (1983).
24. S. Ashwal, W. Stringer, L. Tomasi, S. Schneider, J. Thompson, and R. Perkin, Cerebral blood flow and carbon dioxide reactivity in children with bacterial meningitis, *J. Pediatr. 117*:523(1990).
25. M. Igarashi, R. C. Gilmartin, B. Gerald, F. Wilburn, and J. T. Jabbour, Cerebral arteritis and bacterial meningitis, *Arch. Neurol. 41*:531, (1984).

26. P. R. Dodge, H. Davis, R. D. Feigin, S. J. Holmes, S. L. Kaplan, D. P. Jubelirer, B. W. Stechenberg, and S. K. Hirsh, Prospective evaluation of hearing impairment as a sequela of acute bacterial meningitis, *N. Engl. J. Med. 311*:869 (1984).
24. A. B. Wolff and S. C. Brown, Demographics of meningitis-induced hearing impairment: Implications for immunization of children against *Haemophilus influenzae* type b, *Am. Ann. Deaf.* 131:26 (1987).
28. B. L. Wiedermann, E. P. Hawkins, G. S. Johnson, L. B. Lamberth, E. O. Mason, and S. L. Kaplan, Pathogenesis of labyrinthitis associated with *Haemophilus influenzae* type b meningitis in infant rats, *J. Infect. Dis. 153*:27(1986).
29. S. L. Kaplan, F. I. Catlin, T. Weaver, and R. D. Feigin, Onset of hearing loss in children with bacterial meningitis, *Pediatrics 73*:575 (1984).
30. S. L. Kaplan, J. Goddard, M. V. Kleeck, F. I. Catlin, and R. D. Feigin, Ataxia and deafness in children due to bacterial meningitis, *Pediatrics 68*:8 (1981).
31. D. L. Goldenberg and J. I. Reed, Bacterial arthritis, *N. Engl. J. Med. 312*:764 (1985).
32. X. Sáez-Llorens, H. S. Jafari, K. D. Olsen, H. Nariuchi, E. J. Hansen, and G. H. McCracken, Jr., Induction of suppurative arthritis in rabbits by *Haemophilus* endotoxin, tumor necrosis factor-α and interleukin-1β, *J. Infect. Dis. 163*:1267 (1991).
33. X. Sáez-Llorens, M. M. Mustafa, O. Ramilo, C. Fink, B. Beutler, and J. D. Nelson, Tumor necrosis factor α and interleukin 1β in synovial fluid of infants and children with suppurative arthritis, *Am. J. Dis. Child. 144*:353 (1990).
34. P. J. Rush, A. Shore, R. Inman, R. Gold, T. Jadavji, and B. Laski, Arthritis associated with *Haemophilus influenzae* meningitis: Septic or reactive? *J. Pediatr. 109*:412 (1986).
35. S. A. Chartrand and C. J. Harrison, Buccal cellulitis reevaluated, *Am. J. Dis. Child. 140*:891 (1986).
36. R. S. Daum and A. L. Smith, Epiglottitis (Supraglottitis), *Textbook of Pediatric Infectious Diseases* (R. D. Feigin and J. D. Cherry, eds.), W. B. Saunders Co, Philadelphia, 1992, p. 197.
37. K. I. Li, S. Kiernan, E. R. Wald, and J. S. Reidly, Isolated uvulitis due to *Haemophilus influenzae* type b, *Pediatrics 74*:1054 (1984).
38. B. I. Asmar, T. L. Slovis, J. O. Reed, and A. S. Dajani, *Haemophilus influenzae* type b pneumonia in 43 children, *J. Pediatr. 93*:389 (1978).
39. C. M. Ginsburg, J. B. Howard, and J. D. Nelson, Report of 65 cases of *Haemophilus influenzae* type b pneumonia, *Pediatrics 64*:283 (1979).
40. A. L. Esposito and J. E. Pennington, Experimental pneumonia due to *Haemophilus influenzae*: Observations on pathogenesis and treatment, *J. Infect. Dis. 149*:728 (1984).
41. A. S. Dajani, B. I. Asmar, and M. C. Thirumoorthi, Systemic *Haemophilus influenzae* disease: An overview, *J. Pediatr. 94*:355 (1979).
42. K. M. Kaplan and F. A. Oski, Anemia with *Haemophilus influenzae* meningitis, *Pediatrics 65*:1101 (1980).

43. R. T. O'Brien, J. I. Santos, L. Glasgow, and S. A. Landaw, Pathophysiologic basis for anemia associated with *Haemophilus influenzae* meningitis: Preliminary observations, *J. Pediatr. 98*:928 (1981).
44. R. H. Sills, M. T. Caserta, and S. A. Landaw, Decreased erythrocyte deformability in the anemia of bacterial meningitis, *J. Pediatr. 101*:395 (1982).
45. S. L. Kaplan, J. T. Courtney, and K. A. Kenal, Effect of *Haemophilus influenzae* infection and moxalactam on platelet function in children, *Anitmicrob. Agents Chemother. 31*:467 (1987).
46. J. H. Jorgensen, Update on mechanisms and prevalence of antimicrobial resistance in *Haemophilus influenzae, Clin. Infect. Dis. 14*:1119 (1992).
47. G. R. Istre, J. S. Conner, M. P. Glode, and R. S. Hopkins, Increasing ampicillin-resistance rates in *Haemophilus influenzae* meningitis, *Am. J. Dis. Child. 138*:366 (1984).
48. S. L. Kaplan, E. O. Mason, Jr., and S. J. Kvernland, Effect of prior antibiotics on the susceptibility of *Haemophilus influenzae* type b to ampicillin, *Pediatrics 67*:269 (1981).
49. A. L. Smith, Antibiotic resistance in pediatric pathogens, *Infect. Dis. Clin. North Am. 6*:177 (1992).
50. J. H. Jorgensen, G. V. Doern, C. Thornsberry, D. A. Preston, J. S. Redding, L. A. Maher, and T. Tubert, Susceptibility of multiply resistant *Haemophilus influenzae* to newer antimicrobial agents, *Diagn. Microbiol. Infect. Dis. 9*:27 (1988).
51. G. V. Doern, J. H. Jorgensen, C. Thornsberry, D. A. Preston, T. Tubert, J. S. Redding, and L. A. Maher, National collaborative study of the prevalence of antimicrobial resistance among clinical isolates of *Haemophilus influenzae*, *Antimicrob. Agents Chemother. 32*:180 (1988).
52. J. D. Wenger, A. W. Hightower, R. R. Facklam, S. Gaventa, C. V. Broome, and the Bacterial Meningitis Study Group, Bacterial meningitis in the United States, 1986: Report of a multistate surveillance, *J. Infect. Dis. 162*:1316 (1990).
53. F. H. Kayser, G. Morenzoni, and P. Santanam, The second European collaborative study on the frequency of antimicrobial resistance in *Haemophilus influenzae*, *Eur. J. Microbiol. Infect. Dis. 9*:810 (1990).
54. S. L. Kaplan, Current management of common bacterial meningitides, *Pediatr. Rev. 7*:77 (1985).
55. D. Hatch, G. D. Overturf, A. Kovacs, D. Forthal, and C. Leong, Treatment of bacterial meningitis with ceftazidime, *Pediatr. Infect. Dis. 5*:416 (1986).
56. R. F. Jacobs, G. L. Kearns, A. L. Brown, and D. C. Longee, Cerebrospinal fluid penetration of imipenem and cilastatin (Primaxin) in children with central nervous system infections, *Antimicrob. Agents Chemother. 29*:670 (1986).
57. S. L. Kaplan, Recent advances in bacterial meningitis, *Adv. Pediatr. Infect. Dis. 4*:83 (1989).
58. E. I. Tuomanen, K. R. Powell, M. I. Marks, C. I. Laferriere, D. H. Altmiller, C. M. Sack, and A. L. Smith, Oral chloramphenicol in the treatment of *Haemophilus influenzae* meningitis, *J. Pediatr. 99*:968 (1981).

59. J. G. Vallejo, S. L. Kaplan, and E. O. Mason, Jr., Treatment of meningitis and other infections due to ampicillin-resistant *Haemophilus influenzae* type b in children, *Rev. Infect. Dis. 13*:197 (1991).
60. J. Campos, S. Garcia-Tornel, J. M. Gairi, and I. Fabregues, Multiply resistant *Haemophilus influenzae* type b causing meningitis: Comparative clinical and laboratory study, *J. Pediatr. 108*:897 (1986).
61. U. B. Schaad, S. Suter, A. Gianella-Borradori, J. Pfenninger, R. Auckenthaler, O. Bernath, J.-J. Cheseaux, and J. Wedgwood, A comparison of ceftriaxone and cefuroxime for the treatment of bacterial meningitis in children, *N. Engl. J. Med. 322*:141 (1990).
62. V. K. Wong, H. T. Wright, Jr., L. A. Ross, W. H. Mason, C. B. Inderlied, and K. S. Kim, Imipenem/cilastatin treatment of bacterial meningitis in children, *Pediatr. Infect. Dis. J. 10*:122 (1991).
63. P. Echeverria, E. W. P. Smith, D. Ingram, R. M. Sade, and P. Gardner, *Haemophilus influenzae* type b pericarditis, *Pediatrics 56*:808 (1975).
64. R. Marshall, D. W. Teele, and J. O. Klein, Unsuspected bacteremia due to *Haemophilus influenzae:* Outcome in children not initially admitted to hospital, *J. Pediatr. 95*:690 (1979).
65. P. M. Forman and T. V. Murphy, Reevaluation of the ambulatory pediatric patient whose blood culture is positive for *Haemophilus influenzae* type b, *J. Pediatr. 118*:503 (1991).
66. D. N. Korones, G. S. Marshall, and E. D. Shapiro, Outcome of children with occult bacteremia caused by *Haemophilus influenzae* type b, *Pediatr. Infect. Dis. J. 11*:516 (1992).
67. S. L. Kaplan, Use of home antibiotic therapy for serious infections. Parts 1 and 2, *Semin. Pediatr. Infect. Dis. 1*:295 (1990).
68. M. H. Lebel, B. J. Freij, G. A. Syrogiannopoulos, D. F. Chrane, M. J. Hoyt, S. M. Stewart, B. D. Kennard, K. D. Olsen, and G. H. McCracken, Jr., Dexamethasone therapy for bacterial meningitis. Results of two double-blind, placebo-controlled trials, *N. Engl. J. Med. 319*:964 (1988).
69. C. M. Odio, I. Faingezicht, M. Paris, M. Nassar, A. Baltodano, J. Rogers, X. Sáez-Llorens, K. D. Olsen, and G. H. McCracken, Jr., The beneficial effects of early dexamethasone administrations in infants and children with bacterial meningitis, *N. Engl. J. Med. 324*:1525 (1991).
70. Report of the Committee on Infectious Diseases, American Academy of Pediatrics, Elk Grove Village, IL, 1991, p. 569.
71. U. B. Schaad, U. Lips, H. P. Gnehm, A. Blumberg, J. Wedgwood, and the Meningitis Study Group, Dexamethasone therapy for bacterial meningitis: The Swiss experience, Program and Abstracts of the 32nd ICAAC #71, 1992.
72. S. M. King, B. Law, J. Langley, H. Heurter, D. Bremner, E. Wang, and R. Gold, A randomized controlled trial of dexamethasone versus placebo in children with bacterial meningitis, Programs and Abstracts of the 32nd ICAAC. #72, 1992.
73. E. Wald and the U.S. Meningitis Study Group, Dexamethasone for children

with bacterial meningitis, Program and Abstracts of the 32nd ICAAC. #73, 1992.
74. X. Sáez-Llorens, O. Ramilo, M. M. Mustafa, J. Mertsola, C. Alba, E. Hansen, and G. H. McCracken, Jr., Pentoxifylline modulates meningeal inflammation in experimental bacterial meningitis, *Antimicrob. Agents Chemother. 34*:837 (1990).
75. A. F. Rodriguez, S. L. Kaplan, E. P. Hawkins, and E. O. Mason, Jr., Effect of dexamethasone or HWA-138 in combination with antibiotics in experimental *Haemophilus influenzae* type b infection. *Antimicrob. Agents Chemother. 35*:1980 (1991).
76. R. F. Jacobs, M. K. Sowell, M. M. Moss, and D. H. Fiser, Septic shock in children: Bacteriol etiologies and temporal relationships, *Pediatr. Infect. Dis. J. 9*:196 (1990).
77. E. J. Ziegler, C. J. Fisher, Jr., C. L. Sprung, et al., Treatment of gram-negative bacteremia and septic shock with HA-1A human monoclonal antibody against endotoxin. A randomized, double-blind, placebo-controlled trial, *N. Engl. J. Med. 324*:429 (1991).
78. R. C. Bone, A critical evaluation of new agents for the treatment of sepsis, *JAMA 266*:1686 (1991).
79. M. J. Romano, G. L. Kearns, S. L. Kaplan, et al., Single dose pharmacokinetics and safety of HA-1A, a human IgM antilipid A monoclonal antibody, in pediatric patients with sepsis syndrome. *J. Pediatr. 122*:974 (1993).

21

Infection in Adults Due to *Haemophilus influenzae*

Daniel Musher

Baylor College of Medicine and Veterans Affairs Medical Center, Houston, Texas,

Maria Rodriguez-Barradas

Baylor College of Medicine, Houston, Texas

1. INTRODUCTION

Haemophilus influenzae is a major cause of lower respiratory infection and sinusitis in adults. Otitis media occurs much less commonly in adults than in children, and etiological agents are less well studied, although it is reasonable to believe that *H. influenzae* plays a prominent role. Bacterial meningitis is also uncommon in adults relative to its incidence in children, and *H. influenzae* is implicated much less frequently than *Streptococcus pneumoniae, Neisseria meningitis,* or even *Listeria monocytogenes*. Whereas *H. influenzae* type b (Hib) is the overwhelmingly common cause of bacteremic *Haemophilus* infection in children, it is a relatively uncommon cause of infection in adults. This might reflect the low rate of colonization rather than an exceptionally high prevalence of immunity, although immunity expressed at mucosal surfaces may contribute to the infrequent colonization. In contrast, nontypable *H. influenzae* (NTHI) frequently colonizes and causes the majority of serious *Haemophilus* infections in adults. Most healthy adults have antibody that kills and opsonizes NTHI; disease results from anatomical derangements such as those occurring in chronic lung disease that enable bacteria to overwhelm local immune mechanisms and/or conditions that compromise responses rather than from immunological naivete. Antibodies to certain outer membrane proteins (OMP) have been shown to emerge during acute infection caused by NTHI, although the protective capacity of such antibodies is uncertain. Widespread vaccination of adults to prevent NTHI or Hib infection is not, therefore, likely at present to have a substantial impact on health care although for different reasons.

II. EPIDEMIOLOGY

Nontypable *H. influenzae* can be isolated from the nasopharynx in about one half of healthy adults and in a higher proportion (approaching 85%) of those who have chronic bronchitis. Because of this prevalence, the view was long held in England that NTHI is the cause of chronic bronchitis. It is now believed that exposure to irritative factors, together with genetically determined predisposing factors (largely undefined, except for alpha-1 antitrypsinase deficiency), are the causes of chronic lung disease, but that acute infectious exacerbations, especially when associated with fever and leukocytosis, are commonly a result of infection by NTHI and/or pneumococci. Chodosh (1) has given guidelines based on semi-quantitative interpretation of Gram stains that help to distinguish colonization of the lower airways from infection; our observations have been very similar to his. Chodosh states that the finding of $\geq$10–20 bacteria per oil immersion field (1000 × magnification) in gram-stained sputum suggests active disease. In our laboratory, using thick sputum specimens, we regularly observe $> 10^2$ gram-negative coccobacilli per oil immersion field from patients who are acutely infected, a finding that is consistent with our quantitative studies showing 10^7–10^9 NTHI CFU per ml. In contrast, uninfected, colonized subjects have only $\leq$1–2 organisms per field. *Haemophilus influenzae* type b, in contrast, is only rarely isolated from normal adults; a prevalence of $\leq$2% has been given.

Haemophilus influenzae is second only to *Streptococcus pneumoniae* as the cause of bacterial pneumonia leading to hospitalization of adults. In earlier studies of pneumonia in adults [summarized in Fang et al. (2)], *Haemophilus* was implicated one-tenth to one-half as frequently as *S. pneumoniae.* At our Veterans Affairs Medical Center we have had the impression that, in the past few years, the ratio of *Haemophilus* to pneumococcal pneumonia is about 1:1.5, an incidence similar to that reported by Fang et al. (2). One or both of these organisms are implicated in about 75% of patients who are admitted to our hospital for pneumonia and are able to provide a sputum specimen for microbiological study, a proportion nearly double that found by Fang et al. [2]. The vast majority of pulmonary infections caused by *Haemophilus* in adults are caused by nontypable strains. In a prospective study of 30 consecutive patients who had *Haemophilus* pneumonia (3), the causative organism, when studied by counterimmunoelectrophoresis, was NTHI in 26 (87%). In 14 patients with acute febrile tracheobronchitis, a syndrome that was nearly identical to pneumonia except for the absence of a distinctive pulmonary infiltrate by x-ray and the absence of bacteremia, all infections were due to NTHI strains. In studies of all *Haemophilus* infections in which the organism was isolated from ordinarily sterile sources, one half to two thirds of cases were due to nontypable organisms (4,5).

Most adults who have *Haemophilus* pneumonia have one or more serious underlying diseases that contribute to the susceptibility to infection. Chronic obstructive pulmonary disease is highly prevalent (Table 1), being found in more than three quarters of persons with NTHI pneumonia and in nearly all patients who have acute purulent tracheobronchitis. Many of our patients also had other underlying diseases such as malnutrition, alcoholism, cirrhosis, rheumatoid arthritis (medicated with glucocorticosteroids), and hematological malignancies. A recent population-based study of cases in which *H. influenzae* was isolated from normally sterile sites (5) found a

Table 1 Underlying Disease in Adults with Severe Infection Caused by *Haemophilus influenzae*[a]

	Pneumonia[b] (*n* = 30)	Febrile purulent bronchitis[b] (*n* = 14)	Normally sterile site[c] (*n* = 47)
Chronic lung disease	80	79	36
Malignancy	20	0	15
Pregnancy	—[d]	—	15
Diabetes	7	0	11
Severe alcoholism	27	36	9
Nosocomial	13	0	NR
Steroids	NR	NR	13
Dementia	NR	NR	6
Splenectomy	0	0	4
IV drug use	3	0	4
HIV infection	—[d]	—	4
Miscellaneous	23	27	99

[a]Data are presented as percentage of patients who had each underlying condition.
[b]From Ref. 3.
[c]From Ref. 5.
[d]This series of cases was from a Veterans Affairs Medical Center in 1981–2. Pregnant women are not seen at this hospital, and AIDS was in its early stages of recognition.
NR, Not recorded.

total of 59 predisposing conditions in 47 adults with serious *H. influenzae* infection (Table 1). Fifteen percent of cases occurred in pregnant women, an identical proportion to that found earlier by Wallace et al. (4). The incidence of *Haemophilus* pneumonia in HIV-infected persons is greatly increased (6)—perhaps as much as 10- to 20-fold over that in the population at large and even more so when compared to an age-matched population. Nontypable isolates are three to four times as common as type b isolates in this setting.

Haemophilus influenzae is a not-uncommon cause of bacteremia. We (4) have shown that two thirds of isolates from normally sterile sites were nontypable, a finding that has been confirmed by numerous subsequent investigators. We (4) also found that nearly all blood isolates from infected women around the time of delivery were nontypable, and, in fact, most isolates could be placed into biogroup IV. Recent studies (7) have suggested that a unique clone of organisms within the genus *Haemophilus* is responsible; such work is likely eventually to provide the basis for identification of new species. The majority of *Haemophilus* isolates from cerebrospinal fluid of adults with meningitis have also been nontypable, a finding that might have been predicted based on the high degree of association with sinus disease or prior trauma to the head.

III. PATHOGENESIS

Host factors play a major permissive role in the pathogenesis of bronchopulmonary infection caused by NTHI. As noted above, we (3) found that 24 of 30 (80%) patients with pneumonia and 11 of 14 (79%) with acute febrile tracheobronchitis had chronic obstructive pulmonary disease, a syndrome characterized by excessive production of mucus and diminished clearance mechanisms together with bronchiolar dilatation. The majority of these patients also had at least one underlying disease that contributed to a general increase in susceptibility to infection, including all 9 (100%) who lacked evidence for chronic obstructive pulmonary disease and 20 of the 35 (57%) who had chronic lung disease. Chronic colonization of the upper airways by a single strain of NTHI is the general rule in adults who have pulmonary disease. Bacteria are thought to gain entrance to the lower airways and lungs as a result of micro- or macro-aspiration, especially occurring at a time of depressed cough reflex, for example, during sleep. With diminished clearance, aspirated organisms find a suitable environment for replication in areas of puddling of mucus in dilated bronchioles. Although acute or subacute *Haemophilus* infections may be associated with acquisition of a new strain, as is usually the case in children who have otitis media (8), in the majority of instances in adults a persistent strain is responsible (9).

The finding that nearly all strains of NTHI isolated from children have fimbriae (or pili) (10) has led to the suggestion that these protrusions from bacterial cells are important virulence factors. However, substantial adherence of NTHI to tracheal cells occurs in an organ culture without regard to the presence or absence of fimbriae (11) and the presence of fimbriae does not enhance adherence either to normal or damaged cells in a tracheal organ culture (12). In fact, the principal findings from these in vitro studies help to focus attention on host factors, since a constant finding has been that NTHI adhere more avidly to damaged than to normal tissue-cultured cells. Further damage and invasion can then occur, sometimes associated with bacterial penetration of epithelial cells (11). On balance, it seems likely that NTHI adhere to epithelial cells in the trachea and bronchi, perhaps mediated by fimbriae, with a preferential attachment to damaged cells. Nonfimbrial adhesins may also play a role (13). These observations help to explain the association of NTHI with chronic obstructive pulmonary disease.

Some degree of direct damage is caused by bacterial lipooligosaccharide (LOS), especially if invasion of cells has occurred. Host mechanisms, however, are probably responsible for the bulk of the actual damage. Bacterial LOS activates the complement cascade, leading to the release of C5a and other potent chemotaxins that attract inflammatory cells. These cells ingest bacteria and release substances such as leukotrienes (14) that further amplify the inflammatory response. The subsequent release of bacterial and cell constituents as a result of the breakup of cells causes still greater inflammation. In fact, when *H. influenzae* causes pneumonia, the immune reaction is, in effect, the disease process, just as is the case with *S. pneumoniae*. Neither genus is notable for producing toxins that cause tissue necrosis, and the material that fills alveoli causing extensive consolidation, hypoxia and, in some instances, death is a result of the inflammatory response. In support of this observation is the demonstration of only scanty radiographic abnormalities in patients who develop pneumonia while granulocytopenic.

Antibodies (IgG or IgM) directed against NTHI may be bactericidal or may opsonize these bacteria for phagocytosis by PMN. Protective antibody may be directed toward outer membrane proteins, LOS, or both. The P2 OMP, which is responsible for about one half of OMP by weight, and the less prominent protein P6 have each been shown to elicit antibody responses. Furthermore, antibody to P6 is bactericidal in vitro (15) and protects experimental animals against infection with NTHI (16). If antibody to P2 is essential for protection, the capacity of this protein to undergo slight antigenic shift (17) might help to explain the capacity of a single strain to continue to inhabit the airways and even to cause repeated bouts of infection.

Still elusive, however, is the relationship between the numerous antibodies present in serum of healthy adults or those who have chronic lung disease and the susceptibility to infection (18). We (3) have shown, for example, that serum obtained from patients at the time they were hospitalized for pneumonia caused by NTHI has enormous bactericidal and substantial opsonic activity. Three weeks later, the bactericidal activity is unchanged, but the capacity to opsonize the infecting NTHI for phagocytosis has increased. In a preliminary study (19), we suggested that antibody to identifiable OMP might be involved. Despite intensive efforts by several groups of investigators, it is still unclear whether natural emergence of antibody to any specific component of NTHI confers immunity. A much clearer view of this relationship can be seen in otitis media in children because acquisition of new strains can be documented in longitudinal studies and there is not such a long background of antigen exposure (see Chapter 8). It is important to emphasize that, once chronic obstructive pulmonary disease is established, there is such an extensive degree of local anatomical damage that, even if serum antibody is present, it may not be effective in clearing the infection. Complement may not be operative, conditions may not be conducive for phagocytosis, and inability of the lungs to clear dead and dying white cells and bacteria may further compromise the natural response.

In the case of meningitis caused by NTHI (20), nearly all adults have had some anatomic factor that predisposes to infection of the central nervous system, generally a history of serious trauma to the head, a documented cerebrospinal fluid leak, or otitis media. *Haemophilus influenzae* is second to *S. pneumoniae* as a bacterial cause for recurring bacterial meningitis, a syndrome that is associated with a dural tear, often with a connection between the nasopharynx or sinuses and subarachnoid space.

IV. TREATMENT

Haemophilus influenzae was originally regarded by Fleming as penicillin-resistant. This may have been true by comparison to streptococci and staphylococci, but until the rise to prominence of beta-lactamase–producing isolates in the 1970s, 2–4 μg/ml of penicillin or 0.5–1 μg/ml of ampicillin uniformly inhibited typable or nontypable isolates of *H. influenzae*. The most common mechanism of penicillin resistance in these species is the production of a TEM-1 beta-lactamase (21), but production of another novel beta-lactamase has also been described (22). Non–beta-lactamase–mediated resistance mechanisms such as alteration of the penicillin-binding proteins or decreased cell wall permeability also occur (23) and typically impart only an intermediate level of resistance (21).

The prevalence of resistance to ampicillin has increased both in Hib and NTHI. In 1986 in the United States 21% of Hib strains and 12.1% of NTHI were beta-lactamase producers, with a lower incidence of beta-lactamase production in NTHI isolates obtained from patients older than 25 years (<8.6%) and from respiratory isolates (12.8%). Only 3 years previously we had found almost no resistance (<5%) among isolates from older adults. For the same year, in nine European countries participating in a collaborative study (24), the overall resistance was 10%, with a marked variation observed from country to country (1.6–30.6%). At present the incidence of beta-lactamase–producing strains in the United States has increased to about 40% among Hib and 20% among NTHI.

Several problems with current recommendations for susceptibility testing (25) may be responsible for underdetection of ampicillin resistance. Most prominent is that many laboratories test *Haemophilus* only for beta-lactamase production and do not measure zones of inhibition; as a result, ampicillin-resistant isolates that are non–beta-lactamase producers are likely to be reported erroneously as susceptible.

Ampicillin or, at present, amoxicillin, which has better parenteral absorption and a longer half-life, remains the drug of choice to treat infection caused by susceptible strains of *Haemophilus.* For ampicillin-resistant strains, a number of effective oral and parenteral antibiotics are available. Ampicillin or amoxicillin, combined with a substance that covalently binds beta-lactamase, such as clavulanic acid or sulbactam, is active against beta-lactamase–producing strains. *Haemophilus influenzae* is intrinsically resistant to the first-generation cephalosporins. Some second-generation cephalosporins, such as cefaclor, are active against *Haemophilus,* but not all beta-lactamase–producing strains are susceptible (26). Most of the widely used third-generation cephalosporins are highly active against ampicillin-resistant strains (27,28), including those that do not produce beta-lactamase (21); resistance has not been reported to date. Good to moderate activity has been described for imipenem and aztreonam (29).

Nontypable *H. influenzae* has remained uniformly susceptible to trimethoprim/sulfamethoxazole (TM/SMX) and chloramphenicol and nearly so to tetracycline. Resistance of *Haemophilus* to erythromycin is widespread, approaching 100% in some studies (30), which may reflect, in part, problems existing in testing and interpreting results (31). Newer macrolides such as clarithromycin and azythromycin are effective against *Haemophilus,* but cross-resistance to these antibiotics is predicted for erythromycin-resistant strains (32). Quinolones are highly active against all *H. influenzae* strains (33).

In the treatment of *H. influenzae* infection in adults, the selection of antibiotics should be based on the clinical diagnosis, the proper examination of clinical specimens, the severity of disease, and the prevalence of antibiotic-resistant isolates in the population in question. The sicker the patient and the higher the prevalence of resistance, the greater should be the desire to be certain of using an effective agent, although there is still a substantial degree of latitude in the specific antibiotic selected. Ampicillin or amoxicillin is probably no longer appropriate therapy for initial therapy of a serious *Haemophilus* infection except under the unusual circumstance in which the physician knows that the organism is susceptible; in contrast, combinations of a penicillin and a compound that binds beta-lactamase are excellent choices. In the treatment of acute purulent bronchitis due to *Haemophilus,* oral agents such as amoxicillin/clavulanic acid, TM/SMX, tetracycline or doxycycline, and the quinolones are reasonable choices. Because of its effectiveness against pneumococci, which may also be present, amoxacillin/clavulanic acid may be preferred to these other agents, but this advantage needs to be balanced against the greater cost of this combination.

Many physicians believe they can treat community-acquired lower respiratory tract infections "empirically," by which they mean without examination of a gram-stained sputum or culture. This is, of course, not true. Erythromycin is often used on the theory that it is effective against *S. pneumoniae, H. influenzae,* and *Legionella pneumophila,* the most frequent etiological agents of community-acquired pneumonia. In fact, erythromycin is not effective against *H. influenzae.* On the other hand, it is difficult to be enthusiastic about the use of TM/SMX or tetracycline in pneumonia because of the increasing incidence of resistant *S. pneumoniae.* Ciprofloxacin, which is highly effective against *Haemophilus,* provides borderline serum antibiotic levels required to inhibit *S. pneumoniae.* Very expensive newer agents such as clarithromycin and azithromycin are effective against *H. influenzae, S. pneumoniae,* and other pathogens, but one imagines that physicians would be reluctant to prescribe these agents for themselves if they had to pay for their own prescriptions.

In the case of bacteremic and/or severe disease, puerperal sepsis, or meningitis, treatment should be started with a third-generation cephalosporin until antibiotic susceptibility studies are completed. Chloramphenicol is an equally effective alternative. Ampicillin/sulbactam is another reasonable choice, but sulbactam does not cross the blood-brain barrier sufficiently well to allow this combination to be reliable in treating meningitis.

V. PROPHYLAXIS

Vaccination against Hib, with the capsular Hib polysaccharide vaccine, PRP, does not play an important role in adult immunization as it does in children. Most healthy adults have humoral immunity against Hib (34) and colonization is infrequent, explaining the rarity of invasive disease due to this organism. Adults respond to PRP or conjugate vaccination with a substantial production of IgM and IgG. As might be expected, IgG1 and IgG2 subclasses predominate, although their proportion varies from one individual to another (35). Vaccination with the Hib conjugate vaccine induces a more vigorous antibody response, but does not change the pattern of IgG subclasses (35), and healthy adults seem to respond equally well to different conjugate preparations (36).

Because HIV-infected subjects have an increased susceptibility to disease caused by common bacterial pathogens, the CDC recommends that all such persons receive 23-valent pneumococcal polysaccharide vaccine; some authors (37) have extended this recommendation to include PRP. As might be predicted, however, the response of such subjects to polysaccharide antigens is less than optimal (38,39). Steinhoff et al. (37) evaluated the antibody response of HIV-infected individuals, in different stages of the disease, to PRP or the HbOC conjugate vaccine; HIV-infected individuals had a lower antibody response to either preparation than did controls. Healthy controls, HIV-infected asymptomatic persons, and patients with AIDS-related complex (ARC) responded better to the Hib conjugate vaccine than to PRP; for unclear reasons, however, the opposite occurred in the patients with AIDS. In HIV-infected individuals the antibody response to the conjugated vaccine correlated with the clinical status (asymptomatic > ARC > AIDS) and the CD4 count (for those with a CD4 count of >200 vs. >200 cells/mm^3). About one quarter of *H. influenzae* isolated from AIDS patients are type b. Routine vaccination of all HIV-infected persons against *H. influenzae* type b would be benign and might offer protection to a relatively small number of persons. If done, it should be done early in the course of the HIV disease. Vaccination might also offer limited protection to persons whose spleens have been removed and patients with hematological malignancies or sickle cell disease.

Prophylaxis of *H. influenzae* infection in adults with chronic bronchitis needs a different approach, since most of the isolates responsible for disease in this population are nontypable. Against a backdrop of numerous earlier, unconvincing attempts [summarized in Turk and May (40)], Clancy et al. (41) and Lehmann et al. (42) have recently studied the effect of an oral vaccine in patients with chronic obstructive pulmonary disease and appeared to show a diminution in the number of episodes of acute bronchitis (41,42) but not of pneumonia (42) and a decrease in the mean concentration of *H. influenzae* in the sputum (42) but not in the rate of colonization in vaccinees when compared with the placebo group (41,42). The significance of these results and the role of immunization with this preparation remain unclear, at best. More promising might be the use of surface-exposed antigens of NTHI as potential vaccine components (43). A potential candidate is P6, a low-molecular-weight lipoprotein of *H. influenzae* present in all NTHI and *H. influenzae* type b isolates, antigenically invariable, and shown to elicit bactericidal and protective antibodies (43,44). Clearly, much more work needs to be dedicated to the development of an effective vaccine against NTHI infection, especially because ample antibody is already present at the time infection is diagnosed (3). In the meantime, we are probably not able to protect against this infection as can reasonably be done against other respiratory pathogens such as *S. pneumoniae* and influenza viruses.

REFERENCES

1. S. Chodosh, B. Eichel, C. Ellis, and T. C. Medici, Comparison of trimethoprim-sulfamethoxazole with ampicillin in acute infectious exacerbations of chronic bronchitis: a double-blind crossover study, *Rev Infect Dis. 4:*517 (1982).
2. G.-D. Fang, M. Fine, J. Orloff, D. Arisumi, V. L. Yu, W. Kapoor, J. T. Grayston, S. P. Wang, R. Kohler, R. R. Muder, Y. C. Yee, J. D. Rihs, and R. M. Vickers, New and emerging etiologies for community-acquired pneumonia with implications for therapy: a prospective multicenter study of 359 cases, *Medicine 69:*307 (1990).
3. D. M. Musher, K. R. Kubitshchek, J. Crennan, and R. Bauhgn, Pneumonia and acute febrile tracheobronchitis due to *Haemophilus influenzae, Ann. Intern. Med. 99:*444 (1983).
4. R. J. Wallace Jr., D. M. Musher, E. J. Septimus, J. McGowan J. E., F. Quinones, K. Wiss, P. H. Vance, and P. A. Trier, *Haemophilus influenzae* infections in adults: Characterization of strains by serotypes, biotypes and β-lactamase production, *J. Infect. Dis. 144:*101 (1981).
5. M. M. Farley, D. S. Stephens, P. S. Brachman Jr., C. Harvey, J. D. Smith, J. D. Wenger, and CDC Meningitis Surveillance Group, Invasive *Haemophilus influenzae* disease in adults: A prospective, population-based surveillance, *Ann. Intern. Med. 116:*806 (1992).
6. H. T. Schlamm and S. R. Yancovitz, Hemophilus influenzae pneumonia in young adults with AIDS, ARC or risk of AIDS, *Am. J. Med. 86:*11 (1989).
7. R. Quentin, A. Goudeau, R. J. Wallace Jr., A. L. Smith, R. K. Selander, and J. M. Musser, Urogenital, maternal, and neonatal isolates of *Haemophilus influenzae:* identification of unusually virulent serologically nontypable clone families and evidence for a new *Haemophilus* species, *J. Gen. Microbiol. 136:*1203 (1990).
8. B. G. Loos, J. M. Bernstein, D. M. Dryja, T. F. Murphy, and D. P. Dickinson, Determination of the epidemiology and transmission of nontypeable *Haemophilus influenzae* in children with otitis media by comparison of total genomic DNA restriction fingerprints, *Infect. Immun. 57:*2751 (1989).

9. K. Groeneveld, L. van Alphen, P. P. Eijk, G. Visschers, H. M. Jansen, and H. C. Zanen, Endogenous and exogenous reinfections by *Haemophilus influenzae* in patients with chronic obstructive pulmonary disease: the effect of antibiotic treatment on persistence, *J. Infect. Dis. 161:*512 (1990).
10. L. O. Bakaletz, B. M. Tallan, T. Hoepf, T. F. DeMaria, H. G. Birck, and D. J. Lim, Frequency of fimbriation of nontypable *Haemophilus influenzae* and its ability to adhere to chinchilla and human respiratory epithelium, *Infect. Immun. 56:*331 (1988).
11. J. W. St. Geme III. and S. Falkow, *Haemophilus influenzae* adheres to and enters cultured human epithelial cells, *Infect. Immun. 58:*4036 (1990).
12. R. C. Read, R. Wilson, A. Rutman, V. Lund, H. C. Todd, A. P. R. Brain, P. K. Jeffery, and P. J. Cole, Interaction of nontypable *Haemophilus influenzae* with human respiratory mucosa in vitro, *J. Infect. Dis. 163:*549 (1991).
13. S. J. Barenkamp and E. Leininger, Cloning, expression, and DNA sequence analysis of genes encoding nontypeable *Haemophilus influenzae* high-molecular-weight surface-exposed proteins related to filamentous hemaglutinin of *Bordetella pertussis, Infect. Immun. 60:*1302 (1992).
14. R. Garofalo, H. Faden, S. Sharma, and P. L. Ogra, Release of leukotriene B4 from human neutrophils after interaction with nontypeable *Haemophilus influenzae, Infect. Immun. 59:*4221 (1991).
15. B. A. Green, B. J. Metcalf, T. Quinn-Dey, D. H. Kirkley, S. A. Quataert, and R. A. Deich, A recombinant non-fatty acylated form of the Hi-PAL (P6) protein of *Haemophilus influenzae* elicits biologically active antibody against both nontypeable and type b *H. influenzae, Infect. Immun. 58:*3272 (1990).
16. R. S. Munson Jr. and D. M. Granoff, Purification and partial characterization of outer membrane proteins P5 and P6 from *Haemophilus influenzae* type b, *Infect. Immun. 49:*544 (1985).
17. L. van Alphen, P. Eijk, L. Geelen-van den Broek, and J. Dankert, Immunochemical characterization of variable epitopes of outer membrane protein P2 of nontypeable *Haemophilus influenzae, Infect. Immun. 59:*247 (1991).
18. T. F. Murphy and S. Sethi, Bacterial infection in chronic obstructive pulmonary disease, *Am. Rev. Respir. Dis.* (in press).
19. M. V. Hansen, D. M. Musher, and R. E. Baughn, Outer membrane proteins of nontypable *Haemophilus influenzae* and reactivity of paired sera from infected patients with their homologous isolates, *Infect. Immun. 47:*843 (1985).
20. P. J. Spagnuolo, J. J. Ellner, P. I. Lerner, M. C. McHenry, F. Flatauer, P. Rosenberg, and M. S. Rosenthal, *Haemophilus influenzae* meningitis: the spectrum of diseases in adults, *Medicine 61:*74 (1982).
21. C. A. Needham, *Haemophilus influenzae:* Antibiotic susceptibility, *Clin. Microbiol. Rev. 1:*218 (1988).
22. L. G. Rubin, R. Yolken, A. Medeiros, and E. R. Moxon, Ampicillin treatment failure of apparently beta-lactamase-negative *Haemophilus influenzae* type B meningitis due to novel beta-lactamase, *Lancet ii:*1008 (1981).
23. P. M. Mendelman, D. O. Chaffin, T. L. Stull, C. E. Rubens, K. D. Mack, and A. L. Smith, Characterization of non-B-lactamase-mediated ampicillin resis-

tance in *Haemophilus influenzae, Antimicrob. Agents Chemother. 26:*235 (1984).
24. J. Levy, Antibiotic resistance in Europe and the current use of antibiotics in severe pediatric infections, *Scand. J. Infect. Dis. 73:*23 (1990).
25. P. M. Mendelman, E. A. Wiley, T. L. Stull, C. Clausen, D. O. Chaffin, and O. Onay, Problems with current recommendations for susceptibility testing of *Haemophilus influenzae, Antimicrob. Agents Chemother. 34:*1480 (1990).
26. G. V. Doern, J. H. Jorgensen, C. Thornsberry, D. A. Preston, T. Tubert, J. S. Redding, and L. A. Maher, National Collaborative study of the prevalence of antimicrobial resistance among clinical isolates of *Haemophilus influenzae, Antimicrob. Agents Chemother. 32:*180 (1988).
27. H. J. Dabernat and C. Delmas, Comparative activity of cefotaxime and selected β-lactam antibiotics against *Haemophilus influenzae* and aerobic gram-negative bacilli, *Rev. Infect. Dis. 4:*401 (1982).
28. P. Simard and M. G. Bergeron, Inoculum size effect on the MIC of cefoperazone, moxalactam, cefotaxime, cefoxitin and cephalotin for 118 strains of *Haemophilus influenzae* including "tolerant" microorganisms, *J. Antimicrob. Chemother. 10:*397 (1982).
29. A. T. Cerami and D. L. Shungu, Comparative in vitro activity of imipenem against *Haemophilus influenzae* and *Haemophilus parainfluenzae, Antimicrob. Agents Chemother. 30:*179 (1986).
30. D. J. Hurst, A comparison of cefaclor and tetracycline in the treatment of bacterial bronchitis, *Clin. Ther. 6:*163 (1984).
31. D. M. Musher and R. J. Wallace Jr., Treatment of infections due to *Haemophilus influenzae, Antimicrob. Agents Annu. 2:* 383 (1987).
32. S. C. Piscitelli, L. H. Danziger, and K. A. Rodvold, Clarithromycin and azithromycin: New macrolide antibiotics, *Clin Pharm. 11:*137 (1992).
33. J. S. Wolfson and D. C. Hooper, The fluoroquinolones: structure, mechanism of action and resistance, and spectra of activity in vitro, *Antimicrob. Agents Chemother. 28:*581 (1985).
34. D. M. Musher, A. Goree, T. Murphy, A. Chapman, J. Zahradnik, M. Apicella, and R. Baughn, Immunity to *Haemophilus influenzae* type b in young adults: correlation of bactericidal and opsonizing activity of serum with antibody to polyribosylribitol phosphate and lipooligosaccharide before and after vaccination, *J. Infect. Dis. 154:*935 (1986).
35. O. Makela, P. Mattila, N. Rautonen, I. Seppala, J. Eskola, and H. Kayhty, Isotype concentrations of human antibodies to *Haemophilus influenzae* type b polysaccharide (Hib) in young adults immunized with the polysaccharide as such or conjugated to a protein (diphteria toxoid), *J. Immunol. 139:*1999 (1987).
36. H. Kayhty, J. Eskola, H. Peltola, P.-R. Ronnberg, E. Kela, V. Karanko, and L. Saarinen, Antibody responses to four *Haemophilus influenzae* type b conjugate vaccines, *Am. J. Dis. Child. 145:*223 (1991).
37. M. C. Steinhoff, B. S. Auerbach, K. E. Nelson, D. Vlahov, R. L. Becker, N. M. H. Graham, D. H. Schwartz, A. H. Lucas, and R. E. Chaisson, Antibody

response to *Haemophilus influenzae* type b vaccines in men with human immunodeficiency virus infection, *N. Engl. J. Med. 325:*1837 (1991).
38. A. J. Pinching, Antibody responses in HIV infection, *J. Exp. Immunol. 84:*181 (1991).
39. M. C. Rodriguez-Barradas, D. M. Musher, C. Lahart, C. Lacke, J. Groover, D. Watson, R. Baughn, T. Cate, and G. Crofoot, Antibody to capsular polysaccharides of *Streptococcus pneumoniae* after vaccination of human immunodeficiency virus-infected subjects with 23-valent pneumococcal vaccine, *J. Infect. Dis. 165:*553 (1992).
40. D. Turk and R. May, Haemophilus influenzae: *Its Clinical Importance,* English Universities Press, Ltd., London, 1967.
41. R. Clancy, A. Cripps, K. Murree-Allen, S. Yeung, and M. Engel, Oral immunisation with killed *Haemophilus influenzae* for protection against acute bronchitis in chronic obstructive lung disease, *Lancet* 1395 (1985).
42. D. Lehmann, K. J. Coakley, C. A. Coakley, V. Spooner, J. M. Montgamery, A. Michael, I. D. Riley, T. Smith, R. L. Clancy, A. W. Cripps, and M. P. Alpers, Reduction in the incidence of acute bronchitis by an oral *Haemophilus influenzae* vaccine in patients with chronic bronchitis in the highlands of Papua New Guinea, *Am. Rev. Respir. Dis. 144:*324 (1991).
43. B. A. Green, B. J. Metcalf, T. Quinn-Dey, D. H. Kirkley, S. A. Quataert, and R. A. Deich, A recombinant non-fatty acylated form of the Hi-PAL (P6) protein of *Haemophilus influenzae* elicits biologically active antibody against both nontypeable and type b *Haemophilus influenzae, Infect. Immun. 58:*3272 (1990).
44. T. F. Murphy, L. C. Bartos, P. A. Rice, M. B. Nelson, K. C. Dudas, and M. A. Apicella, Identification of a 16,600 dalton outer membrane protein on nontypable *Haemophilus influenzae* as a target for human bactericidal antibody, *J. Clin. Invest. 78:*1020 (1986).

22

Effect of Vaccination on Oropharyngeal Carriage

Aino K. Takala

National Public Health Institute, Helsinki, Finland

I. INTRODUCTION

Haemophilus influenzae type b (Hib) is a strictly human pathogen. Droplet spread followed by oropharyngeal (OP) colonization with Hib bacteria is the mode of transmission (1,2). Via unknown mechanisms, colonization may proceed to invasive infections such as meningitis, epiglottitis, arthritis, pneumonia, or septicemia. Thus, an ideal way to prevent invasive Hib disease would be the prevention of the initial colonization step. If efficacious, this might ultimately lead to eradication of the bacteria.

A. Factors Affecting OP Colonization with Hib

OP carriage of Hib (see Table 1) is generally rare during the first months of life; it was reported to be 0.7% among Caucasian infants in the United States who were less than 6 months of age and 2.8% among those 6–11 months of age (3). Among infants less than 1 year of age the carriage rate has been reported to be 0.5–2% (2–5). The highest rates (3–5%) have been documented among healthy preschool- and school-aged children, whereas carriage is rare among adults (2–6). This timing may, however, differ between different geographic areas and populations: among Navajo and Apache Indian infants, carriage rates of 3% occur among infants as young as 3 months of age (7), which is in accordance with the high incidence rate of invasive Hib infections early in infancy in this population

Table 1 Factors Affecting OP Colonization with Hib

Factors	Ref.
Host Factors	
Age	2–7
Immunological and host defense factors	
Humoral antibodies	14,16
Mucosal antibodies	15–17
Breast milk	19,34,35
Concurrent viral respiratory infection	3,5,7
Antimicrobial treatment	14,36–41
Increased possibility of transmission	
Day-care attendance	12,26,27
Number of siblings	28
Contact with patient with Hib disease	14,29,30
Season	5
Bacterial factors	
Certain clones according to outer membrane protein (OMP) subtypes	33

(8–10). Detailed age-specific rates of colonization are not available from other populations with high incidences of invasive Hib disease.

Following colonization, Hib bacteria may remain in the pharynx and asymptomatic carriage may continue up to 6 months (11,12). Long-term carriers are probably themselves not at increased risk of invasive Hib infection, but they are an important reservoir of Hib bacteria and can transmit the organism to susceptible individuals (13).

Not much is known about immunological and host defense mechanisms that influence OP carriage of Hib. Colonization with Hib bacteria induces both serum and mucosal antibody responses to the Hib capsular polysaccharide, PRP (14–17). Although the mucosal antibody response, primarily lgA, is believed to afford local protection, its mechanism is not known precisely. Surface proteins such as pili or fimbriae are believed to mediate adherence and colonization of Hib (1,18), which can be prevented by antipili antibodies (18). It is, however, not clear how antibodies to PRP (anti-PRP) would interfere with this step. It seems possible that such antibodies could sterically interfere with the association of non-PRP ligands with epithelial cells. A second possible mode of function of mucosal anti-PRP is complement-mediated bactericidal capacity, or opsonization for phagocytosis. This mechanism would, however, operate best for IgG antibodies and would require a sufficient complement concentration or number or phagocytes on the oropharyngeal mucosa.

It has been suggested that breast milk could prevent adherence of Hib bacteria and, thus, breast feeding could prevent colonization and/or delay onset of colonization (19). It may be that this mechanism plays a role in the preventive effect of breast feeding against development of invasive Hib disease (19–23).

Concurrent viral respiratory infections have in some studies been shown to increase the risk for OP carriage of *Haemophilus influenzae* (5) and Hib (7). Although this association was not found in studies conducted by Michaels et al. (3), the carriage rate among children with upper respiratory infection was higher (5.7%) than among healthy children (3.6%) but the difference was not statistically significant. Influenza A and other major respiratory viruses have been demonstrated to induce changes in the epithelium of pharyngeal cells (24) and, in human volunteers, influenza A infection has been shown to enhance attachment of Hib to pharyngeal epithelium (25).

Day-care attendence increases the likelihood of transmission of Hib (12,26). In this environment, there are many child contacts. In addition, mouthing of objects such as toys contaminated with Hib may increase transmission. Hib has been described to survive up to 48 hours on such objects (27). The presence of young siblings in a household also increases the risk of OP carriage of Hib (28). OP carriage rates of 30–70% have been described among household contacts of patients with Hib disease (14, 29,30). In addition, similar seasonal patterns to that for invasive Hib disease with peaks during fall-winter and spring (31,32) have been described for OP carriage of Hib (5).

Finally, bacterial factors that relate to risk of OP carriage have been described. Strains with Hib outer membrane protein (OMP) subtype 13L occurred more often among carriers than among cases with invasive Hib disease (33).

B. Methods for Detection of OP Carriage of Hib

Bacterial culture using the Hib antiserum agar (ASA) method (42) has been used as the principal method for detection of carriage of Hib. Comparing the sensitivity of detecting Hib from oropharyngeal and nasopharyngeal swabs, the OP swab has been shown to result in a larger yield than the nasopharyngeal swab (3).

Recently two antigen detection methods for detection of Hib capsular polysaccharide from OP swabs have been described. In a study evaluating OP carriage of Hib among 154 family members of patients with invasive Hib disease, latex agglutination was found to be 100% sensitive and 90% specific compared to the ASA method (30).

An ELISA method was recently used to analyze OP carriage of Hib (H. Käyhty, unpublished data). When 421 OP swabs collected from healthy Navajo and Apache Indian infants and children were analyzed with both the ASA method and the ELISA, ELISA was 83% sensitive and 100% specific compared to the ASA method (7). A similar ELISA method has been previously described for the analysis of Hib capsular polysaccharide cerebrospinal fluid from serum, CSF, and nasopharyngeal secretions (43). Despite the few false-positive readings possibly associated with the two antigen-detection methods, they have an advantage in situations where the fairly laborous and expensive ASA method is impractical. Furthermore, these positive antigen findings may represent true-positive findings since false-negative cultures can result from antimicrobial treatment prior to swabbing (7,30) or from detection of Hib strains that are capable of producing capsular polysaccharide but not excreting it to the extracellular space (44).

II. EFFECT OF Hib CAPSULAR POLYSACCHARIDE VACCINE ON OP CARRIAGE OF Hib

The Hib capsular polysaccharide vaccine PRP has been shown to be immunogenic and protective against invasive Hib disease, provided that the child is at least 18 months of age (45). However, because of its T-cell–independent nature, PRP vaccine did not induce immunological memory, and the final serum antibody concentrations following vaccination were only modest: at most 10 μg/ml among children 5–6 years of age (46,47). Vaccination with PRP was shown to induce IgA antibody responses in saliva among children 18 months to 7 years of age (48). Such mucosal responses were also observed among infants as young as 2 months of age as well as older children following invasive Hib disease (15,17). The mucosal antibody responses among the infants occurred independently from their serum antibody responses (17).

However, vaccination with PRP did not influence OP carriage of Hib. This question was first studied in Finland among 1000 3-month- to 5-year-old children, half of whom received PRP vaccine and half a control vaccine (meningococcal A polysaccharide vaccine). There were no differences in the carriage rate of Hib among the two vaccine groups (carriage rates 7.4% and 7.7%, respectively) (45). In a second study conducted among ≥18-month-old day-care attendees in Dallas, Texas, similar results were obtained (49).

A lack of effect on OP carriage has been observed with other polysaccharide vaccines as well—meningococcal group A and C and several serotypes in the *Streptococcus pneumoniae* polysaccharide vaccine (50–54).

III. EFFECT OF Hib CONJUGATE VACCINES ON OP CARRIAGE OF Hib

The conjugate vaccines have several advantages compared to the polysaccharide vaccine: the former are immunogenic and protective in infancy and are T-cell–dependent antigens and, thus, capable of inducing immunological memory and a booster response upon reimmunization. Serum Hib anticapsular antibody levels after the booster dose of Hib conjugate vaccine are at least 10-fold higher than the levels obtained after PRP vaccine (55,56). Preliminary results from recent studies indicate that conjugate vaccines also are capable of inducing IgA responses in the saliva (57).

To date, the effect of vaccination on OP carriage of Hib has been evaluated for three of the four licensed Hib conjugate vaccines, Hib capsular polysaccharide-diphtheria toxoid conjugate vaccine (PRP-D, Connaught), Hib oligosaccharide conjugate vaccine (HbOC, Praxis Biologics, Inc.), and Hib meningococcal protein conjugate vaccine (CPRP-OMPC, Merck). In addition, from the vaccination program with Hib capsular polysaccharide conjugated to tetanus toxoid (PRP-T, Pasteur-Mérieux) conducted in Finland in 1990 through 1991, there is evidence of its effect on OP carriage of Hib.

A. PRP-D

The effect of PRP-D on OP carriage of Hib was evaluated in two studies conducted among healthy children in Finland and in Dallas, Texas (6,49). In the first study, OP carriage of Hib was evaluated among 725 healthy 3-year-old Finnish children. OP swabs were obtained during routine well-child visits at the local child health centers (seven different locations throughout the country) and cultured within 2 days using the ASA method (42). As controls, *Streptococcus pneumoniae* and non–type b *Haemophilus influenzae* were isolated from the swabs. During the first half of the study period between April 1987 and September 1988, the children (N = 398) had not received PRP-D prior to swabbing. During the latter half of the study period from October 1988 through August 1990, all children (N = 327) had received PRP-D, either three doses in infancy and a booster at 14–18 months of age (N = 190) or one dose at 24 months of age (N = 137). The OP carriage rate of Hib was 3.5% (95% CI, 1.9–5.8%) among the unvaccinated children, but 0% (95% CI, 0–1.1%) among the those who had received PRP-D prior to swabbing (p = 0.0002, Fisher's exact test). No differences were observed between vaccinated and unvaccinated children for OP carriage of non–type b *H. influenzae* or *S. pneumoniae* (Table 2).

Table 2 Studies on the Effect of *Haemophilus influenzae* Type b Conjugate Vaccines on Oropharyngeal Carriage of *Haemophilus influenzae* Type b

Vaccinees		Control group (N)	Population	Age at swab mean (range)	Time since last vaccine dose, mean (range)	Method for detection of Hib	Effect of vaccine compared to control group	Ref.
Vaccine (N)	Schedule (in months)							
PRP-D (190)	3,4,6,14–18	No vaccine (398)	Finnish	36 mo (32–43)	21 mo (6–29)	ASA	Reduction of carriage of Hib	6
PRP-D (137)	24	No vaccine (398)	Finnish	36 mo (32–43)	12 mo (0.3–19)	ASA	Reduction of carriage of Hib	6
PRP-D (89)	⩾18	No vaccine (166)	Texas, predominantly white	33 mo ± 13 mo[a]	3 mo ±3 mo[a]	ASA	Reduction of carriage of Hib	49
HbOC (60)	3,5,9	No vaccine (60)	British	52 mo (NA)	41 mo (NA)	ASA	No overall reduction of carriage Decreased intensity of carriage Serum booster response upon carriage	58
PRP-OMPC Vaccinated according to age at swabbing (498)	2,4, 12–15	Not vaccinated according to age at swabbing (925)	Arizona, Apache and Navajo Indians	9.7 mo (3–56)	4.4 mo (1–36)	ELISA	Reduction of carriage of Hib Concurrent respiratory infection increased risk for carriage	7

[a]SD for the mean

The second study was conducted among 283 children 18–59 months of age, attending three different day-care centers in Dallas, Texas (49). Children were primarily Caucasian (93%). The mean age at the first culture was 34–39 months, depending on the center. Throat swabs were obtained at 2-month intervals (mean number of cultures/child: 4.2) and cultured using the ASA method (42). Prior to swabbing, 89 (31%) of the children had received one dose of conjugate vaccine (94% PRP-D), and 51 (18%) had received one dose of PRP vaccine. The mean duration between vaccination and swabbing was 16 and 3 months, respectively, for the PRP and conjugate vaccine groups. The rest of the children had not received any Hib vaccine prior to swabbing.

The percentage of children colonized was not significantly different between unvaccinated children and those who received PRP vaccine (17% vs. 24%). However, the carriage rate among children who had received PRP-D, 7%, was significantly lower than that of unvaccinated children (13%, $p = 0.02$). In the multivariate analysis, controlling for age at first culture, number of cultures, day-care center assignment, and time between vaccination and first culture, the efficacy of PRP-D to prevent colonization was 64% (95% CI, 5–86%; $p = 0.02$). In a subsequent matched analysis using a nested case-control design to further control for seasonal variation of carriage and classroom assignment, the efficacy was 81% (95% CI, 7–96%; $p = 0.02$) (Table 2).

B. HbOC

The effect of HbOC on OP carriage of Hib was evaluated among 120 4-year-old children in Oxford, UK (58). Sixty of the children had received HbOC at age 3, 5, and 9 months and 60 had not received any Hib vaccine. OP carriage of Hib was evaluated at approximately 52 months of age, i.e., 3.5 years after the last dose of HbOC. Children were visited at home, during which data on potential risk factors, a serum sample, and a throat swab were obtained. Detection of Hib was based on an improved ASA culture method (59).

Overall, the carriage rate of Hib did not differ between vaccinees (8%) and nonvaccinees (5%), nor did risk factors for Hib disease or carriage. However, the intensity of colonization was less among vaccinees than nonvaccinees. There was an inverse relationship between colony counts and the IgG anti-PRP concentration in serum.

Among children who were not OP carriers of Hib, the GMT serum anti-PRP level of the vaccinated children was 0.97 μg/ml, and only moderately lower (0.32 μg/ml) among the unvaccinated children. However, among children who were found to be colonized with Hib, the levels were 53.7 and

2.8 μg/ml, respectively, for vaccinated and unvaccinated children. This difference indicates that vaccination with HbOC had primed the vaccinees, so that upon mucosal challenge with Hib bacteria there was a rapid booster serum antibody response (Table 2).

C. PRP-OMPC

The effect of Hib-OMPC vaccine on OP carriage of Hib was evaluated among Navajo and Apache Indian infants and children residing in the Navajo and Apache reservations in Arizona (7).

A total of 1423 swabs were obtained from 1321 3-month- to 4-year-old children during their well-child visit. Eighty-one percent of the children were Navajo and 15% Apache Indians. Data on vaccination history and symptoms of respiratory infection were collected at swabbing. Of the swabs obtained, 293 were from children prior to administration of any Hib vaccine, 1119 were taken post–primary series of PRP-OMPC, and 11 after the booster dose. The ELISA method was used for detection of OP carriage of Hib (H. Käyhty, manuscript in preparation). For 30% of the swabs, bacterial culture was also performed using the ASA method (6,42).

Forty of 1423 swabs were positive for Hib. Carriers were older than noncarriers (mean age 13 months and 9 months, respectively), and a greater proportion of carriers had symptoms of respiratory infection at swabbing (48%) than did noncarriers (30%). Furthermore, 13% of the carriers had received the PRP-OMPC vaccinations appropriate for age at swabbing, compared to 36% of the noncarriers. All these variables were significantly associated with risk of OP carriage of Hib when incorporated jointly in a logistic regression model. There was no association between the use of antimicrobial treatment and OP carriage of Hib.

For a child not vaccinated according to age at swabbing, the risk of OP carriage of Hib was 2.7-fold greater than for a child who had been vaccinated appropriately according to age at swabbing, controlling for the effect of age and presence of respiratory infection at swabbing. In addition, for a child who had symptoms of respiratory infection, risk of OP carriage of Hib was twofold greater compared to a child without respiratory infection, controlling for vaccination status and age (Table 2).

IV. IMPACT OF LARGE-SCALE VACCINATIONS WITH Hib CONJUGATE VACCINES ON OP CARRIAGE OF Hib

In Finland, efficacy trials with Hib conjugate vaccines were conducted in 1986 through 1991. During the first trial (1986–1987) half of the children received three doses of PRP-D in infancy at 3, 4, and 6 months of age and a booster dose at 14–18 months of age, whereas the other half of the children received one dose at 24 months of age (60). During the second trial (1988–1989) all infants were offered Hib conjugate vaccine randomized as either PRP-D or HbOC at 4, 6, and 14–18 months of age (61). In the last phase, a vaccination program with PRP-T was conducted in 1990–1991, during which all infants were offered PRP-T at 4, 6, and 14–18 months of age (62). Vaccination coverage was 94–98% (60–62), and the prospective surveillance of invasive Hib disease was estimated to be 98% effective (22).

In years 1987 through 1991, OP carriage of Hib was evaluated among healthy 3-year-olds, 6-year-olds, and 6- to 14-month-olds in 10 different child health centers throughout Finland. OP swabs were collected at well-child visits and cultured on ASA plates within 2 days. There was a significant reduction of OP carriage of Hib seen first among 327 3-year-old children who had received PRP-D vaccine (6). Thereafter OP swabs were obtained from 338 additional 3-year-old children between September 1990 and December 1991. None of them carried Hib. Furthermore in 1990–1991, OP carriage of Hib also was reduced among nonvaccinated children: among 6-year-old unvaccinated children OP carriage of Hib (0.3%) was significantly ($p < 0.001$) less than the expected rate of 7.6% recorded for children in Finland during 1974–75 (A. Sivonen, personal communication). Among 6 to 14-month-old children ($N = 109$) who had received PRP-T, none carried Hib (62).

Similarly, an overall reduction of OP carriage of Hib among 0- to 5-year-old children has been reported from Iceland, coinciding with the introduction of general vaccination with PRP-D (63). Also, overall carriage was significantly less than expected in a study evaluating OP carriage of Hib among 600 2- to 5-year-old, primarily black children in metropolitan Atlanta from December 1991 through March 1992 (one positive culture, with a carriage rate of 0.17%). Eighty percent of these children had been adequately vaccinated with Hib conjugate vaccine prior to swabbing (64).

V. MECHANISMS FOR PREVENTION OF OP CARRIAGE OF Hib

Compared to the polysaccharide vaccine that had a marginal if any effect on mucosal carriage, the Hib conjugate vaccines have two immunological properties that may explain their ability to lower OP carriage of Hib.

First, the concentrations of serum Hib anticapsular antibodies achieved by conjugate vaccines are significantly higher than those induced by the PRP vaccine. The high serum antibody concentrations might be expected to lead to higher concentrations of mucosal IgA and IgG antibodies by transudation or active transport from the serum. This phenomenon has been demonstrated for antibodies induced by parenteral pneumococcal polysaccharide vaccine (65) or during *Yersinia* infection (66). Consistent with this hypothesis are the somewhat reduced OP carriage rates of Hib among Navajo Indian children shortly after they received passive immunization with bacterial polysaccharide immunoglobulin (BPIG, see Chapter 17) (M. Santosham, personal communication).

Results from animal studies using the infant rat colonization model also provide supporting evidence: intraperitoneal administration of monoclonal or polyclonal anti-Hib capsular polysaccharide antibodies led to prevention of Hib OP colonization upon intranasal challenge with Hib. The level of serum anti-Hib antibodies in the infant rat needed for this effect was approximately 10 μg/ml (67). These results are supported further by results from the above described human studies: whenever a decrease in OP carriage of Hib was detected (6,7,49), the serum anti-Hib capsular polysaccharide level (GMT) in the respective population or comparable population was high (>1–10 μg/ml) (56,68–70). No decrease was seen when antibody concentrations were lower, as was the case with PRP vaccine (GMT 0.11 μg/ml) (71) or among recipients of HbOC 3.5 years after the last dose of HbOC (GMT 0.97 μg/ml) (58). However, in infants vaccinated with HbOC, acquisition of Hib colonization led to a booster-type serum anticapsular antibody response and the intensity of colonization among vaccinees was greatly decreased compared to that of unvaccinated children (58). It is possible that the risk of natural transmission of Hib is lower among vaccinated children with decreased intensity of colonization compared to that of unvaccinated Hib carriers.

Second, a major difference between the Hib polysaccharide vaccine and the conjugate vaccine is the T-dependent nature of the latter, leading to immunological memory and a booster serum antibody response on revaccination (55,56) or natural exposure to Hib (58). OP contact with Hib may lead secondarily to an increase in mucosa antibody in an individual primed with Hib conjugate vaccine. A rapid booster response to nasal challenge also has been demonstrated with influenza A in animals parenterally primed with influenza A vaccine (72). The same study also indicated that the parenterally administered vaccine had given rise to antibody-producing and memory cells on the nasal mucosa. Preliminary results of antibody analysis in saliva from children immunized with PRP-T or PRP-OMPC indicate that mucosal IgA production takes place locally following immunization (57). For this component, the immunogenic differences between plain PRP and Hib conjugate vaccines, e.g., differences in the priming capacity, may be of importance. In addition, IgG anti-PRP levels in saliva were detected only if serum IgG anti-PRP levels were approximately > 10 μg/ml (57), a result supporting the conclusions from the infant rat studies described above (67).

VI. CONCLUSION

The decrease of OP carriage of Hib following vaccination with Hib conjugate vaccines has implications for prevention of invasive Hib disease as well as development of future conjugate vaccines.

Prevention of invasive Hib disease has been shown to be greater than expected on the basis of individual vaccine trials; a decline in disease among unvaccinated infants was observed when toddlers were vaccinated with Hib conjugate vaccines (62,63,73–76). In addition a decline in the incidence of Hib disease among unvaccinated older children has been observed in Finland (62). This decrease may be a result of a vaccine-induced decrease in OP carriage (6,62).

If the ability to decrease or prevent mucosal colonization is a general property of conjugate vaccines, this property would be a special advantage for the pneumococcal and meningococcal conjugate vaccines that are currently being developed. It may be possible to prevent not only systemic but also mucosal infections such as pneumococcal pneumonia and otitis media.

REFERENCES

1. E. H. Beachey, Bacterial adherence: Adhesin-receptor interactions mediating the attachment of bacteria to mucosal surfaces, *J. Infect. Dis. 143:*325 (1981).
2. D. C. Turk, Naso-pharyngeal carriage of *Haemophilus influenzae* type b, *J. Hygiene 61:*247 (1963).
3. R. H. Michaels, C. S. Pozviak, F. E. Stonebaker, and C. W. Norden, Factors affecting pharyngeal *Haemophilus influenzae* type b colonization rates in children, *J. Clin. Microbiol. 4:*413 (1976).
4. D. B. Hall, M. K. W. Lum, L. R. Knutson, W. L. Heyward, and J. I. Ward, Pharyngeal carriage and acquisition of anticapsular antibody to *Haemophilus influenzae* type in a high-risk population in southwestern Alaska, *Am. J. Epidemiol. 126:*1190 (1987).
5. A. J. Howard, K. T. Dunkin, and G. W. Millar, Nasopharyngeal carriage and antibiotic resistance of *Haemophilus influenzae* in healthy children, *Epidemiol. Inf. 100:*193 (1988).
6. A. K. Takala, J. Eskola, M. Leinonen, H. Käyhty, A. Nissinen, E. Pekkanen, and P. H. Mäkelä, Reduction of oropharyngeal carriage of *Haemophilus influenzae* type b (Hib) in children immunized with an Hib conjugate vaccine, *J. Infect. Dis. 164:*982 (1991).
7. A. K. Takala, M. Santosham, J. Almeido-Hill, M. Wolff, W. Newcomer, R. Reid, H. Käyhty, E. Esko, and P. H. Mäkelä, Vaccination with *Haemophilus influenzae* type b meningococcal protein conjugate vaccine reduces oropharyngeal carriage of Hib among American Indian children, *J. Pediatr. Infect Dis. 12:*593 (1993).

8. G. A. Losonsky, M. Santosham, V. M. Sehgal, et al., *Haemophilus influenzae* disease in the White Mountain Apaches: Molecular epidemiology of a high risk population, *Pediatr. Inf. Dis. 3:*539 (1984).
9. J. L. Coulehan, R. H. Michaels, C. Hallowell, et al., Epidemiology of Haemophilus influenzae type b among Navajo Indians, *Public Health Rep. 99:*404 (1984).
10. M. Santosham, B. Rivin, M. Wolff, R. Reid, W. Newcomer, W. Letson, J. Almeido-Hill, C. Thompson, and G. Siber, Prevention of *Haemophilus influenzae* type b infections in Apache and Navajo children, *J. Infect. Dis. 165*(Suppl.):S144 (1992).
11. R. H. Michaels, and C. W. Norden, Pharyngeal colonization with *Haemophilus influenzae* type b: a longitudinal study of families with a child with meningitis due to *Haemophilus influenzae. J. Infect. Dis. 136:*222 (1977).
12. T. V. Murphy, D. M. Granoff, R. N. Chrane, K. D. Olsen, S. J. Barenkamp, S. F. Dowell, and G. H. McCracken, Pharyngeal colonization with *Haemophilus influenzae* type b in children in a day care center without invasive disease, *J. Pediatr. 106:*712 (1985).
13. E. R. Moxon, The carrier state: *Haemophilus influenzae, J. Antimicrob. Chemother. 18*(Suppl. A):17 (1986).
14. M. P. Glode, R. S. Daum, E. G. Boies, T. L. Ballard, M. Murray, and D. M. Granoff, Effect of rifampin chemoprophylaxis on carriage eradication and new acquisition of *Haemophilus influenzae* type b in contacts, *Pediatrics 76:*537 (1985).
15. J. R. Gilsdorf, and W. M. McDonnell, Mucosal antibodies to *Haemophilus influenzae* type b capsular polysaccharide, *Pediatr. Res. 29:*420 (1991).
16. M. E. Pichichero, and R. A. Insel, Relations between naturally occurring human mucosal and serum antibody to the capsular polysaccharide of *Haemophilus influenzae* type b, *J. Infect. Dis. 148:*243 (1982).
17. M. E. Pichichero, C. B. Hall, and R. A. Insel, A mucosal antibody response following systemic *Haemophilus influenzae* type infection in children, *J. Clin. Invest. 67:*1482 (1981).
18. L. van Alphen, N. van den Berghe, and L. Geelen-van den Broek, Interaction of *Haemophilus influenzae* with human erythrocytes and oropharyngeal epithelial cells is mediated by a common fimbrial epitope, *Infect. Immun. 56:*1800 (1988).
19. B. Andersson, O. Porras, L.Å. Hanson, T. Lagergård, and C. Svanborg-Eden, Inhibition of attachment of *Streptococcus pneumoniae* and *Haemophilus influenzae* by human milk and receptor oligosaccharides, *J. Infect. Dis. 153:*232 (1986).
20. S. L. Cochi, D. W. Fleming, and A. W. Hightower, et al., Primary invasive *Haemophilus influenzae* type b disease: A population-based assessment of risk factors, *J. Pediatr. 108:*887 (1986).
21. G. R. Istre, J. S. Conner, C. V. Broome, A. Hightower, and R. S. Hopkins, Risk factors for primary invasive *Haemophilus influenzae* disease: Increased risk from day-care attendance and school-aged household members, *J. Pediatr. 106:*190 (1985).

22. A. K. Takala, J. Eskola, J. Palmgren, P.-R. Rönnberg, E. Kela, P. Rekola, and P. H. Mäkelä, Risk factors of invasive *Haemophilus influenzae* type b disease among children in Finland, *J. Pediatr. 115:*694 (1989).
23. A. K. Takala, and D. A. Clements, Socio-economic risk factors for invasive *Haemophilus influenzae* type b disease, *J. Infect. Dis. 165*(Suppl. 1):S11 (1992).
24. J. L. Carson, A. M. Collier, and S. S. Hu, Aquired ciliary defects in nasal epithelium of children with acute viral upper respiratory infections, *N. Engl. J. Med. 312:*463 (1985).
25. V. Fainstein, D. M. Musher, and T. R. Cate, Bacterial adherence to pharyngeal cells during viral infection, *J. Infect. Dis. 141:*172 (1980).
26. W. P. Stephenson, G. Doern, N. Ganttz, L. Lipworth, and K. Chapin, Pharyngeal carriage rates of *Haemophilus influenzae* type b and non-b, and prevalence of ampicillin-resistant *Haemophilus influenzae* among healthy day-care children in central Massachusetts, *Am. J. Epidemiol. 122:*868 (1985).
27. T. V. Murphy, J. F. Clements, M. Petroni, S. Conry, and L. Stetler, *Haemophilus influenzae* type b in respiratory secretions, *Pediatr. Infect. Dis. J. 8:*148 (1989).
28. A. K. Takala, M. Mäkelä, P.-R. Rönnberg, E. Kela, and J. Eskola, Increased risk of primary invasive *Haemophilus influenzae* type b disease in twins, *Pediatr. Infect. Dis. J. 8:*799 (1989).
29. K. Li, B. Dashefsky, and E. R. Wald, *Haemophilus influenzae* type b colonization in household contacts of infected and colonized children enrolled in day-care, *Pediatrics 78:*15 (1986).
30. R. Heikkilä, A. K. Takala, H. Käyhty, and M. Leinonen, Latex agglutination text for the screening of *Haemophilus influenzae* type b carriers, *J. Clin. Microbiol. 25:*1131 (1987).
31. A. K. Takala, J. Eskola, H. Peltola, and P. H. Mäkelä, Epidemiology of invasive *Haemophilus influenzae* type b disease among children in Finland before vaccination with *Haemophilus influenzae* type b conjugate vaccine, *Pediatr. Infect. Dis. J. 8:*297 (1989).
32. J. I. Ward, M. K. Lum, D. B. Hall, et al., Invasive *Haemophilus influenzae* type b in Alaska: Background epidemiology for a vaccine efficacy trial, *J. Infect. Dis. 153:*17 (1986).
33. C. M. Hampton, S. J. Barenkamp, and D. M. Granoff, Comparison of outer membrane protein subtypes of *Haemophilus influenzae* type b isolates from healthy children in the general population and from diseased patients, *J. Clin. Microbiol. 18:*596 (1983).
34. M. E. Pichichero, A. E. Sommerfelt, M. C. Steinhoff, and R. A. Insel, Breast milk antibody to the capsular polysaccharide of *Haemophilus influenzae* type b, *J. Infect. Dis. 142:*694 (1980).
35. R. A. Insel, M. Amstey, and M. E. Pichichero, Postimmunization antibody to the *Haemophilus influenzae* type capsule in breast milk, *J. Infect. Dis. 152:*407 (1985).
36. D. M. Granoff and J. I. Ward, Current status of prophylaxis for *Haemophilus influenzae* infections, *Current Clinical Topics in Infectious Diseases,* (J.

S. Remington and M. N. Swartz, eds.), McGraw-Hill, New York, 1984, pp. 290–315.
37. J. W. Ogle, G. P. Rabalais, and M. P. Glode, Duration of pharyngeal carriage of *Haemophilus influenzae* type b in children hospitalized with systemic infections, *Pediatr. Infect. Dis. 5:*509 (1986).
38. J. Gilsdorf, Dynamics of nasopharyngeal colonization with *Haemophilus influenzae* b during antibiotic therapy, *Pediatrics 77:*242 (1986).
39. J. Gilsdorf, D. Granoff, C. Gessert, et al., *Haemophilus influenzae* type b (HIB) infection in a day care center (DCC): Eradication of carrier state by rifampin, *Pediatr. Res. 12:*491 (1978).
40. J. I. Ward, G. Goreman, C. Phillips, et al., *Haemophilus influenzae* type b disease in a day care center, *J. Pediatr. 92:*713 (1978).
41. E. Shapiro, and E. Wald, Efficacy of rifampicin in eliminating pharyngeal carriage of *Haemophilus influenzae* type b, *Pediatrics 66:*5 (1980).
42. R. H. Michaels, F. E. Stonebaker, and J. B. Robbins, Use of antiserum agar for detection of *Haemophilus influenzae* type b in the pharynx, *Pediatr. Res. 9:*513 (1975).
43. S. V. Rosales, L. J. LaScolea Jr., and P. L. Ogra, Development of respiratory mucosal tolerance during *Haemophilus influenzae* type b infection in infancy, *J. Immunol. 132:*1517 (1984).
44. L. N. Brophy, J. S. Kroll, J. P. Ferguson, and R. E. Moxon, Capsulation gene loss and 'rescue' mutations during the Cap+ to Cap− transition *Haemophilus influenzae* type b, *J. Gen. Microbiol. 137:*2571 (1991).
45. H. Peltola, H. Käyhty, A. Sivonen, and P. H. Mäkelä, *Haemophilus influenzae* type b capsular polysaccharide vaccine in children: A double-blind field study of 100,000 vaccinees 3 months to 5 years of age in Finland, *Pediatrics 60:*730 (1977).
46. P. H. Mäkelä, H. Peltola, H. Käyhty, H. Jousimies, O. Pettay, E. Ruoslahti, A. Sivonen, and O.-V. Renkonen, Polysaccharide vaccines of group A *Neisseria meningitidis* and *Haemophilus influenzae* type b: A field trial in Finland, *J. Infect. Dis. 136*(Suppl.):S43 (1977).
47. H. Käyhty, V. Karanko, H. Peltola, and P. H. Mäkelä, Serum antibodies after vaccination with *Haemophilus influenzae* type b capsular polysaccharide and response to reimmunization: No evidence of immunologic tolerance or memory, *Pediatrics 74:*857 (1984).
48. M. E. Pichichero, and R. A. Insel, Mucosal antibody response to parenteral vaccination with *Haemophilus influenzae* type b capsule, *J. Allergy Clin. Immunol. 72:*481 (1983).
49. T. V. Murphy, P. N. Pastor, F. B. Medley, M. T. Osterholm, and D. M. Granoff, Decreased *Haemophilus* colonization in children vaccinated with *Haemophilus influenzae* type b conjugate vaccine, *J. Pediatr. 122:*517 (1993).
50. A. Sivonen, Effect of *Neisseria meningitidis* group A polysaccharide vaccine on nasopharyngeal carrier rates, *J. Infect. 3:*266 (1981).
51. W. R. Sanborn, Z. Bencic, B. Cvjetanovic, E. C. Gotschlich, T. M. Pollack, and J. E. Sippel, Trial of a serogroup A meningococcus polysaccharide vaccine in Nigeria, *Progr. Immunobiol. Stand. 5:*497 (1972).

52. B. M. Greenwood, M. Hassan-King, and H. C. Whittle, Prevention of secondary cases of meningococcal disease in household contacts by vaccination, *Br. Med. J. 1:*1317 (1978).
53. C. Rosen, P. Christensen, B. Hovelius, and K. Prellner, A longitudinal study of the nasopharyngeal carriage of Pneumococci as related to pneumococcal vaccination in children attending day-care centres, *Acta Otolaryngol. 98:*524 (1984).
54. E. Herva, J. Luotonen, M. Timonen, M. Sibakov, P. Karma, and P. H. Mäkelä, The effect of polyvalent pneumococcal polysaccharide vaccine on nasopharyngeal and nasal carriage of *Streptococcus pneumoniae, Scand. J. Infect. Dis. 12:*97 (1980).
55. H. Käyhty, J. Eskola, H. Peltola, M. Stout, J. S. Samuelson, and L. K. Gordon, Immunogenicity in infants of a vaccine composed of *Haemophilus influenzae* type b capsular polysaccharide mixed with DTP or conjugated to diphtheria toxoid, *J. Infect. Dis. 155:*100 (1987).
56. H. Käyhty, J. Eskola, H. Peltola, L. Saarinen, and P. H. Mäkelä, High antibody responses to booster doses of either *Haemophilus influenzae* capsular polysaccharide or conjugate vaccine after primary immunization with conjugate vaccine, *J. Infect. Dis. 165*(Suppl. 1):S165 (1992).
57. M. Kauppi, P.-R. Rönnberg, L. Saarinen, E. Pekkanen, J. Eskola, and H. Käyhty, Mucosal antibody concentrations after immunization with *Haemophilus influenzae* type b (Hib) conjugate vaccine, 7th International Congress of Mucosal Immunity, Aug. 16–20, 1992, Prague, Czechoslovakia.
58. M. L. Barbour, R. Booy, D. W. Crook, H. Griffiths, H. Chapel, E. R. Moxon, and R. T. Mayon-White, *Haemophilus influenzae* type b; carriage and immunity four years after conjugate vaccine, Abstract 978, 32nd Interscience Conference on Antimicrobial Agents and Chemotherapy, Anaheim, CA, 11–14 October, 1992.
59. M. L. Barbour, D. W. Crook, and R. T. Mayon-White, An improved antiserum agar method for detecting carriage of *Haemophilus influenzae* type b, *Eur. J. Clin. Microbiol. Infect. Dis. 12:*215 (1993).
60. J. Eskola, H. Käyhty, A. K. Takala, H. Peltola, P.-R. Rönnberg, E. Kela, E. Pekkanen, P. WcVerry, and P. H. Mäkelä, A randomized, prospective field trial of a conjugate vaccine in the protection of infants and young children against invasive *Haemophilus influenzae* type b disease, *N. Engl. J. Med. 323:*1381 (1991).
61. H. Peltola, J. Eskola, H. Käyhty, A. K. Takala, E. Kela, E. Pekkanen, P.-R. Rönnberg, and P. H. Mäkelä, Protection achieved by Clinical efficacy of the PRP-D vs HbOC conjugate vaccines against *Haemophilus influenzae* type b (Hib), Abstract 975, 32nd Interscience Conference on Antimicrobial Agents and Chemotherapy, Anaheim, CA, 1992.
62. J. Eskola, A. K. Takala, H. Käyhty, E. Koskenniemi, H. Peltola, and P. H. Mäkelä, Protection achieved by *Haemophilus influenzae* type b (Hib)conjugate vaccines is better than expected on the basis of efficacy trials, Abstract 979, 32nd Interscience Conference of Antimicrobial Agents and Chemotherapy, Anaheim, CA, 1992.
63. K. E. Jonsdottir, O. Steingrimsson, and O. Olafsson. Immunization of infants in Iceland against *Haemophilus influenzae* type b, *Lancet 340:*252 (1992).

64. J. Mohle-Boetani, G. Ajello, E. Breneman, K. Deaver, C. Harvey, M. Farley, D. Stephens, and J. Wenger, Oropharyngeal carriage of *Haemophilus influenzae* type b in a heavily vaccinated population of 2–5-year-olds, Abstract 1729, 32nd Interscience Conference on Antimicrobial Agents and Chemotherapy, Anaheim, CA, 11–14 October, 1992.
65. M. Koskela, Antibody response of young children to parenteral vaccination with pneumococcal capsular polysaccharides: A comparison between antibody levels in serum and middle ear effusion, *Pediatr. Infect. Dis. J. 5:*431 (1986).
66. E. Grönblad and O. Mäkelä, Salivary and serum antibodies in patients with *Yersinia enterocolitica* infection, *Microb. Pathog. 1:*565 (1986).
67. M. Kauppi, L. Saarinen, and H. Käyhty, Anti-capsular polysaccharide antibodies reduce nasopharyngeal colonization by *Haemophilus influenzae* type b in infant rats, *J. Infect. Dis. 167:*365 (1993).
68. J. S. Holmes, T. V. Murphy, R. S. Anderson, S. L. Kaplan, E. P. Rothstein, V. N. Gan, and D. M. Granoff, Immunogenicity of four *Haemophilus influenzae* type b conjugate vaccines in 17- to 19-month-old children, *J. Pediatr. 118:*364 (1991).
69. M. Santosham, M. Wolff, R. Reid, et al., The efficacy in Navajo infants of a conjugate vaccine consisting of *Haemophilus influenzae* type b polysaccharide and *Neisseria meningitidis* outer-membrane protein complex, *N. Engl. J. Med. 324:*1767 (1991).
70. M. Santosham, J. Almeido-Hill, M. Wolff, et al., Safety and immunogenicity of a *Haemophilus influenzae* type b conjugate vaccine in a high risk American Indian population, *Pediatr. Infect. Dis. J. 10:*113 (1991).
71. C. D. Berkowitz, J. I. Ward, Chung-E-Chiu, S. M. Marcy, L. Gordon, J. O. Hendley, K. Meier, C. D. Marchant, and P. McVerry, Persistence of antibody and booster response to reimmunization with *Haemophilus influenzae* type b polysaccharide and polysaccharide diphtheria toxoid conjugate vaccines in children initially immunized at 15 to 24 months of age, *Pediatrics 85:*288 (1990).
72. R. Ganguly and R. H. Waldman, T-and-B cell memory on mucosal surfaces, In: *The Secretory Immune System,* Ann N.Y. Acad Sc New York *409:*603 (1983).
73. S. B. Black, H. Shinefield, and the Kaiser Permanente Pediatric Vaccine Study Group, Immunization with oligosaccharide conjugate *Haemophilus influenzae* type b (HbOC) vaccine on a large health maintenance organization population: Extended follow-up and impact on *Haemophilus influenzae* disease epidemiology, *Pediatr. Infect. Dis. J. 11:*610 (1992).
74. W. G. Adams, K. A. Deaver, S. L. Cochi, B. D. Plikalytis, E. R. Zell, C. V. Broome, and J. D. Wenger, Decline of childhood *Haemophilus influenzae* type b (Hib) disease in the Hib vaccine era, *JAMA 269:*221 (1993).
75. T. V. Murphy, K. E. White, P. Pastor, L. Gabriel, F. Medley, D. M. Granoff, and M. T. Osterholm, Declining incidence of *Haemophilus influenzae* type b disease since introduction of vaccination, *JAMA 269:*246 (1993).
76. L. E. Broadhurst, R. L. Erickson, and P. W. Kelley, Decreases in invasive *Haemophilus influenzae* diseases in US army children, 1984 through 1991, *JAMA 269:*227 (1993).

23

Conclusions from Immunogenicity Studies, Efficacy Trials, and Large-Scale Use of Vaccines

Juhani Eskola and Helena Käyhty

National Public Health Institute, Helsinki, Finland

I. INTRODUCTION

Haemophilus influenzae type b (Hib) conjugate vaccines are chemically and immunologically well characterized. This knowledge is, however, not sufficient for public health authorities who have to decide whether a vaccine should be used in large scale, which vaccine to choose, and what would be the best schedule of using it. Important information can be obtained from immunogenicity and efficacy trials, but the final test of the usefulness of a vaccine is demonstration of its ability to reduce the incidence of the target disease safely with reasonable cost.

Careful analysis of the current experience can provide guidance for future decisions. In this chapter, we will discuss which immunological properties are important for protective efficacy, what benefits can be expected from large-scale vaccinations, whether the Hib vaccines are safe, and what would be their optimal use.

II. IMMUNOLOGICAL PROPERTIES PREDICTING PROTECTION

A. General Properties

The four presently available Hib conjugate vaccines (PRP-D, HbOC, PRP-OMPC, and PRP-T) differ chemically from each other. Although all these vaccines contain the capsular polysaccharide of Hib bacteria, the size of the polysaccharide varies, as does the protein carrier and the linkage method (1,2).

However, the important immunological property common to all of them and lacking from the polysaccharide vaccine is the ability to induce protective antibodies in infants and in high-risk patients who do not respond to Hib polysaccharide vaccine (3–15). The Hib conjugate vaccines are also able to induce a strong and rapid, IgG-dominated antibody response when a primed child is revaccinated later in life (16).

In addition to the clearly higher concentration of antibodies induced by the conjugates, a considerable amount of data speaks for qualitative differences in the immune response to Hib conjugate vaccines compared to the polysaccharide vaccine. Conjugate vaccines behave as T-cell–dependent immunogens and thus induce the development of immunologic memory. Antibodies evoked by conjugate vaccines are also functionally different from those induced by the polysaccharide vaccine or those occurring naturally (17,18).

In contrast to what has been seen after immunization with polysaccharide vaccines, mucosal carriage of Hib bacteria is also reduced in children vaccinated with Hib conjugates (19–22). All these properties might be important for the ability of Hib conjugate vaccines to protect from invasive infection.

B. Antibody Concentration

Earlier clinical trials with the Hib polysaccharide vaccine produced data to suggest that the antibody concentration of 0.15 μg/ml in vaccinated children predicted short-term protection, whereas a concentration of 1 μg/ml was required for long-term protection (23,24). Although considerably higher antibody concentrations can often be seen in most infants after primary immunization with Hib conjugate vaccines, a significant number of vaccinated children remain below these concentrations. In one comparative immunogenicity study, the percentage of infants with an antibody concentration of at least 1 μg/ml after three doses of vaccine was 29% for PRP-D, 75% for HbOC, 55% for PRP-OMPC, and 83% for PRP-T (25).

In the first efficacy trial with PRP-D, 70% of the vaccinated infants had antibody concentrations above 0.15 μg/ml and only 40% above 1 μg/ml. In 15% of the postvaccination samples the antibody concentration was too low to be detected, while the clinical protection was 90% (26). This suggests that the correlation between the antibody response and clinical protection is more complicated than just a direct one between the antibody concentration and the rate of protection.

C. Immunological Memory

The development of immunological memory and its significance have been demonstrated in several studies. Characteristics of the immune response after vaccination of children who have received a Hib conjugate vaccine are typical to a secondary response: the increase of antibody concentration is rapid and higher than after the first dose of the same vaccine given at the same age (Fig. 1), and the antibodies are mainly of the IgG class. Even those children who do not respond to the primary immunization show this secondary response suggesting that they have been primed although no response in serum antibodies can be demonstrated in the initial phase [26]. The good clinical protection afforded by the Hib conjugate vaccines seems to correlate fairly well with the extent to which they induce immunologic memory.

All Hib conjugates prime for a secondary type response later in life. However, the increase in antibody concentration after subsequent doses of PRP-OMPC is not as marked as with other conjugates. The explanation might be that the PRP-OMPC is not as strongly T-cell dependent as the others, and in fact has many features of a T-cell–independent type-1 antigen (27).

It is important to note that the booster effect can be seen also if a child who has been primed with a conjugate vaccine receives a dose of polysaccharide (28). By analogy it can thus be expected that when a vaccinated child encounters Hib bacteria, a rapid booster response will ensue.

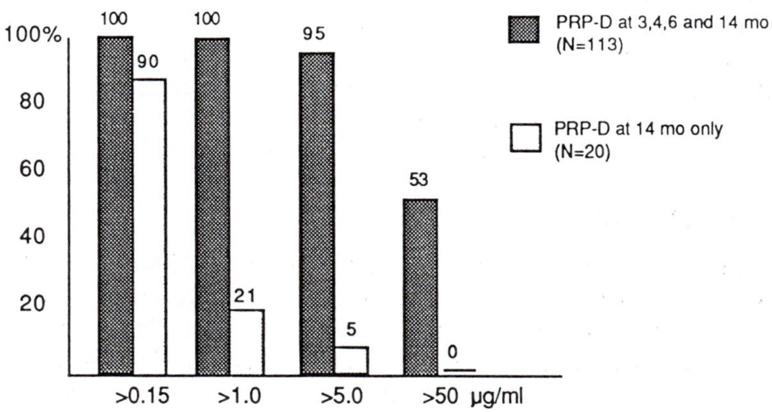

Figure 1 Percentage of 15-month-old children with the indicated serum concentration of anti-Hib polysaccharide 1 month after PRP-D. Dark bars show the distribution in children who had been immunized in infancy and boosted at 14 months; light bars represent children vaccinated at 14 months only.

More evidence for the importance of priming comes from children who became asymptomatic carriers of Hib bacteria after vaccination with a Hib conjugate vaccine. They demonstrate a booster-type antibody response (21). Spontaneous high antibody responses have also been recorded during the follow-up of children vaccinated earlier with Hib conjugates (5).

D. Functional Activity of the Antibodies

Several studies have shown that all Hib conjugate vaccines induce anti-PRP that are functionally active; they are bactericidal (29–31) opsonizing (32–34), and protect animals from bacteremia and meningitis (5,8,35) after challenge with Hib. The most compelling evidence of the activity of anti-PRP comes, however, from studies that show that these vaccines are clinically protective in humans.

There are qualitative differences between the antibodies induced by the conjugate vaccines and those induced by the polysaccharide vaccine (17). Antibodies induced by conjugate vaccines were more effective than polysaccharide-induced antibodies in supportinng neutrophil-mediated killing of an Hib strain (18). Also the protective efficacy in an infant rat infection model was significantly greater with the PRP-D–induced antisera than with the polysaccharide vaccine–induced antisera, when the same concentrations of anti-PRP were given passively.

Schlesinger et al. have compared the average avidity of antibodies evoked in infants by PRP-T, PRP-OMPC, and HbOC (36). In this study the avidity of antibodies evoked by HbOC was the highest and of those evoked by PRP-OMPC the lowest. Even though this study did not compare the functional activity of all antibodies directly, it could show that serum bactericidal activity correlated positively with the avidity of antibodies. This suggests that antibodies evoked by PRP-OMPC conjugate vaccines might have lower protective capacity than antibodies evoked by PRP-T or HbOC.

E. Mucosal Immunity

After vaccination with a Hib conjugate vaccine, specific IgG and IgA antibodies can be found in saliva (37). Both these antibodies have been shown to reduce colonization in an infant rat model (38). The salivary IgA response does not correlate with the serum response, but instead correlates with the presence of the secretory component, suggesting that the IgA in saliva are locally produced. In contrast, the concentration of salivary IgG anti-PRP correlates with the concentration of anti-PRP in serum, a finding consistent with passive transudation of IgG antibodies from the serum.

At present, it is still unknown to what extent this mucosal immunity contributes to protection from invasive Hib infections. However, it is clear that by reducing oropharyngeal carriage, vaccination can decrease transmission of Hib bacteria in the population. This should lead to increased efficacy of vaccination on the population level.

III. PROTECTION FROM INVASIVE Hib INFECTION

A. Efficacy in Clinical Trials

The protective efficacy of Hib conjugate vaccines in preventing invasive Hib infection has been evaluated both in prospective field trials conducted in the prelicensure period and in postlicensure case-control studies. In addition, evidence for protective efficacy has been collected in studies in which changes in the incidence of Hib disease have been compared in the vaccinated and nonvaccinated groups.

Most prospective studies have demonstrated a high rate of efficacy of the Hib conjugates in young infants. PRP-D was 90% efficacious (95% confidence interval [CI]: 70–96%) in Finland (26), HbOC 100% efficacious (95% CI: 68–100%) in Northern California (39), and PRP-OMPC 93% efficacious (95% CI: 53–98%) in Arizona (40). No final results are at present available from the efficacy of PRP-T, but preliminary findings from an English trial suggest a similarly high efficacy for this vaccine (point estimate 100%, 95% CI: 47–100%) (41). This is supported by data from three trials: one in California (42), another in North Carolina (data cited Ref. 7), and the third in Finland (43).

In the PRP-D study, the study group consisted of a socioeconomically and genetically homogeneous Scandinavian population, and in the HbOC study, of a mixed U.S. general population. The results from those studies can thus be generalizable to other industrialized countries with a low or moderate risk of invasive Hib disease. The efficacy trial with PRP-OMPC was conducted in a population with an exceptionally high incidence of Hib disease. Since a high level of protection was achieved even in those difficult circumstances, at least as good protection can be expected in circumstances in which infection pressure is lower. On the basis of these efficacy trials, PRP-D, HbOC, and PRP-OMPC have been licensed for general use both in Europe and America (44). Based on good immunogenicity data and the efficacy experience cited above, PRP-T has also been licensed in European countries and the United States (see Chapter 24) (7).

Questions relating to the efficacy of PRP-D have been raised on the basis of results from a prospective, placebo-controlled study conducted in high-risk settings among the Alaskan Native population; no significant protection could be demonstrated in this study (point estimate 35%, 95% CI: −57 to 73%) (45). There are several potential explanations for the apparently contradictory results in the Finnish (26) and Alaskan studies (46). In our opinion, the most probable ones are differences in the epidemiology of invasive Hib disease (higher incidence in Alaska and different age distribution of the disease both suggesting a high infection pressure) (47,48), differences in socioeconomical factors relating to chances of infection (household composition, duration of breast feeding) (49,50), and differences in the timing of vaccinations in the studies.

Studies on the efficacy of PRP-D have also been published after the licensure of the vaccine for use in children aged 18–59 months in the United States. The protection observed has been better than after Hib polysaccharide vaccine but not complete. In these case-control studies, the point estimates for efficacy varied from 74 to 88% (51,53). These data, together with the result of the Alaskan trial, suggest that the protection achieved by PRP-D is less than ideal at least in settings in which the risk of infection is great.

B. Reduction of Oropharyngeal Carriage

In addition to prevention of invasive infection, Hib conjugate vaccines have an effect on the mucosal carriage of Hib bacteria. The first data were obtained from a surveillance of the effects of PRP-D. In a Finnish study (19), oropharyngeal carriage of Hib was demonstrated in 14 out of 398 3-year-old children who had not been vaccinated, a rate comparable to that reported in the literature (54). Instead, none of the 327 vaccinated children carried Hib. Reduced carriage rate or intensity of colonization has also been recorded in preliminary results from other studies with PRP-D, HbOC, or PRP-OMPC (20–22).

C. Impact of Large-Scale Vaccinations

Large-scale vaccinations with Hib conjugate vaccines in infancy have been carried out in Finland since 1986, in Iceland since 1989, and in United States, Canada, Switzerland, and Germany since 1990. The first experiences of the public health impact of these vaccination programs are now available.

A sharp decline in the incidence rate of invasive Hib disease was seen during the years 1986–1991 in Finland when all infants were vaccinated as part of the efficacy trials with either PRP-D, HbOC, or PRP-T (Fig. 2) [43]. In 1991 there were only two cases among children less than 5 years of age in the whole country compared to the 120–180 cases seen annually before the vaccinations started.

Iceland was the second country to start nationwide vaccinations. Also there the disease has nearly disappeared during the years of vaccination and carriage of Hib bacteria has been reduced. Since 1989, no cases of Hib

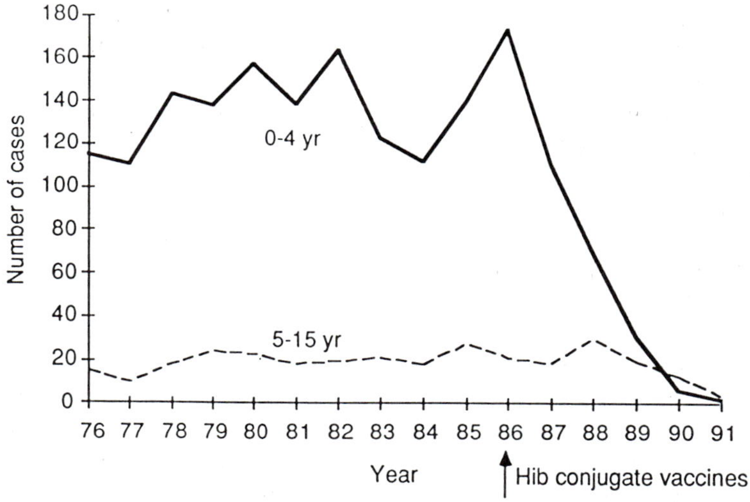

Figure 2 Number of invasive Hib infections in Finland in 1976–1991 among children aged 0–4 years (solid line) and among those older than 5 years (dotted line). Childhood vaccinations with Hib conjugate vaccines started in 1986 in the whole country.

meningitis have occurred, and only two cases of other bacteremic infections caused by Hib occurring beyond neonatal period have been confirmed in Iceland (55).

The vaccination and follow-up in Northern California have been continued after the efficacy trial with HbOC was completed. A 94% reduction was recorded in the number of Hib cases in 1991 compared to figures from the years 1984 to 1987 (56). A significant reduction has also been recorded in the U.S. national meningitis reporting system, with an estimated 9900 cases prevented per year by 1992 (57).

The decline in the incidence of invasive Hib infections has as a rule started in the vaccinated age groups but also has been seen later in older children and in infants. This finding speaks for the effect of the vaccination on the carriage of Hib, leading to reduced transmission, and also for herd immunity created by extensive vaccination.

IV. SAFETY OF THE VACCINES

As Hib conjugate vaccines are among the chemically purest vaccines in use, it is no surprise that their reactogenicity is low compared with most other vaccines. The reported rates of adverse reactions have varied a lot, and the results are difficult to interprete because of variable definitions and methods in recording symptoms. However, the conclusion is that Hib conjugate vaccines are safe, and the reported reactions have in most cases not been clinically very significant.

Since Hib conjugate vaccines in practice are administered simultaneously with other childhood vaccines, mainly with diphtheria-tetanus-pertussis (DTP) or polio vaccines, their direct contribution to the observed rate of adverse reactions is difficult to define. However, in several studies, the character and rate of adverse effects in children receiving Hib conjugate vaccines simultaneously with DTP have been quite similar to those in children receiving DTP only. Most investigators have therefore concluded that there is no substantial increase in adverse events if Hib conjugate vaccines are used simultaneously with other vaccines (5,7,8,58).

Since Hib conjugates are a totally new type of vaccine, their potential for rare serious reactions has also been evaluated. In a study of approximately 30,000 children vaccinated with PRP-D, the rate of both local and systemic reactions observed within 48 hours of vaccination was low. Hospitalizations and seizures occurring within 1 month of immunization appeared to be unrelated to vaccination (59). Another study with HbOC confirmed this finding (60). Further postlicensure studies are currently being conducted.

The above results of specific studies are supported by experience from routine vaccinations. The Finnish experience after approximately 927,000 doses of Hib conjugate vaccines suggests that there are no major differences between the reported adverse reaction rates of various vaccines (Table 1). By fall 1992, approximately 50 million doses of Hib conjugate vaccines had been distributed and used in various countries. Surveillance by vaccine manufacturers or public health authorities has to our knowledge not revealed any signs of severe unexpected reactions related to Hib conjugate vaccines.

Table 1 Frequency of Adverse Reactions (Reports/100,000 Doses Administered in Infancy) Associated with Hib Conjugate Vaccines (data based on 927,000 doses of vaccine given in Finland)

	Frequency of adverse reactions[a]				
Vaccine	Total	Local reaction	Fever	Rash	Irritability
PRP-D	14.1	5.3	6.3	4.4	2.9
HbOC	17.8	7.7	8.9	8.3	—
PRP-T	15.9	6.2	5.9	2.8	2.4

[a]One child may have more than one symptom.

V. CURRENT USE OF Hib CONJUGATE VACCINES

Current recommendation is that vaccination with Hib conjugates can be started during the first months of life; in practice national authorities usually recommend 2–4 months as the starting age. In no place does the routine schedule at present start below the age of 6 weeks. In some countries, e.g., the United States, PRP-D has been licensed only for use at the age of 15 months and older (44), whereas in other countries, e.g., Germany and Iceland, it is successfully used in infancy. HbOC, PRP-OMPC, and PRP-T are licensed and used from infancy on.

Especially for developing countries and populations in which the risk of Hib disease is high and most cases occur very early in life, it would be beneficial if vaccinations could be started during the neonatal period. Unfortunately, preliminary results from two studies are not promising (61,62). At present, the only advice for such high-risk situations is therefore to choose a vaccine with a good immune response very early, preferably already after the first immunization. A clear-cut antibody response can be seen after the first dose in infants vaccinated with PRP-OMPC (8). In some but not all series, PRP-T has also induced an antibody response after the first dose in early infancy (25,63).

Based on results of published efficacy studies, two or three doses of the Hib conjugate vaccines should be used in infancy. A booster dose during the second year of life is included in most routine schedules to ensure a long-term persistence of anti-PRP concentrations high enough for protection. This is a safe practice, although perhaps even fewer doses might be enough (64). Understandably, reduction of the number of vaccine doses is difficult before better serological correlates for protection have been found, and the simplification of the vaccination schedule can be done without fear of losing protective efficacy.

One practical question related to the availability of several Hib conjugate vaccines in the market is whether one can start with one vaccine and give subsequent doses or the booster dose with another. This question was partially answered when it was shown that Hib polysaccharide vaccine can booster the response after any of the conjugate vaccines (28). In no cases has a conjugate vaccine been a less effective immunogen than the polysaccharide. On this basis it is very likely that any conjugate vaccine would be good for eliciting a booster response in a primed child. However, before formal recommendations can be given, results from ongoing studies testing such combined schedules must be awaited.

An advantage of all Hib conjugate vaccines is that they can be given simultaneously with other childhood vaccines. There is a short period of only a few months in infancy when several vaccines should be administered, and if simultaneous administration would not be possible, obstacles for wide use would be significant. Fortunately, Hib conjugate vaccines have been administered for years simultaneously with DTP, polio vaccines, and measles-mumps-rubella vaccines without impairment of the immune response to any of the vaccine components or increase in adverse effects. Thus far the vaccines have been administered as separate injections, but during recent years, mixtures of DTP or inactivated polio vaccine and Hib conjugate vaccines (PRP-D, HbOC, or PRP-T) have also been tested (65–69). A combination vaccine of PRP-D and DTP is already licensed in Canada as is HbOC and DTP in the United States.

VI. COST-EFFECTIVENESS

The vaccination program should also be efficacious in economic terms. The cost effectiveness of immunization of U.S. children with Hib polysaccharide vaccine was evaluated when this was available (70). A recent study compared the direct costs of Hib disease and the vaccinations in infancy in five Western countries (Australia, Finland, Israel, Switzerland, and United Kingdom). In spite of variations in the incidence of the disease and a different health care system in each country, the cost-effectiveness could clearly be demonstrated. The break-even cost of a vaccination program to prevent 90% of Hib disease was estimated to vary from $22 to $84 per child (71). Using similar calculations, the estimate for the United States was considerably higher—$301 per child—because of a higher incidence of disease and higher cost of hospitalization.

VII. CONCLUSIONS

The results of the immunogenicity and efficacy trials with Hib conjugate vaccines show that these vaccines meet the expectations formulated at the beginning of the 1980s. They are highly immunogenic in infants, safe to use, and efficacious in protecting from invasive Hib disease. The cost of vaccination is acceptable. The experience accumulated from several countries after years of large-scale use shows that the clinical protection is even better than expected, probably because the vaccine reduces carriage of Hib bacteria and induces herd immunity.

Continual surveillance of the immune status in the population and the epidemiology of Hib disease is, however, needed for years. There are no data on the long-term duration of immunity and no data on the consequences of potential disappearance of Hib bacteria, although the fact that Hib colonization in unvaccinated populations is less than 10% suggests that it is not an important part of the normal flora. Thus, we do not know yet whether booster doses of Hib vaccine would be needed later in life; this can be decided in time on the basis of both epidemiological and population-based antibody data.

Although some questions remain, practical conclusions can be drawn from existing knowledge. Public health authorities should pay attention to the immunological properties of different Hib conjugate vaccines in addition to the epidemiological situation in their country in order to choose the best vaccine and appropriate vaccination schedule. However, in most cases, the success of vaccination is dependent on how actively the vaccine is used, i.e., on the vaccination coverage. The vaccines now available are good enough to prevent Hib disease if used on a large scale.

REFERENCES

1. J. B. Robbins and R. Schneerson, Polysaccharide-protein conjugates: A new generation of vaccines, *J. Infect. Dis. 161*:821 (1990).
2. G. A. Weinberg and D. M. Granoff, Polysaccharide-protein conjugate vaccines for the prevention of *Haemophilus influenzae* type b disease, *J. Pediatr. 113*:621 (1988).
3. J. Eskola, H. Käyhty, H. Peltola, et al., Antibody levels achieved in infants by course of *Haemophilus influenzae* type b polysaccharide/diphtheria toxoid conjugate vaccine, *Lancet 1*:1184 (1985).
4. M. S. Einhorn, G. A. Weinberg, E. L. Anderson, et al., Immunogenicity in infants of *Haemophilus influenzae* type b polysaccharide in a conjugate vaccine with *Neisseria meningitidis* outer-membrane protein, *Lancet 2*:299 (1986).
5. D. V. Madore, C. L. Johnson, D. C. Phipps, et al., Safety and immunologic response to *Haemophilus influenzae* type b oligosaccharide-CRM_{197} conjugate vaccine in 1- to 6-month-old infants, *Pediatrics 85*:331 (1990).
6. B. A. Claesson, R. Schneerson, J. B. Robbins, et al., Protective levels of serum antibodies stimulated in infants by two injections of *Haemophilus influenzae* type b capsular polysaccharide-tetanus toxoid conjugate, *J. Pediatr. 114*:97 (1989).
7. B. Fritzell and S. Plotkin, Efficacy and safety of a *Haemophilus influenzae* type b capsular polysaccharide-tetanus protein conjugate vaccine, *J. Pediatr. 121*:355 (1992).
8. V. I. Ahonkhai, L. J. Lukacs, L. C. Jonas, et al., *Haemophilus influenzae* type b conjugate vaccine (meningococcal protein conjugate) (Pedvax HIB): Clinical evaluation, *Pediatrics 85*:676 (1990).
9. J. F. Marcinak, A. L. Frank, R. L. Labotka, et al., Immunogenicity of *Haemophilus influenzae* type b polysaccharide-diphtheria toxoid conjugate vaccine in 3- to 17-month-old infants with sickle cell diseases, *J. Pediatr. 118*:69 (1991).
10. A. L. Frank, R. J. Labotka, S. Rao, et al., *Haemophilus influenzae* type b immunization of children with sickle cell disease, *J. Pediatr. 82*:571 (1988).

11. D. M. Granoff, G. A. Weinberg, and P. G. Shackelford, IgG subclass response to immunization with *Haemophilus influenzae* type b polysaccharide-outer membrane protein conjugate vaccine, *Pediatr. Res. 24*:180 (1988).
12. M. C. Steinhoff, B. S. Auerbach, K. E. Nelson, et al., Antibody responses to *Haemophilus influenzae* type b vaccines in men with human immunodeficiency virus infection, *N. Engl. J. Med., 325*:1837 (1991).
13. L. C. Schneider, R. A. Insel, G. Howie, et al., Response to a *Haemophilus influenzae* type b diphtheria CRM_{197} conjugate vaccine in children with a defect of antibody production to *Haemophilus influenzae* type b polysaccharide, *J. Allergy Clin. Immunol. 85*:948 (1990).
14. R. A. Insel and P. W. Anderson, Response to oligosaccharide-protein conjugate vaccine against *Haemophilus influenzae* b in two patients with IgG_2 deficiency unresponsive to capsular polysaccharide vaccine, *N. Engl. J. Med. 315*:499 (1986).
15. A. Barra, C. Cordonnier, M.-P. Preziosi, et al., Immunogenicity of *Haemophilus influenzae* type b conjugate vaccine in allogeneic bone marrow recipients, *J. Infect. Dis. 166*:1021 (1992).
16. H. Käyhty, J. Eskola, H. Peltola, et al., Immunogenicity in infants of a vaccine composed of *Haemophilus influenzae* type b capsular polysaccharide mixed with DPT or conjugated to diphtheria toxoid, *J. Infect. Dis. 155*:100 (1987).
17. O. Mäkelä, P. Mattila, N. Rautonen, et al., Isotype concentrations of human antibodies to *Haemophilus influenzae* type b polysaccharide as such or conjugated to a protein (diphtheria toxoid), *J. Immunol. 139*:1999 (1987).
18. A. Deveikis, K. S. Kim, and J. I. Ward, Prevention of *Haemophilus influenzae* type b in infant rats by human antibody induced by the capsular polysaccharide and polysaccharide-conjugate vaccines, *Vaccine 6*:14 (1988).
19. A. K. Takala, J. Eskola, M. Leinonen, et al., Reduction of oropharyngeal carriage of *Haemophilus influenzae* type b (Hib) in children immunized with an Hib conjugate vaccine, *J. Infect. Dis. 164*:982 (1991).
20. T. V. Murphy, P. N. Pastor, F. B. Medley, et al., Decreased *Haemophilus* colonization in children vaccinated with *Haemophilus influenzae* type b conjugate vaccine, *J. Pediatr. 122*:517 (1993).
21. M. L. Barbour, R. Booy, D. W. Crook, et al., *Haemophilus influenzae* type b; carriage and immunity four years after conjugate vaccination, *Program and Abstracts of the 32nd ICAAC*, Anaheim, CA, 1992, p. 273.
22. A. K. Takala, M. Santosham, J. Almeido-Hill, et al., Effect of *Haemophilus influenzae* type b (Hib) meningococcal protein conjugate vaccine (Hib-OMP) on oropharyngeal (OP) carriage of Hib among American Indian infants and children, *Programs and Abstracts of the 32nd ICAAC*, Anaheim, CA, 1992, p. 274.
23. H. Käyhty, H. Peltola, V. Karanko, et al., The protective level of serum antibodies to the capsular polysaccharide of a *Haemophilus influenzae* type b, *J. Infect. Dis. 147*:1100 (1983).
24. P. Anderson, The protective level of serum antibodies to the capsular polysaccharide of *Haemophilus influenzae* type b, *J. Infect. Dis. 149*:1034 (1984).
25. M. D. Decker, K. M. Edwards, R. Bradley, et al., Comparative trial in infants

of four conjugate *Haemophilus influenzae* type b vaccines, *J. Pediatr. 120*:184 (1992).
26. J. Eskola, H. Käyhty, A. K. Takala, et al., A randomized, prospective field trial of a conjugate vaccine in the protection of infants and young children against invasive *Haemophilus influenzae* type b disease, *N. Engl. J. Med. 323*:1381 (1990).
27. K. E. Stein, Thymus-independent and thymus-dependent responses to polysaccharide antigens, *J. Infect. Dis. 165*:49 (1992).
28. H. Käyhty, J. Eskola, H. Peltola, et al., High antibody responses to booster doses of either *Haemophilus influenzae* capsular polysaccharide or conjugate vaccine after primary immunization with conjugate vaccines, *J. Infect. Dis. 165*:165 (1992).
29. K. L. Cates, K. H. Marsh, and D. M. Granoff, Serum opsonic activity after immunization of adults with *Haemophilus influenzae* type b-diphtheria toxoid conjugate vaccine, *Infect. Immun. 48*:183 (1985).
30. P. W. Anderson, M. E. Pichichero, R. A. Insel, et al., Vaccines consisting of periodate-cleaved oligosaccharides from the capsule of *Haemophilus influenzae* type b coupled to a protein carrier: Structural and temporal requirements for priming in the human infant, *J. Immunol. 137*:1181 (1986).
31. P. Anderson, M. Pichichero, K. Edwards, et al., Priming and induction of *Haemophilus influenzae* type b capsular antibodies in early infancy by Dpo20, an oligosaccharide-protein conjugate vaccines, *J. Pediatr. 111*:644 (1987).
32. D. M. Musher, D. A. Watson, M. L. Lepow, et al., Vaccination of 18-month-old children with conjugated polyribosyl ribitol phosphate stimulates production of functional antibody to *Haemophilus influenzae* type b, *Pediatr. Infect. Dis. J. 7*:156 (1988).
33. B. M. Gray, Opsonophagocidal activity in sera from infants and children immunized with *Haemophilus influenzae* type b conjugate vaccine (meningococcal protein conjugate), *J. Pediatr. 85*:694 (1990).
34. P. P. Vella, J. M. Staub, J. Armstrong, et al., Immunogenicity of a new *Haemophilus influenzae* type b conjugate vaccine (meningococcal protein conjugate vaccine) (Pedvax HIB^{TM}), *Pediatrics 85*:668 (1990).
35. R. Schneerson, J. B. Robbins, C. Y. Chu, et al., Serum antibody responses of juvenile and infant rhesus monkeys injected with *Haemophilus influenzae* type b and pneumococcus type 6A capsular polysaccharide-protein conjugates, *Infect. Immunol. 45*:582 (1984).
36. Y. Schlesinger, D. M. Granoff, the Vaccine Study Group, Avidity and bactericidal activity of antibody elicited by different *Haemophilus influenzae* type b conjugate vaccines, *JAMA 267*:1489 (1992).
37. M. Kauppi, P.-R. Rönnberg, L. Saarinen, et al., Mucosal antibody concentrations after immunization with *Haemophilus influenzae* type b (Hib) conjugate vaccines, 7th International Congress of Mucosal Immunology, Prague, Czechoslovakia, August 16–20, 1992.
38. M. Kauppi, L. Saarinen, and H. Käyhty, Anti-capsular polysaccharide anti-

bodies reduce nasopharyngeal colonization by *Haemophilus influenzae* type b in infant rats, *J. Infect. Dis. 167:*365 (1993).

39. S. B. Black, H. R. Shinefield, B. Fireman, et al., Efficacy in infancy of oligosaccharide conjugate *Haemophilus influenzae* type b (HbOC) vaccine in a United States population of 61 080 children, *Pediatr. Infect. Dis. J. 10*:97 (1991).
40. M. Santosham, M. Wolff, R. Reid, et al., The efficacy in Navajo infants of a conjugate vaccine consisting of *Haemophilus influenzae* type b polysaccharide and *Neisseria meningitidis* outer-membrane protein complex, *N. Engl. J. Med. 324*:1767 (1991).
41. R. Booy, E. R. Moxon, J. A. MacFarlane, et al., Efficacy of *Haemophilus influenzae* type b conjugate vaccine in Oxford region, *Lancet 340*:847 (1992).
42. D. P. Greenberg, C. M. Vadheim, M. S. Marcy, et al., Evaluation of the safety, immunogenicity and efficacy of *Haemophilus influenzae* type b PRP-T conjugate vaccine in a prospective, randomized and placebo-controlled trial in young infants, *Programs and Abstracts of the 31st ICAAC*, Chicago, IL, 1991, p. 109.
43. J. Eskola, A. K. Takala, H. Käyhty, et al., Protection achieved by *Haemophilus influenzae* type b (Hib) conjugate vaccines is better than expected on the basis of efficacy trials, *Programs and Abstracts of the 32nd ICAAC*, Anaheim, CA, 1992, p. 273.
44. American Academy of Pediatrics, *Haemophilus influenzae* type b conjugate vaccines: recommendations for immunization of children 2 months of age and older: Update, *Pediatrics 88*:169 (1991).
45. J. Ward, G. Brenneman, G. W. Letson, et al., Limited efficacy of a *Haemophilus influenzae* type b conjugate vaccine in Alaska native infants, *N. Engl. J. Med. 323*:1393 (1990).
46. J. I. Ward, Prevention of invasive *Haemophilus influenzae* type b disease: Lessons from vaccine efficacy trials, *Vaccine 9*:17 (1991).
47. J. I. Ward, H. S. Margolis, M. K. Lum, et al., *Haemophilus influenzae* disease in Alaskan Eskimos: Characteristics of a population with an unusual incidence of invasive disease, *Lancet 1*:1281 (1981).
48. A. K. Takala, J. Eskola, H. Peltola, et al., Epidemiology of invasive *Haemophilus influenzae* type b disease among children in Finland before vaccination with *Haemophilus influenzae* type b conjugate vaccine, *Pediatr. Infect. Dis. J. 8*:297 (1989).
49. G. M. Petersen, D. R. Silimperi, C.-Y. Chiu, et al., Effects of age, breast feeding, and household structure on *Haemophilus influenzae* type b disease risk and antibody acquisition in Alaskan Eskimos, *Am. J. Epidemiol. 134*:1212 (1991).
50. A. K. Takala, J. Eskola, J. Palmgren, et al., Risk factors of invasive *Haemophilus influenzae* type b disease among children in Finland, *J. Pediatr. 115*:694 (1989).
51. D. P. Greenberg, C. M. Vadheim, N. Bordenave, et al., Protective efficacy of *Haemophilus influenzae* type b polysaccharide and conjugate vaccines in children 18 months of age and older, *JAMA 265*:987 (1991).

52. J. D. Wenger, R. Pierce, K. A. Deaver, et al., Efficacy of *Haemophilus influenzae* type b polysaccharide-diphtheria toxoid conjugate vaccine in US children aged 18–59 months, *Lancet 338*:395 (1991).
53. A. M. Loughlin, C. D. Marchant, S. Lett, et al., Efficacy of *Haemophilus influenzae* type b vaccines in Massachusetts children 18 to 59 months of age, *Pediatr. Infect. Dis. J. 11*:374 (1992).
54. R. H. Michaels, C. S. Pozviak, F. E. Stonebaker, et al., Factors affecting pharyngeal *Haemophilus influenzae* type b colonization rates in children, *J. Clin. Microbiol. 4*:413 (1976).
55. K. E. Jonsdottir, O. Steingrimsson, and O. Olafsson, Immunization of infants in Iceland against *Haemophilus influenzae* type b, *Lancet 340*:252 (1992).
56. S. B. Black, H. R. Shinefield, The Kaiser Permanente Pediatric Vaccine Study Group, Immunization with oligosaccharide conjugate *Haemophilus influenzae* type b (HbOC) vaccine on a large health maintenance organization population: Extended follow-up and impact on *Haemophilus influenzae* disease epidemiology, *Pediatr. Infect. Dis. J. 11*:610 (1992).
57. W. G. Adams, K. Deaver, S. Cochi, et al., Decline of childhood *Haemophilus influenzae* type b (Hib) disease in the vaccine era, *Programs and Abstracts of the 32nd ICAAC*, Anaheim, CA, 1992, p. 273.
58. J. Eskola, H. Käyhty, L. K. Gordon, et al., Simultaneous administration of *Haemophilus influenzae* type b capsular polysaccharide-diphtheria toxoid conjugate vaccine with routine diphtheria-pertussis-tetanus and inactivated polio vaccinations of childhood, *Pediatr. Infect. Dis. J. 7*:480 (1988).
59. C. M. Vadheim, D. P. Greenberg, S. M. Marcy, et al., Safety evaluation of PRP-D *Haemophilus influenzae* type b conjugate vaccine in children immunized at 18 months of age and older: follow-up of 30 000 children, *Pediatr. Infect. Dis. J. 9*:555 (1990).
60. S. Black, H. R. Shinefield, D. Lampert, et al., Safety and immunogenicity of oligosaccharide conjugate *Haemophilus influenzae* type b (HbOC) vaccine in infancy, *Pediatr. Infect. Dis. J. 10*:92 (1991).
61. S. Kurikka, H. Peltola, L. Saarinen, et al., Immunogenicity and tolerability of *Haemophilus influenzae* conjugate vaccine in neonates, *Frontiers in Vaccine Research*, abstracts of an International Symposium at Hanasaari, Espoo, Finland, 1991.
62. J. I. Ward, L. Bulkow, R. Wainwright, et al., Immune tolerance and lack of booster responses to *Haemophilus influenzae* (Hib) conjugate vaccination in infants immunized beginning at birth, *Program and Abstracts of the 32nd ICAAC*, Anaheim, CA, 1992, p. 274.
63. H. Käyhty, J. Eskola, H. Peltola, et al., Antibody responses to four *Haemophilus influenzae* type b conjugate vaccines, *Am. J. Dis. Child. 145*:223 (1991).
64. H. Käyhty, L. Saarinen, A. K. Takala, et al., One dose *Haemophilus influenzae* type b (Hib) conjugate vaccine in infancy, Abstract of APS-SPR-APA Annual Meeting 1992, Baltimore, 1992.
65. H. Shinefield, S. Black, T. Adelman, et al., Safety and immunogenicity of DTaP-HbOC—a combined oligosaccharide conjugate (HbOC, HibTITER[R])

Haemophilus influenzae type b and acellular DTP vaccine (DTaP) in toddlers, *Program and Abstracts of the 32nd ICAAC*, Anaheim, CA, 1992, p. 161.

66. P. Paradiso, D. Madore, D. Hogerman, et al., Immunogenicity of DTaP-HbOC in toddlers primed by DTP and HbOC as separate injections or DTP-HbOC combination vaccine, *Program and Abstracts of the 32nd ICAAC*, Anaheim, CA, 1992, p. 162.
67. A. Kovel, E. R. Wald, N. Guerra, et al., Safety and immunogenicity of acellular diphtheria-tetanus-pertussis and Haemophilus conjugate vaccines given in combination or at separate injection sites, *J. Pediatr. 120*:84 (1992).
68. C. Ferreccio, J. Clements, A. Avendano, et al., The clinical and immunologic response of Chilean infants to *Haemophilus influenzae* type b polysaccharide-tetanus protein conjugate vaccine coadministered in the same syringe with diphtheria-tetanus toxoids-pertussis vaccine at two, four and six months of age, *Pediatr. Infect. Dis. J. 10*:764 (1991).
69. N. Watemberg, R. Dagan, Y. Arbelli, et al., Safety and immunogenicity of Haemophilus type b-tetanus protein conjugate vaccine, mixed in the same syringe with diphtheria-tetanus-pertussis vaccine in young infants, *Pediatr. Infect. Dis. J. 10*:758 (1991).
70. S. L. Cochi, C. V. Broome, and A. W. Hightower, Immunization of US children with *Haemophilus influenzae* type b polysaccharide vaccine: A cost-effectiveness model of strategy assessment, *JAMA 253*:521 (1985).
71. D. A. Clements, R. Booy, R. Dagan, et al., A comparison of epidemiology and cost of *Haemophilus influenzae* type b (Hib) disease in five Western countries, *Pediatr. Infect. Dis. J. 12*:362 (1993).

24

Regulatory Perspectives in Vaccine Licensure

Carl E. Frasch

Center for Biologics Evaluation and Research, Bethesda, Maryland

I. INTRODUCTION

The first licensed *Haemophilus influenzae* type b (Hib) vaccine consisted of the purified capsular polysaccharide and was approved in 1985. The first Hib conjugate vaccine was approved 2 years later. The clinical and immunological studies required for approval of conjugate vaccines were based, in part, upon the existing database used for approval of the polysaccharide vaccine. The Hib polysaccharide vaccine was conceptually the same as the meningococcal and pneumococcal polysaccharide vaccines, which were first licensed about 10 years earlier, in that the immunological properties of the *Haemophilus* polysaccharide could be predicted based upon the vaccine's purity and molecular size. In contrast, conjugate vaccines represented a new application of a biotechnological process developed more than 60 years earlier (1). Each of the now licensed conjugate vaccines is different, having its own specifications and immunological characteristics. At the time of the first Hib conjugate vaccine there was no prior experience for guidance in establishment of product specifications. For example, what physical-chemical properties could be used to predict clinical potency? With virtually all polysaccharide vaccines there is a clear correlation between molecular size and immunogenicity. However, for the conjugates no such size correlation exists.

In the United States, clinical evaluation of a new vaccine begins with submission to the Food and Drug Administration (FDA) of an Investigational New Drug (IND) application. The IND application is the mechanism that allows investigational products, including vaccines, to be exempted from the licensing requirements so that they may be studied in humans for evidence of safety and effectiveness. Studies conducted under an IND can generally be divided into Phase I, Phase II, and Phase III. Phase I studies are conducted in relatively small numbers of individuals and are designed to show whether a vaccine does or does not have serious safety problems and to establish the best vaccine formulation. Phase II studies involve larger numbers of subjects and establish the optimal dosage and immunization schedule based upon antibody measurements. During Phase II studies the manufacturer is expected to demonstrate both clinical and manufacturing consistency. Finally, in well-designed controlled Phase III trials the efficacy of the vaccine is demonstrated as measured by disease prevention. Once the manufacturer has sufficient evidence for the safety and efficacy of the vaccine, a Product License Application (PLA) is filed, approval of which permits marketing of the new product.

After the different phases of vaccine evaluation under an IND or similar application are near completion and the sponsor believes the vaccine to be effective for its indication, a PLA and an Establishment License Application (ELA) are prepared by the manufacturer for submission to the national control authority for biological products. The PLA or its equivalent would include the detailed manufacturing process, proposed product specifications, product stability information, and all clinical studies supporting the safety and effectiveness of the product. The ELA or its equivalent contains information concerning the manufacturing facilities, including rooms, work areas, equipment, and personnel involved in production of the vaccine described in the PLA. The ELA must show that the product is being produced using good manufacturing practices such as those described in the U.S. Code of Federal Regulations, series 21, part 211.

This chapter will present the regulatory process that led to approval of the different Hib conjugate vaccines. It views the process from the perspective of U.S. FDA scientists, who were involved throughout the approval procedure for each Hib vaccine. The focus of this chapter will be the types of information used by the FDA to determine whether and how each Hib conjugate vaccine was demonstrated to be safe and effective. The World Health Organization has published requirements for Hib conjugate vaccines (2) as a guide for vaccine manufacturers and the national control authorities of countries using these vaccines.

II. Hib POLYSACCHARIDE VACCINE

Although the first Hib conjugate vaccine was approved in December of 1987, a review of the process leading to its approval must begin with the Hib polysaccharide vaccine, first licensed in April 1985 for use in children 24 months to 6 years of age. This is because the first conjugate vaccines were approved based upon clinical comparisons with the polysaccharide. A new manufacturer, Praxis Biologics, was first to market the polysaccharide, and by the end of 1985 two additional manufacturers, Connaught Laboratories, Inc. and Lederle Laboratories, were licensed.

Between 1973 and 1977 a blinded efficacy trial was conducted in Finland in over 100,000 children to determine whether a group A meningococcal polysaccharide vaccine could prevent group A meningococcal disease in infants and children. As a control for this trial, an Hib polysaccharide vaccine was administered in a dose of 12.7 μg to 49,000 children 3 months to 6 years of age (3). The trial was designed to demonstrate efficacy of the group A vaccine, which it did. Sufficient Hib disease was present in the population to measure the protective efficacy of the control polysaccharide. This trial would, almost 10 years later, become the basis for the demonstration of the efficacy of Hib polysaccharide vaccines.

A. Safety

The record of safety for the meningococcal polysaccharide vaccines provided some assurance regarding the safety of purified polysaccharide vaccines. However, the Hib polysaccharide would be the first polysaccharide vaccine to be given routinely to large numbers of young U.S. children. At the time of approval different Hib polysaccharide vaccines had been given to more than 60,000 children, most during the Finnish efficacy studies. An Hib polysaccharide was administered to 9000 children in Mecklenberg County, North Carolina (4), in which no serious adverse reactions were reported. Studies of the Praxis Biologics vaccine indicated that about 2% of children would have local reactions, and another 2% fever over 38°C, substantially less than for diptheria-tetanus-pertussis vaccine (DTP). The lower levels of local and systemic reactions can be attributed to the substantially reduced levels of endotoxin present in the polysaccharide compared to DTP. Thus, these data provided the needed safety data for approval. Since it was not practical to look for the occurrence of rarer adverse reactions before approval, the manufacturers were required to conduct post-marketing surveillance for immediate and, importantly, delayed adverse reactions. Praxis, working with the Northern California Kaiser Permanente HMO, established an electronic tracking system to follow up for a period of 30 days 100,000 children receiving the Hib polysaccharide vaccine (5). The design and tracking system of this postmarketing study became the basis for several subsequent postmarketing studies with other vaccines.

B. Efficacy

Licensure of the polysaccharide vaccine depended upon evidence showing that the vaccine manufactured in 1985 had physical and chemical characteristics comparable to the vaccine shown to be efficacious in the Finnish efficacy trial and had equivalent immunogenicity. The problem was that there was little published information concerning the physical and chemical properties of the earlier Finnish vaccine, although studies on immunogenicity of the vaccine had been published (3). Approval, therefore, depended heavily on demonstration of equivalent immunogenicity and upon the knowledge that the polysaccharide should be of high molecular weight.

There have been several attempts to estimate the amount of anti-Hib polysaccharide antibody required for protection against invasive Hib disease. Studies by Robbins et al. (6) estimated that 0.1 μg/ml of anti-Hib polysaccharide antibody was protective based upon the amount of antibody present in sera from adults and in agammaglobulinemic children receiving immunoglobulin therapy. Later studies by the Finnish investigators showed that 1 μg/ml or more of antipolysaccharide antibody 3–4 weeks after immunization was indicative of long-term protection (7). The 1 μg/ml value was used by the FDA not so much as a measure of protection but as a benchmark for comparison of vaccines. The most important measure was not the overall geometric mean titer (GMT), but the percent of children responding to the vaccine with >0.15 and >1.0 μg/ml. Using this measure the new polysaccharide vaccine induced immune responses equivalent to the Finnish vaccine.

C. Manufacturing

Purity of the Hib polysaccharide was based, in part, upon the requirements established for the meningococcal polysaccharide vaccines, in that it had to contain less than 1% nucleic acid and 1% protein. An important difference was the requirement for much less endotoxin (40 times less) than was permitted in the meningococcal vaccines. The purity requirement set for the polysaccharide vaccine was retained for the saccharide portion of each of the Hib conjugate vaccines.

III. THE FIRST *HAEMOPHILUS* CONJUGATE VACCINE (PRP-D)

The lower-than-expected efficacy of the Hib polysaccharide vaccine in the United States (8) increased the pressure on the manufacturers to develop

Table 1 Chronology of Approvals for Vaccines Against *H. influenzae* Type b

Date approved	Manufacturer	Type of vaccine	Trade name	Name used in paper	Age at first dose (months)
Apr. 12, 1985	Praxis	Polysaccharide	B-CAPSA I™	PRP	24
Dec. 20, 1985	Connaught	Polysaccharide	HIB-VAX™	PRP	24
Dec. 20, 1985	Lederle	Polysaccharide	Hib-Immune™	PRP	24
Dec. 22, 1987	Connaught	Conjugate	ProHIBit™	PRP-D	18[a]
Dec. 21, 1988	Praxis	Conjugate	HibTITER™	PRP-CRM	18[a]
Dec. 20, 1989	Merck	Conjugate	PedvaxHIB™	PRP-OMPC	15
Oct. 4, 1990	Praxis	Conjugate	HibTITER™	PRP-CRM	2
Dec. 13, 1990	Merck	Conjugate	PedvaxHIB™	PRP-OMPC	2
Mar. 30, 1993	Pasteur-Mérieux	Conjugate	ActHIB™	PRP-T	2

[a]Approved on November 2, 1989 for immunization of children ≥15 months of age.

more effective Hib vaccines and for the FDA to expedite the approval process. In 1980 Schneerson et al. (9) published the first description of an Hib conjugate vaccine, and shortly thereafter scientists at Connaught Laboratories used this methodology to produce the first commercial conjugate vaccine. In December 1987, Connaught Laboratories became the first manufacturer to receive a product license for a Hib conjugate vaccine (Table 1). The proper name for their vaccine is Hib Conjugate Vaccine (Diphtheria Toxoid Conjugate), but it is often referred to as PRP-D. The vaccine is a liquid and formulated to contain 25 μg of Hib polysaccharide conjugated to 18 μg of diphtheria toxoid per 0.5-ml dose.

A. Safety

Inasmuch as PRP-D was the first conjugate vaccine to be tested in humans, extensive studies were requested starting with immunization of adults. By the time the vaccine had been approved it had been administered in U.S. studies to approximately 350 children between 16 and 24 months of age and to 720 children between 7 and 14 months. In addition, the vaccine had been administered to over 31,000 infants in Finland. Side effects were minimal, consisting of mild local reactions or low-grade fever. In a placebo-controlled trial in almost 900 children between 7 and 14 months of age, local and systemic reactions including fever occurred with equivalent frequencies in the PRP-D and placebo groups.

Although the vaccine appeared to elicit no serious immediate adverse reactions, as a requirement for licensure the FDA requested that a postmarketing study be conducted for unexpected adverse reactions in at least 10,000 children. A 30-day follow-up for serious adverse reactions, defined as requiring the parent to seek medical attention for the child, was conducted in more than 50,000 children (10). These Phase IV studies revealed a number of less common adverse reactions, including urticaria and febrile seizure, but no cause-and-effect relationship could be established.

B. Efficacy

Approval of the Connaught Hib conjugate vaccine for use in children as young as 18 months of age was derived from the Finnish polysaccharide vaccine efficacy trial, which established an antibody correlate of efficacy. Eighteen months was the youngest age that protection was found in Finland using the polysaccharide vaccine. The Connaught Hib conjugate vaccine was therefore approved for use in 18-month-olds based upon demonstration of better immunogenicity compared to the licensed polysaccharide vaccine (11,12). The GMT response of 24-month-olds to the polysaccharide was approximately 1 μg/ml compared to 3 μg/ml for PRP-D in 18- to 21-month-olds. More importantly, the rates of seroconversion to 1 μg/ml for the polysaccharide and conjugate vaccine were about 45% and 70%, respectively. Interestingly about 13% of children failed to show any response to the polysaccharide (<0.15 μg/ml preimmunization and less than twofold increase after immunization), compared to 2% of 18-month-olds for PRP-D. Subsequent postmarketing studies showed that PRP-D was significantly more effective in U.S. children than the polysaccharide vaccine (13,14).

It was important to know that conjugate-induced antibodies are biologically active. Antibodies induced by PRP-D were shown to be functionally equivalent to those induced by the polysaccharide (15). In direct comparisons between antisera obtained after immunization of children with the two vaccines, the bactericidal antibodies induced were functionally equivalent on a weight basis. The conjugate-induced antibodies were also compared in an infant rat model. The rats were passively protected by both polysaccharide- and conjugate-induced antibodies (16).

C. Manufacturing

PRP-D consists of somewhat size-reduced Hib polysaccharide attached through a six-carbon spacer, adipic hydrazide, to diphtheria toxoid as described by Schneerson et al. (9). The spacer was attached to the protein, followed by reaction with cyanogen bromide–activated polysaccharide. This resulted in a conjugate having a protein to polysaccharide ratio of approximately 0.7. Studies by Connaught clearly showed that the polysaccharide must be attached to the protein for it to be immunogenic in animals and that the ratio of protein to polysaccharide affected the immunogenicity of the conjugate.

As a condition for approval, the manufacturer was asked to demonstrate that their conjugate vaccine could be consistently prepared to the same specifications. To do so, they needed to prepare three consecutive lots and submit them to the FDA for analysis along with manufacturing test results on these lots. The three lots need to be produced in the manufacturing facility by the same manufacturing process for which a license is being sought. The lots need not be produced to full manufacturing scale but should make use of all pieces of equipment to be used in the full-scale process. Any changes in the method of manufacture should be reported, and any change that results in a new manufacturing step should be approved by the national control authority. The consistency lots must meet all lot release specifications (see Ref. 2).

Specifications are set for each of the important product components, based upon the physical and chemical characteristics of vaccine lots shown to be effective. The ratio of polysaccharide to protein, the amount of unconjugated Hib saccharide and protein in the vaccine, as well as the degree of conjugation are important product specifications (2). The specification limits are set based upon the analytical results on vaccine lots with the desired immunological characteristics and the reproducibility of the assay methods used.

It was reasoned that only saccharide attached to protein would be immunogenic in young children. FDA scientists therefore requested that methods be devised to specifically quantitate free saccharide, in part as a measure of vaccine stability. An excellent method was developed by Connaught Laboratories based on the strong affinity of the diphtheria toxoid for phenyl sepharose. The unconjugated saccharide that fails to attach to the phenyl sepharose is quantified. PRP-D has a specification of not more than 37% free saccharide at the start of the dating period. It was found that free saccharide accumulated at a rate of about 1% a month. However, when vaccine lots, stored for 1–4 years at 2–8°C with free saccharide contents ranging from 50 to 80%, were clinically evaluated, the older lots were found to have comparable immunogenicity in children to recently manufactured vaccine. A dating period of 24 months was established for this vaccine.

IV. PRP-CRM OLIGOSACCHARIDE VACCINE

The Hib conjugate vaccine manufactured by Lederle-Praxis is unique in that it does not contain the Hib polysaccharide, but oligosaccharides of about 25 repeat units attached directly to Diphtheria CRM_{197} protein. The CRM_{197} protein is a naturally nontoxic variant of diphtheria toxin. The proper name of the vaccine is Hib conjugate vaccine (diphtheria CRM_{197} protein conjugate) and is referred to as PRP-CRM, or HbOC. PRP-CRM is a liquid formulation containing 10 μg of Hib oligosaccharide and 25 μg of CRM_{197} protein per dose. The vaccine was licensed in December 1988 for immunization of children 18 months to 6 years of age.

A. Safety

At the time PRP-CRM was licensed, PRP-D had been on the market for a year and over a million doses had been administered with few reported serious adverse reactions. Although concern for the overall safety of conjugate vaccines was reduced, PRP-CRM was tested in over 1000 children. Side effects associated with use of the vaccine were minimal and similar to those reported for PRP-D. Twenty-four hours after immunization, about 2% of children had erythema, 1% had swelling, and 2% had local tenderness. About 2% of the children had mild systemic reactions. Safety data from ongoing efficacy trials in more than 25,000 infants provided further assurance for the safety of PRP-CRM.

B. Efficacy

Efficacy of the Praxis vaccine in children beginning at 18 months of age was supported by the same polysaccharide efficacy trial as PRP-D. PRP-CRM induced much higher antibody levels in toddlers than the polysaccharide. Thus, PRP-CRM was approved based upon superior immunogenicity in 18-month-old children compared to the polysaccharide in 24- to 26-month-olds.

Three lots of the vaccine were examined in multicenter trials for clinical consistency. The GMT antibody responses of 287 children 15–23 months of age increased from 0.2 to 13.4 μg/ml after a single dose of vaccine. Ninety-nine percent of these children had 1 μg/ml or more of anti-Hib polysaccharide antibody. Interestingly, when the antibody responses of 15- to 17-month-old children were examined separately, the GMT was 12.5 μg/ml, and again 99% had >1 μg/ml of antibody.

Inasmuch as over 50% of invasive Hib disease occurs in children under 18 months of age, there was a desire to protect a greater number of children. From the standpoint of the ability to respond to the conjugate vaccine, the 18-month recommendation was an arbitrary cut-off but was based on the minimum age at which the polysaccharide had elicited protection in Finland. The FDA advisory committee had clearly stated that efficacy studies were required for use of conjugate vaccines in infants, but children between 12 and 18 months of age were in a gray zone. The FDA requested data on the age-specific ability to respond to a single dose of conjugate vaccine. The Connaught vaccine, PRP-D, had been approved based on 70–75% seroconversion to 1 μg/ml at 18 months of age. When PRP-CRM and the Merck conjugate vaccines (see below) were compared, both reached the 70–75% seroconversion rate by 12 months of age. Furthermore, the age-related ability to repond to the Praxis vaccine peaked by 15 months of age. In July of 1989 the FDA Vaccines and Related Biological Products Advisory Committee was asked their opinion on lowering the age of immunization to 12 or 15 months of age. The committee recommended 12 months, but concerns about interference with ongoing infant efficacy trials led the FDA to approve in November 1989 a reduction of the minimum age for immunization to 15 months of age, as an interim measure until an infant recommendation could be approved.

C. Manufacturing

The methodology used to produce the PRP-CRM vaccine is based upon studies by Porter Anderson (17). A vaccine prepared from short oligosaccharides, from a conceptual standpoint, should be very reproducible. The first of the oliogosaccharide-CRM vaccines was prepared using oligosaccharides obtained by acid hydrolysis of the *Haemophilus* polysaccharide, but later studies showed that a more immunogenic vaccine could be prepared by use of periodate-hydrolyzed polysaccharide, because this produced oligosaccharides, activated at both ends, which were able to covalently interact by reductive amination with the protein (18). Praxis Biologics chose the CRM_{197} protein because of carrier priming by DTP vaccine and because more lysine amino groups were available to interact with the oligosaccharides, since the protein was not detoxified with formalin. Earlier studies by Anderson showed that the number of oligosaccharides per protein, i.e., the packing density, was critical for an optimal antibody response (18). From these observations, we considered the protein-to-saccharide ratio an important measure of potency. The average protein-to-saccharide ratio for PRP-CRM is 2.5, compared to 0.7 for PRP-D.

Because the oligosaccharides are activated at both ends, they cross-link CRM_{197} molecules to produce high-molecular-weight aggregates (17). The size of these aggregates is controlled. Stability studies demonstrate little increase in free saccharide during storage at the recommended temperature of 2–8°C and little change in the elution profile on Sepharose 4B.

V. Hib CONJUGATE VACCINE UTILIZING A MEMBRANE VESICLE CARRIER

Compared to the other conjugate vaccines, the Merck conjugate vaccine has a number of unique properties. The protein carrier is not a component of the DTP vaccine, but lipopolysaccharide-depleted meningococcal outer membrane vesicles. Unlike the other vaccines, the Merck vaccine induces a strong immune response in infants after the first dose. Recent studies suggest that the unique immunological properties are probably related to the nature of the protein carrier (20,21). The proper name of the vaccine is Hib conjugate vaccine (meningococcal protein conjugate), and it is commonly referred to as PRP-OMP or PRP-OMPC. The vaccine is a freeze-dried product to be reconstituted with the aluminum hydroxide diluent provided. Each dose of the reconstituted vaccine contains 15 μg of Hib polysaccharide covalently bound to 250 μg of meningococcal protein, for a protein-to-polysaccharide ratio of about 17. The vaccine was licensed in December 1989 for immunization of children 15 months and older.

A. Safety

The safety profile of PRP-OMPC was of special concern, because the vaccine contained more LPS than the other Hib conjugates due to the LPS present in the OMPC. However, essentially all of the increased LPS was membrane bound, and animal studies have shown such LPS to be about 100-fold less toxic than free LPS (22). In preliminary clinical studies in children, PRP-OMPC was evaluated after reconstitution with either saline or aluminum hydroxide (23). Children in both groups had equivalent immune responses, but those who received the aluminum hydroxide-reconstituted vaccine had fewer adverse reactions.

At the time of approval, PRP-OMPC had been administered to more than 2100 children 2–71 months of age, all actively followed for adverse reactions. Approximately 1000 of the children were over 1 year of age, and those under 1 year of age received two doses of vaccine. In the older age group 4% of the individuals had fevers of >38.3°C, compared to 2–4% of younger children. Induration/swelling > 2.5 cm in diameter was observed in 1–2% of vaccinees. Additional adverse experiences reported included nausea, vomiting, diarrhea, rash, and high-pitched crying, but no serious adverse reactions requiring medical attention were reported. These data provided the safety database needed to approve the vaccine for use in children 15 months of age and older.

B. Efficacy

The vaccine was licensed for use in children 15–71 months of age based upon its ability to induce antibodies in 15-month-old children superior to those induced by the polysaccharide vaccine in 24- to 26-month-olds. A single dose of PRP-OMPC induced approximately 4 μg/ml in 15- to 18-month-olds, and 85% had 1 μg/ml or more of antipolysaccharide antibodies. The age-related maturation in ability to respond to a single dose plateaued between 18 and 20 months of age, somewhat older than for PRP-CRM. As with the other conjugate vaccines, PRP-OMPC–induced antibodies in children were shown to be mostly IgG1 and to be both bactericidal and opsonic.

C. Manufacturing

The Merck Hib conjugate vaccine is composed of markedly size-reduced polysaccharide (about 75 repeat units compared to over 400 in the native polysaccharide) attached to lipopolysaccharide-depleted outer membranes from *Neisseria meningitidis* through a bigeneric spacer using methodology described by Marburg et al. (24). In this process the polysaccharide and OMPC are separately derivatized, and then the two components covalently linked creating a unique amino acid, S-carboxymethylhomocysteine (S-CHMC). Use of a bigeneric spacer allows precise quantitation of the number of functional groups added to the polysaccharide and covalent links created during the final conjugation. Measurements of these compounds is a critical part of the lot release testing performed by the manufacture.

The polysaccharide is derivatized by addition of bromacetyl groups, and these are quantitated in relation to the polysaccharide to determine the degree of side-chain loading. Over derivatization of the polysaccharide could be expected to reduce its immunogenicity. Thus, there was a specification for the amount of bromacetyl groups. The OMPC is derivatized by reaction with *N*-acetylhomocysteine thiolactone. Acid hydrolysis of the conjugate releases S-CHMC which, when measured in relation to the ribose content, provides an important measure of polysaccharide loading onto the OMPC.

The protein carrier of PRP-OMPC is not a single protein, but membrane vesicles containing three or four major surface exposed proteins of the meningococcal outer membrane. These proteins all become thiolated and contribute to conjugate formation. Though there are several proteins in the membrane, they are consistently present in similar proportions in different membrane preparations.

The manufacturing process removes nearly all of the unreacted polysaccharide, and measurements of stability include monitoring for release of free saccharide and immunogenicity in BALB/c mice (23). The free saccharide levels and mouse immunogenicity remain stable throughout the dating period.

VI. AN INFANT INDICATION

A Hib conjugate vaccine was first approved for routine immunization of infants in October 1990. Three vaccines, PRP-D, PRP-CRM and PRP-OMPC, were entered into infant efficacy trials (25–28), but only the last two were approved for use in infants.

The Connaught vaccine, PRP-D, was the first vaccine to complete efficacy trials, one in Finland, the other in Alaska (25,26). In January 1989 the FDA's Vaccines and Related Biological Products Advisory Committee heard conflicting results from the two efficacy studies. The Finnish trial had an efficacy rate of 90%, but the Alaska trial failed to demonstrate efficacy. In the Finnish trial the GMT antibody level was 0.53 μg/ml after three doses, with 40% having 1 μg/ml or more, compared to a GMT of only 0.11 μg/ml in the Alaska trial. Protection in Finland was seen in the presence of lower-than-expected antibody levels. An explanation for these conflicting results was proposed by Robbins and Schneerson (29). Thus, failure of the 1974 Finnish polysaccharide vaccine trial results to accurately predict efficacy of the polysaccharide in the United States, indicating a possible difference in the epidemiology of Hib disease between the two countries, and failure of PRP-D to protect in a high-risk U.S. population made it very difficult to justify approval of PRP-D for infant administration in the United States. Although never approved for use in U.S. infants, PRP-D has been to be excellent as a booster in toddlers who were primed as infants with another Hib conjugate vaccine (30).

PRP-CRM was approved for infant immunization based upon an efficacy trial in northern California using a three-dose primary immunization schedule at 2, 4, and 6 months of age (27). This trial, conducted in over 50,000 infants (22,124 received the vaccine and 30,558 were controls), showed the vaccine to be both safe and effective with an estimated efficacy of 100%. The trial was not placebo-controlled, but one in which the control group comprised two populations: those not offered the vaccine (excluded by day of birth) and those who were offered the vaccine but refused. The mean follow-up was less than one year. These features of trial design caused some problems in statistical analysis, but the complete absence of disease in infants receiving the full three-dose immunization series was compelling.

The Merck efficacy study was a double-blind placebo-controlled trial in Navajo Indian children, a population with an incidence of Hib disease approximately 10 times higher than that of the general U.S. population, permitting a much smaller study population (28). There was, however, some concern about a trial in such a high-risk population since PRP-D had failed to protect in a similar population in Alaska. Children were immunized with PRP-OMPC at 2 and 4 months and followed for disease occurrence until 18 months of age. In the trial 2056 children received the vaccine and 2105 received the aluminum hydroxide placebo. Efficacy was analyzed after the primary two-dose series. There was one case of disease in the vaccinated children compared to 14 in the placebo group, for an estimated efficacy of 93%. This study thus provided the efficacy data and some of the necessary safety data that led to approval of an infant indication in December 1990.

A decision was made to require a booster immunization at 15 months of age for infants receiving PRP-CRM and at 12 months of age (later changed to 12–15 months) for those receiving the PRP-OMPC vaccine. This decision was based on several considerations. Vaccine failures have occurred a year or more after the primary immunization series in children who did not receive a booster. As part of the approval process the manufacturers were asked to provide evidence for antibody persistence up to 2 years of age. There was decline in vaccine-induced antibodies, but the decline in antibodies following PRP-OMPC was much more rapid than for PRP-CRM. By 12–15 months of age the GMT in PRP-OMPC–vaccinated children was only about 0.3 μg/ml. However, there were data indicating that a booster dose with any Hib conjugate vaccine would induce a marked anamnestic response (30).

During the first 20 months following approval of the Hib conjugate vaccines for routine infant immunization, over 30,000,000 doses were administered, most frequently along with the DTP and oral polio vaccines. Attempts to assess the presence of possible rare adverse events in children receiving the Hib conjugate vaccine is compounded by the fact the vaccine is being administered with the much more reactogenic DTP vaccine, but also that the vaccines are administered at an age coinciding with the peak incidence of sudden infant death syndrome (SIDS) and appearance of neurological problems. SIDS has a peak incidence between 3 and 5 months of age and occurs with a frequency of about 1/500 live births (31). Thus, the probability is high that SIDS will occur shortly after immunization with any vaccine and will therefore be reported to the FDA as vaccine associated. More studies will be required to evaluate these associations.

VII. ANTIBODY SURROGATES FOR APPROVAL OF A NEW Hib CONJUGATE VACCINE

A. An Immunological Surrogate

Once a vaccine is approved it becomes ethically very difficult to design an acceptable blinded clinical trial to demonstrate efficacy of another conjugate vaccine. Immunological surrogates must be used, therefore, to demonstrate equivalence between a new vaccine and the existing licensed vaccines for the same indication. Approval of the Lederle-Praxis Hib conjugate vaccine for use in infants in October 1990 resulted in termination of two ongoing efficacy trials with the Hib conjugate vaccine manufactured by Pasteur Mérieux, referred to here as PRP-T.

Some immunological surrogates of an effective Hib conjugate vaccine are presented in Table 2. Studies of four different Hib conjugate vaccines have shown a number of common features that clearly differentiate the immune responses to conjugate vaccines from those to the unconjugated Hib polysaccharide. These include induction of antibodies in infants at an age when they do not respond to the free polysaccharide, induction of higher levels of IgG1 relative to IgG2, and priming of infants for a booster response to the native polysaccharide. However, conjugate vaccines differ from one another in the magnitude and duration of the initial response after the recommended two- or three-dose immunization series. Protection against Hib disease is associated with opsonic and bactericidal antibodies

Table 2 Some Immunological Surrogates of an Effective Hib Conjugate Vaccine to Be Considered in Evaluation of New Vaccines

1. Randomized comparative immunogenicity studies with currently licensed vaccines in infants.
2. Measurement of antibody persistence after the primary immunization series out to age of the recommended booster dose.
3. Determination of whether the conjugate vaccine primes infants for a subsequent booster response to the native polysaccharide given 6 months or more after primary immunization.
4. Comparison of IgG, IgM, and IgG subclasses following the primary immunization series to those reported for licensed vaccines.
5. Demonstration of functional capacity of conjugate-induced antibodies in infants by measurement of opsonic or bactericidal activity.

directed against the capsular polysaccharide. It is likely that opsonic activity alone is sufficient because individuals with deficiencies in the late complement components appear not to be at increased risk of Hib disease, as they are for meningococcal disease. Bactericidal and opsonic antibody levels to Hib have been shown to correlate with one another (32). It was the opinion of the FDA Vaccines and Related Biological Products Advisory Committee in September 1991 that immunological criteria as shown in Table 2 could be used as the basis for demonstrating clinical efficacy of a new Hib conjugate vaccine.

B. Approval of a New Hib Conjugate Vaccine

The Hib conjugate vaccine produced by Pasteur-Mérieux, Lyon, France (PRP-T), was approved for use in infants in March 1993. The proper name of the vaccine is Hib Conjugate Vaccine (Tetanus Toxoid Conjugate).

1. The Vaccine

Pasteur-Mérieux used a conjugation procedure developed in the laboratory of John Robbins (33). Adipic acid dihydrazide was used to add a six-carbon spacer molecule to the polysaccharide, which is then conjugated in presence of EDAC to purified tetanus toxoid. Free polysaccharide and other unconjugated reactants are removed by zonal centrifugation, resulting in a product substantially free of unconjugated materials. The vaccine is lyophilized and, when reconstituted with saline, contains 10 μg of polysaccharide and 24 μg of tetanus toxoid. The dried vaccine shows good stability when stored at 2–8°C, with no measurable change in the molecular size of the conjugate.

2. Safety of PRP-T

The Pasteur-Mérieux vaccine has been administered to more than 11,000 U.S. infants using a three-dose primary immunization series. The vaccine was frequently administered simultaneously with DTP and OPV. In comparative studies administration of PRP-T concurrently with DTP resulted in no increased local or systemic reactions compared to DTP alone. Children who received PRP-T alone had rates of adverse reactions comparable to those seen with the other Hib conjugate vaccines. Safety of PRP-T was also evident from studies in a number of countries including Chile, England, Finland, and France.

3. Immunological Correlates

PRP-T was evaluated against the immunological correlates shown in Table 2. It was compared for immunogenicity to the licensed Hib conjugate vaccines (34,35). In the Granoff study (34) the GMT antibody response of

PRP-T was not statistically different from either PRP-CRM or PRP-OMPC. After the full primary immunization series, the seroconversion rates to 1μg/ml for PRP-OMPC, PRP-CRM, and PRP-T were, respectively, 85, 90, and 97%. The decline in antibody levels for PRP-CRM and PRP-T were comparable, with a GMT of about 1 μg/ml at time of booster.

It is important to demonstrate that the primary immunization series will prime the infant for a subsequent booster response to the native polysaccharide alone as a surrogate for natural exposure. Finnish children who received the polysaccharide at 14 months of age after PRP-T at 4 and 6 months of age responded with an anamnestic response and a GMT of 29 μg/ml, compared to about 3 μg/ml when polysaccharide was given to unimmunized 14-month-olds (unpublished data).

The initial antibody response to all Hib conjugates, including PRP-T, includes both IgM and IgG. On reimmunzation the response becomes predominantly IgG, with proportionately more IgG1 (36,37). It is important to demonstrate that vaccine-induced antibodies are functionally active and comparable to that of licensed conjugates. Studies show that the avidity of conjugate-induced antibodies vary between different conjugates with PRP-CRM inducing overall higher avidity antibodies (38). Higher avidity antibodies on a weight basis are more bactericidal. PRP-T induced antibodies of higher avidity than PRP-OMPC.

Based on satisfactory demonstration that PRP-T met each of the antibody surrogates shown in Table 2, the vaccine became the first conjugate to be licensed using immunological surrogates of efficacy.

REFERENCES

1. O. T. Avery and W. F. Goebel, Chemo-immunological studies on conjugated carbohydrate-proteins. II. immunological specificity of synthetic sugar-proteins, *J. Exp. Med. 60*:533 (1929).
2. Requirements for Haemophilus type b conjugate vaccines (requirements for biological substances No. 46), WHO Technical Report Series, Geneva, No. 814, 1991.
3. H. Peltola, H. Makela, H. Kayhty, H. Jousimies, E. Herva, K. Hallstrom, A. Sivonen, O. V. Renkonen, O. Pettay, V. Karanko, P. Ahvonen, and S. Sarna, Clinical efficacy of meningococcus group A capsular polysaccharide vaccine in children three months to five years of age, *N. Engl. J. Med. 297*:686 (1977).
4. J. C. Parke Jr, R. Schneerson, J. B. Robbins, and J. J. Schlesselman, Interim report of a controlled field trial of immunization with capsular polysaccharides of *Haemophilus influenzae* type b and group C *Neisseria meningitidis* in Mecklenberg county, North Carolina (March 1974–March 1976), *J. Infect. Dis. 136*:s51 (1977).

5. S. B. Black, H. R. Shinefield, and the Northern California Permenente Medical Care Program Departments of Pediatrics Vaccine Study Group b-CAPSA I *Haemophilus influenzae*, type b capsular polysaccharide vaccine safety, *Pediatrics 79*:321 (1987).
6. J. B. Robbins, J. C. Parke Jr., R. Schneerson, and J. K. Whisnant, Quantitative measurement of "natural" and immunization induced *Haemophilus influenzae* type b capsular polysaccharide antibodies, *Pediatr. Res. 7*:103 (1973).
7. H. Kayhty, H. Peltola, V. Karanko, and P. H. Makela, The protective level of serum antibodies to the capsular polysaccharide of *Haemophilus influenzae* type b, *J. Infect. Dis. 147*:1100 (1983).
8. E. D. Shapiro and A. T. Berg, Protective efficacy of *Haemophilus influenzae* type b polysaccharide vaccine, *Pediatrics 85* (Suppl.):643 (1990).
9. R. Schneerson, O. Barrera, A. Sutton, and J. B. Robbins, Preparation, characterization, and immunogenicity of *Haemophilus influenzae* type b polysaccharide protein conjugates, *J. Exp. Med. 152*:361 (1980).
10. Connaught Laboratories, Inc., package circular, ProHIBiT Hib conjugate vaccine (diphtheria toxoid conjugate), Swiftwater, PA, February 1990.
11. C. D. Berkowitz, J. I. Ward, K. Meier, J. O. Hendley, P. A. Brunell, R. A. Barkin, J. M. Zahradnik, J. Samuelson, and L. Gordon, Safty and Immunogenicity of *Haemophilus influenzae* type b polysaccharide and polysaccharide diphtheria toxoid conjugate vaccines in children 15 to 24 months of age, *J. Pediatr. 110*:509 (1987).
12. J. O. Hendley, J. G. Wenzel, K. M. Ashe, and J. S. Samuelson, Immunogenicity of *Haemophilus influenzae* type b capsular polysaccharide vaccines in 18-month-old infant, *Pediatrics 80*:351 (1987).
13. A. M. Loughlin, C. D. Marchant, S. Lett, and E. D. Shapiro, Efficacy of *Haemophilus influenzae* type b vaccines in Massachusetts children 18 to 59 months of age, *Pediatr. Infect. Dis. J. 11*:374 (1992).
14. C. E. Frasch, E. E. Hiner, and T. P. Gross, Hib disease after vaccination with Hib polysaccharide or conjugate vaccine, *Am. J. Dis. Child. 145*:1379 (1991).
15. K. L. Cates, Serum opsonic activity for *Haemophilus influenzae* type b in infants immunized with polysaccharide-protein conjugate vaccines, *J. Infect. Dis. 152*:1076 (1985).
16. D. M. Granoff, E. G. Boies, and R. S. Munson, Immunogenicity of *Haemophilus influenzae* type b polysaccharide-Diphtheria toxoid conjugate vaccine in adults, *J. Pediatr. 105*:22 (1984).
17. P. W. Anderson, M. E. Pichichero, R. A. Insel, R. Betts, R. Eby, and D. H. Smith, Vaccines consisting of periodate-cleaved oligosaccharides from the capsule of *Haemophilus influenzae* type b coupled to a protein carrier: structural and temporal requirements for priming in the human infant, *J. Immunol. 137*:1181 (1986).
18. P. W. Anderson, M. E. Pichichero, E. C. Stein, S. Porcelli, R. F. Betts, D. M. Connuck, D. Korones, R. A. Insel, J. M. Zahradnik, and R. Eby, Effect of oligosaccharide chain length, exposed terminal group, and hapten loading on the antibody response of human adults and infants to vaccines consisting of

Haemophilus influenzae type b capsular antigen uniterminally coupled to the diphtheria protein CRM197, *J. Immunol. 142*:2464 (1989).
19. K. E. Stein, Thymus-independent and Thymus-dependent responses to polysaccharide antigens, *J. Infect. Dis. 165* (Suppl.):S49 (1992).
20. M. A. Liu, A. Friedman, A. I. Oliff, J. Tai, D. Martinez, R. R. Deck, J. T. C. Shieh, T. D. Jenkins, J. J. Donnelly, and L. A. Hawe, A vaccine carrier derived from *Neisseria meningitidis* with mitogenic activity for lymphocytes, *Proc. Natl. Acad. Sci. USA 89*:4633 (1992).
21. D. M. Ambriosino, D. Bolon, H. Collard, R. van Etten, M. V. Kanchana, and R. W. Finberg, The effect of *Haemophilus influenzae* polysaccharide outer membrane protein complex vaccine on macrophages, *J. Immunol. 149*:3978 (1992).
22. C. M. Tsai, C. E. Frasch, E. Rivera, and H. D. Hochstein, Measurement of lipopolysaccharide endotoxin in meningococcal protein and polysaccharide preparations for vaccine usage, *J. Biol. Stand. 17*:249 (1989).
23. P. P. Vella, J. M. Staub, J. Armstrong, K. T. Dolan, C. M. Rusk, S. Szymanski, W. E. Greer, S. Marburg, P. J. Kniskern, T. L. Schofield, R. L. Tolman, F. Hartner, S. Pan, R. J. Gerety, and R. W. Ellis, Immunogenicity of a new *Haemophilus influenzae* type b conjugate vaccine (meningococcal protein conjugate) (PedvaxHIB), *Pediatrics 85*(Suppl.):668 (1990).
24. S. Marburg, D. Jorn, R. L. Tolman, B. Arison, J. McCauley, P. J. Kniskern, A. Hagopian, and P. P. Vella, Bimolecular chemistry of macromolecules: synthesis of bacterial polysaccharide conjugates with *Neisseria meningitidis* membrane protein, *J. Am. Chem. Soc. 108*:5282 (1987).
25. J. Eskola, H. Peltola, A. K. Takala, H. Kayhty, M. Hakulinen, V. Karanko, E. Kela, P. Rekola, P.-R. Ronnberg, J. S. Samuelson, L. K. Gordon, and P. H. Makela, Efficacy of *Haemophilus influenzae* type b polysaccharide-diphtheria toxoid vaccine in infancy, *N. Engl. J. Med. 317*:717 (1987).
26. J. Ward, G. Brenneman, G. W. Letson, W. L. Heyward, and Alaska H. influenzae Vaccine Group, Limited efficacy of a *Haemophilus influenzae* type b conjugate vaccine in Alaska Native infants, *N. Engl. J. Med. 323*:1393 (1990).
27. S. B. Black, H. R. Shinefield, B. Fireman, R. Hiatt, M. Polen, E. Vittinghoff, and North CA Kaiser Perm Vaccine Sty Ctr, Efficacy in infancy of oligosaccharide conjugate *Haemophilus influenzae* type b (HbOC) vaccine in a United States population of 61 080 children, *Pediatr. Infect. Dis. J. 10*:97 (1991).
28. M. Santosham, M. Wolff, R. Reid, M. Hohenboken, M. Bateman, J. Goepp, M. Cortese, D. Sack, J. Hill, W. Newcomer, L. Capriotti, J. Smith, M. Owen, S. Gahagan, D. Hu, R. Kling, L. Lukacs, R. W. Ellis, P. P. Vella, G. Calandra, H. Matthews, and V. Ahonkhai, The efficacy in Navajo infants of a conjugate vaccine consisting of Haemophilus influenzae type b polysaccharide and Neisseria meningitidis outer-membrane protein complex, *N. Engl. J. Med. 324*:1767 (1991).
29. J. B. Robbins and R. Schneerson, Evaluating the *Haemophilus influenzae* type b conjugate vaccine PRP-D, *N. Engl. J. Med. 323*:1415 (1990).

30. M. D. Decker, K. M. Edwards, P. Palmer, and R. Bradley, Booster response to four *Haemophilus influenzae* b (Hib) conjugate vaccines, *Pediatr. Res. 31*:90A (1992).
31. S. B. Black, H. R. Shinefield, D. Lampert, B. Fireman, R. H. Hiatt, M. Polen, E. Vittinghoff, and The Northern California Kaiser Permanente Vaccine Study Center Pediatrics Group, Safety and immunogenicity of oligosaccharide conjugate *Haemophilus influenzae* type b (HbOC) vaccine in infancy, *Pediatr. Infect. Dis. J. 10*:92 (1991).
32. K. L. Cates, K. H. Marsh, and D. M. Granoff, Serum opsonic activity after immunization of adults with *Haemophilus influenzae* type b-diphtheria toxoid conjugate vaccine, *Infect. Immun. 48*:183 (1985).
33. C. Chu, R. Schneerson, J. B. Robbins, and S. C. Rastogi, Further studies on the immunogenicity of *Haemophilus influenzae* type b and pneumococcal type 6A polysaccharide-protein conjugates, *Infect. Immun. 40*:245 (1983).
34. D. M. Granoff, E. L. Anderson, M. T. Osterholm, S. J. Holmes, J. E. McHugh, R. B. Belshe, F. Medley, and T. V. Murphy, Differences in the immunogenicity of three *Haemophilus influenzae* type b conjugate vaccines in infants, *J. Pediatr. 121*:187 (1992).
35. M. D. Decker, K. M. Edwards, R. Bradley, and P. Palmer, Comparative trial in infants of four conjugate *Haemophilus influenzae* type b vaccines, *J. Pediatr. 120*:184 (1992).
36. D. M. Ambrosino, S. K. Sood, M. C. Lee, D. Chen, H. R. Collard, D. L. Bolon, C. Johnson, and R. S. Daum, IgG1, IgG2 and IgM responses to two *Haemophilus influenzae* type b conjugate vaccines in young infants, *Pediatr. Infect. Dis. J. 11*:855 (1992).
37. J. C. Parke, Jr., R. Schneerson, C. Reimer, C. Black, S. Welfare, D. Bryla, L. Levi, D. Pavliakova, T. Cramton, D. Schulz, M. Cadoz, and J. B. Robbins, Clinical and immunologic responses to *Haemophilus influenzae* type b-tetanus toxoid conjugate vaccine in infants injected at 3, 5, 7, and 18 months of age, *J. Pediatr., 118*:184 (1991).
38. Y. Schlesinger, D. M. Granoff, and Vaccine Study Group, Avidity and bactericidal activity of antibody elicited by different *Haemophilus influenzae* type b conjugate vaccines, *JAMA 267*:1489 (1992).

25

New Approaches to Polysaccharide Vaccines

Alexander H. Lucas

Children's Hospital Oakland Research Institute, Oakland, California

I. INTRODUCTION

The development of protein-conjugated *Haemophilus influenzae* type b (Hib) polysaccharide vaccines represents a major advance in pediatric immunization. Since the introduction in 1990 of the Hib conjugate vaccines for the immunization of infants starting at 2 months of age, the incidence of invasive Hib disease is already reported to be diminishing rapidly (1–4). This decrease in disease can be attributed directly to the ability of the conjugate vaccines to prime for and induce protective anti-Hib capsular polysaccharide (polyribosylribitol phosphate, PRP) antibody responses in infants (5–14). In addition, conjugate vaccination appears to lower Hib carriage rates, and this feature also may contribute to decreasing infections in susceptible populations (15,16).

The primary immunological problem encountered in developing an effective Hib vaccine is the maturational delay associated with immune responsiveness to PRP. The ability to produce serum antibodies in response to vaccination with plain PRP does not fully mature until after 2 years of age (17,18). The design strategy of the Hib conjugate vaccines was based upon empirical observations that polysaccharide immunogenicity could be increased by covalent attachment of protein carriers (19–21). Thus, an important milestone was achieved with the demonstration that protein carrier-linked PRP was immunogenic in 2-month-old infants (5). This fundamental observation not only validated the conjugate vaccine approach, but also demonstrated that PRP-specific B cells were actually present in early infancy. This latter point, which is prerequisite to any vaccination strategy, and which may appear obvious in retrospect, was not always apparent. Indeed, one hypothesis to explain the anergy of infants to polysaccharide vaccination posited that polysaccharide-specific B cells were not present in the infant because the appropriate immunoglobulin genes had not yet been assembled (22,23). Although this hypothesis can be rejected, at least in general for the PRP repertoire, it remains to be determined whether it may be true for other antipolysaccharide antibody repertoires whose expression is maturationally delayed.

The physiological basis underlying the requirement for protein carrier coupling to achieve polysaccharide immunogenicity in the infant is poorly understood. The attachment of a protein carrier to the polysaccharide is thought to convert the polysaccharide from a T-cell–independent antigen into a T-cell–dependent antigen. Presumably, carrier-reactive T cells are required to promote the activation and differentiation of PRP-specific B cells in the infant. This requirement for T-cell help appears to diminish with age, since older children and adults do produce antibodies after vaccination with plain PRP.

Despite our ignorance concerning mechanism, the success of the Hib conjugate vaccines validates the suitability of the empirical approach and its applicability to the development of new polysaccharide conjugate vaccines for other clinically relevant pathogens. However, the existing Hib conjugate vaccines differ in their immunological properties, and these differences may be important in the design of new conjugates. In the first part of this article, I will review this topic, and then consider future polysaccharide conjugate vaccines. Finally, I discuss some new approaches that may be applicable to polysaccharide vaccine design.

II. POLYSACCHARIDE CONJUGATE VACCINES

A. Immunological Differences Between the Hib Conjugate Vaccines

Three Hib conjugate vaccines are licensed presently in the United States for use beginning in 2-month-old infants: PRP oligomers coupled to CRM_{197}, a nontoxic mutant diphtheria toxin (HbOC); PRP coupled to the outer membrane protein complex of group B *Neisseria meningitidis* (PRP-OMPC); and PRP coupled to tetanus toxoid (PRP-T). These vaccines differ structurally (for detailed discussion see Chapters 3 and 6) and immunologically

Table 1 Immunological Differences Between the Hib Conjugate Vaccines

Characteristic	Example	Ref.
Immunogenicity	PRP-OMPC stimulates primary antibody response in 2-month-old infants, whereas HbOC and PRP-T do not	5, 14
Anamnestic response	Following 2nd and 3rd injections, HbOC stimulate markedly elevated serum antibody levels, whereas PRP-OMPC gives modest increases	10, 14
Carrier priming requirement	Vaccination with DT enhances anti-PRP response induced by PRP-T and HbOC in rhesus monkeys; in human infants, little anti-PRP response occurs following HbOC in absence of DT immunization, whereas PRP-OMPC is immunogenic in absence of DT immunization	27–29
Antibody avidity	Mean serum anti-PRP avidity following three injections: HbOC > PRP-T > PRP-OMPC	35
Idiotype/Light-chain Variable region expression	HbOC and PRP-T stimulate predominantly HibId-1/VκII-A2 antibodies, whereas PRP-OMPC stimulates both HibId-1/VκII-A2 and HibId-2/VλVII	37

(Table 1). A notable functional difference between the HbOC vaccine and the PRP-OMPC vaccine is their immunogenicity. The PRP-OMPC vaccine elicits serum PRP-specific antibody after one injection in 2-month-old infants, but generates only modest increases in serum antibody levels after two subsequent injections (5,10,14). The HbOC vaccine does not elicit detectable anti-PRP following a single injection in 2-month-old infants but primes for an anamnestic response as antibody production is stimulated upon two further immunizations at intervals of 1–2 months (10,14). Thus, the OMPC conjugate can stimulate a primary PRP-specific antibody response, but the CRM conjugate cannot. These differences in immunogenicity suggest that these vaccines elicit antibody responses by different mechanisms. Although the OMPC carrier contains T-cell epitopes and functions as a T-helper cell–inducing protein carrier (24), this property probably does not account fully for its ability to induce a primary response, since the CRM carrier also is thought to have effective T-cell–priming capability. Rather, the ability of the OMPC conjugate to elicit serum antibody in 2-month-old infants likely results from immunomodulating and adjuvantlike properties of the OMPC, such as its B-cell mitogenic (25) and macrophage-stimulating ability (26).

Thus, conversion of the polysaccharide into a T-cell–dependent antigen appears not to be the sole mechanism by which anti-PRP responses can be generated in infants.

Another difference between the Hib conjugate vaccines is the effect of carrier priming on immunogenicity. Studies in rhesus monkeys show that immunization with diphtheria and tetanus toxoids (DT) enhances the anti-PRP response to PRP-T and HbOC (27,28). Similarly, in human infants HbOC is minimally immunogenic in the absence of DT immunization (29). In contrast, PRP-OMPC vaccine, which has a carrier immunologically unrelated to DT, is immunogenic in infant rhesus monkeys and human infants irrespective of DT priming (28,29). Studies in mice show that carrier priming can either enhance or suppress the antibody response to haptens or polysaccharides coupled to the carrier (30–32). Similarly, in human infants, the consequences of carrier priming may be quite variable depending upon the age at priming. For example, vaccination of newborns with DT does not lead to enhanced, and may even suppress, anti-PRP responses following three injections of either HbOC or PRP-T at 2, 4, and 6 months of age (33). In contrast, vaccination of infants with DT at 1 month of age results in enhanced anti-PRP responses following three injections of either PRP-T or HbOC (34). Multiple mechanisms have been suggested to account for these disparate effects including induction of suppressor T-cell activities (30) and clonal competition by carrier-reactive B cells (31). Given this complexity, it is apparent that as new conjugate vaccines are introduced, careful monitoring of the carrier-priming effects will be required as the conclusions drawn from one conjugate vaccine or one priming schedule may not be generally applicable to another conjugate vaccine.

The Hib conjugate vaccines differ in the quality of the anti-PRP they induce. A comparison of antibody avidities elicited by the conjugate vaccines following three injections in infants showed that HbOC vaccination induced antibodies having the highest average avidity for PRP, whereas vaccination with the OMPC conjugate induced the lowest-avidity antibodies (35). The mean avidity of anti-PRP induced by PRP-T was intermediate between those induced by the HbOC and the OMPC vaccines. These differences in antibody avidity may relate to the size of the PRP moiety utilized in these vaccines. HbOC consists of PRP oligomers, whereas the OMPC and tetanus conjugates consist of higher molecular weight PRP. Conceivably, the oligomeric form of PRP may selectively activate B cells having higher-affinity receptors for PRP. In addition, HbOC and PRP-T may provide more extensive T-cell helper influence than the OMPC vaccine and, thereby, promote more B-cell clonal proliferation, accompanied by somatic mutation and subsequent affinity maturation.

Further evidence that the different Hib conjugate vaccines induce qualitatively different antibodies comes from idiotypic analyses. Two idiotypes have been defined that serve as markers for two light-chain variable regions used in anti-PRP: HibId-1 is a marker for the ϰII-A2 region (36), and HibId-2 is a marker for a λVII region (37). Anti-PRP bearing the HibId-1/VϰII-A2 region predominate the serum response of older children and adults immunized with either plain or protein-conjugated PRP (36,38). In contrast, serum anti-PRP having the HibId-2 idiotype are minimally represented in older children and adults (38) (see Chapter 10). When the serum expression of HibId-1 and HibId-2 anti-PRP was evaluated in infants who had received three injections of conjugate vaccine at 2, 4, and 6 months of age, a striking association between vaccine formulation and idiotype expression was observed (37). HibId-1 antibodies were present in 68 and 64% of infants immunized with either HbOC or PRP-T, respectively, whereas only 33% of infants vaccinated with PRP-OMPC produced HibId-1 antibodies. In contrast, HibId-2 antibodies were present in 47% of PRP-OMPC-vaccinated infants but in only 18 and 10% of infants vaccinated with HbOC or PRP-T, respectively. Furthermore, in this same study, a correlation was observed between anti-PRP avidity and idiotype expression. Infants who were immunized with either PRP-T or PRP-OMPC and who produced HibId-1 antibodies had higher avidity antibodies than infants not producing HibId-1 antibodies. On the other hand, infants immunized with HbOC produced high-avidity antibodies irrespective of idiotype expression.

These data indicate fundamental differences among the Hib conjugate vaccines in both the variable region composition and the functional activity of the antibodies they induce. Further study is required to determine whether these differences affect protective efficacy. In vitro studies show that higher-avidity anti-PRP are significantly more active in complement-mediated bactericidal and opsonic activities than lower-avidity antibodies (35,39), a result suggesting that vaccines that elicit higher-avidity antibodies, such as HbOC, may offer greater protection against invasive Hib disease, especially in those situations where low levels of anti-PRP antibodies are present.

B. Future Polysaccharide Conjugate Vaccines

The Hib conjugate vaccine strategy is being applied to the development of other polysaccharide vaccines for encapsulated bacteria that cause significant disease and that are poor immunogens in the young, the elderly, or other susceptible populations. It seems reasonable to expect success using the strategy of enhancing polysaccharide immunogenicity by conjugation of protein carriers. However, even the few Hib conjugate vaccines developed to date differ in their immunological properties, and, therefore, similar immunological variability likely will be encountered as more polysaccharide conjugate vaccines are developed.

New polysaccharide conjugate vaccines are being synthesized and evaluated individually. As the number of new vaccines increases, it will be of practical importance to determine whether different vaccines can be combined together in a single dose. For pediatric vaccination it is desirable to minimize the number of office visits as well as the number of separate injections administered at each visit and to integrate new vaccines into established vaccination schedules. A combination vaccine has been developed by Lederle-Praxis that consists of HbOC vaccine mixed with DTP vaccine. Immunogenicity studies indicate that the antibody responses to the individual components induced by the combination vaccine are comparable to the antibody responses induced by separate injection of the vaccines (40). A combination vaccine consisting of PRP-T and DTP is also being evaluated. Another practical issue, which is relevant to the existing Hib conjugate vaccines and which will become even more important as new conjugate vaccines are developed, is to determine whether vaccines utilizing the same or similar polysaccharide but linked to different carriers can be interchanged during the course of the injection series. Recent data suggest that infants vaccinated at 2 months of age with PRP-OMPC produce PRP-specific antibodies following two subsequent vaccinations with the HbOC vaccine (41). Indeed, the anti-PRP levels achieved after the third injection in this group exceeded the antibody levels achieved in infants receiving three injections of HbOC. Although somewhat surprising as one might have predicted that priming and booster injections with homologous vaccine would be superior to heterologous booster vaccination, these results are encouraging, for they suggest that vaccine "matching" may not be required during the vaccination regimen in order to achieve effective antipolysaccharide antibody responses. Similar studies will have to be undertaken with each new polysaccharide conjugate vaccine to ensure that these findings are generally applicable.

Conjugate vaccines for pneumococcal, group B streptococcal, *Salmonella typhimurium*, and *N. meninigitidis* polysaccharides are being formulated using the protein carriers that have proven suitable for Hib conjugate vaccines (42). In the future, one could envision a combination vaccine consisting, for example, of a mixture of tetanus toxoids that have been individually modified with different polysaccharides. To avoid high protein doses, the concentrations of the individual components may have to be decreased and the minimum immunogenic dose for each polysaccharide component determined empirically. The development of new adjuvants may facilitate this objective. Alternatively, a vaccine could be formulated that consists of a single carrier protein multiply conjugated with different polysaccharides. This strategy may suffer from difficulties in controlling and evaluating the extent of conjugation of the individual component polysaccharides. As the number of polysaccharides coupled to a carrier molecule increases, the probability of antigenically compromising the carrier by overmodification likewise increases.

Bacterially-derived proteins have served as adequate carriers for polysaccharide antigens. They have proven to be effective, relatively safe, and nontoxic. Elegant conjugation chemistries have been designed to modify proteins covalently with polysaccharides (43,44), but the sites on the carrier protein that are being modified remain for the most part ill-defined. Although the polysaccharide loading number can be monitored, the uniformity of particular peptidyl site modification between vaccine lots is generally not known. Since proteins may contain an hierarchy of T-cell epitopes, only a few of which may dominate in the immune response (45), any lot-to-lot variations in the modification of these putative immunodominant epitopes might result in variable carrier efficacy.

The lack of chemical definition of the carrier in conventional polysaccharide-protein conjugates could be circumvented if T-cell peptide epitopes could be identified and used as carriers in place of the full-sized native or toxoided protein. This strategy would have to take into account the potential for genetic restrictions or so-called immune response gene effects that operate at the level of major histocompatibility complex (MHC)-restricted presentation of peptides to T cells. Certain alleles of MHC class II may bind and present a particular peptide to specific T cells, whereas other class II alleles may not. Panina-Bordignon and colleagues identified a tetanus toxin peptide spanning amino acid residues 830 to 844 that promiscuously bound to human MHC class II and also functioned as a T-cell immunogen in all subjects studied (46). They suggested that this peptide might serve as a "universal" T-cell epitope. This tetanus peptide epitope also functioned in mice as a genetically unrestricted carrier for a *Plasmodium falciparum* merozoite antigenic peptide (47). Thus, the use of synthetic peptides as carrier determinants for polysaccharide vaccines merits further study.

Assuming that several promiscuous T-cell peptide epitopes could be identified for human use, there are several other design features that would have to be considered for a polysaccharide-vaccine utilizing synthetic peptide. To fullfill the need for "linked recognition," covalent linkage of the T-cell peptide determinant and the B-cell polysaccharide determinant would be required. This modification should not compromise either antigenic determinant. For example, it would have to be demonstrated that polysaccharide attachment to the peptide does not interfere with MHC presentation of the peptide to specific T cells. One potential configuration that would serve to link the two determinants utilizes a synthetic peptide scaffold. Using solid-phase peptide synthesis, Tam devised a multiple antigen peptide system (MAP) consisting of a core matrix of oligolysines that served as a scaffold to incorporate synthetic peptide antigens (48). In the original description, Tam demonstrated that a MAP containing peptides of 9–16 amino acid residues elicited specific antibodies reactive with the corresponding native proteins (48). The MAP system has been utilized in a malarial vaccine consisting of a MAP scaffold to which a B-cell peptide epitope and a T-cell peptide epitope of *Plasmodium berghei* were attached. This entirely synthetic vaccine was effective in protecting mice from infection with *P. berghei* sporozoites (49). The V3 loop of the gp120 protein of human immunodeficiency virus (HIV) also has been incorporated into a MAP (50). The MAP system as applied to peptide antigens has the advantages of the synthetic approach: a homogeneous molecularly-defined entity lacking the chemical ambiguities of traditional carrier-based vaccines and having flexibility in design elements such as size, molecular spacing, and branching. Application of the MAP system for the construction of a polysaccharide vaccine is illustrated in Figure 1. In this example, a single universal promiscuous T-cell peptide epitope and a single polysaccharide oligomer are attached at different sites to the oligolysine scaffold. One could envision variations on this theme such as attachment of multiple T-cell peptidyl epitopes and multiple B-cell polysaccharide determinants. The MAP system might be modified to include peptide sequences in the scaffold itself that serve as target sites favored by endosomal proteases. Engineering such sites into the scaffold would serve to facilitate intracellular processing of the molecule such that disjunction occurs between the polysaccharide epitope and the T-cell epitope, thus favoring association of the peptidyl moiety with MHC-II.

Other design criteria for new conjugate vaccines will have to be tailored to specific polysaccharides. For example, the choice between oligomers or higher-molecular-weight polysaccharide will be dictated largely by the antigenic requirements of particular polysaccharides. Anderson and colleagues have shown that oligosaccharide chain length is important in priming capability and immunogenicity of Hib conjugate vaccines in infants (51). Paoletti et al. also have demonstrated that a tetanus toxoid conjugate vaccine containing intermediate-sized oligosaccharides of group B streptococcus type III were superior to either smaller or larger oligo-

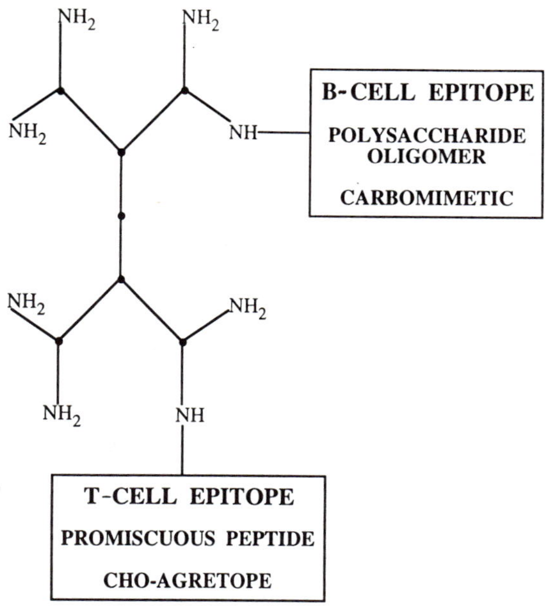

Figure 1 "Polysaccharide" vaccine construct. An oligolysine core matrix, as devised by Tam (48), covalently modified to contain a B-cell epitope (either a polysaccharide oligomer or a carbomimetic) and a T-cell epitope (either a promiscuous peptide or a carbohydrate [CHO]-peptidyl agretope).

saccharide conjugates in their ability to induce protective antibodies in rabbits (52). Undoubtedly oligosaccharide size will be critical in the design of other conjugate vaccines, especially those using polysaccharide such as the group B meningococcal (53,54) or pneumococcal type 14 (55), which require extended chain lengths in order to assemble conformational antigenic determinants.

The advent of recombinant DNA technology and the refinement of synthetic peptide chemistry have permitted the realization of recombinant vaccines for hepatitis B, malaria, and rabies. These vaccines contain epitopes capable of stimulating both T and B lymphocytes. Since the chemical synthesis of complex polysaccharides is still at an early stage (56), it is unlikely that a totally synthetic polysaccharide-protein conjugate vaccine will be developed in the near future. Nonetheless, combining the power of synthetic chemistry with our increasing knowledge of antigen recognition will lead to novel strategies for the design of future polysaccharide conjugate vaccines.

III. CARBOHYDRATE-SPECIFIC T CELLS

Although the cellular basis for the carrier effect remains to be fully elucidated, it is commonly accepted that one mechanism by which the attachment of a protein carrier enhances the immunogenicity of a polysaccharide involves conversion of the polysaccharide into a T-cell–dependent antigen. Implicit in this model is the notion that polysaccharides themselves are are not capable of directly sensitizing specific T cells, i.e., they are T-cell–independent antigens. Considerable evidence from studies of murine systems indicates that anticarbohydrate antibody responses in mature animals can occur in the relative absence of T lymphocytes (57), and this general notion may be true in humans as well. The lack of anamnestic antibody responses in adults to vaccination with purified polysaccharides has been taken as evidence of T-cell independence (58), and a recent study of patients with acquired immunodeficiency syndrome who were deficient in CD4 T cells (T-helper cells) showed that the antibody response to HbOC was impaired to a greater extent than the response to the plain polysaccharide (59).

T-cell receptors for antigen are generally thought not to be capable of directly recognizing polysaccharide antigens. Although studies of the murine response to SIII polysaccharide have implicated a type of T-suppressor/regulatory activity that is induced by SIII immunization (60), the specificity of these T cells for the SIII polysaccharide has not been demonstrated. Also, some studies suggest that immunization with carbohydrates or glycopeptides may induce T-cell–mediated cellular immune responses, but again, the specificity of the T cells has not been defined (61–63). If, however, carbohydrate antigens themselves could be made to be "T-cell recognizable," then this approach would offer a new strategy for the design of polysaccharide vaccines.

T-helper cells recognize fragments of protein antigens presented in the context of MHC class II molecules. Proteins are taken up by antigen presenting cells, proteolytically degraded and processed in the endocytic compartment, and subsequently presented on the cell surface in the peptide-binding groove of MHC class II molecules, where they then can be recognized by T-cell receptors. One explanation to account for the inability of carbohydrate antigens to sensitize T cells is that carbohydrate antigens are not presented to T cells in an MHC context, either because carbohydrates are not enzymatically processed in such a way as to allow their intracellular association with MHC and/or they intrinsically lack the structural properties required for binding to the MHC groove. Alternatively, T-cell receptors themselves may be intrinsically incapable of recognizing carbohydrate epitopes, although this explanation seems less likely given the similarities between T-cell receptor and immunoglobulin variable domains at both the genetic and protein levels. Thus, in principle, T-cell variable domains might be able to accommodate some carbohydrate epitopes as long as the epitope was presented in the appropriate MHC context.

Two recent studies suggest that T cells may indeed be capable of carbohydrate recognition. Ishioka and colleagues examined murine T-cell proliferative responses to *N*-acetyl-glucosamine (GlcNAc)–substituted analogs of an ovalbumin peptide known to be a dominant T-cell epitope (64). Comparisons between the ability of GlcNAc-substituted and -unsubstituted analogs to stimulate T cells indicated that in some instances the GlcNAc moiety was an integral part of the determinant being recognized by the T cell. Singhal and colleagues also have obtained data consistent with T-cell recognition of carbohydrate (65). They found that murine CD4-positive T cells proliferated and secreted interleukin-2 in vitro in response to a mucin from adenocarcinoma cells containing high levels of O-linked *N*-acetyl-galactosamine. T-cell responses were much lower to the deglycosylated form of the mucin. The involvement of peptidyl determinants in T-cell recognition could not be ruled out in either of these two studies. This caveat notwithstanding, these findings together suggest that T-cell receptors can, under appropriate conditions, recognize and respond to carbohydrate epitopes. Thus, a silent repertoire of carbohydrate-specific T cells may be present but rarely expressed, possibly as a result of constraints in antigen processing and/or MHC associability. This putative latent repertoire potentially represents a rich source of T-effector cells that could be tapped for therapeutic use.

One prerequisite for designing MHC-associable, T-cell–recognizable carbohydrate epitopes relies upon the identification of particular peptide sequences or sequence motifs responsible for the binding of peptide fragments to human MHC class II molecules. These areas of contact between peptides and MHC molecules have been termed agretopes, to distinguish them from epitopes, which are the regions of the peptide molecule directly recognized by the T-cell receptor variable domain. A single MHC molecule can potentially bind a large number of peptides, and different allelic forms of MHC class II may bind distinct repertoires of peptides. Therefore, a single agretope sequence may not be sufficiently promiscuous to bind all MHC class II molecules, although a region within the tetanus peptide discussed above is a possible candidate. Ogasawara and coworkers have identified what appears to be an agretope from pidgeon cytochrome c that associates with both the A^k and A^b alleles of murine MHC-II (66). This peptide sequence served as a cassette into which a synthetic peptide comprising a T-cell epitope of influenza virus hemagglutinin was inserted. Although no single agretope consensus sequence or particular motif has yet been identified, this area is an active field of study. Rapid progress is being made in the understanding of MHC recognition of protein antigens. Crystal structures of several MHC molecules are providing clues into the structure of the MHC peptide binding groove and the nature of the contacts between MHC and peptides (67–71). This structural information, in combination with immunological functional analysis, should lead in the future to general principles of agretope design (66,72,73).

Thus in the future, it may be possible to construct a "carrier determinant" containing a T-cell carbohydrate epitope attached to a peptidyl agretope. Figure 2 shows a cartoon of how this T-cell recognition may occur. The agretope peptide anchors the carbohydrate into the MHC-II binding groove and orients the carbohydrate epitope for engagement to the T-cell receptor. The viability of this approach will depend upon the identification of promiscuous agretopes that bind to a wide array of human MHC

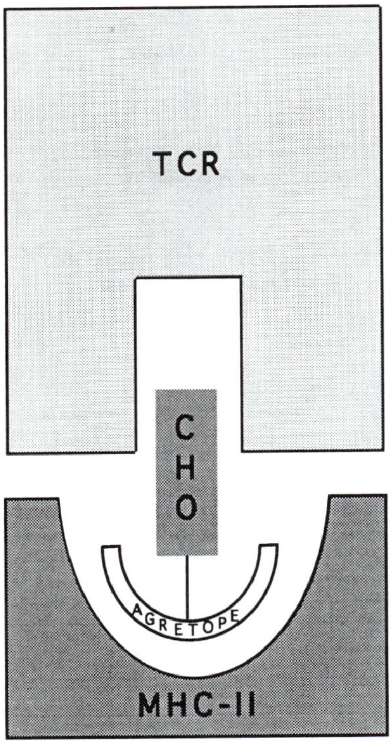

Figure 2 Hypothetical depiction of T-cell recognition of a carbohydrate (CHO) epitope. A peptide capable of MHC-II binding (agretope) is covalently linked to a CHO moiety. The agretope anchors the CHO in the MHC-II groove, allowing the T-cell receptor (TCR) to engage the CHO epitope.

alleles and the definition of the structural requirements of T-cell carbohydrate epitopes. A polysaccharide vaccine utilizing this type of T-cell determinant would of course still have to contain B-cell polysaccharide epitopes. Perhaps the MAP system could be used to linked these two entities. This approach avoids classic carrier coupling methods and the involvement of conventional carrier-reactive T cells and, thus, would avoid potential problems attendant with the use of conventional carriers such as carrier-priming effects and epitope suppression.

IV. CARBOMIMETICS: PEPTIDYL REPRESENTATIONS OF CARBOHYDRATE EPITOPES

Technologies based upon molecular genetic (74–77) and chemical synthesis techniques (78–81) have been developed that permit the construction of highly diverse peptide libraries. For example, one approach uses recombinant bacteriophage as a vehicle for expressing a diverse array of peptides on the surface of bacteriophage coat proteins (77). Peptide libraries, constructed either chemically or biologically and constituting millions of different peptidyl sequences, have been screened for biological activities, and peptidyl ligands have been identified that react with binding sites specific for biotin (76), methyl α-D-mannopyranoside (82,83), β-endorphin (75), and a peptide from interleukin 1β (84), to name a few.

This approach has great potential for drug discovery, and also may be useful for the identification of peptides that mimic carbohydrate epitopes. Geysen, who introduced the approach of using synthetic peptides as mimetics of antigenic determinants (mimotopes) (78), identified small peptides reactive with antibodies specific for the blood group A polysaccharide (85). More recently, two studies have shown that peptides can be isolated from a bacteriophage library that bind to the mannose-binding lectin concanavalin A (82,83). These peptides shared a common sequence motif, bound to methyl α-D-mannopyranoside with a Kd similar to concanavalin A, and they inhibited the precipitation reaction between dextran and concanavalin A. Mannose is a relatively simple sugar, and it may be premature to extrapolate these results to more complex polysaccharide antigenic determinants. Nonetheless, despite the lack of direct evidence for the ability of peptides to mimic three-dimensionally carbohydrate structures, these studies suggest that screening peptide libraries for reactivity with anticarbohydrate antibodies may identify carbomimetics, i.e., peptides that mimic carbohydrate antigenic determinants.

Rapid advances are being made in the construction of peptide libraries that may increase the likelihood of discovering carbomimetics. Longer peptides are being engineered, and they are being assembled in the context of tethering regions or minidomains that serve to constrain the peptide conformation and permit the expression of potentially complex, discontinuous peptide determinants. The recent work of Pessi et al. elegantly demonstrates this technology (86). Using a totally synthetic chemistry, they constructed a 61-amino-acid β-protein which they termed a minibody. The minibody was adapted from the structure of an immunoglobulin variable heavy domain and contained both framework sequences as well as two hypervariable sequences. Based upon the zinc-binding properties of carbonic anhydrase, they grafted histidine residues into the minibody hypervariable regions and generated a minibody with zinc-binding properties similar to carbonic anhydrase.

Immunoglobulins themselves have been used as scaffolds for grafting foreign residues. Zanetti and colleagues introduced the concept of "antigenizing" antibodies by inserting oligopeptides into the third hypervariable loop of the heavy-chain variable region (87). A peptide B-cell epitope of *Plasmodium falciparum* was grafted in this manner, and immunization of rabbits and mice with the antigenized antibody elicited antibodies that reacted with the native parasite antigen and inhibited parasite infectivity in vitro (88). Zaghouani et al. mutagenized the third hypervariable loop of a mouse antibody heavy chain to contain a helper T-cell epitope of the PR8 influenza virus hemagglutinin (89). When paired with its native light chain, this chimeric murine heavy chain was able to prime mice for a virus-specific T-helper cell response. Dose-response analysis showed that the chimeric heavy chain was one or more orders of magnitude more efficient at stimulating T-helper cells in vitro than the hemagglutinin peptide itself, presumably due to the efficient internalization of the chimeric immunoglobulin by Fc receptors on antigen-presenting cells. Thus, MHC-associable, foreign T-cell helper determinants can be generated from the processing of self-immunoglobulin molecules. This finding is consistent with studies showing that T-helper cells can recognize idiotypic determinants derived from the processing of endogenous immunoglobulins (90,91). Zaghouani et al. suggest several advantages to using immunoglobulins as hosts for foreign antigenic determinants (89). These include extended half-life, low toxicity, and strong immunogenicity.

The proposition that some carbohydrate epitopes could be mimicked by peptide sequences assumes that peptides can assume a three-dimensional structure similar to that formed by a carbohydrate epitope, or by a more complex conformationally dependent polysaccharide epitope. The display of peptide epitopes, in either synthetic minibodies or in natural immunoglobulin domains, provides an efficient means to screen for carbomimetics. One strategy to isolate a carbomimetic is to screen a bacteriophage peptide library against a well-defined anticarbohydrate monoclonal antibody. Since a single antibody combining site may be multispecific in the sense that it may be able to bind more than one ligand (92–94), a peptide-expressing phage particle could be isolated which may bind to a particular carbohydrate-specific combining site, but the peptide structure itself may have no direct relevance to the nominal carbohydrate determinant. However, the mimetic fidelity of the peptide could be tested by immunizing animals with the bacteriophage displaying the peptide on its surface and determining whether anticarbohydrate antibodies of the appropriate specificity are induced. Alternatively, the peptide could be synthesized and coupled to a carrier protein to determine its immunogenicity. The isolation of a true carbomimetic would be a significant accomplishment. Carbomimetics could be easily synthesized and incorporated into a scaffold such as MAP, or possibly they could be used to "antigenize" human immunoglobulins so as to provide an immunogenic complex. One could conceive of a "polysaccharide" vaccine consisting entirely of peptidyl determinants: a peptide that mimics the B-cell polysaccharide determinant combined with another peptide that functions as a promiscuous T-helper cell determinant (Fig. 1). As discussed below, there may be some "natural" situations where immunoglobulins mimic carbohydrate epitopes through their idiotopes.

V. IDIOTYPE VACCINES

The antigen-binding domain of antibody molecules is formed by the association of the heavy- and light-chain variable (V) regions. V regions consist of framework residues having relatively little amino acid sequence variability and complementarity determining residues (CDR), or hypervariable regions, having a high degree of sequence polymorphism. The CDRs of the heavy- and light-chain V regions impart shape and character to the combining site and confer antigen-binding specificity to the V domain (95,96). Antigenic determinants associated with immunoglobulin V domains are called idiotypes. Anti-idiotypic antibodies can be prepared that react with different portions of the V domain. For example, antibodies specific for particular framework sequences have been used as reagents to type antibody V regions according to their family or subgroup, irrespective of their antigen-binding specificity (97). Antibodies also can be prepared against V region epitopes that are determined for the most part by the CDRs of the heavy and light chains, either in combination or individually (98). Frequently, a tight correspondence between expression of a particular idiotype and a particular antigen-binding specificity is observed. Idiotypes may serve as serological markers for particular V regions having a common genetic origin. For example, the HibId-1 and HibId-2 idiotypes discussed earlier are markers for anti-PRP having light-chain V regions derived from either the κII-A2 gene or the λVII gene, respectively (36,37).

When two different antibodies bind to one another via their V domains, one is considered to be the anti-idiotype and the other is considered the target idiotype. In conventional systems, such as the anti-PRP–associated idiotypes, it is clear that the human anti-PRP antibody is expressing a target idiotype that is recognized by a murine monoclonal anti-idiotypic antibody. In other systems, however, the distinction between which antibody is functioning as the idiotype and which is the anti-idiotype is not always apparent. The term anti-idiotype is defined *operationally*; one immunizes with an antibody specific for antigen X, and a complementary anti-(anti-X) antibody is isolated, which is referred to as the anti-idiotype. In some situations, the so-called anti-idiotype antibody may actually be expressing an idiotype that resembles, at least immunochemically, the nominal antigen X. These types of anti-idiotypic antibodies are said to express the internal image of antigen X (99–102). Thus, it has been proposed that the repertoire of idiotypic internal images might be exploited to produce idiotypic vaccines (103–106).

Idiotypic internal images are not simply defined. The use of the term is not uniform, and various criteria, extending from the structural to the functional levels, have been used to define an internal image (107–110). Idiotypic mimicry of a "foreign" peptidyl epitope, based upon the sharing of primary amino acid sequence, has been demonstrated for an epitope of reovirus hemagglutinin molecule (110,111), the group-specific "a" determinant of human hepatitis B virus surface antigen (112–114), the rabbit a-1 allotypic determinant (115), and an epitope of the synthetic polymer, Glu-Ala-Tyr (116). In these cases, amino acid sequences in the CDRs of the anti-idiotypic antibodies corresponded to amino acid sequences in the respective antigens being mimicked. However, shared primary structure is not prerequisite for shared conformational structure (117,118). For example, hemoglobins are heme-containing, oxygen-carrying proteins that phylogenetically show extreme differences in primary sequence while maintaining remarkably similar three-dimensional structures as determined by x-ray crystallography (117). The serine proteases and the cytochromes represent further examples of proteins that can be grouped into families having highly similar conformational structures but quite divergent amino acid sequences (118). Thus, similar conformational structure and biological function do not require similar primary structure. By analogy, idiotypes need not share primary sequence with the molecule they are mimicking. This is one explanation of how anti-idiotypic antibodies might be able to mimic steroid, lipids, and polysaccharides. Similarly, the isolation of peptidomimetics that functionally behave like mannose (82,83) and biotin (76) represent situations where peptides may be structurally mimicking nonprotein molecules. Indeed, the notion of carbomimetics suggests that some peptide sequences (idiotopes), when assembled in an appropriate scaffold such as a minibody or an immunoglobulin CDR, are capable of assuming conformations that structurally resemble carbohydrate epitopes. The use of constrained peptide libraries to express epitopes can be thought of as a synthetic approach that recreates an internal image type of idiotope. The aforementioned work using immunoglobulin molecules as scaffolds for introducing foreign antigenic determinants into the CDRs formally demonstrates the synthesis of an internal image idiotope (87–89). The operational distinction between these synthetic approaches and the anti-idiotype approach is that with anti-idiotypic immunization one tries to select naturally derived internal images by exploiting the diversity and complementarity of the antibody V region repertoire.

Over the past 20 years, an extensive body of experimental evidence has shown that (anti-idiotypic) antibodies can *functionally* mimic a variety of molecules including protein antigens of viruses, parasites, and tumors, as well as nonprotein antigens such as steroids, lipids, catecholamines, and carbohydrates (110,119). Table 2 lists examples of carbohydrate-specific antibody responses that have been induced by anti-idiotypic immunization. In some cases, the anti-idiotypes appear to functionally mimic carbohydrate epitopes. Westerinck and colleagues prepared an anti-idiotypic antibody against a murine monoclonal antibody specific for the *Neisseria meningitidis* group C polysaccharide (127–129). This anti-idiotype inhibited group C polysaccharide binding of both murine as well as human antibodies. This result indicates that the anti-idiotype was not genetically restricted, a property consistent with an internal image antibody. Immunization of mice with the anti-idiotype elicited boosterable, T-cell–dependent group C polysaccharide-specific IgM and IgG antibody responses. In contrast, the murine antibody response to the group C polysaccharide was primarily IgM, T-cell independent, and not boosterable. Moreover, a single injection of the anti-idiotype was able to protect neonatal mice from meningococcal bacteremia, whereas immunization with the group C polysaccharide was ineffective. Schreiber and colleagues have obtained similar data in their studies of *Pseudomonas* polysaccharides. They have demonstrated that anti-idiotypic antibodies can function in mice as surrogate antigens for the *Pseudomonas aeruginosa* lipopolysaccharide O-specific side chain (124,125) and the mucoid exopolysaccharide (126). Antibodies to the O-specific side chain, which were induced in mice by anti-idiotypic immunization, were capable of fixing complement to the bacterial surface and protecting neutropenic mice from pesudomonas sepsis. Importantly, the anti-idiotype also reacted with human antibodies to

Table 2 Examples of Carbohydrate-Specific Antibody Responses Induced by Anti-Idiotypic Antibodies

Carbohydrate antigen	Anti-idiotypic antibody[a]	Finding	Ref.
Escherichia coli K13 polysaccharide	Mouse monoclonal	Injection of anti-idiotype into neonatal mice primed for protection against lethal *E. coli* K13 challenge	120
β (2-6) Fructosan (levan)	Mouse polyclonal	Injection of anti-idiotype into neonatal mice induced normally silent anti-β (2-6) fructosan B-cell clones to be expressed after levan immunization	121
Streptococcus pyogenes Group A polysaccharide	Mouse monoclonal	Differential effects depending upon particular anti-idiotype; some anti-idiotypes (coupled to hemocyanin) directly stimulated anti-group A antibody response in adult mice, whereas other anti-idiotypes primed for enhanced antibody response following group A polysaccharide challenge	122
Streptococcus pyogenes Group A polysaccharide	Mouse monoclonal	Anti-idiotype (coupled to agarose beads and in presence of T-cell supernatant) stimulated human B cells to secrete IgM antibodies to group A polysaccharide in vitro	123
Pseudomonas aeuroginosa LPS O-specific polysaccharide	Mouse monoclonal	Injection of anti-idiotype into mice stimulated anti-O polysaccharide antibodies that protected neutropenic mice from lethal *Pseudomonas* sepsis	124,125
Pseudomonas aeuroginosa exopolysaccharide	Mouse monoclonal	Injection of anti-idiotype into mice stimulated complement fixing and opsonic anti-exopolysaccharide antibodies	126
Neisseria meningitidis Group C polysaccharide	Mouse monoclonal	Injection of anti-idiotype into neonatal and adult mice stimulated anti-group C polysaccharide antibody response and protected mice from meningococcal bacteremia	127–129
Trypanosoma cruzi glycoprotein (GP 72)	Rabbit polyclonal	Anti-idiotype immunization of mice, rabbits, and guinea pigs induced GP72-specific antibodies; anti-idiotype reacted with human anti-GP72 antibodies	130

[a]In these studies, the anti-idiotypic antibodies were made against antibodies specific for the carbohydrate antigen listed in the first column.

the O-specific side chain, a result consistent with an internal image. Exopolysaccharide-specific antibodies also could be induced by anti-idiotypic immunization, and they were functionally active in opsonizing mucoid pseudomonas for killing by human neutrophils in the presence of complement.

These studies demonstrate the ability of anti-idiotypic antibodies functionally to mimic polysaccharides by inducing biologically relevant antibody responses. Anti-idiotypic immunization also has been applied successfully to other bacterial antigens. Kohler and colleagues developed a protective idiotypic vaccine for pneumococcus, based upon the induction of protective antibodies reactive with phosphorylcholine (131). Su et al. produced an anti-idiotypic antibody that recognized an idiotype present on mouse, rabbit, and chicken antibodies specific for lipid A (132). They demonstrated that this anti-idiotype functioned as a surrogate antigen for lipid A, since immunization with this anti-idiotype coupled to hemocyanin, protected mice against gram-negative bacteremia and endotoxinemia (133). These results, as well as the findings discussed above with anti-idiotypic polysaccharide mimics, can be interpreted in two ways. On one hand, the anti-idiotype could be recognizing an interspecies idiotype present on a structurally conserved V region that has been maintained in the germline throughout evolution perhaps because of its selective advantage. On the other hand, the broad reactivity of the anti-idiotype could be accounted for by its expression of a structural mimic of lipid A. Distinguishing between these two possibilities is important for understanding the mechanism(s) of idiotypic vaccination and for rational vaccine design (107,134,135). However, from a practical point of view, it may be sufficient to demonstrate that an anti-idiotypic antibody is immunogenic in most human subjects and elicits durable, protective immunity.

What is the likelihood that idiotypic-based vaccines will be developed for polysaccharides or other microbial antigens? The success of the Hib polysaccharide-protein conjugate vaccines has verified the application of this strategy for developing new polysaccharide vaccines and, thus, for most polysaccharide antigens, has diminished the need for the idiotypic approach. Nonetheless, one could envision several advantages to using idiotypic vaccines. First, a monoclonal antibody–based idiotypic vaccine might be cheaper to produce than a polysaccharide-protein conjugate. Second, the vaccine would be relatively homogeneous, molecularly well defined, and potentially more stable than the present conjugate vaccines. Third, an idiotype vaccine, especially a humanized version (see below), might be extremely safe and nontoxic. Fourth, idiotypic vaccination might be considered in those situations where the relevant polysaccharide or other microbial antigen is poorly immunogenic, difficult to isolate, poorly defined, or toxic. This latter point is particularly relevant to producing a vaccine for the prevention of gram-negative sepsis. Use of a lipid A idiotypic mimic would relieve the problem of toxicity associated with the use of lipopolysaccharide (133). Idiotypic vaccines share some properties with the current polysaccharide-protein conjugate vaccines. The former act in many cases as T-cell–dependent antigens, and they are able to prime and/or induce specific antibody in immature animals (Table 2). Thus, there may be situations where anti-idiotypic vaccination might be indicated, for example, in individuals who fail conventional vaccination (136,137), in populations who are low responders to polysaccharide conjugate vaccines (138, 139), or as a priming stimulus prior to conventional vaccination.

Even if a strong rationale could be made for developing an idiotypic vaccine, several important issues would have to be addressed. Presumably the anti-idiotypic antibody would have to be primarily of human origin. Although the use of a murine monoclonal antibody vaccine might be efficacious as a priming stimulus for the nominal antigen, repeated injection would lead to human antimouse antibody responses that could both neutralize the vaccine and lead to harmful allergic reactions. Humanization of monoclonal antibodies, by grafting murine CDRs onto human immunoglobulin framework scaffolds, can now be accomplished readily using recombinant DNA technology (95,96). The anti-idiotypic antibody presumably would provide the stimulus for antigen-specific B cells. Whether a humanized idiotype vaccine would require attachment of foreign T-cell carrier determinants is more problematic. The aforementioned studies showing that immunoglobulins engrafted with foreign antigenic determinants are strongly immunogenic in syngeneic species suggest that the coupling of heterologous carrier determinants may not be necessary. Furthermore, the studies of Thanavala and colleagues have demonstrated that an anti-idiotypic antibody mimicking the group-specific "a" determinant of human hepatitis B virus contains idiotopes/epitopes capable of activating both T and B cells (114). Finally, the dose and the isotype of the anti-idiotypic vaccine will require considerable investigation, as studies in experimental animals have shown that both these variables play a role in determining whether anti-idiotype injection results in enhancement or suppression of immune responsiveness to the nominal antigen (140).

VI. AUGMENTING VACCINE IMMUNOGENICITY

The development of better and refined adjuvants that are suitable for human use will play an important role in vaccine development (141). Immune stimulating complexes (ISCOMS) (142), liposomes (143), biodegradable microspheres (144), and the development of new immunomodulating molecules (141,145) represent some of the major areas of study in this burgeoning field. Review of this topic is beyond the scope of this chapter. Rather, I would like to discuss briefly some recent novel developments that are likely to influence vaccine design in the near future.

One area in which rapid progress is being made is the field of cytokine biology. It is becoming apparent that collaboration between B and T cells is mediated in part by cytokines, and that particular cytokines or the balance between different cytokines play a pivotal role in determining T-cell effector activities, immunoglobulin isotype, and, ultimately, the directionality (e.g., cell-mediated versus humoral) of an immune response (146–148). Cytokines may have potent stimulatory effects when administered with antigens (149,150), and many of the well-known adjuvant effects of bacterial products may actually be cytokine mediated. A novel strategy of combining the cytokine, granulocyte-macrophage colony-stimulating factor, and an idiotypic antigen into a single molecular construct recently was shown to markedly increase the immunogenicity of the idiotype (151). The immunogenicity of this fusion protein exceeded that of conventional carrier-conjugated idiotype. Presumably, coupling the antigen with the cytokine resulted in direct targeting of the cytokine to antigen-presenting cells, and, possibly, idiotype-specific B cells. The idea of fusing cytokines with antigens may be directly applicable to polysaccharide vaccine design. Perhaps the protein carrier requirement for polysaccharide immunogenicity in the infant reflects the requirement for T-cell–derived (or other) cytokines for efficient antigen processing and/or B-cell activation and differentiation. A fusion construct, consisting of the appropriate cytokine coupled to a polysaccharide oligomer, might bypass T-cell dependency and render the polysaccharide immunogenic in infants, thereby relieving the need for conventional carrier coupling.

Other novel means of augmenting immunogenicity have appeared recently in the literature. Gosselin and colleagues demonstrated that the coupling of Fc receptor–specific antibodies to tetanus toxoid enhanced presentation in vitro of tetanus antigen to human T cells 100-fold (152). This strategy might be adopted into a vaccine consisting of an Fc receptor–specific domain grafted onto a MAP or minibody construct. Rhodes and coworkers have designed a unique adjuvant based upon their observation that Schiff base formation (carbonyl-amino condensation) between cell surface ligands appears essential in the interaction of antigen-presenting cells and T cells (153). To favor Schiff base formation, they incorporated the enzymes galactose oxidase and neuraminidase into an aqueous mixture with various antigens including HIV glycoprotein 120, the P69 subunit of *Bordetella pertussis*, and the major malarial merozoite surface antigen. In all cases, this adjuvant system was equivalent to or superior to Freund's adjuvant in priming antigen-specific T cells (154).

VII. CONCLUDING REMARKS

Presently, vaccinology is more art than science. The empirical approach has served well for development of Hib conjugate vaccines and can be expected to yield further rewards as new polysaccharide conjugate vaccines are developed. In the future, the need for alternate design strategies may become greater, especially for difficult problems such as HIV and parasitic diseases (155). Even with polysaccharide antigens, the development of new strategies based upon synthetic chemistry or unconventional modes of antigen recognition may ultimately provide more uniform, better-defined, cheaper, and, possibly, more universally efficacious vaccines.

Although the design of vaccines based upon mechanistic understanding is still in its infancy, we may expect to see the insights gained from basic science studies applied toward the development of better vaccines. As our knowledge of immune system physiology increases, so will our ability to design vaccines based upon a rational approach. For example, our understanding of the carrier requirement for polysaccharide immunogenicity in infants is minimal, and this phenomenon clearly reflects something important about immune system ontogeny. Delineating this mechanism will undoubtedly contribute to designing better pediatric vaccines. The time may not too far off when we will be able to apply our knowledge so that we may tailor the immune response by specificity, by antibody class and affinity, and by effector cell type.

ACKNOWLEDGEMENTS

The author thanks Dan Granoff and Don Reason for their critical review of the manuscript, Mark Scott for help with computer graphics, and Wally Brill for essential reagents. The work in the author's laboratory was supported by NIH grant AI25008.

REFERENCES

1. H. Peltola, T. Kilpi, and M. Anttila, Rapid disappearance of *Haemophilus influenzae* type b meningitis after routine childhood immunisation with conjugate vaccines, *Lancet 340*:592 (1992).
2. T. V. Murphy, K. E. White, P. Pastor, L. Gabriel, F. Medley, D. M. Granoff, and M. T. Osterholm, Declining incidence of *Haemophilus influenzae* type b disease since introduction of vaccination, *JAMA 269*:246 (1993).
3. S. B. Black and H. R. Shinefield, Immunization with oligosaccharide conjugate *Haemophilus influenzae* type b (HbOC) vaccine on a large health maintenance

organization population: Extended follow-up and impact on *Haemophilus influenzae* disease epidemiology. The Kaiser Permanante Pediatric Vaccine Study Group, *Pediatr. Infect. Dis. J. 11*:610 (1992).
4. S. Black, H. Shinefield, N. Lewis, P. Ray, B. Fireman, and R. Hiatt, Dramatic reduction in invasive Hib disease in a large California population following HbOC conjugate vaccine in infancy, *Pediatr. Res. 33*:163A (1993).
5. M. S. Einhorn, G. A. Weinberg, E. L. Anderson, P. D. Granoff, and D. M. Granoff, Immunogenicity in infants of *Haemophilus influenzae* type b polysaccharide in a conjugate vaccine with *Neisseria meningitidis* outer-membrane protein, *Lancet ii*:299 (1986).
6. P. Anderson, M. E. Pichichero, and R. A. Insel, Immunization of 2-month-old infants with protein-coupled oligosaccharides derived from the capsule of *H. influenzae* type b, *J. Pediatr. 107*:346 (1985).
7. J. C. Parke, R. Schneerson, C. Reimer, C. Black, S. Welfare, D. Bryla, L. Levi, D. Paviliakova, T. Crampton, D. Schultz, M. Cadoz, and J. B. Robbins, Clinical and immunological responses to *Haemophilus influenzae* type b-tetanus toxoid conjugate vaccine in infants injected at 3, 5, 7 and 18 months of age, *J. Pediatr. 118*:184 (1991).
8. S. J. Holmes, T. V. Murphy, R. S. Anderson, S. L. Kaplan, E. P. Rothstein, V. N. Gan, and D. M. Granoff, Immunogenicity of four *Haemophilus influenzae* type b conjugate vaccines in 17- to 19-month-old children, *J. Pediatr. 118*:364 (1991).
9. A. A. Lenoir, P. D. Granoff, and D. M. Granoff, Immunogenicity of *Haemophilus influenzae* type b polysaccharide-*Neisseria meningitidis* outer membrane protein conjugate vaccine in 2- to 6-months old infants, *Pediatrics 80*:283 (1987).
10. D. M. Granoff, E. L. Anderson, M. T. Osterholm, S. J. Holmes, R. B. Belshe, F. Medley, and T. V. Murphy, Differences in the immunogenicity of three *Haemophilus influenzae* type b conjugate vaccines in infants, *J. Pediatr. 121*:187 (1992).
11. P. Anderson, Antibody responses to *Haemophilus influenzae* type b and diphtheria toxin induced by conjugates of oligosaccharides of the type b capsule with the nontoxic protein CRM197, *Infect. Immun. 39*:233 (1983).
12. D. V. Madore, C. L. Johnson, D. C. Phipps, Pennridge Pediatric Associates, L. A. Popejoy, R. Eby, and D. H. Smith, Safety and immunologic response to *Haemophilus influenzae* type b oligosaccharide-CRM_{197} conjugate vaccine in 1- to 6-month-old infants, *Pediatrics 85*:331 (1990).
13. J. Eskola, H. Käyhty, A. K. Takala, H. Peltola, P.-R. Rönnberg, E. Kella, E. Pekkanen, P. H. McVerry, and P. H. Mäkelä, A randomized, prospective field trial of a conjugate vaccine in the protection of infants and young children against invasive *Haemophilus influenzae* type b disease, *N. Engl. J. Med. 323*:1381 (1990).
14. M. D. Decker, K. M. Edwards, R. Bradley, and P. Palmer, Comparative trial in infants of four conjugate *Haemophilus influenzae* type b vaccines, *J. Pediatr. 120*:184 (1992).

15. T. V. Murphy, P. Pastor, F. Medley, M. T. Osterholm, D. M. Granoff, Decreased *Haemophilus* colonization in children vaccinated with *Haemophilus influenzae* type b conjugate vaccine, *J. Pediatr. 122*:517 (1993).
16. A. K. Takala, J. Eskola, M. Leininen, H. Käyhty, A. Nissinen, E. Pekkanen, and P. H. Mäkelä, Reduction of oropharyngeal carriage of *Haemophilus influenzae* type b (Hib) in children immunized with an Hib conjugate vaccine, *J. Infect. Dis. 164*:982 (1991).
17. P. Anderson, G. Peter, R. B. Johnston Jr., L. H. Wetterlow, and D. H. Smith, Immunization of humans with polyribophosphate, the capsular antigen of *Haemophilus influenzae*, type b, *J. Clin. Invest. 51*:39 (1972).
18. D. H. Smith, G. Peter, D. L. Ingram, A. L. Harding, and P. Anderson, Responses of children immunized with the capsular polysaccharide of *Haemophilus influenzae*, type b, *Pediatrics 52*:637 (1973).
19. O. T. Avery and W. F. Goebel, Chemo-immunological studies on conjugated carbohydrate-proteins. II. Immunological specificity of synthetic sugar-protein antigens, *J. Exp. Med. 50*:533 (1929).
20. W. F. Goebel, The immunological properties of an artificial antigen containing cellobiuronic acid, *J. Exp. Med. 68*:469 (1939).
21. R. Schneerson, O. Barrera, A. Sutton, and J. B. Robbins, Preparation, characterization, and immunogenicity of *H. influenzae* type b polysaccharide-protein conjugates, *J. Exp. Med. 152*:361 (1980).
22. F. W. Alt, T. K. Blackwell, and G. D. Yancopoulos, Development of the primary antibody repertoire, *Science 238*:1079 (1987).
23. H. W. Schroeder, J. L. Hilson, and R. M. Perlmutter, Early restriction of the human antibody repertoire, *Science 238*:791 (1987).
24. J. J. Donnelly, R. R. Deck, and M. A. Liu, Immunogenicity of a *Haemophilus influenzae* polysaccharide-*Neisseria meningitidis* outer membrane protein complex conjugate vaccine, *J. Immunol. 145*:3071 (1990).
25. M. A. Liu, A. Friedman, A. I. Olif, J. Tai, D. Martinez, R. R. Deck, J. T. C. Shieh, T. D. Jenkins, J. J. Donnelly, and L. A. Hawe, A vaccine carrier derived from *Neisseria meningitidis* with mitogenic activity for lymphocytes, *Proc. Natl. Acad. Sci. USA 89*:4633 (1992).
26. D. M. Ambrosino, D. Bolon, H. Collard, R. Van Etten, M. V. Kanchana, and R. W. Finburg, Effect of *Haemophilus influenzae* polysaccharide outer membrane protein complex conjugate vaccine on macrophages, *J. Immunol. 149*:3978 (1992).
27. R. Schneerson, J. B. Robbins, C. Chu, A. Sutton, W. Vann, J. C. Vickers, W. T. London, B. Curfman, M. C. Hardegree, J. Shiloach, and S. C. Rastogi, Serum antibody responses of juvenile and infant rhesus monkeys injected with *Haemophilus influenzae* type b and pneumococcus type 6A capsular polysaccharide-protein conjugates, *Infect. Immun. 45*:582 (1984).
28. P. P. Vella, and R. W. Ellis, Immunogenicity of *Haemophilus influenzae* type b conjugate vaccine in infant rhesus monkeys, *Pediatr. Res. 29*:10 (1991).
29. D. M. Granoff, M. H. Rathore, S. J. Holmes, P. D. Granoff, and A. H. Lucas, Effect of immunity to the carrier protein on antibody responses to *Haemophilus influenzae* type b conjugate vaccines, *Vaccine 11*:S46 (1993).

30. L. A. Herzenberg, T. Tokuhisa, and K. Hayakawa, Epitope-specific regulation, *Ann. Rev. Immunol. 1*:609 (1983).
31. M.-P. Schutze, E. Deriaud, G. Przewlocki, and C. LeClerc, Carrier-induced epitopic suppression is initiated through clonal dominance, *J. Immunol. 142*:2635 (1989).
32. C. C. A. Peeters, A.-M. Tenbergen-Meekes, J. T. Poolman, M. Beurret, B. J. M. Zeegers, and G. T. Rijkers, Effect of carrier priming on immunogenicity of saccharide-protein conjugate vaccines, *Infect. Immun. 59*:3504 (1991).
33. J. M. Liberman, D. P. Greenberg, V. F. Wong, S. M. Marcy, S. Partridge, S.-J. Chang, C.-Y. Chiu, and J. I. Ward, Does newborn immunization with diphtheria-tetanus toxoid (DT) prime for enhanced antibody responses to *H. influenzae* type b (Hib) conjugate vaccines? *Pediatr. Res. 33*:174A (1993).
34. D. M. Granoff, S. J. Holmes, R. B. Belshe, and E. L. Anderson, The effect of carrier priming on the anti-capsular (PRP) antibody responses to *Haemophilus influenzae* type b (Hib) conjugate vaccines, *Pediatr. Res. 33*:169A (1993).
35. Y. Schlesinger, D. M. Granoff, and the Vaccine Study Group, Avidity and bactericidal activity of antibody elicited by different *Haemophilus influenzae* type b conjugate vaccines, *JAMA 267*:1489 (1992).
36. A. H. Lucas, R. J. Langley, D. M. Granoff, M. H. Nahm, M. Y. Kitamura, and M. G. Scott, An idiotypic marker associated with a germ-line encoded κ light chain variable region that predominates the human antibody response to the *Haemophilus influenzae* b polysaccharide, *J. Clin. Invest. 88*:1811 (1991).
37. D. M. Granoff, P. G. Shackelford, S. J. Holmes, The Vaccine Collaborative Study Group, and A. H. Lucas, Variable region expression in the antibody responses of infants vaccinated with *Haemophilus influenzae* type b polysaccharide-protein conjugates. Description of a new λ light chain-associated idiotype and the relation between idiotype expression, avidity, and vaccine formulation, *J. Clin. Invest. 91*:788 (1993).
38. A. H. Lucas, F. H. Azmi, C. M. Mink, and D. M. Granoff, Age-dependent V region expression in the human antibody response to the *Haemophilus influenzae* type b polysaccharide, *J. Immunol. 150*:2056 (1993).
39. J. Amir, X. Liang, and D. M. Granoff, Variability in the functional activity of vaccine-induced antibody to *Haemophilus influenzae* type b, *Pediatr. Res. 27*:358 (1990).
40. Combined diphtheria, tetanus, pertussis and *Haemophilus influenzae* type b conjugate vaccines: Recommendations for use in infants and children, *MMWR* (in press).
41. D. P. Greenberg, J. M. Liberman, S. M. Marcy, S. Partridge, S.-J. Chang. C.-Y. Chiu, and J. I. Ward, Safety and immunogenicity of mixed sequences of *Haemophilus influenzae* type b (Hib) conjugate vaccines in infants, *Pediatr. Res. 33*:169A (1993).
42. R. Z. Dintzis, Rational design of conjugate vaccines, *Pediatr. Res. 32*:376 (1992).
43. S. Marburg, D. Jorn, R. L. Tolman, B. Arison, J. MacCauley, P. J. Kniskern, A. Hagopian, and P. P. Vella, Biomolecular chemistry of macromolecules:

synthesis of bacterial polysaccharide conjugates with *Neisseria meningitidis* membrane protein, *J. Am. Chem. Soc. 108*:5282 (1986).
44. W. E. Dick and M. Burret, Glycoconjugates of bacterial carbohydrate antigens: A survey and consideration of design and preparation factors, *Conjugate Vaccines. Contrib. Microbiol. Immunol.* (J. M. Cruse and R. E. Lewis, Jr., eds.), Karger, Basel, Vol. 10, 1989, p. 48.
45. E. E. Sercarz, P. V. Lehmann, A. Ametani, G. Benichou, A. Miller, and K. Moudgil, Dominance and crypticity of T cell antigenic determinants, *Ann. Rev. Immunol. 11*:729 (1993).
46. P. Panina-Bordignon, A. Tan, A. Termijtelen, S. Demotz, G. Corradin, and A. Lanzavecchia, Universally immunogenic T cell epitopes: Promiscuous binding to human MHC class II alleles and promiscuous recognition by T cells, *Eur. J. Immunol. 19*:2237 (1989).
47. A. Kumar, R. Arora, P. Kaur, V. S. Chauhan, and P. Sharma, "Universal" T helper cell determinants enhance immunogenicity of a *Plasmodium falciparum* merozoite surface antigen peptide, *J. Immunol. 148*:1499 (1992).
48. J. P. Tam, Synthetic peptide vaccine design: Synthesis and properties of a high-density multiple antigenic peptide system, *Proc. Natl. Acad. Sci. USA 85*:5409 (1988).
49. J. P. Tam, P. Clavijo, Y. Lu, V. Nussenzweig, R. Nussenzweig, and F. Zavala, Incorporated of T and B epitopes of the circumsporozoite protein in a chemically defined vaccine against malaria, *J. Exp. Med. 171*:299 (1990).
50. B. Nardelli, Y.-A. Lu, D. R. Shiu, C. Delpierre-Deffort, A. T. Profy, and J. P. Tam, A chemically defined synthetic vaccine model for HIV-1, *J. Immunol. 148*:914 (1992).
51. P. W. Anderson, M. E. Pichichero, E. C. Stein, S. Procelli, R. F. Betts, D. M. Connuck, D. Korones, R. A. Insel, J. M. Zahradnik, and R. Eby, Effect of oligosaccharide chain length, exposed terminal group, and hapten loading on the antibody response of human adults and infants to vaccines consisting of *Haemophilus influenzae* type b capsular antigen uniterminally coupled to the diphtheria protein CRM197, *J. Immunol. 142*:2463 (1989).
52. L. C. Paoletti, D. L. Kasper, F. Michon, J. DiFabio, H. J. Jennings, T. D. Toteson, and M. R. Wessels, Effects of chain length on the immunogenicity in rabbits of group B streptococcus type III oligosaccharide-tetanus toxoid conjugates, *J. Clin. Invest. 89*:146 (1991).
53. H. J. Jennings, R. Roy, and F. Michon, Determinant specificities of the groups B and C polysaccharides of *Neisseria meningitidis, J. Immunol. 134*:2651 (1984).
54. R. Yamasaki and B. Bacon, Three-dimensional structural analysis of the group B polysaccharide of *Neisseria meningitidis* 6275 by two-dimensional NMR: The polysaccharide is suggested to exist in helical conformations in solution, *Biochemistry 30*:851 (1991).
55. M. R. Wessels and D. L. Kasper, Antibody recognition of type 14 pneumococcal capsule. Evidence for a conformational epitope in a neutral polysaccharide, *J. Exp. Med. 169*:2121 (1989).

56. S. J. Danishefsky, K. F. McClure, J. T. Randolph, and R. B. Ruggeri, A strategy for the solid-phase synthesis of oligosaccharides, *Science, 260*:1307 (1993).
57. K. E. Stein, Thymus-independent and thymus-dependent responses to polysaccharide antigens, *J. Infect. Dis. 165*:S49 (1992).
58. H. Käyhty, V. Karanko, H. Peltola, and P. H. Mäkelä, Serum antibodies after vaccination with *Haemophilus influenzae* type b capsular polysaccharide: No evidence of immunologic tolerance or memory, *Pediatrics 74*:857 (1984).
59. M. C. Steinhoff, B. S. Auerbach, K. E. Nelson, D. Vlahov, R. L. Becker, N. M. H. Graham, D. H. Schwartz, A. H. Lucas, and R. E. Chaisson, Antibody responses to *Haemophilus influenzae* type b vaccines in men with human immunodeficiency virus infection, *N. Engl. J. Med. 325*:1837 (1991).
60. P. J. Baker, T cell regulation of the antibody response to bacterial polysaccharide antigens: Examination of some general characteristics and their implications, *J. Infect. Dis. 165*:S44 (1992).
61. C. M. Henningsson, S. Selvaraj, G. D. MacLean, M. R. Suresh, A. A. Noujaim, and B. M. Longnecker, T cell recognition of a tumor-associated glycoprotein and its synthetic carbohydrate epitopes: Stimulation of anticancer T cell immunity *in vivo, Cancer Immunol. Immunother. 25*:231 (1987).
62. A. Bellamy, A. N. Davidson, and M. Feldman, Derivation of ganglioside-specific T cell lines of suppressor or helper phenotype from cerebrospinal fluid from multiple sclerosis patients, *J. Neuroimmunol. 12*:107 (1986).
63. P. L. Black, E. S. Vitetta, J. Forman, C.-Y. Kang, R. D. May, and J. W. Uhr, Role of glycosylation in the H-2 restricted cytolysis of virus-infected cells, *Eur. J. Immunol. 11*:48 (1981).
64. G. Y. Ishioka, A. G. Lamont, D. Thompson, N. Bulbow, F. C. A. Gaeta, A. Sette, and H. M. Grey, MHC interaction and T cell recognition of carbohydrates and glycopeptides, *J. Immunol. 148*:2446 (1992).
65. A. Singhal, M. Fohn, and S. Hakemori, Induction of α-N-acetylgalactosamine-O-serine/threonine (Tn) antigen-mediated cellular immune response for active immunotherapy in mice, *Cancer Res. 51*:1406 (1991).
66. K. Ogasawara, H. Naruse, Y. Itoh, T. Gotohda, J. Arikawa, H. Kida, R. A. Good, and K. Onoé, A strategy for making synthetic peptide vaccines, *Proc. Natl. Acad. Sci. USA 89*:8995 (1992).
67. P. J. Bjorkman, M. A. Saper, B. Samraoui, W. S. Bennett, J. L. Strominger, and D. C. Wiley, Structure of the human class I histocompatability antigen, HLA-A2, *Nature 329*:506 (1987).
68. D. H. Fremont, M. Matsumura, E. A. Stura, P. A. Peterson, and I. A. Wilson, Crystal structures of two viral peptides in complex with murine MHC class I H-2K^b, *Science 257*:919 (1992).
69. M. Matsumura, D. H. Fremont, P. A. Peterson, and I. A. Wilson, Emerging principles for the recognition of peptide antigens by MHC class I molecules, *Science 257*:927 (1992).
70. P. Parham, Deconstructing the MHC, *Nature 360*:300 (1992).
71. M. Barinaga, Getting some "backbone:" How MHC binds peptides, *Science 257*:880 (1992).

72. D. F. Hunt, H. Michel, T. A. Dickinson, J. Shabanowitz, A. L. Cox, K. Sakaguchi, E. Appella, H. M. Grey, and A. Sette, Peptides presented to the immune system by the murine class II major histocompatability complex molecule I-A^d, *Science 256*:1817 (1992).
73. A. Sette, J. Sidney, M. Albertson, C. Miles, S. M. Colon, T. Pedrazzini, A. G. Lamont, and H. M. Grey, A novel approach to the generation of high affinity class II-binding peptides, *J. Immunol. 145*:1809 (1990).
74. J. K. Scott and G. P. Smith, Searching for peptide ligands with an epitope library, *Science 249*:386 (1990).
75. S. E. Cwirla, E. A. Peters, R. W. Barrett, and W. J. Dower, Peptides on phage: A vast library of peptides for identifying ligands, *Proc. Natl. Acad. Sci. USA 87*:6378 (1990).
76. J. J. Devlin, L. C. Panganiban, and P. E. Devlin, Random peptide libraries: a source of specific protein binding molecules, *Science 249*:404 (1990).
77. G. P. Smith and J. K. Scott, Libraries of peptides and proteins displayed on filamentous phage, *Meth. Enzymol. 217*:228 (1993).
78. H. M. Geysen, R. H. Melven, and S. J. Barteling, Use of peptide synthesis to probe viral antigens for epitopes to a resolution of a single amino acid, *Proc. Natl. Acad. Sci. USA 81*:3998 (1984).
79. S. P. Fodor, J. L. Read, M. C. Pirrung, L. Stryer, A. T. Lu, and D. Solas, Light-directed, spatially addressable parallel chemical synthesis, *Science 251*: 767 (1991).
80. K. S. Lam, S. E. Salmon, E. M. Hersh, V. J. Hruby, W. M. Kazmierski, and R. J. Knapp, A new type of synthetic peptide library for identifying ligand-binding activity, *Nature 354*:82 (1991).
81. R. A. Houghten, C. Pinilla, S. E. Blondelle, J. R. Appel, C. T. Dooley, and J. H. Cuervo, Generation and use of synthetic peptide combinatorial libraries for basic research and drug discovery, *Nature 354*:84 (1991).
82. K. R. Oldenburg, D. Loganathan, I. J. Goldstein, P. G. Schultz, and M. A. Gallop, Peptide ligands for a sugar-binding protein isolated from a random peptide library, *Proc. Natl. Acad. Sci USA 89*:5393 (1992).
83. J. K. Scott, D. Loganathan, R. B. Easley, X. Gong, and I. J. Goldstein, A family of concanavalin A-binding peptides from a hexapeptide epitope library, *Proc. Natl. Acad. Sci. USA 89*:5398 (1992).
84. F. Felici, L. Castagnoli, A. Musacchio, R. Jappelli, and G. Cesareni, Selection of antibody ligands from a large library of oligopeptides expressed on a multivalent exposition vector, *J. Mol. Biol. 222*:301 (1991).
85. H. M. Geysen, R. MacFarlan, S. J. Rodda, G. Tribbick, T. J. Mason, and P. Shoofs, Peptides which mimic carbohydrate antigens, *Towards Better Carbohydrate Vaccines* (R. Bell and G. Torrigiani, eds.), John Wiley & Sons, Ltd., 1987, p. 103.
86. A. Pessi, E. Bianchi, A. Crameri, S. Venturini, A. Tramontano, and M. Sollazzo, A designed metal-binding protein with a novel fold, *Nature 362*:367 (1993).
87. M. Zanetti, Antigenized antibodies, *Nature 355*:476 (1992).

88. R. Billetta, M. R. Hollingdale, and M. Zanetti, Immunogenicity of an engineered internal image antibody, *Proc. Natl. Acad. Sci. USA 88*:4713 (1991).
89. H. Zaghouani, R. Steinman, R. Nonacs, H. Shah, W. Gerhard and C. Bona, Presentation of a viral T cell epitope expressed in the CDR3 region of a self immunoglobulin molecule, *Science* (Wash. D.C.) *259*:224 (1993).
90. B. Bogen, B. Malissen, and W. Haas, Idiotype-specific T cell clones that recognize syngeneic immunoglobulin fragments in the context of class II molecules, *Eur. J. Immunol. 16*:1373 (1986).
91. A. Y. Rudensky, and V. L. Yurin, Immunoglobulin-specific T-B cell interaction. I. Presentation of self immunoglobulin determinants by B lymphocytes, *Eur. J. Immunol. 19*:1677 (1989).
92. F. F. Richards, W. H. Konigsberg, R. W. Rosenstein, and M. Varga, On the specificity of antibodies, *Science* (Wash. D.C.) *187*:130 (1975).
93. R. L. Rubin, R. S. Balderas, E. M. Tan, F. J. Dixon, and A. N. Theofilopoulos, Multiple autoantigen binding capabilities of mouse monoclonal antibodies selected for rheumatoid factor activity, *J. Exp. Med. 159*:1429 (1984).
94. A. B. Edmundson and K. R. Ely, Binding of N-formylated chemotactic peptides in crystals of the Mcg light chain dimer: Similarities with neutrophil receptors, *Mol. Immunol. 22*:463 (1985).
95. P. T. Jones, P. H. Dear, J. Foote, M. S. Neuberger, and G. Winter, Replacing the complementarity-determining regions in a human antibody with those from a mouse, *Nature 321*:522 (1986).
96. G. Winter and C. Milstein, Man-made antibodies, *Nature 349*:293 (1991).
97. G. J. Silverman and A. H. Lucas, Variable region diversity in human circulating antibodies specific for the capsular polysaccharide of *Haemophilus influenzae* type b: Preferential usage of two types of VH3 heavy chains, *J. Clin. Invest. 88*:911 (1991).
98. J. M. Davie, M. V. Seiden, N. S. Greenspan, C. T. Lutz, T. L. Bartholo, and B. L. Clevinger, Structural correlates of idiotypes, *Ann. Rev. Immunol. 4*:147 (1986).
99. J. Lindenmann, Speculations on idiotypes and homobodies, *Ann. Immunol.* (Paris) *124C*:171 (1973).
100. J. Lindenmann, Homobodies: Do they exist? *Ann. Immunol.* (Inst. Pasteur) *130C*:311 (1973).
101. N. K. Jerne, Towards a network theory of the immune system, *Ann. Immunol.* (Paris) *125C*:373 (1974).
102. N. K. Jerne, J. Roland, and P. A. Cazenave, Recurrent idiotopes and internal images, *EMBO J. 1*:243 (1982).
103. A. Nisonoff and E. Lamoyi, Implications of the presence of an internal image of the antigen in anti-idiotypic antibodies: Possible application to vaccine production, *Clin. Immunol. Immunopath. 21*:397 (1981).
104. I. M. Roitt, A. Cooke, D. K. Male, F. C. Hay, G. Guarnotta, P. M. Lydyard, L. P. De Carvalho, Y. Thanavala, and J. Ivanyi, Idiotypic networks and their possible exploitation for manipulation of the immune response, *Lancet i*:1041 (1981).

105. J. R. Hiernaux, Idiotypic vaccines and infectious diseases, *Infect. Immun. 56*:1407 (1988).
106. A. G. Dagliesh and R. C. Kennedy, Anti-idiotypic antibodies as immunogens: Idiotype-based vaccines, *Vaccine 6*:215 (1988).
107. N. S. Greenspan, Antigen mimicry with anti-idiotypic antibodies, *Structure of Antigens* (M. H. V. Van Regenmortel, ed.), CRC Press, Boca Raton, FL, 1992, p. 55.
108. W. V. Williams, D. B. Weiner, T. Kieber-Emmons, and M. I. Greene, Antibody geometry and form: Three dimensional relationships between anti-idiotypic antibodies and external antigens, *Trends Biotechnol. 8*:256 (1990).
109. D. C. Poskitt, M. J. B. Jean-Francois, S. Turnbull, L. Macdonald, and D. Yasmeen, Internal image (Ab2β) anti-idiotype vaccines: Theoretical and practical aspects, *Vaccine 9*:792 (1991).
110. G. N. Gaulton and M. I. Greene, Idiotypic mimicry of biological receptors, *Ann. Rev. Immunol. 4*:253 (1986).
111. R. Taub and M. I. Greene, Functional validation of ligand mimicry by anti-receptor antibodies: Structural and therapeutic implications, *Biochemistry 31*:7431 (1992).
112. Y. M. Thanavala, A. Bond, R. Tedder, F. C. Hay, and I. M. Roitt, Monoclonal 'internal image' anti-idiotypic antibodies of hepatitis B surface antigen, *Immunology 55*:197 (1985).
113. Y. M. Thanavala, S. E. Brown, C. R. Howard, I. M. Roitt, and M. W. Steward, Surrogate hepatitis B virus antigenic epitope represented by a synthetic peptide and an internal image anti-idiotype antibody, *J. Exp. Med. 164*:227 (1986).
114. M. W. Pride, H. Shi, J. M. Anchin, D. S. Linthicum, P. T. LoVerde, A. Thakur, and Y. Thanavala, Molecular mimicry of hepatitis B surface antigen by an anti-idiotype-derived synthetic peptide, *Proc. Natl. Acad. Sci. USA 89*:11900 (1992).
115. V. H. Van Cleave, C. W. Naeve, and D. W. Metzger, Do antibodies recognize amino acid side chains of protein antigens independently of the carbon backbone? *J. Exp. Med. 167*:1841 (1988).
116. P. Ollier, J. Rocca-Serra, G. Sommé, J. Theze, and M. Fougereau, The idiotypic network and the internal image: possible regulation of a germ-line network by paucigene encoded Ab2 (anti-idiotypic) antibodies in the GAT system, *EMBO J. 4*:3681 (1985).
117. B. F. Erlanger, Some thoughts on the structural basis of internal imagery, *Immunol. Today 10*:151 (1989).
118. T. E. Creighton, *Proteins,* 2nd ed. W. H. Freeman and Co., 1993.
119. N. S. Greenspan and C. Bona, Idiotypes: Structure and immunogenicity, *FASEB J. 7*:437 (1993).
120. K. E. Stein and T. Söderström, Neonatal administration of idiotype or anti-idiotype primes for protection against *Escherichia coli* K13 infection in mice, *J. Exp. Med. 160*:1001 (1984).

121. L. J. Rubinstein, B. Goldberg, J. Hiernaux, K. E. Stein, and C. A. Bona, Idiotype-antiidiotype regulation. V. The requirement for immunization with antigen or monoclonal antiidiotypic antibodies for the activation of β2-6 and β2-1 polyfructosanreactive clones in BALB/c mice treated at birth with minute amounts of anti-A48 idiotype antibodies, *J. Exp. Med. 158*:1129 (1983).
122. W. J. Monafo, N. S. Greenspan, J. A. Cebra-Thomas, and J. M. Davie, Modulation of the immune response to streptococcal group A carbohydrate by immunization with monoclonal anti-idiotope, *J. Immunol. 139*:2702 (1987).
123. A. Bloem, G. Zenke, K. Eichman, and F. Emmrich, Human immune response to group A streptococcal carbohydrate (A-CHO). II. Antigen-independent stimulation of IgM anti-A-CHO production in purified B cells by a monoclonal anti-idiotopic antibody, *J. Immunol. 140*:277 (1988).
124. J. R. Schreiber, M. Patawaran, M. Tosi, J. Lennon, and G. B. Pier, Anti-idiotype-induced lipopolysaccharide-specific antibody response to *Pseudomonas aeruginosa, J. Immunol. 144*:1023 (1990).
125. J. R. Schreiber, K. L. Nixon, M. F. Tosi, G. B. Pier, and M. B. Patawaran, Anti-idiotype induced, lipopolysaccharide-specific antibody response to *Pseudomonas aeruginosa*: II. Isotype and functional activity of the anti-idiotype-induced antibodies, *J. Immunol. 146*:188 (1991).
126. J. R. Schreiber, G. B. Pier, M. Grout, K. Nixon, and M. Patawaran, Induction of opsonic antibodies to *Pseudomonas aeruginosa* mucoid exopolysaccharide by anti-idiotypic monoclonal antibody, *J. Infect. Dis. 164*:507 (1991).
127. M. A. J. Westerinck, A. A. Campagnari, M. A. Wirth, and M. A. Apicella, Development and characterization of an anti-idiotype antibody to the capsular polysaccharide of *Neisseria meningitidis* serogroup C, *Infect. Immun. 56*:1120 (1988).
128. M. A. J. Westerinck, P. C. Giardina, A. A. Campagnari, and M. A. Apicella, The thymus dependent nature of the murine antibody response to a monoclonal anti-idiotypic antibody to the *Neisseria meningitidis* serogroup C polysaccharide, *Microb. Pathog. 8*:411 (1990).
129. M. A. J. Westerinck and P. C. Giardina, Anti-idiotype induced protection against *Neisseria meningitidis* serogroup C bacteremia, *Microb. Pathog. 12*:19 (1992).
130. D. L. Sacks, L. V. Kirchoff, S. Hieny, and A. Sher, Molecular mimicry of a carbohydrate epitope on a major surface glycoprotein of *Trypanosoma cruzi* by using anti-idiotypic antibodies, *J. Immunol. 135*:4155 (1985).
131. M. K. McNamara, R. E. Ward, and H. Kohler, Monoclonal idiotope vaccine against *Streptococcus pneumoniae* infection, *Science* (Wash. D.C.) *226*:1325 (1984).
132. S. Su, M. M. Ward, M. A. Apicella, and R. E. Ward, Analysis of the immune response to lipopolysaccharide. Existence of an interspecies cross-reactive idiotype associated with anti-lipid A antibodies, *J. Immunol. 145*: 2994 (1990).

133. S. Su, M. M. Ward, M. A. Apicella, and R. E. Ward, A nontoxic, idiotope vaccine against gram-negative bacterial infections, *J. Immunol. 148*:234 (1992).
134. H.-L. Cheng, A. K. Sood, R. E. Ward, T. Kieber-Emmons, and H. Kohler, Structural basis of stimulatory anti-idiotypic antibodies, *Mol. Immunol.*:33 (1988).
135. J.-Y. Huang, R. E. Ward, and H. Kohler, Biologic mimicry of antigenic stimulation: Analysis of the *in vivo* responses induced by monoclonal anti-idiotypic antibodies, *Immunology 63*:1 (1988).
136. D. M. Granoff, A. Chako, K. R. Lottenbach, and K. E. Sheetz, Immunogenicity of *Haemophilus influenzae* type b polysaccharide-outer membrane protein conjugate vaccine in patients who acquired *Haemophilus* disease despite previous vaccination with type b polysaccharide vaccine, *J. Pediatr. 114*:925 (1989).
137. S. J. Holmes, A. H. Lucas, M. T. Osterholm, J. E. Froeschle, D. M. Granoff and the Collaborative Study Group, Immunoglobulin deficiency and idiotype expression in children developing *Haemophilus influenzae* type b disease after vaccination with conjugate vaccine, *J. Am. Med. Assoc. 266*:1960 (1991).
138. G. R. Siber, M. Santosham, G. R. Reid, C. Thompson, J. Almeido-Hill, A. Morell, G. deLange, J. K. Ketcham, and E. H. Callahan, Impaired antibody response to *Haemophilus influenzae* type b polysaccharide and low IgG2 and IgG4 concentrations in Apache children, *N. Engl. J. Med. 323*:1387 (1990).
139. J. Ward, G. Brenneman, G. W. Letson, W. L. Heyward, and the Alaska *H. influenzae* Vaccine Study Group, Limited efficacy of a *Haemophilus influenzae* type b conjugate vaccine in Alaska native infants, *N. Engl. J. Med. 323*:1393 (1990).
140. K. Rajewsky and T. Takemori, Genetics, expression, and function of idiotypes, *Ann. Rev. Immunol. 1*:569 (1983).
141. G. Gregoriadis, A. C. Allison, and G. Poste (eds.), *Immunological Adjuvants and Vaccines*, Plenum, New York, 1989.
142. A. M. Mowat and A. M. Donachie, ISCOMS—a novel strategy for mucosal immunization, *Immunol. Today 12*:383 (1991).
143. N. M. J. Garcon and H. R. Six, Universal vaccine carrier. Liposomes that provide T-dependent help to weak antigens, *J. Immunol.* β:3697 (1991).
144. J. H. Eldridge, J. K. Staas, J. A. Meulbroek, T. R. Tice, and R. M. Gilley, Biodegradable and biocompatible poly(DL-lactide-co-glycolide) microspheres as an adjuvant for staphylococcal enterotoxin B toxoid which enhances the level of toxin-neutralizing antibodies, *Infect. Immun. 59*:2978 (1991).
145. R. Schneerson, A. Fattom, S. C. Szu, D. Bryla, J. T. Ulrich, J. A. Rudbach, G. Schiffman, and J. B. Robbins, Evaluation of monophosphoryl lipid A (MPL) as an adjuvant. Enhancement of the serum antibody response in mice to polysaccharide-protein conjugates by concurrent injection with MPL, *J. Immunol. 147*:2136 (1991).
146. E. Maggi, P. Parronchi, R. Manetti, C. Simonelli, M. Piccinni, F. S. Rugiu, M. De Carli, M. Ricci, and S. Romagnani, Reciprocal regulatory effects of

IFN-γ and IL-4 on the *in vitro* development of Th1 and Th2 clones, *J. Immunol. 148*:2142 (1992).

147. T. R. Mosmann and R. L. Coffman, TH1 and TH2 cells: Different patterns of lymphokine secretion lead to different functional properties, *Ann. Rev. Immunol. 7*:145 (1989).

148. C.-S. Hsieh, S. E. Macatonia, C. S. Tripp, S. F. Wolf, A. O'Garra, and K. M. Murphy, Development of TH1 $CD4^+$ T cells through IL-12 produced by *Listeria*-induced macrophages, *Science* (Wash. D.C.) *260*:547 (1993).

149. M. F. Good, D. Pombo, M. N. Lunde, W. L. Maloy, R. Halenbeck, K. Koths, L. H. Miller, and J. A. Berzofsky, Recombinant human IL-2 overcomes genetic nonresponsiveness to malarial sporozoite peptides Correlation of effect with biologic activity, *J. Immunol. 141*:972 (1988).

150. T. Yin, P. Schendel and Y. C. Yang, Enhancement of *in vitro* and *in vivo* antigen-specific antibody responses by interleukin 11, *J. Exp. Med. 175*:211 (1992).

151. M.-H. Tao and R. Levy, Idiotype-granulocyte-macrophage-colony stimulating factor fusion protein as a vaccine for B-cell lymphoma, *Nature 362*:755 (1993).

152. E. J. Gosselin, K. Wardwell, D. R. Gosselin, N. Alter, J. L. Fisher, and P. M. Guyre, Enhanced antigen presentation using Fcγ receptor (monocyte/macrophage)-specific immunogens, *J. Immunol. 149*:3477 (1992).

153. J. Rhodes, Evidence for an intercellular covalent reaction essential in antigen-specific T cell activation, *J. Immunol. 143*:1482 (1989).

154. B. Zheng, S. J. Brett, J. P. Tite, M. R. Lifely, T. A. Brodies, and J. Rhodes, Galactose oxidation in the design of immunogenic vaccines, *Science 256*:1560 (1992).

155. R. Arnon and M. H. V. Van Regenmortel, Structural basis of antigenic specificity and design of new vaccines, *FASEB J. 6*:3265 (1992).

Index

About the Editors

RONALD W. ELLIS is Executive Director of Virus & Cell Biology at Merck Research Laboratories, West Point, Pennsylvania. The author or coauthor of over 100 articles and 20 review chapters in the fields of vaccines, infectious diseases, molecular and cellular biology, virology, and experimental oncology, Dr. Ellis is the editor of *Hepatitis B Vaccines in Clinical Practice* (Marcel Dekker, Inc.) and *Vaccines: New Approaches to Immunological Problems*. A member of the American Society for Microbiology, he received the B.A. degree (1974) in biology from the University of Chicago, Illinois, the Ph.D. degree (1979) in biology from Cornell University, Ithaca, New York, and the M.B.A. degree (1981) from the University of Maryland, College Park.

DAN M. GRANOFF is Executive Director of Biocine Clinical Research, Chiron Corporation, Emeryville, California, and a Research Scientist at Children's Hospital Oakland Research Institute, Oakland, California. Formerly a Professor of Pediatrics and Director of Pediatric Infectious Diseases at Washington University School of Medicine, St. Louis, Missouri, Dr. Granoff is the author or coauthor of over 100 professional articles in fields related to infectious diseases, immunology, and the clinical development of polysaccharide conjugate vaccines. He is a Fellow of the Infectious Diseases Society of America and the American Academy of Pediatrics, as well as a member of the American Pediatric Society, the Society for Pediatric Research, and the American Society for Clinical Investigation, among others. He received the A.B. degree (1963) in biology and the M.D. degree (1968) from Johns Hopkins University, Baltimore, Maryland.